EXERCISE AND SPORTS CARDIOLOGY

EXERCISE AND SPORTS CARDIOLOGY

EDITOR

Paul D. Thompson, M.D.
*Director of Preventive Cardiology and
    Cardiovascular Research*
Hartford Hospital
Hartford, Connecticut
Professor of Medicine
University of Connecticut Medical Center
Farmington, Connecticut

Foreword by Eric J. Topol

McGRAW-HILL

Medical Publishing Division

*New York   St. Louis   San Francisco
Auckland   Bogotá   Caracas   Lisbon
London   Madrid   Mexico City   Milan
Montreal   New Delhi   San Juan
Singapore   Sydney   Tokyo   Toronto*

McGraw-Hill

A Division of The McGraw·Hill Companies

EXERCISE AND SPORTS CARDIOLOGY

123456789 DOCDOC 09876543210

ISBN 0-07-134773-9

This book was typeset in Times New Roman
by Rainbow Graphics.
The editors were Darlene Barela Cooke, Susan R.
Noujaim, and Karen Davis.
The production supervisor was Richard Ruzycka.
The text designer was Joan O'Connor.
The cover designer was Amieé Nordin.
The index was prepared by Angie Wiley.
RR Donnelley & Sons, Inc. was printer and binder.
This book is printed on acid-free paper.

Library of Congress Cataloging-in-Publication Data

Exercise and sports cardiology / editor, Paul D. Thompson.
      p. ; cm.
   Includes bibliographical references and index.
   ISBN 0-07-134773-9 (alk. paper)
     1. Heart. 2. Sports—Physiological aspects. 3. Exercise—Physiological aspects. 4.
Cardiovascular system—Diseases—Exercise therapy. I. Thompson, Paul D., M.D.
     [DNLM: 1. Sports. 2. Cardiovascular Diseases—prevention & control. 3.
Exercise—physiology. 4. Risk Factors. QT 260 S7625 2001]
   RC1236.H43 S665 2001
   612.1'7'088796—dc21

                                                                  00-029217

*This book is dedicated
to my parents,
Dorothy Davis Thompson and
the Reverend Owen D. Thompson,
and to my wife's parents,
Suzanne and Earle Bessey, Jr.*

Contents

Contributors

Gary J. Balady, M.D.
Section of Cardiology
Boston University Medical Center
Boston, Massachusetts

Randy W. Braith, Ph.D.
Associate Professor
Director, Clinical Exercise Physiology
Center for Exercise Science
College of Health and Human Performance
College of Medicine
University of Florida
Gainesville, Florida

J. Timothy Bricker, M.D.
Professor and Chief
The Lillie Frank Abercrombie Section of
*   Cardiology*
Department of Pediatrics
Baylor College of Medicine and Texas Children's
*   Hospital*
Chief of Pediatric Cardiology Department
Texas Heart Institute
Houston, Texas

Jirayos Chintanadilok, M.D.
Fellow in Geriatric Medicine
Geriatric Research, Education and Clinical
*   Center*
Veterans Affairs Medical Center
University of Florida College of Medicine
Gainesville, Florida

Jeffrey Alan Conwell, M.D.
Director of Pediatric Cardiology
Department of Pediatrics
Naval Medical Center
Assistant Clinical Professor
University of California, San Diego
San Diego, California

Pamela S. Douglas, M.D.
Director of Noninvasive Cardiology
Cardiovascular Division
Beth Israel Medical Center
Associate Professor of Medicine
Harvard Medical School
Boston, Massachusetts

J. Larry Durstine, Ph.D.
Professor
Director of Clinical Exercise Programs
Department of Exercise Science
The University of South Carolina
Columbia, South Carolina

N. A. Mark Estes III, M.D.
Chief, Cardiac Arrhythmia Service
Professor of Medicine
Tufts University School of Medicine
New England Medical Center
Boston, Massachusetts

Cynthia M. Ferguson, B.S.
Research Associate
Palo Alto VA Health Care System
Medical Student
Stanford University
Palo Alto, California

Victor F. Froelicher, M.D.
Professor of Medicine
Stanford University
Director, ECG and Exercise Laboratory
Palo Alto VA Health Care System
Palo Alto, California

Andrew W. Gardner, Ph.D.
Department of Medicine
Division of Gerontology
University of Maryland
Geriatric Research, Education and Clinical
  Center
The Baltimore Veterans Affairs Medical Center
Baltimore, Maryland

Helene L. Glassberg, M.D.
Section of Cardiology
Boston University Medical Center
Boston, Massachusetts

Bret H. Goodpaster, M.D.
Instructor of Medicine
Division of Endocrinology/Metabolism
University of Pittsburgh
Pittsburgh, Pennsylvania

Munther Homoud, M.D.
Director, New England Cardiac Arrhythmia
  Monitoring Center
New England Cardiac Arrhythmia Center
Assistant Professor of Medicine
Tufts University School of Medicine
Boston, Massachusetts

David E. Kelley, M.D.
Associate Professor of Medicine
Division of Endocrinology/Metabolism
University of Pittsburgh
Pittsburgh, Pennsylvania

I-Min Lee, M.B.B.S., Sc.D.
Associate Professor of Medicine
Harvard Medical School
Assistant Professor of Epidemiology
Harvard School of Public Health
Brigham and Women's Hospital
Boston, Massachusetts

Benjamin D. Levine, M.D.
Director, Institute for Exercise and
  Environmental Medicine
S. Finley Ewing Jr. Chair for Wellness at
  Presbyterian Hospital of Dallas
Harry S. Moss Heart Chair for Cardiovascular
  Research
Associate Professor of Medicine
University of Texas Southwestern Medical Center
  at Dallas
Dallas, Texas

Joseph R. Libonati, Ph.D.
Human Performance Laboratory
Department of Cardiopulmonary Sciences
Bouvé College of Health Professions
Northeastern University
Boston, Massachusetts

Mark S. Link, M.D.
Director, Center for the Evaluation of Athletes
New England Cardiac Arrhythmia Center
Assistant Professor of Medicine
Tufts University School of Medicine
Boston, Massachusetts

David T. Lowenthal, M.D., Ph.D.
*Director, Geriatric Research, Education
  and Clinical Center*
Veterans Affairs Medical Center
Director of Hypertension
*Division of Nephrology, Hypertension
  and Transplantation*
*Professor of Medicine, Pharmacology
  and Exercise Science*
University of Florida College of Medicine
Gainesville, Florida

Barry J. Maron, M.D.
Cardiovascular Research
Minneapolis Heart Institute Foundation
Minneapolis, Minnesota

Niall M. Moyna, Ph.D.
Division of Cardiology
Hartford Hospital
Hartford, Connecticut

Jonathan Myers, Ph.D.
Director of Research
Exercise Laboratory
Palo Alto VA Health Care System
Palo Alto, California

Ralph S. Paffenbarger, Jr., M.D., Dr.P.H.
Professor Emeritus (Active) of Epidemiology
Stanford University School of Medicine
Stanford, California
Adjunct Professor of Epidemiology
Harvard School of Public Health
Boston, Massachusetts

Antonio Pelliccia, M.D.
Institute of Sports Science
Department of Medicine
Italian Olympic Committee
Rome, Italy

James C. Puffer, M.D.
Professor and Chief
Division of Sports Medicine
*University of California, Los Angeles Division
  of Family Medicine*
Los Angeles, California

Reed E. Pyeritz, M.D., Ph.D.
*Professor of Human Genetics, Medicine and
  Pediatrics*
Chair, Department of Human Genetics
MCP Hahnemann School of Medicine
Director, Center for Medical Genetics
Allegheny General Hospital
Pittsburgh, Pennsylvania

Lisa R. Thomas, M.D.
Cardiovascular Division
Beth Israel Medical Center
Boston, Massachusetts

Paul D. Thompson, M.D.
*Director of Preventive Cardiology and
  Cardiovascular Research*
Hartford Hospital
Hartford, Connecticut
Professor of Medicine
University of Connecticut Medical Center
Farmington, Connecticut

Paul J. Wang, M.D.
Division of Criscitiello Heart Station
New England Cardiac Arrhythmia Center
Associate Professor of Medicine
Tufts University School of Medicine
Boston, Massachusetts

Foreword

In evaluating patients with heart disease, perhaps the most frequently neglected part of long-term management is the practice of prescribing and managing patients' exercise programs. Without question, appropriate exercise has emerged as a cornerstone of preventive cardiology, and, in this book, *Exercise and Sports Cardiology,* Dr. Paul Thompson has masterfully edited a comprehensive approach that embodies virtually all aspects of exercise and sports in cardiovascular medicine. The insightful and systemic approach takes on many dimensions. All aspects of heart disease are addressed including congenital, valvular, and coronary artery disease, and cardiomyopathy (hypertrophic). The impact of comorbidities is carefully probed with chapters on diabetes, hypertension, peripheral arterial disease, and connective tissue disease.

In the 21st century, there is no question about the prominence of exercise for improving a patient's quality of life and even promoting survival. Mechanistic studies have pointed toward the potential of exercise to reduce inflammation beyond the expected improvement in lipoprotein abnormalities. Further clinical investigation in the years ahead will undoubtedly unravel other key pathways by which exercise promotes cardiovascular health.

This book fits an unmet need in cardiovascular medicine today. There is no textbook that has been previously assembled that presents the field in toto by the recognized experts in the field. I wholeheartedly recommend it to all practicing cardiologists, nurse practitioners, exercise physiologists, and health care professionals engaged in cardiac rehabilitation and preventive cardiology.

Eric J. Topol, M.D.
Chairman and Professor, Department
of Cardiology
Director, Joseph J. Jacobs Center for Thrombosis
and Vascular Biology
The Cleveland Clinic Foundation
Cleveland, Ohio

Preface

I agreed to edit *Exercise and Sports Cardiology* because I have had a lifelong interest in competitive distance running and because I thought I could learn quite a lot by selecting excellent contributors and by reviewing their contributions. I was right. I learned a great deal from editing this text and am certain that you will as well.

The text is divided into five sections. The first section reviews normal exercise physiology and provides an overview of exercise testing and the physiological adaptations that accompany chronic exercise training. One chapter, unique to a medical text, is entitled "Principles of Exercise Training for Physicians." The author is Niall Moyna, Ph.D. and he knows his subject well. Dr. Moyna is an exercise physiologist, coaches several successful distance runners, and was himself the Irish National Champion in the 800-m race for 3 successive years. The second section addresses the risks of exercise. Physicians in all specialties are frequently required to evaluate individuals for exercise programs and must have a clear concept of the potential cardiac risks of exercise. The third section deals with special clinical issues in athletes such as the advisability of exercise for children following repair of congenital cardiac lesions and how to advise patients with valvular heart disease about their exercise risk. The fourth section is confined to the use of exercise as adjunctive therapy for such conditions as congestive heart failure, coronary artery disease, and claudication. I am repeatedly impressed with the magnitude of improvement exercise can provide selected patients with each of these conditions. This section provides an overview of that topic written by individuals who have experience in both the clinical and research aspects of their subject. The final section discusses the use of exercise in preventing cardiovascular disease. It also discusses the value of exercise in managing diabetes, lipid disorders, and hypertension.

The breadth of the text should make it useful to a wide variety of practicing clinicians. I often feel that exercise is the Rodney Dangerfield of medical interventions: It "just can't get any respect." In some cases this is appropriate because the public and clinicians can overestimate the therapeutic benefits of exercise and underestimate its risks. This text seeks to keep these conflicting viewpoints in balance. Consequently, the text is of use to those clinicians who are strong advocates of an active lifestyle, as well as to those whose primary need for exercise knowledge is to advise patients seeking medical clearance for exercise. Similarly, the text provides useful information for physicians caring for individuals at the extremes of exercise performance: patients who are competitive athletes and patients with advanced cardiovascular disease. The text should also be useful to clinicians who provide wellness and preventive medicine services to their communities and to researchers interested in the broad topic of clinical exercise, its risks, and benefits.

I hope you enjoy reading this text as much as I enjoyed editing it. Part of my pleasure came from working with old and new friends who are also outstanding clinicians and investigators. Some, such as Barry Maron, are household names in the sports cardiology community. Others are not, but I am sure you will understand why I selected them as authors once you read their chapters. I have learned much from such colleagues and their research. I now look forward to learning from you, and so I welcome your comments and questions about the book by e-mail at pthomps@harthosp.org.

I want to thank the authors who contributed; my family for their patience during these last months of missed deadlines; McGraw-Hill for taking on this project, especially Darlene Barela Cooke, Executive Editor, and Susan R. Noujaim, Development Editor, in the Medical Publishing Division at McGraw-Hill; and the organizations that have helped support our research on the relationship of exercise and health, including the American Heart Association, the National Institutes of Health, The Miriam and Hartford Hospitals' Research Funds, the Althea and Richard B. Nye Family Trust, and the McNulty, Jakober, and Haire families. Finally, I thank you for sharing with me an interest in exercise and sports cardiology.

EXERCISE AND SPORTS CARDIOLOGY

PART I

NORMAL EXERCISE PHYSIOLOGY

Chapter 1

EXERCISE PHYSIOLOGY FOR THE CLINICIAN

Benjamin D. Levine, M.D.

Exercise physiology, and its practical application during exercise testing, is an essential tool for quantifying the functional capacity of patients and examining the integrity of the cardiorespiratory system. As such, it plays an important role for clinicians in optimizing the quality of life, independent of its ability to "diagnose" coronary artery disease.

OXYGEN UPTAKE AND THE OXYGEN CASCADE

In order to perform physical work, the uptake and transport of oxygen is required for oxidative phosphorylation and the efficient production of adenosine triphosphate (ATP) to support the metabolic demands of the body.

A simplified diagram of the components of the "oxygen cascade," or the steps of the respiratory chain through which oxygen must pass from the atmosphere to the mitochondria, is shown in Figure 1.1. This includes:

3

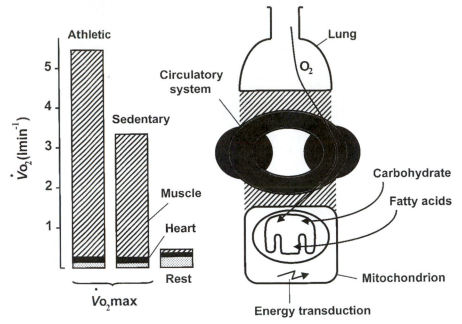

FIGURE 1.1. *The figure on the right represents a stylized depiction of the essential elements of the "oxygen cascade." Oxygen, the partial pressure of which is determined by the ambient altitude, enters the body via pulmonary ventilation; it then diffuses across the pulmonary capillary where it binds to hemoglobin and is transported by bulk flow via the cardiovascular system; a second diffusion step occurs at the muscle capillary where O_2 passes into the muscle cell and then is transported intracellularly to the mitochondria where it is used for oxidative phosphorylation and energy transduction. The left side of the figure demonstrates the large variation in oxygen uptake ($\dot{V}O_2$) from rest (right bar), to peak exercise in either a sedentary (middle bar) or athletic (left bar) human. Note that the majority of the increase in oxygen uptake during exercise comes from skeletal muscle.* From Ref. 1.

1. Atmospheric partial pressure of oxygen determined by the environment
2. The interface between the environment and the body via the lungs and ventilation
3. Diffusion across the pulmonary capillary into the blood
4. Allosteric binding of oxygen to hemoglobin
5. Bulk transport of oxygen via the cardiovascular system
6. Diffusion at the muscle capillary into skeletal muscle
7. Oxidation in the mitochondria for energy production[1]

At rest, this metabolic demand is dominated by the relatively high aerobic requirements of tissues such as the brain, heart, and kidney. For most individuals, on average, resting metabolic rate is approximately 3.5 ml O_2/min/kg, which has been termed *1 MET,* or *metabolic equivalent.* Resting skeletal muscle has a very low metabolic demand and consequently a very low resting blood flow. However, during exercise, skeletal muscle has the capacity to augment its metabolic demand > 10-fold (> 20-fold in endurance athletes; Fig. 1.1), leading to a large increase in systemic oxygen flux.

As the *external* work performed by skeletal muscle increases (e.g., speed and grade on a treadmill, or Watts on a cycle ergometer), the amount of oxygen that passes along the oxygen cascade is increased, and the rate of ventilatory

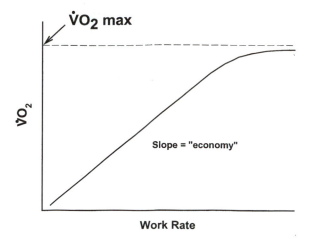

FIGURE 1.2. Idealized representation of the relationship between work rate (speed and grade on a treadmill, Watts on a cycle ergometer) and oxygen uptake ($\dot{V}O_2$). When work rate is increased, oxygen uptake increases with a slope equal to the economy of the particular activity. When work rate increases, but oxygen uptake can no longer increase, $\dot{V}O_2$ max is achieved.

oxygen uptake, or $\dot{V}O_2$, can be measured (Fig. 1.2).

The slope of the line relating $\dot{V}O_2$ to work rate is termed the *economy* and is very different for different types of exercise. For example, walking is very economical, as is cycling, and the economy of these activities varies relatively little among individuals. In contrast, running is less efficient, and activities such as swimming may convert only 10% of energy production into useful work.[2,3] Eventually, there reaches a point beyond which further increases in work rate do not lead to additional increases in oxygen uptake, and this value represents $\dot{V}O_2$, max, or the maximal rate of ventilatory oxygen uptake.[4]

$\dot{V}O_2$, max is the best objective measure of fitness and is a widely used index of the integrity of cardiovascular function.[5] According to the Fick Principle, $\dot{V}O_2$, is the product of cardiac output multiplied by the arteriovenous oxygen difference across the body. Thus, there are both central (oxy-

gen delivery) and peripheral (oxygen extraction) factors that determine systemic oxygen transport. However, except in some disease states that impair the ability of skeletal muscle to utilize oxygen,[6] the single most important factor that limits $\dot{V}O_2$, max in normal individuals at sea level is the maximal cardiac output.[7]

One of the most inviolate relationships in all of exercise physiology is that between oxygen uptake and cardiac output. Regardless of age, gender, or the presence of various disease states, in general, about 6 L of cardiac output are required for every liter of oxygen uptake above rest[8] (Fig. 1.3). When this relationship breaks down, it may be a sign of severe underlying disease with impending decompensation. For example, in patients with heart failure, regardless of any other clinically measured variable, the maintenance of a normal relationship between cardiac output and oxygen uptake identifies patients with relatively good short-term prognosis.[9] In contrast, when the relationship breaks down, urgent transplantation may be required.[9] Thus, the measure of maximal exercise capacity, or $\dot{V}O_2$, max, may be viewed as a surrogate for the measure of maximal cardiac output.

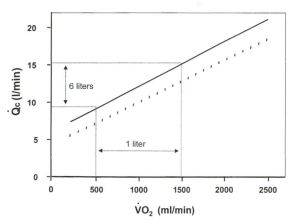

FIGURE 1.3. This figure represents one of the key principles in exercise physiology: that is, the remarkably constant relationship between the increase in oxygen uptake ($\dot{V}O_2$) and the corresponding increase in cardiac output ($\dot{Q}c$), which in most cases is 6/1.

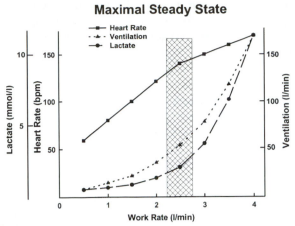

FIGURE 1.4. *Graph shows the increase in heart rate, ventilation, and lactate during incremental increases in work rate. At a specific physiological work rate, shown as a hatched bar, the rate of increase in heart rate slows (heart rate break point), ventilation increases out of proportion to oxygen uptake (ventilatory threshold), and lactate begins to accumulate in the blood (lactate threshold). Because exercise intensities beyond this work rate cannot be sustained for prolonged periods of time, it is termed the "maximal steady state."*

SUBMAXIMAL EXERCISE AND THE MAXIMAL STEADY STATE

Important clues to functional capacity and the ability to perform and sustain tasks of daily living also can be found in the submaximal responses to exercise (Fig. 1.4).

The most common and easy to measure variable is heart rate, which increases linearly with oxygen uptake. The slope of this line is dependent on a number of factors, particularly cardiorespiratory fitness. In unfit subjects, there is a more rapid increase in heart rate at low levels of work than more fit individuals for whom this increase is substantially delayed. Moreover, the relationship may be importantly affected by medications such as beta blockers, or calcium channel blockers, which will blunt the heart rate response to exercise. Conversely, diseases that diminish the diastolic reserve and limit the ability to increase stroke volume during exercise (see later) will also influence

the heart rate response since the relationship between oxygen uptake and cardiac output is relatively fixed. As exercise intensity increases, there comes a point at which the rate of increase of heart rate begins to slow as maximal exercise capacity is approached. This is termed the heart rate *break point,* or *Conconi* heart rate.[10,11]

What can also be measured is ventilation ($\dot{V}e$), and it is relatively low at low levels of exercise. As exercise intensity increases, there is a point beyond which the rate of increase in $\dot{V}e$ is greater than the rate of increase in $\dot{V}o_2$.[12] This point is most precisely termed the *ventilatory threshold.*

Although the regulation of breathing during exercise is beyond the scope of this chapter, a few points deserve comment. First of all, there is substantial reserve in the pulmonary system, both structurally and functionally, so that in normal individuals at sea level the pulmonary system rarely provides any limitations to oxygen transport.[1,13]

In Figure 1.5, the left graph shows a typical flow-volume loop at rest (small, inside loop) and during exercise (middle loop) in a normal,

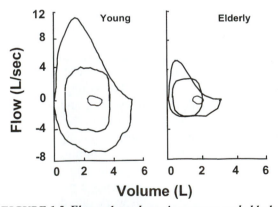

FIGURE 1.5. *Flow-volume loops in a young and elderly individual at rest (small inside loop), and at peak exercise (middle loop); both loops are subtended by a maximal flow volume loop. Note that for the young individual, there is substantial inspiratory and expiratory reserve, even at peak exercise. However for the elderly person, there is prominent flow limitation on both the inspiratory and expiratory side, as well as markedly reduced peak flows.*

healthy individual. This demonstrates a decrease in end-expiratory lung volume and an increase in end-inspiratory lung volume during exercise, both of which are well within the reserve capacity of the maximal flow-volume loop (outer loop). In contrast to this young individual, the curve on the right shows what happens to an elderly individual during exercise. Although little difference is evident at rest, the elderly individual during exercise cannot decrease end-expiratory lung volume due to decreased maximal expiratory flow and reduced lung volumes. Thus, in order to increase ventilation sufficiently during exercise, end-inspiratory lung volume must increase markedly, using virtually all the inspiratory reserve available to this individual and resulting in a prominent sensation of dyspnea, even without hypoxemia. These curves demonstrate a common misconception among clinicians—that if arterial oxyhemoglobin saturation is normal, then exertional dyspnea cannot be pulmonary in origin. This conclusion is not true and for many patients, particularly the elderly, those with emphysema, or even obese patients, pulmonary limitations to exercise performance become manifest and lead to prominent dyspnea.[14–16]

Similar to the ventilatory response during exercise, as shown in Figure 1.4, blood lactate, the product of glycolytic metabolism, remains near resting levels at low-to-moderate intensities of exercise because lactate production is balanced by clearance in active and inactive skeletal muscle as well as heart and liver.[17] However, during graded exercise protocols in which lactate production increases more rapidly than disposal mechanisms can compensate, a certain exercise intensity is reached at which the blood lactate concentration begins to rise. This inflection in blood lactate concentration during graded exercise protocols is most precisely termed the *lactate threshold,* or the *o*nset of *b*lood *l*actate *a*ccumulation (OBLA). The term *anaerobic threshold* has been applied to this level of exercise intensity and has achieved widespread, popular appeal.[18,19] However, current understanding of the biochemistry of exercise has made it clear

that there is *not* a "threshold" where a shift from "aerobic" to "anaerobic" metabolism occurs.[20–22] Rather, at high rates of energy requirements, substrate level phosphorylation (ATP production via glycolysis, creatine kinase, adenylate kinase, and succinyl-CoA synthetase) plays an increasingly important role in supplying ATP for contractile function, even though the rate of energy supply via oxidative phosphorylation is not exceeded.[23,24] As opposed to a shift from oxidative to glycolytic pathways, the lactate threshold during progressive exercise protocols is due to (a) the energetics of substrate utilization, which by mass action lead to an increased rate of pyruvate production and thus inevitably result in lactate production as both a product of glycolysis and for direct oxidation via the lactate shuttle; (b) an increased rate of glycolytic flux as exercise intensity increases; and (c) the efficiency of lactate clearance mechanisms.[25,26] Hence, from an organ-systems perspective, the rise in blood lactate provides useful information on compensatory mechanisms possessed by sets of distributed, but interrelated, functions. It must also be recognized that maximal or near-maximal levels of oxidative flux continue during exercise at intensities that equal or even exceed maximal oxygen uptake. Moreover, with the rapid initiation of exercise of any intensity, substrate level phosphorylation is required for energy supply. Thus, the concept of an "anaerobic threshold" is not correct and more physiological terminology should be encouraged.

Regardless of terminology, however, it is important to recognize that there *does* exist a level of exercise intensity for every individual, beyond which exercise cannot be sustained for prolonged periods of time. The term *maximal steady state* is, therefore, preferred when focusing on this clinically relevant level of activity. This work rate can be identified by any of the techniques mentioned earlier (i.e., Conconi heart rate, ventilatory threshold, onset of blood lactate accumulation) and represents a discrete physiological substrate (hatched bar in Fig. 1.4) which occurs when a certain percentage of maximal oxygen uptake is reached.[11,21] For most normal individuals, it usually occurs at 50 to 70% of maximal oxygen uptake, though in elite athletes, it may be as high as 90 to 95% of $\dot{V}O_2$ max. The maximal steady state is an important physiological parameter to identify since most sustained activities in nonathletes are performed substantially below maximal capacity. Moreover, the majority of exercise prescribed for patients for training purposes should take place at intensities below the maximal steady state.

Although an "anaerobic threshold" does not exist, maximal capacity for glycolytic flux, or "anaerobic capacity," which can be considered to mean the rate and magnitude of the absolute quantity of energy available through substrate level phosphorylation, plays an important role in high-intensity, short-duration activities lasting 1 to 2 min in duration and may be an extremely important characteristic to identify in sprint or middle-distance athletes. Although the optimal method to measure this characteristic is still a matter of some debate, probably the best approach is that described by Medbo et al,[27] which employs the maximal accumulated oxygen deficit. In essence, if high intensity exercise at an intensity above that which can be supported by maximal oxygen uptake is initiated suddenly, substrate level phosphorylation will be required to generate ATP for muscular contraction and, particularly within the first minute of exercise, will provide the dominant source of energy. The difference between the energy that would be required if all the exercise were performed "aerobically," or with energy supplied by oxidative sources, and the actual oxygen uptake is termed the *oxygen deficit*. Such high intensity effort can rarely be sustained for more than 2 to 4 min, and the total oxygen deficit achieved during exhaustive effort is termed the *anaerobic capacity*.[27–29] If the (a) maximal oxygen uptake; (b) economy; (c) maximal steady state; and (d) anaerobic capacity are measured, a comprehensive evaluation of performance capability of any competitive or recreational athlete can be obtained.

CLINICAL APPLICATION OF MAXIMAL OXYGEN TRANSPORT DURING EXERCISE TESTING

The primary unit of oxygen uptake is liters of oxygen per minute (L/min), and, in absolute terms, is a direct function of body size. However, as a measure of work capacity, or the ability to move a human body through space, it is usually normalized to body mass, and in its most familiar form is expressed as milliliters per kilogram per minute (ml/kg/min). Clinically, $\dot{V}O_2$ is normalized again to metabolic equivalents, which, as described earlier, represents an average value of resting energy expenditure of 3.5 ml/kg/min. The amount of fitness, or cardiovascular function, required to perform various occupational, recreational, or physical conditioning activities then can be represented by the number of metabolic equivalents, or the systemic oxygen transport above rest required for their pursuit (Table 1.1). Thus, both the achievable and sustainable metabolic equivalents are key factors in determining a patient's functional capacity.

Maximal oxygen uptake changes with respect to a number of variables such as training status, gender, and age.[5] On average, $\dot{V}O_2$ max normalized to total body weight decreases by approximately 10% per decade (0.4–0.5 ml/min/kg per year),[30,31] though this decline may be slowed by maintaining both a high level of physical activity and ideal body weight.[32,33] When absolute $\dot{V}O_2$ max is considered, or it is normalized to fat-free mass (FFM), the decline is much less (4–5% per decade, or 0.2 ml/min/kg FFM per year). The American Heart Association has established gender and age-specific guidelines that can be used to broadly characterize a patient's functional capacity (Table 1.2).

Not only is the $\dot{V}O_2$ max, or maximal metabolic equivalent level, a key variable in determining functional capacity, it has inherent clinical relevance (Table 1.3). For example, most activities of daily living require energy expenditures ≤ 4 METs.[34,35] For a patient with congestive heart failure, if this level of oxygen transport exceeds

TABLE 1.1. AMOUNT OF OXYGEN UPTAKE/ENERGY PRODUCTION REQUIRED FOR VARIOUS ACTIVITIES

Category	Self-Care or Home	Occupational	Recreational	Physical Cond.
Very light < 3 METS < 10 ml/kg/min < 4 kcal	Washing, shaving, dressing Desk work, writing Washing dishes Driving auto	Sitting (clerical, assembly) Standing (store clerk, bartender) Driving truck Operating crane	Shuffleboard Horseshoes Bait casting Billiards Archery Golf (cart)	Walking (2 mi/h) Stationary bicycle (very low resistance) Very light calisthenics
Light 3–5 METS 11–18 ml/kg/min 4–6 kcal	Cleaning windows Raking leaves Weeding Power lawn mowing Waxing floors (slow) Painting Carrying objects (15–30 lb)	Stocking shelves (light objects) Light welding Light carpentry Machine assembly Auto repair Paper hanging	Dancing (social and square) Golf (walking) Sailing Horseback riding Volleyball (6-man) Tennis (doubles)	Walking (3–4 mi/h) Level bicycle (6–8 mi/h) Light calisthenics
Moderate 5–7 METS 18–25 ml/kg/min 6–8 kcal	Easy digging in garden Level hand lawn mowing Climbing stairs (slow) Carrying objects (30–60 lb)	Carpentry (exterior home building) Shoveling dirt Using pneumatic tools	Badminton (comp.) Tennis (singles) Snow skiing (downhill) Light backpacking Basketball Football Skating (ice/roller) Horseback riding (glp)	Walking (4.5–5 mi/h) Bicycle (9–10 mi/h) Swimming (breast stroke)
Heavy 7–9 METS 25–32 ml/kg/min 8–10 kcal	Sawing wood Heavy shoveling Climbing stairs (mod.) Carrying objects (60–90 lb)	Tending furnace Digging ditches Pick and shovel	Canoeing Mountain climbing Fencing Paddleball Touch football	Jog (5 mi/h) Swim (crawl stroke) Rowing machine Heavy calisthenics Bicycling (12 mi/h)
Very Heavy > 9 METS > 32 ml/kg/min > 10 kcal	Carrying loads upstairs Carrying objects (> 90 lb) Climbing stairs (fast) Shoveling heavy snow Shoveling 10 min (16 lb)	Lumberjack Heavy laborer	Handball Squash Ski touring over hills Vigorous basketball	Running (6 +) Bicycling (13 + or up steep hill) Rope jumping

$\dot{V}O_2$ max, the short-term prognosis is extremely poor. Heart transplant specialists use this level as a critical determinant of whether a patient is in imminent need of cardiac transplantation.[36] In contrast, for a patient with coronary heart disease, the ability to exercise to 10 METs without ischemia places the patient in an extremely low-risk subgroup, with a 1-year mortality of < 2%.[37] A maximal exercise capacity of 13 METs, regardless of other comorbidities or the presence and extent of ischemia, predicts a similarly excellent short-term prognosis.

Thus, the ability to measure exercise capacity precisely is an essential component of an exercise tolerance test. Unfortunately, habit and economics have conspired to reduce the precision with which most clinical exercise tests provide this information, based on the widespread use of the Bruce protocol for exercise tolerance testing. Developed by Robert Bruce at the University of Washington in the late 1960s,[38] the speeds and grades used in the protocol were not determined by reasonable consideration and physiological principles, but by the fixed gear ratios available

TABLE 1.2. GUIDELINES CHARACTERIZING FUNCTIONAL CAPACITY

Cardiorespiratory Fitness Classification

Age (years)	Maximum Oxygen Uptake (ml/min/kg)				
	Low	Fair	Average	Good	High
Women					
20–38	< 24	24–30	31–37	38–48	49+
30–39	< 20	20–27	28–33	34–44	45+
40–49	< 17	17–23	24–30	31–41	42+
50–59	< 15	15–20	21–27	28–37	38+
60–69	< 13	13–17	18–23	24–34	35+
Men					
20–29	< 25	25–33	34–42	43–52	53+
30–39	< 23	23–30	31–38	39–48	49+
40–49	< 20	20–26	27–35	36–44	45+
50–59	< 18	18–24	25–33	34–42	43+
60–69	< 16	16–22	23–30	31–40	41+

Adapted with permission from American Heart Association: *Exercise Testing and Training of Apparently Healthy Individuals: A Handbook for Physicians,* 1972, p. 15.

on the treadmill used for the initial development and validation of the concept. The biggest problem with using the Bruce protocol for testing of

TABLE 1.3. MAXIMAL METABOLIC EQUIVALENT LEVEL IN DETERMINING FUNCTIONAL CAPACITY

MET	Functional Capacity
• 1	Resting
• 2	Level walking at 2 mi/h
• 3	Level walking at 4 mi/h
• < 4	Poor prognosis; usual limit immediately after MI; peak cost of basic activities of daily living
• 10	Prognosis with medical therapy as good as coronary artery bypass surgery
• 13	Excellent prognosis regardless of other exercise responses
• 18	Endurance athletes
• > 20	World class athletes

MI, myocardial infarction.

Adapted with permission from Fletcher GF, Balady G, Froelicher VF, et al: Exercise Standards: A statement of healthcare professionals from the American Heart Association. Writing Group. *Circulation* 20:684–696, 1997.

patients with cardiovascular disease is the relatively large increments in $\dot{V}O_2$ required to make the transitions between the early stages. Why is this such an important issue?

It is an inherent principle in medicine and science that the sampling frequency of any measure determines the maximal resolution of the measuring instrument (Nyqvist limit). A well-known example of this phenomenon is shown in Figure 1.6 which depicts the visual resolution ability of the human eye to determine the direction of motion of an airplane propeller.

As the rate of rotation of the propeller increases to the point where it makes slightly less than a full rotation during a single sampling period (1/35 s for the human eye, points 5–6), the propeller looks as if it changes direction. This process is called *aliasing* and represents the loss of discriminatory power of the technique.

For exercise testing, one of the most important pieces of clinical information comes from the ability to discriminate at least 1 MET increments in functional capacity. Especially at low levels of physical activity, 1 MET may be a substantial fraction of a patient's maximal aerobic power. Simplified examples of some common clinical protocols are shown in Figure 1.7.[35]

The Bruce protocol is unique among these by beginning at about 4 METs and progressing with relatively large increments in aerobic requirements of 3 METs every 3 min by an increase in both speed and grade. The first change in stage thus involves nearly a doubling of the work requirements (from 4–7 METs) and is not very useful in determining true functional capacity at the level that most patients with cardiovascular disease can achieve. Alternative protocols shown in the figure begin at different intensities and walking speeds, which can be estimated by watching the patient walk into the treadmill room. Each, in general, involves a fixed walking speed, with increments in grade that add approximately 1 MET every 2 min. Such protocols should be the rule rather than the exception, unless the patient is young, fit, and the clinical expectation is that his or her exercise capacity exceeds 10 METs. For

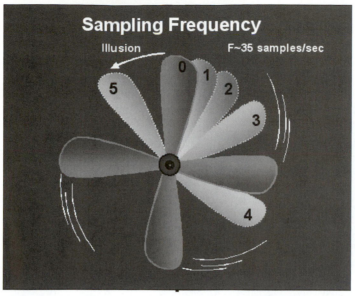

FIGURE 1.6. Demonstration of the principle of aliasing of an airplane propeller, as described in the text. When the speed of the rotation of the propeller exceeds the sampling interval of the human eye so that more than half of a rotation is completed before the next sample, the propeller appears to rotate backward. This figure demonstrates the importance of sampling frequency (must be greater than twice the interval of interest) relative to the capacity of the measurement instrument for scientific observations.

the testing of competitive athletes, similar considerations apply. Thus, an initial speed should be chosen. This speed should reflect a comfortable base training pace (e.g., 9–10 mi/h for collegiate middle-distance runners with a $\dot{V}O_2$ max of 65–75 ml/kg/min), with increments in grade of 2% every 2 min. Such protocols invariably result in exhaustion in 10 to 12 min and provide an appropriate testing environment for the athlete.[39] Finally, since maximal work capacity provides such important, clinically relevant information, clinical exercise tests should never be stopped arbitrarily by the test administrator for fixed endpoints such as a specific work rate or percentage of predicted maximal heart rate.[40] The latter is so variable, with a standard deviation of ± 10 beats per minute, as to be essentially useless for individual patients.[40] Patient-specific criteria, such as fatigue, dyspnea, hemodynamics, development of

signs or symptoms of ischemia, or arrhythmias, are more appropriate endpoints, the threshold for which may be altered depending on the specific clinical situation.

CARDIOVASCULAR REGULATION DURING EXERCISE: FROM EXTERNAL TO INTERNAL WORK

The previous sections of this chapter have focused on the integrative, systemic responses of the body during exercise with an emphasis on oxygen uptake. The majority of the increase in oxygen demand during exercise comes from skeletal muscle,[1,41] which must be met by appropriate increases in oxygen transport along the oxygen cascade. The following section of this chapter will focus on the specific mechanisms by

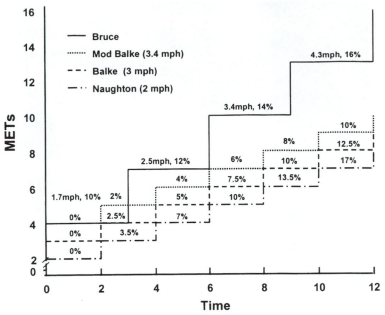

FIGURE 1.7. Idealized representation of common clinical protocols. The Bruce protocol is unique in that large increases in work rate (accomplished by changing both speed and grade on the treadmill) occur with each stage, so that for relatively deconditioned patients, maximal work capacity is rapidly exceeded. Other protocols establish a basic treadmill speed, and increase by approximately 1 MET every 2 minutes exclusively by increases in grade.

which the cardiovascular system mediates this increase in oxygen transport, both to skeletal and cardiac muscle. Neural mechanisms, mediated by the autonomic nervous system, and local mechanisms, mediated by the mechanical function of the heart and regional regulation of vascular resistance are essential to this coordinated response. An overview of the cardiovascular response to exercise is shown diagrammatically in Figure 1.8.

During dynamic exercise, involving rhythmic contractions of large muscle groups (such as running, swimming, or cycling), the cardiovascular response to exercise is initiated by higher order centers in the brain, termed *central command*.[42–44] As exercise continues, both mechanical and metabolic signals from active skeletal muscle provide feedback to cardiovascular centers in the brain to precisely match systemic oxygen delivery with

metabolic demand.[45,46] Vascular resistance decreases to facilitate increases in muscle perfusion, and cardiac output increases proportionate with oxygen uptake, thus allowing the maintenance or even increase in mean arterial pressure.

The cardiovascular responses to dynamic exercise and static exercise are significantly different: Static exercise (high-intensity, sustained muscle contractions limiting muscle blood flow such as weight lifting or isometric exercise) is associated with smaller increases in oxygen uptake, cardiac output, and stroke volume than with dynamic exercise, but with equivalent increases in blood pressure[47] (Fig. 1.9).

Many activities include a combination of both static and dynamic exercise. Under such circumstances, such as rowing, high-resistance cycling, or jumping sports, increases in blood pressure may be particularly dramatic[48,49] (Fig. 1.10).

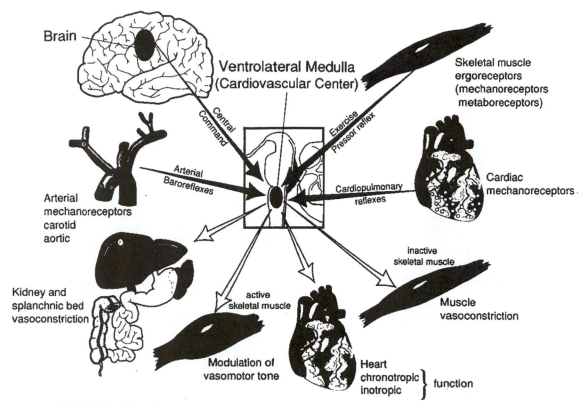

FIGURE 1.8. Pictorial representation of the cardiovascular response to exercise. Central command initiates the exercise pressor response, which is maintained and augmented via feedback from cardiopulmonary and arterial baroreceptors, as well as by stimulation of skeletal muscle mechanically sensitive and metabolically sensitive receptors. After integration in the brain, efferent responses via the parasympathetic (vagal) and sympathetic nervous systems result in increased heart rate and contractility, vasoconstriction in inactive skeletal muscle, and vasodilation in active muscle beds mediated by release of local vasodilating substances ("functional sympatholysis").

BLOOD PRESSURE REGULATION DURING AND AFTER EXERCISE: THE CONCEPT OF THE "TRIPLE PRODUCT"

Arterial pressure is a function of the triple product of heart rate × stroke volume (i.e., cardiac output) × total peripheral resistance.[50] Increases in both heart rate and stroke volume contribute to

the increase in cardiac output, though body posture markedly influences the relative importance of changes in stroke volume.

Gravity plays a critical role in determining the distribution of pressure and volume within the cardiovascular system.[51] In the upright position, stroke volume is only about one-half its value in the supine position, due to peripheral pooling and

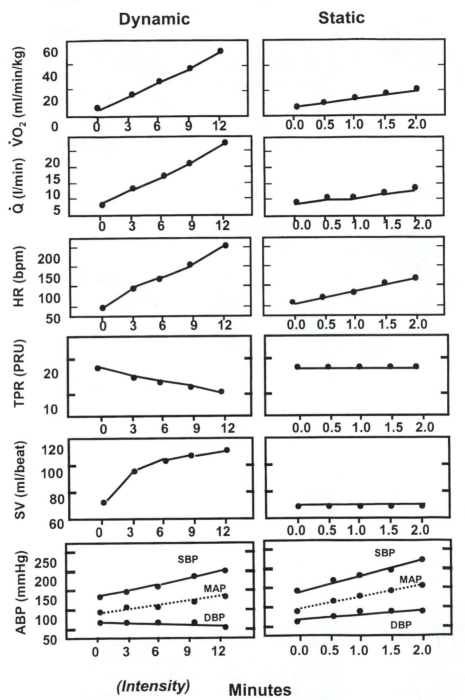

FIGURE 1.9. *Hemodynamic responses to dynamic (regular, rhythmic contraction of large muscle groups), and static (isometric or high intensity sustained contraction) exercise. Figure reproduced from Ref. 47.*

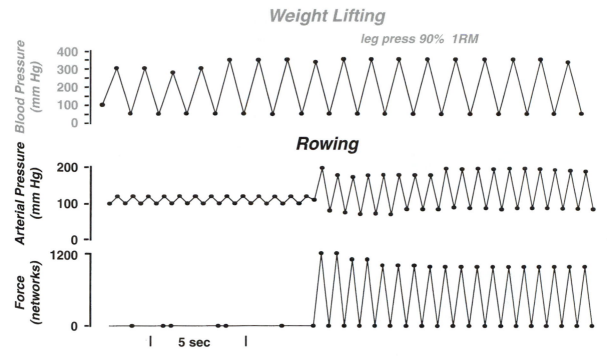

FIGURE 1.10. Top graph shows the dramatic hypertension (systolic blood pressure 300–400 mmHg) which occurs during weight lifting at 90% of a single repetition maximum (1RM) leg press. (From Ref. 48.) Bottom graph shows similar hypertension with mean blood pressures nearly 200 mmHg which occurs during each stroke on a rowing ergometer. From Ref. 49.

a reduction in left ventricular end-diastolic volume. At the onset of exercise, the pumping action of skeletal muscle (Fig. 1.11) acts to augment venous return substantially,[52,53] and stroke volume normally increases > 50% via the Starling mechanism.[54]

Maximal stroke volume is achieved at relatively low levels of exercise intensity (approximately 50% of $\dot{V}O_2$ max), as pericardial constraint serves to limit left ventricular end-diastolic volume. Evidence in support of this concept may be seen during supine exercise, when left ventricular end-diastolic volume and consequently SV (stroke volume) do not increase during graded exercise.[54] Moreover, if the pericardium is surgically removed, maximal stroke volume, maximal cardiac output, and maximal oxygen uptake may be increased in experimental animals.[55] Elite ath-

letes have a marked increase in the ability to use the Starling mechanism during exercise,[56] which is the primary adaptation allowing the very high maximal cardiac outputs and oxygen uptakes of endurance athletes. In contrast, patients with congestive heart failure have diminished diastolic reserve and stroke volume may not increase appreciably, even during upright exercise.[57]

At very high work rates, when a large amount of active muscle mass is engaged, the capacity for muscle vasodilatation may exceed the cardiac pump capacity and blood pressure may decrease unless sympathetically mediated vasoconstriction occurs in active muscle as well as other vascular beds.[7,58,59] If exercise and muscle contraction cease abruptly, the pumping action of skeletal muscle is lost despite a persistent vasodilatation (Fig. 1.12).

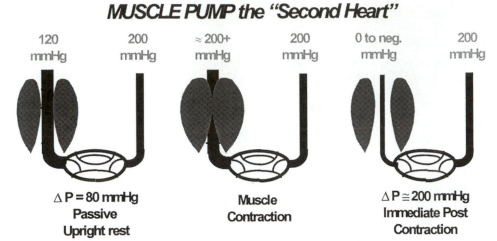

MUSCLE PUMP the "Second Heart"

| 120 mmHg | 200 mmHg | ≈ 200+ mmHg | 200 mmHg | 0 to neg. mmHg | 200 mmHg |

$\Delta P = 80$ mmHg
Passive Upright rest

Muscle Contraction

$\Delta P \cong 200$ mmHg
Immediate Post Contraction

FIGURE 1.11. In the upright position, large hydrostatic gradients exist in the lower extremities with a perfusion pressure of approximately 80 mmHg in leg skeletal muscle. During muscle contraction, the veins are transiently occluded resulting in a rise in pressure (middle figure); when the muscle relaxes, intact venous valves lead to a negative pressure in the veins markedly increasing the effective perfusion pressure. From Ref. 8.

The importance of this redistribution of the cardiac output into the venous capacitance was recognized more than 300 years ago by Lower who wrote in *De Corde* in 1669:

> A defective pulse and languor of the spirit are thus the sequel to over-dilation of these veins—venous dilation anywhere diminishes the movement of the heart very appreciably by diverting the due supply and inflow of blood.[60]

It should be no surprise therefore that blood pressure may fall acutely under such circumstances, and syncope is relatively common in athletes or exercising individuals who stand still immediately *following* a bout of intensive exercise, such as occurs after a road or track race or at the foul line on a basketball court. Originally described by Gordon in 1907,[61] this process of postexercise hypotension was first systematically investigated in the 1940s by Ludwig Eichna, who performed tilt studies on soldiers after marching or treadmill exercise, at the Armored Medical Research Laboratory in Fort Knox, Kentucky.[62] The *key observations* from these studies included the following:

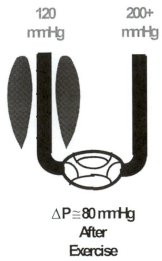

| 120 mmHg | 200+ mmHg |

$\Delta P \cong 80$ mmHg
After Exercise

FIGURE 1.12. During exercise there is a marked redistribution of the cardiac output to skeletal muscle due to metabolic vasodilation. After exercise, without the muscle pump to increase venous return, cardiac filling may fall dramatically due to a reduction in LVEDV and SV, leading to hypotension and syncope.

1. Slightly more than 50% of the soldiers experienced postexertional orthostatic hypotension.
2. Of these, an additional 50% (27% of the total) developed true syncope and were unable to remain in the tilt position for a full 5 min.
3. Repeat testing in susceptible individuals revealed continued syncope and orthostatic hypotension for an average of 1 and 2 h, respectively—in one subject after a 32-mi hike, orthostatic hypotension was still present 12 h after completion of the exercise.
4. Simple maneuvers such as moving the legs were sufficient to restore blood pressure to normal during acute hypotension, emphasizing the importance of both peripheral redistribution of blood volume and the muscle pump.

Studies by Holtzhausen and Noakes[63] before and after an ultramarathon of 80 km (50 mi) revealed that 68% of runners experienced orthostatic hypotension during quiet standing. Although none of their subjects actually became syncopal, 23% had blood pressures below 90 mmHg and all of these had symptoms of dizziness and nausea. Interestingly, the magnitude of the postrace orthostatic hypotension could not be related to the degree of plasma volume lost during the race, despite that on average the runners had lost nearly 5% of body weight. Thus, although dehydration probably contributed to reducing left ventricular filling and orthostatic hypotension, it appears likely that other factors regulating distribution of cardiac output such as thermoregulation may be more important. During severe heat stress, nearly one-third of the cardiac output may be redirected to the skin to facilitate cooling.[64]

HEART RATE REGULATION

At low levels of exercise, heart rate increases almost exclusively via vagal withdrawal, with little evidence for systematic increases in sympathetic nerve activity until the intensity of exercise is at or above the maximal steady state.[65,66] Central command plays an essential role in the increase in heart rate during exercise, in contrast to sympathetic nerve activity and the regulation of systemic vascular resistance, which is adjusted to feedback from muscle metaboreceptors.[44] Three (extensive) lines of evidence support this conceptual framework. First of all, cardioacceleration actually precedes the onset of muscle contraction during voluntary exercise.[42,67] Second, when neuromuscular blocking agents such as curare are administered to reduce muscle force and metabolic stimulation, but subjects are instructed to try to maintain force (increased effort and central command but decreased feedback from exercising muscle), the heart rate response is increased.[44,68] Third, if a blood pressure cuff is inflated to suprasystolic levels at peak exercise and subjects stop exercising, thereby trapping muscle metabolites and sustaining metaboreceptor stimulation but eliminating central command and mechanoreceptor stimulation, heart rate returns immediately to baseline, while blood pressure and sympathetic nerve activity remain high.[69]

The key determinant of the magnitude of the heart rate and blood pressure response to exercise is the *relative intensity*—that is, the fraction of maximal voluntary contraction for static exercise, or the percentage of $\dot{V}O_2$ max for dynamic exercise,[70] as well as the absolute amount of muscle mass engaged.[70,71] For example, consider two different individuals: a 30-year-old competitive marathon runner and a 50-year-old sedentary male executive. If each goes for an easy jog—the marathon runner at 10 mi/h, and the executive at 5 mi/h—each may be running at 70% of $\dot{V}O_2$ max and each might have a heart rate of 150, or 85% of maximal heart rate. In contrast, if the executive tried to run at 10 mi/h, he might easily achieve his maximal heart rate of 180 and be unable to sustain this absolute work rate for more than a few seconds. Similarly, if the marathon runner ran at 5 mi/h, this might be perceived as no more than minimal exertion and heart rate would be only slightly above rest. Moreover, if the executive performed exercise training for 6 months, he would increase his $\dot{V}O_2$ max and be able to run at substantially faster absolute speeds, even though his heart rate would remain 150 at 70% of $\dot{V}O_2$ max. A similar example could be given for static exercise. A 250-lb body builder might be able to lift 500 lb of weight with a maximal voluntary contraction (MVC), while the same executive could only lift 150 lb. However, at 30% of MVC (150 lb for the body builder, 45 lb for the executive), the heart rate and blood pressure response would be essentially the same. Weight training would reduce the relative cardiovascular stress at any given absolute workload in a fashion similar to endurance training as described earlier.

MYOCARDIAL OXYGEN DEMAND AND SUPPLY

The magnitude of the cardiovascular response to exercise will determine the magnitude by which blood flow to the heart must increase to meet its own oxygen requirements, *regardless of the absolute level of external work being performed.* Myocardial oxygen uptake ($\dot{M}O_2$), or the *internal* work of the heart, will depend on the extent to which the well-known determinants of myocardial oxygen requirements increase during exercise (Fig. 1.13). *It is important to emphasize that* the $\dot{M}O_2$, *rather than the* $\dot{V}O_2$ *is what determines the degree to which myocardial blood flow must increase during exercise.*

Although direct measures of $\dot{M}O_2$ are difficult to make, it can be estimated using simple clinical parameters measured during routine exercise tests. Figure 1.14 shows the derivation of the "rate pressure product," which provides a remarkably good estimate of MO_2[72] and which is weighted heavily toward the contribution of heart rate and chronotropic work, but also incorporates the significant contribution of inotropic, pressure, and volume work of the heart.

A form of the Fick equation, similar to that for *systemic* oxygen uptake emphasizes that *myocardial* oxygen uptake ($\dot{M}O_2$) is a function of myocardial blood flow multiplied by the arteriovenous oxygen difference across the heart. However, the heart is unique in that it extracts the majority of oxygen that it receives even at rest. Thus, the ability of the heart to augment oxygen utilization to meet increased energy demands must be met predominantly by increasing myocardial blood flow.

Normally, the coronary blood flow can increase by at least fivefold both via vasodilation of small, peripheral resistance arterioles, as well as

---

DETERMINANTS OF
MYOCARDIAL OXYGEN DEMANDS ($\dot{M}O_2$)

WALL STRESS *(LV PRESSURE * LV VOLUME)*
————————————————
WALL THICKNESS

HEART RATE

CONTRACTILITY

FIGURE 1.13. *The primary determinants of myocardial oxygen demands, including wall stress immediately before the onset of contraction (pre-load), wall stress immediately after and during contraction (after-load), heart rate (chronotropic work), and contractility.*

$$RPP = HR_{max} * SBP_{max}$$
$$HR * (Q_C * TPR)$$
$$HR * (HR * SV) * TP$$
$$RPP \approx HR^2 * SV * TPR$$

FIGURE 1.14. *Derivation of the rate-pressure product (RPP) as an index of myocardial oxygen consumption during exercise. HR = heart rate, SBP = systolic blood pressure, TPR = total peripheral resistance; Qc = cardiac output. Thus the RPP is weighted in favor of chronotropic work, but also includes components reflecting both pressure and volume work of the heart.*

by flow-mediated vasodilation of the large conduit arteries. This process is called *coronary flow reserve* and is the essential physiological factor that determines whether exercise will result in myocardial ischemia in patients with atherosclerosis. When atherosclerosis involves the epicardial vessels, both their conduit function and their vascular responsiveness may be impaired. A waterfall effect begins to become physiologically significant when the total luminal cross-sectional area is reduced approximately 75% (> 50% cross-sectional diameter).[73] In addition, even modest degrees of atherosclerosis may impair the normal endothelium-dependent vasodilation of the coronary arteries leading to vasoconstriction, rather than vasodilation during exercise as shown in Figure 1.15.[74]

Ultimately, if the ability to augment coronary blood flow is inadequate to meet myocardial oxygen demands at a given level of both systemic and myocardial work, then ischemia will develop. Probably the weak link in the interpretation of a clinical exercise test is that it uses a relatively indirect and nonspecific phenomenon to detect the presence of ischemia—shifts in the ST segment of the electrocardiogram (ECG).[35] Such changes

depend on a differential repolarization pattern between the endocardium and the epicardium resulting in shifts of the ST segment that may be detectable on the surface of the heart. However, it is important to emphasize that these shifts occur in a graded fashion and are proportional to the imbalance between $\dot{M}O_2$ and myocardial O_2 supply.[35] More severe and intense ischemia will lead to greater shifts in the ST segment of the ECG.[75] Thus, there is no "magic" associated with the standard clinical criteria of 1-mm ST-segment depression. It is simply a convenient measure that was determined initially from the fact that the recording paper was printed with 1-mm increments and is entirely dependent on the point at which the exercise test is stopped. This critical point has direct clinical relevance as well.

For example, the concept of Bayesian analysis of the exercise tolerance test, in which the pretest probability of disease is a specific determinant of the posttest probability of disease (see Chapter 4 for detailed discussion) is often cited as a limitation of exercise testing. However, this conceptual framework requires an exercise test to be "positive" or "negative" based on a discreet analysis of the exercise ECG (> 1-mm ST depression, posi-

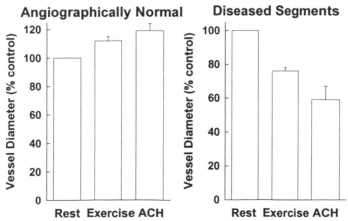

FIGURE 1.15. Change in coronary artery diameter during coronary arteriography in the same patients who have both angiographically normal appearing segments (left graph) and segments heavily involved with atherosclerosis (right graph). In the normal appearing segments, both exercise and acetylcholine infusion (ACH, an endothelium dependent vasodilator) result in vasodilation; in the obviously diseased segments, they cause vasoconstriction. From Ref. 74.

tive; < 1-mm ST depression, negative). Often overlooked in the original description of Bayesian analysis of the exercise ECG[76] is that in addition to the grouped analysis of all tests with ST-segment deviations > 1 mm, separate analyses were also performed of ST-segment deviations in 0.5-mm increments.

This approach is reproduced in Figure 1.16 and confirms the continuous nature of the ECG response during exercise. In this analysis, the posttest probability of angiographically significant coronary artery disease is radically different if there is 1.0- to 1.5-mm ST depression, compared to > 2.0-mm or downsloping ST-segment depression. Even for a very low pretest probability of disease of 20 to 30%, a test with > 2.0-mm or downsloping ST segments would very likely demonstrate > 50% coronary lesions. In fact, more than 20 years ago, the ultimate conclusion from this original presentation of Bayesian analysis was that "the terms 'positive' and 'negative' are inappropriate to describe most stress-test results. Instead, it should be interpreted in terms of a continuum of risk based on the extent of ST-segment depression."[76]

PERSONAL PERSPECTIVE: TOWARD A RATIONAL USE OF THE EXERCISE TEST IN THE MANAGEMENT OF PATIENTS WITH CORONARY HEART DISEASE

The past decade has seen a remarkable change in the management of patients with coronary heart disease. Medical therapy and percutaneous and surgical revascularization have all improved dramatically, including aggressive lipid-lowering therapy, coronary angioplasty and stenting, and new strategies for reducing the risk and prolonging the efficacy of bypass surgery. This revolution in disease management is due in part to fundamental changes in the understanding of the pathophysiology and now the biology of atherosclerosis that has driven mechanism-based changes in therapy.

In contrast to patient treatment, the strategies for patient assessment have not kept up with the progress made in basic science and therapy. One of the reasons for this discrepancy is the preference by most physi-

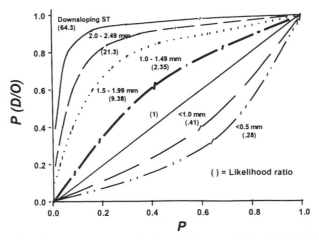

FIGURE 1.16. Graphical representation of Bayes theorem demonstrating the relationship between the pretest probability of disease (P, derived from clinical predictors) and the posttest probability of disease [P(D/O), determined by the presence of at least a 50% lesion in a coronary artery by angiography], and how it is influenced by ST segment depression of graded magnitudes during an exercise test. The likelihood ratio of 1 suggests that there is no difference between the pretest and posttest probability of disease after the test. Adapted from Ref. 76.

cians to have a test that is black and white, with outcomes that are positive or negative, and therefore a disease that is either "present" or "absent." Although this strategy may be useful for clearly discreet conditions, the approach may be more complicated with disorders such as atherosclerotic heart disease.

A consequence of the tendency toward discreet analysis of clinical problems has been a focus on terms such as *sensitivity* and *specificity* for the interpretation of cardiovascular tests.[77,78] Exercise testing has been used for more than 70 years for the evaluation of patients with coronary artery disease.[79] It has become one of the most frequently used diagnostic tests in clinical medicine, accounting for > 800,000 procedures per year. However, the performance of the routine exercise test without adjunctive imaging has been vilified in the literature.[80] Meta-analysis of the ETT (exercise tolerance test) involving 147 studies and > 24,000 patients who had both exercise tests with ECG monitoring and coronary angiography showed that the reported sensitivity ranged from 23% to > 90%, depending on the population being studied, with a mean sensitivity of 68%.[81,82] The specificity was slightly better, with a mean of 77%.[81,82] Such relatively poor test performance has led some investigators to suggest that the routine exercise test is nearly useless for the management of patients with coronary artery disease.[80]

However, in order to follow this approach, two fundamental tenets must be accepted: (a) that an exercise test is either positive or negative; and (b) that coronary artery disease is either present or absent. In the previous sections, it should be evident from a comprehensive understanding of exercise physiology that the former is untenable and that exercise responses are continuous variables that defy simple discreet characterization. Modern understanding of the development and progression of coronary artery disease has also provided evidence that atherosclerosis is similarly continuous.

THE CONTINUOUS NATURE OF CORONARY ARTERY DISEASE

The process of atherosclerosis begins early in life. Early studies of Korean War casualties revealed that a surprisingly high number of young American men between the ages of 18 to 20 already had the early fatty streaks and fibrous plaques that we now know develop into atherosclerotic lesions.[83] A comprehensive evaluation of accident victims in the United States has con-

firmed this finding.[84] A summary of the current understanding of the nature of the progression of coronary artery disease is shown in Figure 1.17.[85]

This figure emphasizes that not only may atherosclerosis progress slowly and continuously leading to the development of ischemia-causing lesions, but it also progresses rapidly and catastrophically leading to rapid changes in vessel diameter, vascular occlusion, and myocardial infarction. In fact, the majority of coronary events occur in blood vessels that are not necessarily heavily stenosed.[86,87] Thus, it should not be much of a surprise that exercise testing, which is designed to detect ischemia, would not be very good at detecting lesions that are not physiologically significant, but ultimately will experience plaque rupture and thrombosis.

This limitation is also present for virtually all routinely available diagnostic tests in cardiovascular medicine. The performance of an exercise test has most often been compared to coronary angiography as a "gold standard" to determine whether disease is present or absent. However, coronary angiography only depicts the lumen of the coronary blood vessels and does not give a clear picture of the presence or absence of atherosclerosis as shown in Figure 1.18.

Moreover, most of the articles examining the performance of exercise testing have relied on visual interpretation of the coronary angiogram for the determination of lesion significance, a technique that is notoriously unreliable. First of all, there is poor inter- and intraobserver variability in the assessment of coronary artery stenoses performed by visual interpretation of coronary angiograms.[88] Furthermore, even when the % diameter stenosis is determined by quantitative coronary angiography, there is poor correlation between the severity of the stenosis on the angiogram and the magnitude of its effect on limiting coronary flow reserve (Fig. 1.18).[89] Particularly in patients with multivessel disease, neither % cross-sectional diameter, nor % area stenosis is particularly good at detecting patients with abnormal coronary flow reserve, though the minimal luminal diameter may be more reliable.[90] Such measures appear to be more accurate when coronary disease is less extensive,[91] because the % area stenosis more closely reflects the minimal luminal diameter. The presence of eccentric, long, or complex lesions may further complicate the relation between angiographic appearance and physiological significance of a lesion (Table 1.4).

One of the most important articles which helps to

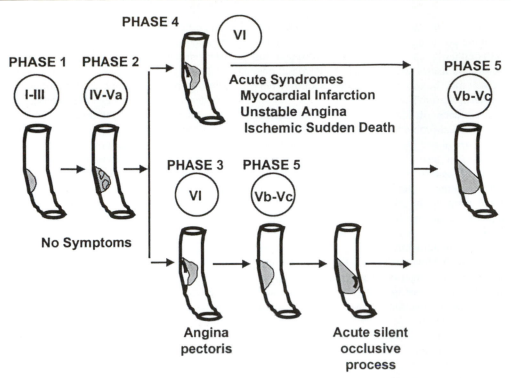

FIGURE 1.17. *Pictorial representation of the current understanding of the progression of athero-sclerosis, which begins at an early age with progressive deposition of atherosclerotic plaque (phase 1) and intermittent plaque fissuring or hemorrhage (phase 2) which are nonocclusive but lead to more rapid changes in plaque size. Angina pectoris develops when the degree of occlusion is sufficient to impair myocardial blood flow (phase 3); acute coronary syndromes develop when the blood vessel is frankly occluded which may occur suddenly and rapidly, even in a noncritical stenosis (phase 4).* Adapted from Ref. 85.

explain the apparent disparity between results of exercise testing and the "presence" of coronary artery disease by coronary angiography was published by Wilson et al in *Circulation* in 1991.[92] These investigators studied 40 patients with single vessel coronary artery disease, a normal resting ECG, and no left ventricular hypertrophy (LVH) or prior myocardial infarction. All patients underwent both graded treadmill exercise testing with ECG monitoring and coronary arteriography with the measurement of lesional severity both by quantitative coronary angiography and by the assessment of coronary flow reserve using a Doppler catheter after the injection of intracoronary papaverine (normal increase in flow velocity > 3.5 above rest). As expected from previous studies by this group, no static measure of lesion severity (percent diameter or percent area) predicted well patients with either ST-segment devia-

tion during exercise or coronary flow reserve. However, the vast majority of patients with no or minimal ST-segment deviation during exercise had normal coronary flow reserve (Fig. 1.19) regardless of lesion severity, confirming the ability of the coronary circulation to augment coronary blood flow to match increases in MO_2 during exercise. In contrast, the majority of patients with abnormal ST-segment deviation during exercise had abnormal flow reserve (Fig. 1.20). Furthermore, 100% of patients with severely reduced flow reserve (peak/resting velocity < 2.5) had significant ST segment depression during exercise (Fig. 1.21). Thus, although this study involved a relatively select patient population, it confirms that ST-segment depression during exercise is directly related to impaired coronary flow reserve, and normal coronary flow reserve, regardless of lesion severity, is usually

Angiographic View (Diameter)

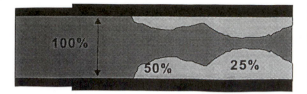
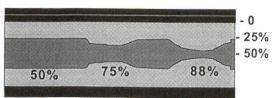

| Max Diameter = 50% ↓ From Normal | Min Diameter = 75% ↓ From Norm But 50% ↓ from Max Diameter in Adjacent Seg | Min Diameter = 88% ↓ From Norm But 75% ↓ from Max Diameter |

Histologic View (Diameter)

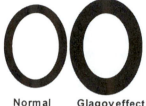
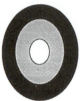

| Normal | Glagov effect "normal lumen" | 50% ↓ Diam. 75% ↓ X-Sec. Area | 75% ↓ Diam. 95% ↓ X-Sect. Area | 50% ↓ Diam. = 75% ↓ X-Sec. Area (Maximal Area) | 75% ↓ Diam. = 95% ↓ X-Sect. Area (20% ↓ from Max X-Sect. Area) | 88% ↓ Diam. = 98% ↓ X-Sect. Area (23% ↓ from Max X-Sect. Area) |

FIGURE 1.18. Demonstration of the difference between the angiographic view of a coronary lumen, and the pathological view of the entire blood vessel. The angiographic view may grossly underestimate the total atherosclerotic burden due to the Glagov effect which induces vascular remodeling at the early stages of atherosclerosis. Moreover, angiography may be hampered by the requirement to compare a lesion to a neighboring vessel which may or may not be involved diffusely with atherosclerosis. From Refs. 89, 90.

associated with the absence of ischemia significant enough to be detected by the surface ECG.

The clinical importance of this analysis is substantial. For example, there are often cases when patients have substantial ST-segment depression during exercise, but < 70% cross-sectional diameter lesions by coronary angiography. Such patients have generally been considered to have a "false positive" exercise test. An alternative interpretation could be, however, that the angiogram underestimated the physiological significance of the lesion (particularly common with diffuse disease) or that during exercise, endothelial dysfunction led to coronary vasoconstriction rather than vasodilation. I would consider such patients to have a "false

negative" catheterization. Similarly, some patients have no evidence of ST-segment depression during exercise, but coronary angiography reveals > 50% stenosis. Such patients have traditionally been considered to have a false negative exercise test. Alternatively, such

TABLE 1.4.   PROBLEMS WITH ANGIOGRAPHY

Poor inter- and intraobserver variability (particularly with 30–60% intermediate lesions)
Eccentric lesions
Diffuse disease
Static, resting measure

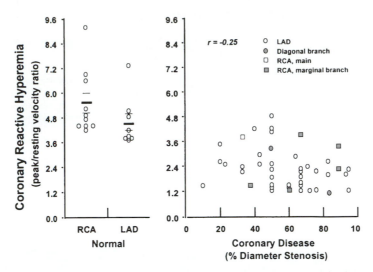

FIGURE 1.19. Vasodilator reserve as measured from reactive hyperemia (with a Doppler catheter in a coronary artery) after infusion of papaverine. A peak/resting velocity ratio, reflecting the peak increase in blood flow velocity compared to baseline of 3.5 or greater is considered normal, as shown on the left graph. The right graph shows that typical visual interpretations of a coronary angiogram assessing coronary disease from the % diameter stenosis do not predict well the vasodilator reserve in the coronary circulation, which is the key factor determining whether or not there will be ischemia during exercise. From Ref. 89.

patients may have normal coronary flow reserve, with an overestimation of the anatomic severity of the lesion (particularly common with visual interpretation of coronary angiograms). I would consider this situation to be a false positive catheterization. It is also possible that the test was stopped prematurely at either a fixed heart rate or work rate and that ischemia simply was not present at the systemic and myocardial work rates achieved on the specific exercise test.

In summary, Tables 1.5 and 1.6 list the goals of an exercise test that can and cannot be accomplished.

Finally, in this day of large-scale clinical trials as the standard for evaluating medical care, it should not be forgotten that statistical theory does not allow the application of population-based statistics to individual cases. Thus, the careful assessment of an individual patient, based on sound physiological understanding of both exercise physiology and coronary heart disease, remains an essential tool for the physician who must manage patients one at a time.

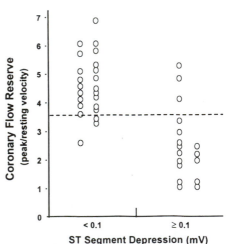

FIGURE 1.20. This figure shows that patients with ST segment depression of < 0.1 mV during an exercise test nearly always have normal coronary flow reserve, as determined by a peak/resting flow reserve ratio of 3.5 (dashed line). In contrast, patients with ≥ 0.1 mV ST depression during exercise nearly always have abnormal coronary flow reserve, regardless of coronary anatomy. From Ref. 92.

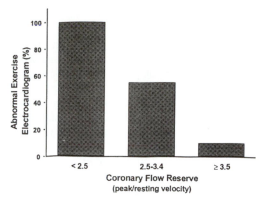

FIGURE 1.21. Quantitative relationship between the magnitude of impairment of coronary flow reserve and the presence of at least 0.1 mV ST depression on an exercise electrocardiogram. Note that virtually 100% of patients with severely impaired coronary flow reserve demonstrate significant ST depression during exercise. From Ref. 92.

ACKNOWLEDGMENTS

I would like to express my appreciation to George Brooks, Ph.D., Loren Bertocci, Ph.D., Tony Babb, Ph.D., and Jeramie Hinojosa, M.S., for their careful reading of this chapter and insightful suggestions.

TABLE 1.5.   GOALS OF EXERCISE TEST

Exercise Testing *Can:*

Determine functional capacity.

Evaluate global hemodynamic and cardiovascular function during physical activity.

Provide a predictable and objective setting for the evaluation of symptoms (chest pain, dyspnea, fatigue) of questionable etiology.

Detect the presence of myocardial ischemia during increasing $\dot{M}O_2$ that is sufficient to cause a shift in the ST segment of the ECG.

Identify a threshold of systemic and myocardial work rates beyond which ischemia is likely to be present.

Provide important clinical information that may assist in the estimation of prognosis (particularly by identifying low-risk subgroups of patients with ischemic heart disease).

TABLE 1.6.   GOALS OF EXERCISE TEST

Exercise Testing *Cannot:*

Determine the structure and composition of an atherosclerotic plaque (i.e., lipid laden-rupture *prone* vs. hard and calcific-rupture *resistant*).

Identify the presence of atherosclerotic plaques that will rupture and cause a myocardial infarction.

Predict the presence or absence of ischemia at work rates *greater* than that achieved on the test.

REFERENCES

1. Hoppeler H, Weibel ER: Limits for oxygen and substrate transport in mammals. *J Exp Biol* 201:1051–1064, 1998.
2. van Ingen Schenau GJ, Cavanagh PR: Power equations in endurance sports. *J Biomech* 23:865–881, 1990.
3. Baudinette RV: The energetics and cardiorespiratory correlates of mammalian terrestrial locomotion. *J Exp Biol* 160:209–231, 1991.
4. Mitchell JH, Blomqvist G: Maximal oxygen uptake. *N Engl J Med* 284:1018–1022, 1971.
5. Snell PG, Mitchell JH: The role of maximal oxygen uptake in exercise performance. *Clin Chest Med* 5:51–62 1984.
6. Lewis SF, Haller RG: Skeletal muscle disorders and associated factors that limit exercise performance. *Exerc Sport Sci Rev* 17:67–113, 1989.
7. Saltin B: Hemodynamic adaptations to exercise. *Am J Cardiol* 55:42D–47D, 1985.
8. Rowell LB: *Human Circulation: Regulation During Physical Stress.* 1st ed. New York: Oxford University Press; 1986.
9. Chomsky DB, Lang CC, Rayos GH, et al: Hemodynamic exercise testing: A valuable tool in the selection of cardiac transplantation candidates. *Circulation* 94:3176–3183, 1996.
10. Conconi F, Ferrari M, Ziglio PG, et al: Determination of the anaerobic threshold by a noninvasive field test in runners. *J Appl Physiol* 52:869–873, 1982.
11. Conconi F, Grazzi G, Casoni I, et al: The Conconi test: Methodology after 12 years of application [see comments]. *Int J Sports Med* 17:509–519, 1996.

12. Whipp BJ, Ward SA: Cardiopulmonary coupling during exercise. *J Exp Biol* 100:175–193, 1982.

13. Dempsey JA, Wagner PD: Exercise-induced arterial hypoxemia. *J Appl Physiol* 87:1997–2006, 1999.

14. O'Donnell DE, Lam M, Webb KA: Measurement of symptoms, lung hyperinflation, and endurance during exercise in chronic obstructive pulmonary disease. *Am J Resp Crit Care Med* 158:1557–1565, 1998.

15. O'Donnell DE: Dyspnea in advanced chronic obstructive pulmonary disease. *J Heart Lung Transpl* 17:544–554, 1998.

16. O'Donnell DE, Bertley JC, Chau LK, et al: Qualitative aspects of exertional breathlessness in chronic airflow limitation: Pathophysiologic mechanisms. *Am J Resp Crit Care Med* 155:109–115, 1997.

17. Brooks GA: Anaerobic threshold: Review of the concept and directions for future research. *Med Sci Sports Exerc* 17:22–34, 1985.

18. Davis JA: Anaerobic threshold: Review of the concept and directions for future research. *Med Sci Sports Exerc* 17:6–21, 1985.

19. Wasserman K: Anaerobiosis, lactate, and gas exchange during exercise: The issues. *Fed Proc* 45:2904–2909, 1986.

20. Connett RJ, Gayeski TE, Honig CR: Lactate accumulation in fully aerobic, working, dog gracilis muscle. *Am J Physiol* 246:H120–H128, 1984.

21. Myers J, Ashley E: Dangerous curves. A perspective on exercise, lactate, and the anaerobic threshold. *Chest* 111:787–795, 1997.

22. Connett RJ, Honig CR, Gayeski TE, et al: Defining hypoxia: A systems view of Vo_2, glycolysis, energetics, and intracellular Po_2. *J Appl Physiol* 68:833–842, 1990.

23. Connett RJ, Sahlin K: *Control of glycolysis and glycogen metabolism.* New York: Oxford University Press for the American Physiological Society; 1996.

24. Katz A, Sahlin K: Regulation of lactic acid production during exercise. *J Appl Physiol* 65:509–518, 1988.

25. Howlett RA, Heigenhauser GJ, Hultman E, et al: Effects of dichloroacetate infusion on human skeletal muscle metabolism at the onset of exercise. *Am J Physiol* 277:E18–E25, 1999.

26. Gibala MJ, MacLean DA, Graham TE, et al: Anaplerotic processes in human skeletal muscle

during brief dynamic exercise. *J Physiol* 502:703–713, 1997.

27. Medbo JI, Mohn AC, Tabata I, et al: Anaerobic capacity determined by maximal accumulated O_2 deficit [see comments]. *J Appl Physiol* 64:50–60, 1988.

28. Medbo JI, Tabata I: Relative importance of aerobic and anaerobic energy release during short-lasting exhausting bicycle exercise. *J Appl Physiol* 67:1881–1886, 1989.

29. Medbo JI, Burgers S: Effect of training on the anaerobic capacity. *Med Sci Sports Exerc* 22:501–507, 1990.

30. Astrand I, Astrand PO, Hallback I, et al: Reduction in maximal oxygen uptake with age. *J Appl Physiol* 35:649–654, 1973.

31. Hodgson JL, Buskirk ER: Physical fitness and age, with emphasis on cardiovascular function in the elderly. *J Am Geriatr Soc* 25:385–392, 1977.

32. Astrand PO, Bergh U, Kilbom A: A 33-yr follow-up of peak oxygen uptake and related variables of former physical education students. *J Appl Physiol* 82:1844–1852, 1997.

33. Kasch FW, Boyer JL, Van Camp S, et al: Cardiovascular changes with age and exercise. A 28-year longitudinal study [see comments]. *Scand J Med Sci Sports* 5:147–151, 1995.

34. Fletcher GF, Balady G, Blair SN, et al: Statement on exercise: Benefits and recommendations for physical activity programs for all Americans. A statement for health professionals by the Committee on Exercise and Cardiac Rehabilitation of the Council on Clinical Cardiology, American Heart Association. *Circulation* 94:857–862, 1996.

35. Fletcher GF, Balady G, Froelicher VF, et al: Exercise standards. A statement for healthcare professionals from the American Heart Association. Writing Group [see comments]. *Circulation* 91:580–615, 1995.

36. Weber KT: What can we learn from exercise testing beyond the detection of myocardial ischemia? *Clin Cardiol* 20:684–696, 1997.

37. DeBusk RF, Blomqvist CG, Kouchoukos NT, et al: Identification and treatment of low-risk patients after acute myocardial infarction and coronary-artery bypass graft surgery. *N Engl J Med* 314:161–166, 1986.

38. Bruce RA, McDonough JR: Stress testing in screening for cardiovascular disease. *Bull N Y Acad Med* 45:1288–1305, 1969.

39. Levine BD, Stray-Gundersen J: "Living high-training low": Effect of moderate-altitude acclimatization with low-altitude training on performance. *J Appl Physiol* 83:102–112, 1997.

40. Myers J, Froelicher VF: Exercise testing. Procedures and implementation. *Cardiol Clin* 11: 199–213, 1993.

41. Knight DR, Poole DC, Schaffartzik W, et al: Relationship between body and leg $\dot{V}o_2$ during maximal cycle ergometry. *J Appl Physiol* 73: 1114–1121, 1992.

42. Victor RG, Secher NH, Lyson T, et al: Central command increases muscle sympathetic nerve activity during intense intermittent isometric exercise in humans. *Circ Res* 76:127–131, 1995.

43. Williamson JW, Olesen HL, Pott F, et al: Central command increases cardiac output during static exercise in humans. *Acta Physiol Scand* 156:429–434, 1996.

44. Mitchell JH, Victor RG: Neural control of the cardiovascular system: Insights from muscle sympathetic nerve recordings in humans. *Med Sci Sports Exerc* 28:S60–S69, 1996.

45. Rowell LB: *Human Circulation: Regulation During Physical Stress.* 2nd ed. New York: Oxford University Press; 1996.

46. Thomas GD, Chavoshan B, Sander M, et al: Invited editorial on "Effect of arterial occlusion on responses of group III and IV afferents to dynamic exercise" [editorial]. *J Appl Physiol* 84: 1825–1826, 1998.

47. Mitchell JH, Haskell WL, Raven PB, et al: Classification of sports. *J Am Coll Cardiol* 24: 864–866, 1994.

48. MacDougall JD, Tuxen D, Sale DG, et al: Arterial blood pressure response to heavy resistance exercise. *J Appl Physiol* 58:785–790, 1985.

49. Clifford PS, Hanel B, Secher NH: Arterial blood pressure response to rowing. *Med Sci Sports Exerc* 26:715–719, 1994.

50. Levine BD, Buckey JC, Fritsch JM, et al: Physical fitness and cardiovascular regulation: Mechanisms of orthostatic intolerance. *J Appl Physiol* 70: 112–122, 1991.

51. Blomqvist CG, Stone HL: Cardiovascular adjustments to gravitational stress. In: Shepherd JT, Abboud FM, eds. *Handbook of Physiology: The Cardiovascular System.* Bethesda, MD: American Physiological Society; 1025–1063, 1983.

52. Richardson RS, Poole DC, Knight DR, et al: High muscle blood flow in man: Is maximal O_2 extraction compromised? *J Appl Physiol* 75:1911–1916, 1993.

53. Sheriff DD, Zhou XP, Scher AM, et al: Dependence of cardiac filling pressure on cardiac output during rest and dynamic exercise in dogs. *Am J Physiol* 265:H316–H322, 1993.

54. Poliner LR, Dehmer GJ, Lewis SE, et al: Left ventricular performance in normal subjects: A comparison of the responses to exercise in the upright and supine positions. *Circulation* 62:528–534, 1980.

55. Stray-Gundersen J, Musch TI, Haidet GC, et al: The effect of pericardiectomy on maximal oxygen consumption and maximal cardiac output in untrained dogs. *Circ Res* 58:523–530, 1986.

56. Levine BD, Lane LD, Buckey JC, et al: Left ventricular pressure-volume and Frank-Starling relations in endurance athletes. Implications for orthostatic tolerance and exercise performance. *Circulation* 84:1016–1023, 1991.

57. Sullivan MJ, Cobb FR: Central hemodynamic response to exercise in patients with chronic heart failure. *Chest* 101:340S–346S, 1992.

58. Secher NH, Clausen JP, Klausen K, et al: Central and regional circulatory effects of adding arm exercise to leg exercise. *Acta Physiol Scand* 100: 288–297, 1977.

59. Saltin B: Capacity of blood flow delivery to exercising skeletal muscle in humans. *Am J Cardiol* 62:30E–35E, 1988.

60. Lower R: Tractatus de corde, item de motu et colore sanguinis, et chyli in eum transitu, in Redmayne J (ed). London: J Allestry; 1669.

61. Gordon GA: Observations on the effect of prolonged and severe exertion on the blood pressure in healthy athletes. *Edin Med J* 22:53–56, 1907.

62. Eichna LW, Horvath SM, Bean WB: Post-exertional orthostatic hypotension. *Am J Med Sci* 213:641–654, 1947.

63. Holtzhausen LM, Noakes TD: The prevalence and significance of post-exercise (postural) hypotension in ultramarathon runners. *Med Sci Sports Exerc* 27:1595–1601, 1995.

64. Rowell LB: Cardiovascular aspects of human thermoregulation. *Circ Res* 52:367–379, 1983.

65. Ray CA, Rea RF, Clary MP, et al: Muscle sympathetic nerve responses to dynamic one-legged exercise: Effect of body posture. *Am J Physiol* 264:H1–H7, 1993.

66. Saito M, Tsukanaka A, Yanagihara D, et al: Muscle sympathetic nerve responses to graded leg cycling. *J Appl Physiol* 75:663–667, 1993.

67. Vissing SF, Scherrer U, Victor RG: Stimulation of skin sympathetic nerve discharge by central command. Differential control of sympathetic outflow to skin and skeletal muscle during static exercise. *Circ Res* 69:228–238, 1991.

68. Leonard B, Mitchell JH, Mizuno M, et al: Partial neuromuscular blockade and cardiovascular responses to static exercise in man. *J Physiol (Lond)* 359:365–379, 1985.

69. Mitchell JH, Kaufman MP, Iwamoto GA: The exercise pressor reflex: Its cardiovascular effects, afferent mechanisms, and central pathways. *Annu Rev Physiol* 45:229–242, 1983.

70. Lewis SF, Taylor WF, Graham RM, et al: Cardiovascular responses to exercise as functions of absolute and relative work load. *J Appl Physiol* 54:1314–1323, 1983.

71. Mitchell JH, Payne FC, Saltin B, et al: The role of muscle mass in the cardiovascular response to static contractions. *J Physiol (Lond)* 309:45–54, 1980.

72. Rooke GA, Feigl EO: Work as a correlate of canine left ventricular oxygen consumption, and the problem of catecholamine oxygen wasting. *Circ Res* 50:273–286, 1982.

73. Gould KL, Lipscomb K, Hamilton GW: Physiologic basis for assessing critical coronary stenosis. Instantaneous flow response and regional distribution during coronary hyperemia as measures of coronary flow reserve. *Am J Cardiol* 33:87–94, 1974.

74. Gordon JB, Ganz P, Nabel EG, et al: Atherosclerosis influences the vasomotor response of epicardial coronary arteries to exercise. *J Clin Invest* 83:1946–1952, 1989.

75. Tavel ME, Shaar C: Relation between the electrocardiographic stress test and degree and location of myocardial ischemia. *Am J Cardiol* 84:119–124, 1999.

76. Rifkin RD, Hood WB, Jr: Bayesian analysis of electrocardiographic exercise stress testing. *N Engl J Med* 297:681–686, 1977.

77. Yerushalmy J: Statistical problems in assessing methods of medical diagnosis, with special reference to x-ray techniques. *Pub Health Rep* 62:1432–1449, 1947.

78. Diamond GA, Forrester JS: Analysis of probability as an aid in the clinical diagnosis of coronary-artery disease. *N Engl J Med* 300:1350–1358, 1979.

79. Master AM, Oppenheimer ET: A simple exercise tolerance test for circulatory efficiency with standard tables for normal individuals. *Am J Med Sci* 177:223, 1929.

80. Borer JS, Brensike JF, Redwood DR, et al: Limitations of the electrocardiographic response to exercise in predicting coronary-artery disease. *N Engl J Med* 293:367–371, 1975.

81. Detrano R, Gianrossi R, Froelicher V: The diagnostic accuracy of the exercise electrocardiogram: A meta-analysis of 22 years of research. *Prog Cardiovasc Dis* 32:173–206, 1989.

82. Gianrossi R, Detrano R, Mulvihill D, et al: Exercise-induced ST depression in the diagnosis of coronary artery disease. A meta-analysis. *Circulation* 80:87–98, 1989.

83. Strong JP. Landmark perspective: Coronary atherosclerosis in soldiers. A clue to the natural history of atherosclerosis in the young. *JAMA* 256:2863–2866, 1986.

84. Strong JP, Malcom GT, McMahan CA, et al: Prevalence and extent of atherosclerosis in adolescents and young adults: Implications for prevention from the Pathobiological Determinants of Atherosclerosis in Youth Study. *JAMA* 281:727–735, 1999.

85. Fuster V: Elucidation of the role of plaque instability and rupture in acute coronary events. *Am J Cardiol* 76:24C–33C, 1995.

86. Little WC, Constantinescu M, Applegate RJ, et al: Can coronary angiography predict the site of a subsequent myocardial infarction in patients with mild-to-moderate coronary artery disease? *Circulation* 78:1157–1166, 1988.

87. Ambrose JA, Tannenbaum MA, Alexopoulos D, et al: Angiographic progression of coronary artery disease and the development of myocardial infarction. *J Am Coll Cardiol* 12:56–62, 1988.

88. Zir LM, Miller SW, Dinsmore RE, et al: Interobserver variability in coronary angiography. *Circulation* 53:627–632, 1976.

89. White CW, Wright CB, Doty DB, et al: Does visual interpretation of the coronary arteriogram predict the physiologic importance of a coronary stenosis? *N Engl J Med* 310:819–824, 1984.

90. Harrison DG, White CW, Hiratzka LF, et al: The value of lesion cross-sectional area determined by quantitative coronary angiography in assessing the

physiologic significance of proximal left anterior descending coronary arterial stenoses. *Circulation* 69:1111–1119, 1984.

91. Wilson RF, Marcus ML, White CW: Prediction of the physiologic significance of coronary arterial lesions by quantitative lesion geometry in patients with limited coronary artery disease. *Circulation* 75:723–732, 1987.

92. Wilson RF, Marcus ML, Christensen BV, et al: Accuracy of exercise electrocardiography in detecting physiologically significant coronary arterial lesions. *Circulation* 83:412–421, 1991.

Chapter 2

OVERVIEW OF THE ATHLETIC HEART SYNDROME

James C. Puffer, M.D.

The ability to perform vigorous physical activity is, to a great extent, a multiorgan system phenomenon. While the response of the body to muscular exercise is dependent upon the integrated functioning of each of these organ systems, the cardiovascular system plays a critical role in mediating strenuous activity. Continuous muscular work ultimately depends upon the transport of oxygen to the periphery to be utilized at the cellular level. Well-conditioned, elite athletes have been noted for the significant increases in oxygen consumption that they sustain at peak exercise; in some instances, this may reach 25 times that noted at rest. While the ability to optimize oxygen consumption relies upon the ability of the lungs to supply oxygen as well as the ability of peripheral tissues to extract oxygen, the most important factor is the ability of the cardiovascular system to supply oxygen to exercising muscle. As a result, the heart undergoes profound changes in response to systematic athletic training. These changes result in morphologic, functional, and electrophysiological alterations, which have collectively been identified and recognized as the athletic heart syndrome.

HISTORICAL PERSPECTIVE

It seems logical to assume that the athlete's heart plays a significant role in the ability to perform maximum muscular work. This was noted as early as the seventeenth century by the father of cardiology, Giovanni Lancisi.[1] In the late nineteenth century, the great Sir William Osler noted, "In the process of training, the getting of wind as it is called, is largely a gradual increase in the capability of the heart . . . the large heart of athletes may be due to the prolonged use of their muscles, but no man becomes a great runner or oarsman who has not naturally a capable if not large heart."[2] Unfortunately, however, many physicians in the late nineteenth and early twentieth centuries felt that athletic activity had deleterious effects on the heart. This resulted from the work of the German cardiologist, Beneke, who published calculations in 1879 explaining that the growth of the left ventricle was disproportionate to the diameter of the ascending aorta in adolescent athletes.[3] This myth persisted for almost 50 years until work done by two Austrian physicians dispelled it.[4]

Felix Deutsch and Emil Kauf systematically studied the hearts of thousands of athletes of all ages at the Vienna Heart Station.[4] The Heart Station was the central location for the examination of Austrian athletes' hearts. Using a technique known as roentgenographic orthodiagraphy, with all subjects in the standing position and the diaphragm held constant, they measured the transverse diameter of the heart and compared these measurements to figures for the normal population. Their data, compiled for male and female athletes in 16 sports, revealed that the average heart size of male competitive swimmers exceeded normal by 30 to 40%, while female competitive swimmers had increases of 4 to 12%. The greatest average increases in heart size were noted in cross-country skiers, followed by oars-

men, cyclists, swimmers, wrestlers, mountain climbers, runners, weight lifters and throwers, soccer players, boxers, and fencers. They followed these athletes at 6-month intervals for the purpose of reexamination and found no serious problem of disproportionate heart size among those athletes who participated in regular, vigorous training. Interestingly, they found that older athletes and those who had trained longer had the largest transverse diameters.

While this seminal piece of work dispelled the notion that vigorous athletic activity was deleterious to health, it raised several interesting questions with respect to heart size and athletic ability. Are championship athletes naturally endowed with large hearts, or do the changes noted in cardiac dimension occur as a result of vigorous physical training? While the work of Deutsch and Kauf could not specifically answer this question, later work has provided insight into the athletic heart syndrome. Before reviewing this, however, it is perhaps useful to review some physiological considerations that play an important role in the manifestations of this syndrome.

PHYSIOLOGICAL CONSIDERATIONS

As mentioned previously, the ability to perform continuous muscular work depends upon the transport of oxygen to exercising muscle. Oxygen consumption can best be appreciated by understanding the Fick Principle. Mathematically, this principle can be expressed as follows:

$$V_{O_2} = (CO)(A-V_{O_2} \text{ difference})$$

The Fick Principle reveals that oxygen consumption is a function of cardiac output multiplied by the difference between oxygen content in arterial and mixed venous blood. Furthermore, this equation demonstrates that there are both central and peripheral mechanisms that are responsible for governing oxygen consumption in the athlete, since the extraction of the oxygen by peripheral tissues is critical in determining $A-V_{O_2}$ difference. Our discussion of the athletic heart syndrome will concentrate on the portion of this equation that deals with central mechanisms responsible for oxygen consumption, namely cardiac output.

It is obvious that the performance of strenuous exercise requires a significant demand for increased cardiac output. The role that cardiac output plays in the determination of peak levels of exercise by well-conditioned athletes can best be appreciated when factors that determine cardiac efficiency are taken into consideration. Astrand and Rodohl have enumerated five factors that significantly influence work efficiency:[5]

1. A given stroke volume can be ejected with the minimum myocardial shortening if the contraction starts at a larger volume.
2. Energy losses in the form of friction and tension developed in the heart wall are also at a minimum in the dilated heart.
3. Stretched muscle fiber can, within limits, provide a higher tension than can the unstretched one.
4. Loss of energy is larger when contraction occurs rapidly, that is, with a high heart rate as compared to a slower one.
5. The greater the volume of the heart, the higher the tension of the myocardial fibers necessary to sustain a particular intraventricular pressure (as a consequence of LaPlace's law).

It is apparent that the first four factors favorably influence work efficiency while the fifth tends to decrease efficiency at maximum workloads. LaPlace's law explains that wall tension is directly related to intraventricular pressure and the radius of the ventricle, and inversely related to wall thickness. This can be expressed in the following way:

$$T = (P)(R/Th)$$

Therefore, it can be seen that increases in chamber size can be moderated by concomitant increases in wall thickness. Therefore, theoretically,

an individual with a high capacity for oxygen transport would best benefit from a heart that was able to produce a large stroke volume and that had a slow heart rate. This was confirmed as early as 1918 by Evans; he demonstrated in isolated heart preparations that an increase in cardiac output, caused by increased stroke volume, markedly improved the efficiency of cardiac work as evidenced by lower myocardial oxygen demands.[6]

MORPHOLOGIC CHANGES

From the discussion earlier, it can be appreciated that changes in cardiac dimension are effected to create significant mechanical advantage when cardiovascular hemodynamics are taken into consideration. The athlete in need of a high capacity for oxygen transport benefits from a large stroke volume, a low heart rate, and a hypertrophied ventricular wall. While the heart maintains its ability to function adequately as a pump by altering heart rate and contractility when a sudden demand is placed upon it, the heart responds to chronic demand by means of dilation and hypertrophy. Therefore, athletes who participate primarily in activities that place chronic volume demands upon the heart would be expected to increase end-diastolic diameter with resultant increases in wall thickness to normalize wall tension. In contrast, athletes who participate in sports that place chronic pressure demands on the heart would be expected to increase wall thickness without corresponding changes in end-diastolic diameter.

Sufficient experimental evidence exists to support these assumptions. Morgenroth and colleagues utilized echocardiography to assess left ventricular dimensions in 56 athletes.[7] They demonstrated that left ventricular end-diastolic volume and mass increased in isotonic athletes (athletes performing work with chronic volume demands) as compared to controls, while isometric athletes (athletes performing work that required chronic pressure demand) had increased left ventricular mass but normal end-diastolic volume. On average, wall thickness was greater in the isometric athletes.

Further evidence demonstrates that these changes in the dimensions of the heart, in fact, are responsible for performance. Turpeinen and colleagues used magnetic resonance imaging and echocardiography to assess cardiac dimensions in 9 male endurance athletes and 8 sedentary controls. As would be expected, they demonstrated that the trained subjects had evidence of significant increases in left ventricular mass as well as increased long axis left ventricular diameter. Most importantly, however, they demonstrated that maximum oxygen consumption significantly correlated with long axis left ventricular diameter.[8]

As mentioned earlier, one of the critical questions that could not be answered by reviewing the Deutsch and Kauf data was whether athletes were naturally endowed with large hearts or whether their hearts changed in response to exercise. Work by Ehsani and colleagues has answered this question.[9] They performed a longitudinal study in which cardiac dimension was assessed in response to training and detraining in competitive swimmers over a 12-week period. During the 9-week training session, left ventricular end-diastolic diameter increased significantly from 48.7 mm at baseline to 52 mm. Correspondingly, left ventricular free-wall thickness increased significantly from 9.4 mm at baseline to 10.1 mm at the end of the training session. After 3 weeks of detraining, echocardiographic measurements were again performed revealing evidence of significant regression in all of the athletes studied.

The degree to which wall thickness changes in response to exercise is highly variable. Perhaps the largest series of athletes whose cardiac dimensions have been studied noninvasively has been performed by Pelliccia and colleagues.[10] He used echocardiography to measure left ventricular dimensions in 947 elite, male athletes.[10] Wall thickness varied from less than 7 mm to as much as 16 mm. Sixteen athletes had wall thicknesses greater than or equal to 13 mm, and 15 of the athletes with the greatest wall thicknesses were rowers or canoeists. This group collected similar data from elite, female athletes.[11] Using echocardiography, they assessed cardiac dimension in 600 elite, female athletes compared with 65 sedentary controls. Left ventricular end-diastolic diameter and wall thickness were greater in the athletes as compared to the controls by 6 and 14%, respectively. Left ventricular end-diastolic diameter exceeded 54 mm in 47 women. The data are represented in Figures 2.1 and 2.2.

Considerable evidence has been presented to support the notion that the changes in cardiac dimension that occur in athletes are a normal adaptive response to strenuous exercise. The work of Sugishita and colleagues should be reviewed[12] to compare and contrast the normal changes that occur in the athlete's heart in response to training from the abnormal changes that occur in response to pathological conditions in the heart. They assessed cardiac morphology echocardiographically in 31 runners and 17 judo athletes and compared this data with that obtained from 15 patients with aortic regurgitation, 13 patients with hypertension, 14 patients with dilated cardiomyopathy, 11 patients with hypertrophic cardiomyopathy, and 25 controls. They found that the ratio of left ventricular radius to wall thickness was normal in runners but increased in patients with aortic regurgitation and dilated cardiomyopathy. Therefore, the changes that occurred in response to the chronic volume demands placed upon the long-distance runners' hearts could clearly be distinguished from the abnormal changes in those patients with pathological volume overload states.

FUNCTIONAL CHANGES

The advent of positron emission tomography (PET) has provided new technology to further assess the properties of the athletic heart noninvasively. Nuutila and coworkers have assessed metabolic function in the hearts of endurance athletes using this new imaging technology.[13] They evaluated insulin-stimulated glucose uptake in the heart and skeletal muscle of 7 male endurance

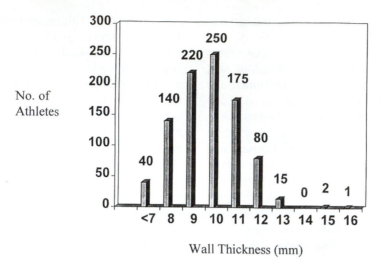

FIGURE 2.1. Left ventricular wall thickness in 947 elite male athletes measured by echocardiography. *Adapted with permission from Pelliccia A, Maron BJ, Spataro A, et al: The upper limit of physiologic cardiac hypertrophy in highly trained elite athletes. N Engl J Med 324:295–301, 1991.*

athletes and 7 sedentary controls. While glucose uptake was enhanced in the whole body and skeletal muscle in the athletes as compared to the controls, myocardial glucose uptake was reduced. This suggests that the athlete's heart either has altered energy requirements or alternatively may use a different substrate for meeting energy de-

mands. Turpeinen and colleagues demonstrated with PET that fatty acid oxidation was not used preferentially as an alternative energy source.[8] While these data suggest that the energy requirements for the athlete's heart may, in fact, be unique, no data to date have been published looking at coronary perfusion reserve in the athletic

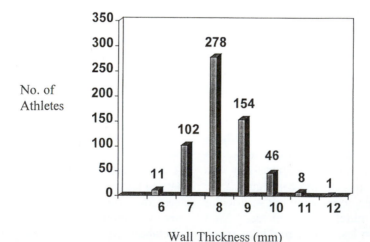

FIGURE 2.2. Left ventricular wall thickness in 600 elite female athletes measured by echocardiography. *Adapted with permission from Pelliccia A, Maron BJ, Culasso F, et al: Athlete's heart in women. JAMA 276:211–215, 1996.*

heart. We have undertaken a pilot study using N-13 ammonia and PET before and after dipyridamole administration in competitive athletes and age-matched controls. Resting echocardiograms and maximum oxygen consumption were obtained prior to evaluation. Data from a small number of subjects suggest that regional myocardial blood flow is similar in both the athletes' and controls' hearts and that the coronary reserve is normal-to-increased after dipyridamole administration. No relation has been demonstrated between left ventricular wall thickness and blood flow or coronary reserve.[14]

THE ELECTROCARDIOGRAM

A number of common electrocardiographic findings have been documented in athletes. These changes include alterations in rhythm, conduction, repolarization, and precordial voltage. Most of these effects can be attributed to an increase in vagal tone or to an alteration in the total neural input to the heart resulting in downregulation in sympathetic drive. Alternatively, denervation studies, performed either surgically or chemically induced with atropine and propranolol, have revealed that trained subjects consistently demonstrate lower intrinsic heart rates than sedentary controls, whether at rest or during exercise. This suggests an intrinsic cardiac component to these changes.[15] In all likelihood, the effect of training on both autonomic input and intrinsic pacemaker adaptation most likely account for the majority of the electrocardiographic changes which will be described later.

By far the most frequent finding in the electrocardiogram (ECG) of well-conditioned athletes is resting sinus bradycardia. This has been noted in over one-half of all dynamic athletes, with a recorded resting rate as low as 25.[16] However, sinus arrhythmia occurs almost as commonly. Several studies have documented the presence of this rhythm in 13.5 to 69% of athletes studied; a rate that is significantly higher than the 2.4% found in the general population.[15] A wandering atrial pacemaker has been found less frequently but does appear to occur more commonly in athletes than in sedentary controls. All of these rhythms extinguish with exercise as sympathetic drive is increased. Conduction abnormalities also occur commonly in well-conditioned athletes. First-degree atrioventricular block occurs with a frequency of anywhere between 10 and 33%, which is again significantly higher than the 0.65% found in the general population.[15] Interestingly, in athletes in whom first-degree heart block is absent, relative prolongation of the PR interval is frequently noted.[17] As might be expected, the PR interval normalizes or shortens following exercise.

Second-degree atrioventricular block has also been reported in well-conditioned athletes. While the frequency of Möbitz type I and II heart block in an asymptomatic population is less than 0.003%, Möbitz I block has been reported in 2.4 to 10% of athletes.[15] Zeppilli and coworkers investigated 10 athletes with Möbitz I second-degree heart block.[18] They found that a Valsalva maneuver normalized conduction in 7, while exertion resulted in normal conduction in 9. The administration of atropine corrected this conduction abnormality in all 10. They noted that complete remission occurred following cessation of training. Several of the athletes demonstrated variation in the degree of block on previous ECGs, which was primarily related to the intensity of the training. Five additional cases, as well as two cases of third-degree heart block were reported from a pool of 12,000 athletes.[19] Sympathetic inducing maneuvers normalized the conduction in all of these athletes, and again sinus rhythm was restored when training stopped. Nine years of follow-up did not reveal evidence of progression of heart block.

Junctional rhythm, which is present in only 0.06% of the general population, has been reported with a frequency varying between 0.31 to 7% in athletes.[15] Postexercise junctional rhythm has been observed in well-trained athletes as well. While a complete bundle branch block has been described in a small number of athletes, there is no reliable evidence to suggest that it occurs more frequently in athletes or is induced by training. A summary of these finding is found in Table 2.1.

Studies in which electrocardiographic comparisons of athletes and nonathletes have been obtained from routine 12-lead ECG tracings are somewhat problematic in that only a few seconds of cardiac electrical activity is recorded on these tracings. Depending on the relative balance between sympathetic and parasympathetic activity at the moment of measurement, many abnormalities may be missed. The easiest way to avoid this problem is with the use of ambulatory electrocardiographic technology, which captures electrical activity over a prolonged period of time. A study by Hanne-Paparo and Kellerman demonstrated that athletes had consistently lower heart rates, higher incidence of first- and second-degree block, and more frequent and longer sinus pauses then a group of controls.[20] The incidence of ventricular premature beats was similar, while two controls had short runs of ventricular tachycardia compared to none of the athletes. These findings have been duplicated in subsequent studies with similar methodology.

Alterations in repolarization also occur frequently in athletes and can be categorized into four distinct patterns:[15]

1. ST-segment elevation of 0.5 mm or greater (frequently with upward concavity) accompanied by elevated J-points or terminal slurring of the R wave, rapid QRS transition, and precordial peaked T waves
2. Rare J-point depression with depressed ST segments, which may be horizontal or upsloping, and T waves, which are either positive, low-amplitude or isoelectric, or biphasic
3. "Juvenile T waves" (i.e., biphasic with terminal negativity) in leads V_1–V_4
4. Terminal T-wave inversion in the lateral precordium with or without ST-segment changes

By far the most common ST-segment and T-wave changes seen in athletes are those of early repolarization as described earlier in the first subgroup. The literature describes varying prevalences of this phenomenon with frequencies varying from 10 to 100% in a number of cross-sectional studies. In nonathletes, the physiological basis for this phenomenon is thought to be nonhomogeneous repolarization of the ventricles with the epicardium repolarizing first. It is more commonly noted in African Americans and is usually most prominent in leads V_2–V_4 with reciprocal changes in the inferior leads. J-point elevation is usually present, and occasionally T-wave inversion or tall, peaked T waves can be seen. The increased frequency of early repolarization seen in competitive athletes has been related to a training-induced decrease in resting sympathetic tone, which then uncovers an inherent asymmetry of repolarization in those so inclined.[21] This theory is consistent with the fact that normalization of ST segments occurs with exercise and disappears

TABLE 2.1.   RHYTHM CHANGES IN THE ATHLETIC HEART

Arrhythmia	Frequency in Population (%)	Frequency in Athletes (%)
Sinus bradycardia	23.7	50–85
Sinus arrhythmia	2.4–20	13.5–69
Wandering atrial pacemaker	—	7.4–19
First-degree heart block	0.65	6–33
Second-degree heart block		
Möbitz I	0.003	0.125–10
Möbitz II	0.003	Not Reported
Third-degree heart block	0.0002	0.017
Junctional rhythm	0.06	0.031–7.0

with detraining; in both instances it would be expected that increased sympathetic tone would override resting asymmetric repolarization, thereby equalizing action potential duration. It should be noted, however, that normalization does not always occur after deconditioning, and, therefore, this theory must still be considered speculative. Furthermore, ST-segment normalization with exercise can be seen with cardiomyopathies, and, therefore, exercise-induced normalization of ST-segment elevation does not always necessarily rule out an underlying pathological basis for this phenomenon. ST-segment depression is found much less frequently than the changes of early repolarization. One large review found a 0.1 mV depression in 3% of bicyclists studied.[22] With exertion, the ST segment will usually return to baseline. However, in one small study of 3 athletes, ST-segment normalization did not occur with exertion.[23] In the case of these athletes, the depressed segments remained as long as 10 years after cessation of competition without adverse effects. Since pretraining ECGs were not available for review, it could not be concluded that these changes had occurred as a result of physical training.

Alteration in the T wave can occur in one of two ways. Either the T wave is tall and peaked or it may be inverted. Tall, peaked T waves are frequently seen as part of the early repolarization syndrome that has been described earlier. Unfortunately, the literature does not document whether tall, peaked T waves can occur in the absence of ST-segment changes, although my personal experience has shown this to be the case. It is known that T-wave amplitude is not related to hyperkalemia since the amplitude of the T wave decreases as serum potassium rises following exertion. It has been demonstrated that amplitude rises in the precordial leads as training progresses, but this occurs with ST-segment elevation as well; as mentioned previously, normalization of the ST segment and decreased T-wave amplitude occur after cessation of training.[24] Therefore, tall, peaked T waves occur concomitantly with physical training, but they are clearly not an isolated finding. The increased amplitude may be a reflection of repolarization changes or may be merely secondary to repolarization of increased ventricular mass.

Frank T-wave inversion occurring across the precordium and/or in the limb leads has been well documented in a number of cross-sectional studies; normalization of these inversions occurs following maximal exertion or other sympathetic maneuvers, and they disappear with cessation of training.[15] A comparison of athletes with and without T-wave inversion has been reported.[25] All of the athletes had normal thallium treadmill tests. Those with inverted T waves were shown to have impressive increases in precordial QRS voltage, interventricular septal thickness, left ventricular posterior wall thickness, and calculated left ventricular mass. Whether these inverted T waves were due to increased ventricular mass *per se* or whether the T waves were simply a reflection of appropriate adaptation to training could not be answered. It has been suggested that T-wave inversion results from differences in action potential duration of myocardial cells.[26] Increasing the sympathetic stimulus could normalize a wave by equalizing the duration of depolarization. This would explain why T-wave inversion occurs, why it can normalize with exertion, and subsequently disappear with deconditioning.

A variation of frank T-wave inversion is the presence of biphasic or terminal negativity, which typically occurs in leads V_3–V_5. Whether this is a training-induced effect or simply a part of a "juvenile pattern" is unclear. While no evidence exists that the frank or terminal T-wave inversion that arises as a result of training is an indicator of pathology, care must be exercised in the evaluation of deep T-wave inversions, which are accompanied by symmetric T-wave contour, ST depression, prolonged QT interval, or absence of normal septal Q waves. These patterns are more likely to signal the presence of significant underlying pathology.

Voltage changes in the QRS complex are commonly seen on ECGs of athletes. Since the diagnostic criteria for left and right ventricular hypertrophy have not been standardized in various studies, it is difficult to compare frequencies in athletes versus nonathletes. The reported prevalence in athletes varies from 8 to 76%.[27] Six studies have been published comparing the average precordial voltage summations of athletes versus control subjects.[15] The deflections of SV_1 and RV_5 average more than 35 mm in 5 of the 6 studies. Many authors have used this as a method for assessing left ventricular hypertrophy on the ECG, although it is known that this criteria may be falsely positive in young adults. Further review of this data reveals that dynamic athletes demonstrate consistently greater voltages than athletes who participate in static activities such as weightlifting.

Similarly, 4 large surveys have found frequencies of 18 to 69% for right ventricular hypertrophy with the summation of RV_1 and SV_5 greater than 10.5 mm.[15] As with criteria for left ventricular hypertrophy, this was met more often in dynamic than static athletes.

Voltage increases of 25% have been noted after only 11 weeks of training and decreases in voltage are witnessed following deconditioning, although it occurs more slowly.[15] The QRS axis progressively becomes more vertical as athletic conditioning improves and an incomplete right bundle branch block pattern is not uncommon. This has been attributed to an increase in muscle mass of the apex of the right ventricle and has been noted to resolve after cessation of training. Miscellaneous findings include increased P-wave amplitude and notching, as well as prominent U waves.

To summarize the findings seen on the ECG of well-trained athletes, it is apparent that sinus bradycardia, sinus arrhythmia, first-degree heart block, Möbitz I type heart block, and junctional rhythm can be found with higher frequency in athletes than in nonathletes. ST-segment elevation, tall and peaked T waves, or biphasic T waves are common; less commonly, ST depression or isolated T-wave inversion is seen. Increased P-wave amplitude and QRS voltage is seen, while frequently utilized criteria for left ventricular hy-

pertrophy and right ventricular hypertrophy are frequently surpassed. The QRS axis rotates toward the right and becomes more vertical. An incomplete right bundle branch block can be seen. Insufficient data exist to suggest that Möbitz type II heart block, third-degree heart block, or frequent ventricular or atrial ectopy are part of the athletic heart syndrome. A representative ECG of an individual with changes characteristic of the athletic heart is shown in Figure 2.3.

CLINICAL CORRELATION

The well-trained athlete demonstrates decreased body fat, increased muscle mass, and various changes in the cardiovascular examination. The pulse is slowed, and its amplitude may be increased secondary to increased stroke volume. The duration of the left ventricular impulse may be prolonged, and its area enlarged. Grade 1–2 systolic murmurs have been commonly noted in dynamic athletes with a frequency of 30 to 50% in a number of studies.[15] These murmurs have the clinical characteristics of benign flow murmurs. Similarly, third and fourth heart sounds are common. The frequency of third heart sounds is generally greater than 50% in dynamic athletes, with a range of 30 to 100% in five studies; fourth heart sounds were found somewhat less frequently in these same studies with a range varying from 20 to 60%.[15]

Occasionally, clinical confusion will surround the differentiation of hypertrophic cardiomyopathy from athletic heart syndrome. This distinction is critical to make since hypertrophic cardiomyopathy is known to account for a significant number of sudden deaths in athletes during physical activity. Maron and colleagues have analyzed 150 sudden deaths in the United States from 1985 to 1995 and found that 46% were due to hypertrophic cardiomyopathy or possible hypertrophic cardiomyopathy.[28] Unlike athletic heart syndrome, which reflects the heart's normal adaptation to strenuous physical activity, hypertrophic cardiomyopathy is a disorder that is characterized

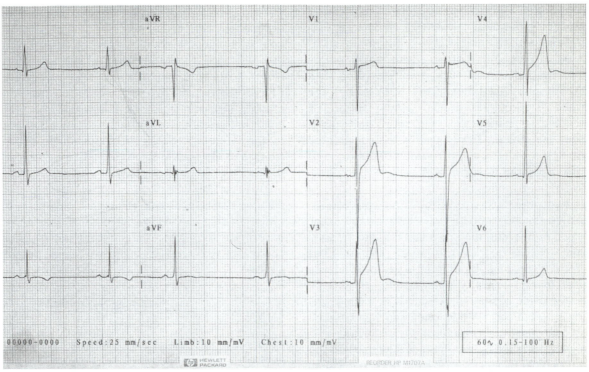

FIGURE 2.3. A representative electrocardiogram with changes characteristic of the athletic heart. Note profound bradycardia, notched P waves, increased QRS voltages, and early repolarization.

by profound hypertrophy, which usually occurs at the expense of the left ventricular cavity, asymmetrical septal hypertrophy, and myofibrillar disarray. This creates an underlying substrate for malignant arrhythmias. Half of all cases are familial and result from mutations in the beta-cardiac myosin heavy chain. Mutations have also been discovered in troponin T, tropomyosin, and myosin-binding protein C. Those mutations of the troponin T moiety, while accounting for only 15% of cases of hypertrophic cardiomyopathy, are important. These mutations are characterized by mild to subclinical hypertrophy but are associated with an extremely high incidence of sudden death.[29]

Problems frequently arise in the noninvasive evaluation of athletes when dimensions of the left ventricular free wall and septum exceed normal limits. As mentioned earlier, Pelliccia's work has demonstrated considerable variability in the dimensions of the left ventricle in well-trained athletes.[10,11] Prior work by other investigators has documented this as well, and, in fact, measurement of the left ventricular posterior free wall exceeds the normal value of 11 mm in up to 60% of athletes.[15] A study of childhood swimmers revealed a thickness above the 95th percentile in 81%.[30] Similarly, septal hypertrophy has been demonstrated in endurance athletes and has been shown to increase as training progresses.[15] Measurements greater than 11 mm have been seen in up to 60% of basketball players and 83% of childhood swimmers.[30,31] As a result of these changes, the ratio of the intraventricular septum to the left ventricular free wall can occasionally exceed the normal ratio of 1:3 and has been reported as high as 2:1 in athletes in several studies.[15] Menapace and colleagues have demonstrated the ability to distinguish the physiological septal hypertrophy that occurs in weight lifters from the pathological changes in individuals with hypertrophic cardiomyopathy.[32] Dividing the width of the intraventricular septum by the left ventricular end-systolic diameter clearly separates the athletes from those with hypertrophic cardiomyopathy. A cut-off value of 0.48 or more (the mean plus 3 standard deviations) is indicative of hypertrophic cardiomyopathy.

Nevertheless, there can be significant overlap demonstrated in athletes who demonstrate either septal or free-wall thickness that fall into the gray zone—values that are not grossly abnormal but clearly exceed the upper limit of normal. In these particular instances, discontinuation of training may provide additional assistance in distinguishing between the athletic heart and hypertrophic cardiomyopathy. Discontinuation of training will result in a rapid and progressive decrement in the morphologic changes that have been previously described, and repeat echocardiography will demonstrate normalized wall thickness. Those individuals with hypertrophic cardiomyopathy will demonstrate no evidence of regression, thereby confirming the diagnosis.

SUMMARY

The athletic heart syndrome represents a constellation of clinical findings that are the result of normal physiological adaptation to strenuous physical activity. Typically, these include increases in the left and right ventricular cavity sizes as well as the interventricular septum and free walls of the ventricles. The left atrium may be dilated and even hypertrophied as well. Stroke volume progressively increases as training progresses. In the isometric, or static, athlete the left and right ventricular cavities do not seem to dilate, although hypertrophy of the ventricular walls is present. A number of characteristic electrocardiographic changes occur; all of which are the

result of increased vagal tone and diminished sympathetic drive. In some instances clinical confusion may exist with respect to distinguishing athletes who have athletic heart syndrome from those with hypertrophic cardiomyopathy. These individuals typically have echocardiographic measurements that fall within the gray zone, but cessation of training will usually result in the ability to clearly distinguish one group from the other as the changes that have occurred in response to physical activity regress. A thorough understanding of the manifestations of the athletic heart syndrome will assist clinicians in differentiating the normal adaptations that occur in response to physical training from pathological conditions that jeopardize the well-being of the athlete.

PERSONAL PERSPECTIVE

I continue to be fascinated by the variety of manifestations of the athletic heart syndrome. Working at a university with a large division I athletic program, I have the opportunity to evaluate hundreds of athletes each year, both for clearance to participate as well as for exercise-related problems. Just when I think that I have seen every variation on the theme, I am surprised by yet another clinical presentation that can be attributed to the athletic heart syndrome.

The most perplexing situation for the clinician is when an athlete has a problem that cannot be attributed to the athletic heart syndrome. The usual clinical situation is one in which exercise-associated collapse, near-syncope, or syncope is the presenting complaint, and a carefully taken history and physical examination are unrevealing. Further workup will usually include an ECG and/or an echocardiogram. If the ECG demonstrates an abnormal rhythm or the echocardiogram reveals septal or wall measurements that fall within the gray zone, the dilemma becomes whether these are characteristic of underlying pathology or whether they are simply manifestations of the athletic heart syndrome.

The great majority of electrocardiographic changes seen in the athletic heart syndrome result from diminished sympathetic drive and enhanced vagal tone, and, therefore, any maneuver that increases sympathetic tone may result in disappearance of the "abnormality."

More concerning are the echocardiographic findings that fall into the gray zone. Are these measurements indicative of hypertrophic cardiomyopathy or simply reflective of the heart's robust response to intense training? In instances in which it is not clear, a period of detraining and reassessment will usually clarify the situation. Obviously, changes reflective of the athletic heart will regress while those of hypertrophic cardiomyopathy will not.

Finally, let me comment on the critical importance of communicating clearly with the athlete and, in instances where he or she is a minor, the parents. Nothing can be more alarming than concern about underlying cardiac disease, and therefore when the evaluation reveals no evidence of significant disease, the clinician must place this in proper perspective for the patient. Reassurance that these findings are a normal response to training will allow the athlete to return to full activity without the concern that "something may be wrong with my heart." Carefully allaying this concern is crucial in optimizing performance.

REFERENCES

1. Lancisi G: quoted by Zuntz and Schumberg in *Studien Zur Physiologie Des Marsches,* Berlin, 1902, from the treatise "On the Motion of the Heart and on the Aneurisms," 1928.
2. Osler W: *The Principles and Practice of Medicine.* New York, D. Appleton and Company, 1892.
3. Beneke cited by Karpovich PV: Textbook fallacies regarding child's heart. *Res Quar* 8:33, 1937.
4. Deutsch F, Kauf E: *Heart and Athletics.* Warfield LM (translator). St. Louis, CV Mosby Company, 1927, pp. 17–103.
5. Astrand P, Rodohl K: *Textbook of Work Physiology.* New York, McGraw-Hill Book Company, 1977, p. 176.
6. Evans CL: The velocity factor in cardiac work. *J Physiol* 62:6, 1918.
7. Morganroth J, Maron BJ, Henry WL, et al: Comparative left ventricular dimensions in trained athletes. *Ann Intern Med* 82:521–524, 1975.
8. Turpeinen AK, Kuikka JT, Vanninen E, et al: Athletic heart: A metabolic, anatomical and functional study. *Med Sci Sports Exerc* 28:33–40, 1996.
9. Ehsani AA, Hagberg JM, Hickson RC: Rapid changes in left ventricular dimensions and mass in response to physical conditioning and deconditioning. *Am J Cardiol* 42:52–56, 1978.
10. Pelliccia A, Maron BJ, Spataro A, et al: The upper limit of physiologic cardiac hypertrophy in highly trained elite athletes. *N Engl J Med* 324:295–301, 1991.
11. Pelliccia A, Maron BJ, Culasso F, et al: Athlete's heart in women. *JAMA* 276:211–215, 1996.
12. Sugishita Y, Koseki S, Matsuda M, et al: Myocardial mechanics of athletic hearts in comparison with diseased hearts. *Am Heart J* 105:273–280, 1983.
13. Nuutila P, Knuuti MJ, Heinonen OJ, et al: Different alterations in the insulin-stimulated glucose uptake in the athlete's heart and skeletal muscle. *J Clin Inves* 93:2267–2272, 1994.
14. Puffer JC, Larson T: Unpublished data, UCLA, 1998.
15. Huston TP, Puffer JC, Rodney WM: The athletic heart syndrome. *N Engl J Med* 313:24–32, 1985.
16. Chapman J: Profound sinus bradycardia in the athletic heart syndrome. *J Sports Med Phys Fit* 22:45–48, 1982.
17. VanGanse W, Versee L, Evlenbosch W, et al: The electrocardiogram of athletes: Comparison with untrained subjects. *Brit Heart J* 32:160–164, 1970.
18. Zeppilli P, Fenici R, Sassara M, et al: Wenkebach second-degree A-V block in top-ranking athletes: An old problem revisited. *Am Heart J* 100:281–293, 1980.
19. Finici R, Caselli G, Zeppilli P, et al: High degree A-V block in 17 well-trained endurance athletes, in Lubick T, Venerando A (eds): *Sports Cardiology,* Bologna, Aulo Gaggi, 1980.
20. Hanne-Paparo N, Kellerman JJ: Long term Holter ECG monitoring of athletes. *Med Sci Sports Exerc* 13:294–298, 1981.
21. Zeppilli P, Pirrami M, Sassara M, et al: T wave abnormalities in top ranking athletes: Effects of isoproterenol, atropine and physical exercise. *Am Heart J* 100:213–222, 1980.
22. Minamitani K, Miyagawa M, Konco M, et al: The electrocardiogram of professional cyclists, in Lubick T, Venerando A (eds): *Sports Cardiology,* Bologna, Aulo Gaggi, 1980.
23. Strauzenberg SE, Olsen G: The occurrences of electrocardiographical abnormalities in athletes: An expression of cardiovascular adaptation or a sign of myocardial lesion? in Lubick T, Venerando A (eds): *Sports Cardiology,* Bologna, Aulo Gaggi, 1980.

24. Saltin B, Grimby G: Physiological analysis of middle-aged and old former athletes. *Circulation* 38:1104–1115, 1968.

25. Nishimura T, Kambara H, Chen C, et al: Noninvasive assessment of T wave abnormalities in precordial electrocardiograms in middle-aged professional bicyclists. *J Electrocardiog* 14:357–363, 1981.

26. Taggart P, Carruthers M, Joseph S, et al: Electrocardiographic changes resembling myocardial ischaemia in asymptomatic men with normal coronary arteriograms. *Brit Heart J* 41:214–225, 1979.

27. Hanne-Paparo N, Drory Y, Schoenfeld Y, et al: Common ECG changes in athletes. *Cardiology* 61:267–278, 1976.

28. Maron BJ, Shirani J, Poliac LC, et al: Sudden death in young competitive athletes. *JAMA* 276:199–204, 1996.

29. Watkins H, McKenna WJ, Thierfelder L, et al: Mutations in the genes for cardiac troponin T and alpha-tropomyosin in hypertrophic cardiomyopathy. *N Engl J Med* 332:1058–1064, 1995.

30. Allen HD, Goldberg SJ, Sahn DJ, et al: A quantitative echocardiographic study of champion childhood swimmers. *Circulation* 55:142–145, 1977.

31. Roeske WR, O'Rourke RA, Klein A, et al: Noninvasive evaluation of ventricular hypertrophy in professional athletes. *Circulation* 53:286–292, 1976.

32. Menapace FJ, Hammer WJ, Ritzer TF, et al: Left ventricular size in competitive weight lifters: An echocardiographic study. *Med Sci Sports Exerc* 14:72–75, 1982.

Chapter 3

ECHOCARDIOGRAPHIC FINDINGS IN ATHLETES

Lisa R. Thomas, M.D.   *Pamela S. Douglas, M.D.*

Regular exercise and athletic training have become an increasing part of daily life for a sizeable portion of the population. Over the last two decades, the popularity of regular exercise has grown with people of all ages participating at all levels, including increased participation by older individuals who are at higher risk of having pathologic cardiovascular disease. In addition to the rise in numbers and ages of people exercising, there has also been an increase in the intensity of exercise with many elite and recreational athletes participating in ultraendurance events. As a result, cardiovascular changes and complications associated with athletic training are becoming more widespread and are commanding the attention of athletes and physicians.

Several adaptations of cardiac shape and function occur with athletic training to improve the heart's function as a pump and thereby increase aerobic capacity. The predominant adaptations include increased left ventricular end-diastolic cavity dimension, increased left ventricular wall thickness, improved diastolic filling, and decreased heart rate. These adaptations are related

43

to gender, age, and race and to the type, duration, and intensity of the sport performed. While the adaptations are usually beneficial and allow the heart to function as a more efficient and powerful pump, there is a process known as "cardiac fatigue" in which reversible systolic and diastolic left ventricular dysfunction have been described after extremely prolonged exercise.

Distinguishing the nonpathologic, adaptive morphologic changes of the athlete's heart from the pathologic structural heart disease that is associated with an increased risk of sudden death is tremendously important. Identification of true structural heart disease may in many cases result in recommendations to stop participating in athletics in order to reduce the risk of sudden death. The ability to distinguish athlete's heart from structural heart disease will help to prevent the unwarranted removal of healthy athletes from playing sports. While echocardiographic screening of all athletes is impractical because it is time-intensive and costly, consensus recommendations and guidelines have been developed for cardiovascular preparticipation screening of competitive athletes.

ECHOCARDIOGRAPHIC FINDINGS IN ATHLETES

The athlete's heart was first described in human beings by Henschen[1] who discovered enlarged hearts in cross-country skiers at the end of the last century. He estimated heart size by carefully performed percussion and concluded that, "skiing results in an enlargement of the heart, the enlarged heart is able to perform an enlarged workload, and therefore a physiological enlargement by sports exists, e.g., an athlete's heart." For years, heart enlargement was identified by physical exam and chest radiography or suggested by electrocardiographic patterns consistent with left ventricular enlargement or hypertrophy.[1–13] The development of M-mode echocardiography in the 1970s allowed for more detailed evaluation of the morphologic and functional changes in the heart in response to chronic training.

Since the first echocardiographic study of athletes by Morganroth et al. in 1975,[14] a substantial number of echocardiographic studies have been performed in a variety of athletic populations.[9,13–71] Most of the studies assessed small numbers of competitive athletes at one point in time (thereby providing only cross-sectional data), included athletes that were predominantly young adult men, and involved only a small number of sports. There have also been a series of studies assessing the morphologic adaptations of the heart to athletic training in a large population of elite athletes of both sexes participating in 27 sports.[68,69,71] The findings of the numerous echocardiographic studies in athletes are remarkably similar and provide a clear picture of the adaptive structural and functional changes in the heart in response to exercise.

In general, echocardiographic studies of athletes compare the resting cardiac dimensions in athletes during an active period of training with the dimensions of an age- and sex-matched group of nonathletic, sedentary control subjects. The values for cardiac dimensions measured by echocardiography in the groups of trained athletes show marked overlap with the matched control subjects. The cardiac dimensions in the athletes are usually only mildly increased over the control subjects and generally remain within, or are increased only slightly above, the accepted normal range.[58,69,70] Nevertheless, while the absolute differences in measurements between the athlete and control dimensions are small, they usually reach statistical significance.

When an acute demand is placed on the heart, it maintains its ability to function as an adequate pump by altering heart rate and contractility. When a chronic demand is imposed on the heart, structural and functional cardiac adaptations occur to maintain adequate pump function. When pressure overload is chronic, septal and free-wall thicknesses increase to normalize myocardial wall stress (LaPlace's law). In chronic volume overload, the left ventricular end-diastolic diameter increases, with a proportional increase in septal and free-wall thicknesses to normalize wall stress.[72] These morphologic changes are appropriate compensation for the mild chronic volume overload involved in most athletic training and allow for sustained increases in cardiac output that are required during competition. Thickening of the septum and posterior free wall without an increase in the left ventricular end-diastolic cavity dimension has been seen in athletes who perform predominantly isometric sports (weight lifters and shot putters), which impose primarily a pressure overload on the heart.[72]

Other factors related to cardiac efficiency contribute to cardiac morphology in athletes.[73] A given stroke volume can be ejected with less myocardial shortening and lower frictional and tension energy losses when the contraction starts at a larger end-diastolic volume. Stretched muscle can provide a higher tension than unstretched fibers. Loss of energy is greater when contraction occurs more rapidly at higher heart rates than it would at lower rates. Hence, low heart rates and increased end-diastolic cavity dimension and volume tend to augment ventricular efficiency in athletes. However, in accordance with LaPlace's law, the greater the volume of the heart, the higher the tension of the myocardial fibers necessary to maintain a given intraventricular pressure. This higher tension in turn increases myocardial oxygen consumption and decreases myocardial efficiency, but it can be compensated for by an increase in myocardial mass. Hence, an athlete who requires a high capacity of oxygen transport benefits from a large stroke volume, an increased left ventricular end-diastolic diameter, a thickened ventricular wall, and a low heart rate.

LEFT VENTRICULAR CAVITY

Echocardiographic studies of athletes have consistently shown an increased left ventricular end-diastolic dimension when compared to age- and sex-matched sedentary, nonathletic controls[9,13–71] (Fig. 3.1). Two exceptions are the studies of Gilbert and colleagues[16] and Granger and co-workers[52] in which distance runners had normal left ventricular diastolic dimensions that were not increased over controls. The elevated dimension reflects a true increase in cavity size that is present even when corrections are made for body surface area and weight.[14,74] The increase in left ventricular cavity dimension in most athletes is modest and does not often exceed the accepted normal range for adults without heart disease.[58,75] The cavity dimension in athletes is increased by an average of 10% over that in matched sedentary control subjects with the average reported end-diastolic dimension in athletes being approximately 54 mm.[14–71] An occasional subject has been reported to have marked left ventricular cavity dilatation, with the largest being 70 mm reported in a professional cyclist; however, it is uncommon for the normal "athlete's heart" to show an increase in left ventricular dimension greater than 60 mm.[58,70,71,76] The increase in left ventricular diastolic dimension is most pronounced and most consistently seen in athletes who perform primarily dynamic (or isotonic) exercise. Studies that have compared athletes who perform isotonic exercise (predominantly endurance runners) with athletes who perform isometric exercise (primarily weight-lifters) have generally demonstrated larger left ventricular diastolic dimension in the endurance athletes.[11,14,36,44,47,54] Pelliccia et al.[71] measured the left ventricular end-diastolic cavity dimension in 1309 highly trained male and female athletes ranging in age from 13 to 59 years and participating in 38 different sports. They found that left ventricular end-diastolic cavity dimension varied substantially—38–66 mm (mean 48 mm) in women and 43–70 mm (mean 55 mm) in men—and was within accepted normal limits ($\leq$ 54 mm) for 725 (55%) of the athletes. It exceeded upper limits of normal ($\geq$ 55 mm) in 584 (45%) of the participants and was substantially enlarged ($\geq$ 60 mm) in 185 of the athletes (14%). The type of sport and body surface area were the variables most significantly associated with left ventricular cavity dimension followed by heart rate, sex, and age. The impact of these variables will be dis-

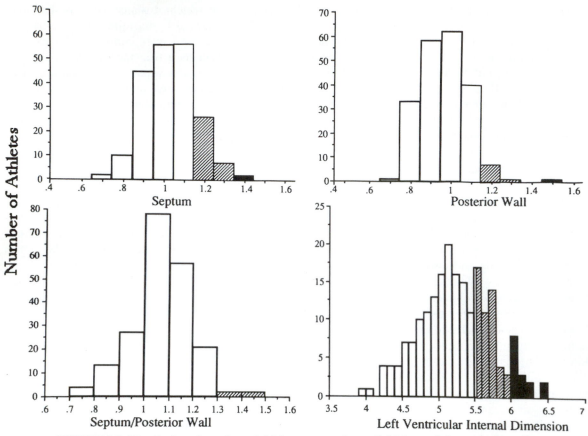

FIGURE 3.1. Distribution plots of septal thickness, posterior wall thickness, left ventricular end-diastolic internal dimension, and septal-to-wall thickness ratio. **Hatched** *and* **black bars** *represent outliers using partition values as follows: mildly increased septal or posterior thickness > 1.1 cm* (**hatched**), *markedly increased ≥ 1.3 cm* (**black**); *mildly increased left ventricular internal diastolic dimension > 5.5 cm* (**hatched**), *markedly increased > 6.0 cm* (**black**); *abnormal septal to posterior wall thickness ratio > 1.3* (**hatched**). *Reprinted from Douglas PS, O'Toole ML, Katz SE, et al: Left ventricular hypertrophy in athletes. Am J Cardiol 80:1386, 1997. Copyright © 1997, with permission from Excerpta Medica Inc. All rights reserved.*

cussed in greater detail later in this chapter. Another interesting finding in the study by Pelliccia et al. was that the athletes with the greatest left ventricular cavity dilatation also had the most pronounced other adaptive changes including increased left ventricular wall thickness, increased left ventricular mass, and left atrial dilatation.

Although left ventricular cavity dimensions are generally not normalized to body size in clinical practice, it is clear that in some groups of athletes (e.g., basketball players), such adjustment is reasonable, if not mandatory. Vasan and colleagues published a distribution and categorization of echocardiographic variables in a population sample of 4957 subjects based on deviation from height- and sex-specific reference limits.[77]

LEFT VENTRICULAR WALL THICKNESS

The thickness of both the interventricular septum and the posterior left ventricular free wall are often increased in athletes when compared to age- and sex-matched sedentary, nonathletic control subjects[14–71] (Fig. 3.1). The increases in both septal and posterior wall thicknesses are typically small, and the absolute values are generally within the normal range or slightly above it. The average value for septal thickness is 10.4 mm, while that for the posterior wall is 10.6 mm.[58,68,70] While these values are well within the accepted normal range, they are 15 to 20% greater than the values reported for matched sedentary control subjects. Pelliccia and colleagues[71] found that ventricular septal thickness ranged from 5 to 15 mm (mean thickness 9.3 + 1.4 mm) and exceeded the generally accepted upper limits of normal (12 mm) in 14 of the 1309 athletes in the study (1.1%). Posterior free-wall thickness ranged from 6 to 14 mm (mean thickness 9.0 ± 1.3 mm) and was greater than the upper limits of normal (12 mm) in 4 athletes (0.3%). A significant correlation was found between left ventricular cavity dimension and wall thickness, and multivariate analysis revealed that the type of sport, gender, age, and body surface area were also all independently related to wall thickness. These factors will be discussed in greater detail later. Other investigators have suggested that physiologic hypertrophy seen with exercise is in part related to the pressure load imposed during exercise.[56,78,79] Douglas et al.[56] demonstrated that left ventricular wall thickness correlated with mean blood pressure and cardiac output during prolonged exercise.

M-mode echocardiographic studies of most athletes show symmetric septal and posterior free-wall thickness with a normal septal to free-wall ratio of < 1:3. Some investigators[15,17,50,70] found a small number of athletes with an elevated septal and free-wall ratio > 1:3, one of the echocardiographic criteria used for diagnosis of hypertrophic cardiomyopathy. However, the absolute thickening of the septum was minimal in these athletes and not diagnostic of hypertrophic

cardiomyopathy. Douglas and colleagues[70] studied 235 triathletes and found that only 4 athletes (2%) had evidence of asymmetry by septal-to-posterior wall ratios of > 1:3. (Fig. 3.2). In addition, calculation of relative wall thickness (mean wall thickness ÷ cavity radius) demonstrated that only 4 athletes (2%) had concentric remodeling (relative wall thickness ≥ 0.45) and 15 athletes (6%) had eccentric remodeling (relative wall thickness < 0.30).

LEFT VENTRICULAR MASS

Echocardiographic studies have shown that the majority of highly trained athletes participating in a variety of sports have an increase in left ventricular mass[14–71] (Fig. 3.3). Ventricular mass can be calculated by using the values for left ventricular end-diastolic dimension and septal and posterior wall thickness measured by M-mode echocardiography.[80,81] Since both left ventricular diameter and wall thickness are increased in athletes, it follows that left ventricular mass is also increased. Pooled data from studies show that left ventricular mass in highly trained athletes is on average 45 to 50% greater than that in sedentary control subjects;[14–71] however, criteria for the diagnosis of left ventricular hypertrophy are met by only 15 to 25% of athletes. Pelliccia and colleagues[71] found that left ventricular mass normalized to body surface area exceeded upper normal limits[82] in 90 men (9%) and 24 women (7%). When left ventricular mass was normalized to height, it exceeded normal limits[83] in 182 men (20%) and 14 women (4%). Douglas et al.[70] evaluated 235 triathletes and found that about one-fourth of the athletes met *sex-specific cutoffs* for left ventricular hypertrophy.[84,85] There were no differences between younger (< 40 years) and older athletes; however, the prevalence of hypertrophy was greater in women regardless of the method of normalization used—that of 36 to 43% in women as opposed to only 17 to 22% of men.

One possible explanation of the increase in left ventricular mass in the athlete's heart is an increase in total body mass. However, measurement

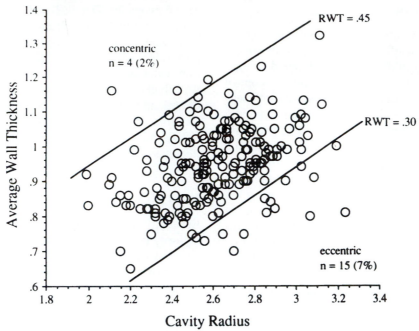

FIGURE 3.2. *Scatter plot of average left ventricular wall thickness (septal plus posterior wall thickness divided by 2) versus cavity radius. Two lines are drawn representing a relative wall thickness (RWT) of 0.45, above which is concentric remodeling (**upper left of graph**), and a relative wall thickness of 0.30, below which is eccentric remodeling (**lower right of graph**). Of 235 participants in the Hawaii Ironman Triathlon, only 4 athletes had concentric remodeling and 15 eccentric remodeling.* Reprinted from Douglas PS, O'Toole ML, Katz SE, et al: Left ventricular hypertrophy in athletes. Am J Cardiol 80:1387, 1997. Copyright © 1997, with permission from Excerpta Medica. All rights reserved.

of left ventricular mass normalized for body surface area or weight has demonstrated a persistently significant increase in athletes compared to sedentary controls.[12,14,16,22,24,27,31,33,41,45,49,50,52,61,70,71]

LEFT VENTRICULAR SYSTOLIC FUNCTION

Fractional shortening, ejection fraction, and velocity of circumferential fiber shortening are the most commonly used echocardiographic variables for the assessment of left ventricular systolic function.[86] Echocardiographic studies have generally demonstrated normal indices of systolic function in athletes at rest, suggesting that intrinsic myocardial contractility remains normal in

athletes despite changes in wall thickness and cavity dimension.[14–71] Exceptions include Blair et al.,[30] who found that 9 of 20 endurance athletes had reduced fractional shortening, but normal velocity of circumferential fiber shortening, and Gilbert et al.,[16] who found a significant reduction in fractional shortening in endurance runners when compared to control subjects. Nishimura et al.[26] found mildly decreased indices of left ventricular contractility in professional cyclists in the 40- to 49-year-old age group who had trained for an average of 27 years. These demonstrations of reduced ventricular systolic function in athletes may be explained in part by the fact that the echocardiographic variables used to assess sys-

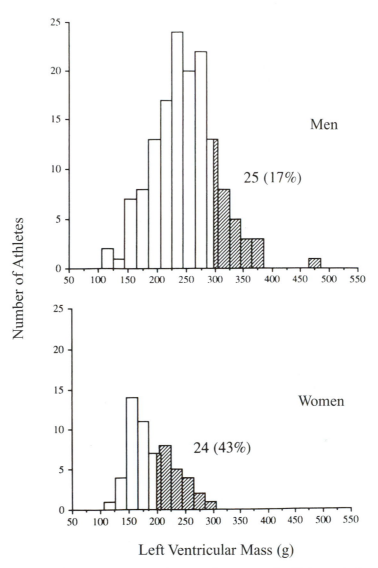

FIGURE 3.3. Distribution plots for men and women for unnormalized left ventricular mass. **Athletes with left ventricular hypertrophy are shown in** **hatched bars,** **determined according to** **partition values of mass > 294 g in men and > 198 g in women.** *Reprinted from Douglas PS, O'Toole ML, Katz SE, et al: Left ventricular hypertrophy in athletes.* Am J Cardiol *80:1387, 1997.* *Copyright © 1997, with permission from Excerpta Medica. All rights reserved.*

tolic performance are somewhat load dependent. In a study by Colan et al.,[61] noninvasive load-independent indices of myocardial contractility were used to assess left ventricular systolic func-

tion in both dynamic and strength-trained athletes. All of the athletes had normal contractile function despite significant changes in cavity dimension and wall thickness.

LEFT VENTRICULAR DIASTOLIC FUNCTION

Diastolic function of the heart is dependent on several factors including heart rate, systolic blood pressure, myocardial perfusion, compliance of the ventricle, left ventricular filling pressure, and left ventricular wall thickness.[87] Abnormalities in diastolic function have been shown in patients with increased left ventricular wall thickness secondary to hypertension, aortic stenosis, and primary myocardial disease.[88–94] Because athletic training results in increased left ventricular wall thickness, many investigators have looked at diastolic function in athletes using both digitized M-mode and Doppler echocardiography.[51,56,59,95–97] These studies have all demonstrated normal indices of diastolic function in both endurance and strength-trained athletes under basal conditions. Some investigators have reported an augmentation of early diastolic filling in athletes.[51,59,96,98–100] Vanoverschelde and colleagues[98] evaluated the potential relation between left ventricular diastolic function and exercise capacity in normal subjects. They assessed resting left ventricular systolic and diastolic function in a population of sedentary and trained subjects using two-dimensional and Doppler echocardiography, and investigated the relation of these indices with $\dot{V}O_2$ max, which was measured separately during a multistage dynamic cycle exercise protocol. They demonstrated that subjects with higher exercise capacity had faster peak early filling velocities (85 ± 8 vs. 56 ± 9 cm/s, $p < 0.0001$) and higher ratios of early-to-late filling velocity (1.90 ± 0.25 vs. 0.95 ± 0.19, $p < 0.0001$) than did subjects with a low exercise capacity. Stepwise multiple regression identified the ratio of early-to-late transmitral filling velocities as the most powerful independent correlate of $\dot{V}O_2$max. Nixon et al.[99] assessed diastolic filling in 10 highly trained basketball players and 10 age- and sex-matched control subjects. Although no significant differences were found in left ventricular diastolic filling indices at rest, a significant augmentation was found in these parameters during exercise. Early peak filling velocity was significantly increased in athletes during exercise at 120 beats per min, and during recovery at 120 and 80 beats per min, and the E/A ratio was consistently significantly higher in athletes at all heart rates during both exercise and recovery. Forman and associates[100] compared transmitral pulsed Doppler inflow spectra in healthy young adults, healthy elderly, sedentary subjects, and healthy, elderly endurance athletes. They demonstrated that, despite an increase in left ventricular mass, early diastolic filling was enhanced in master athletes as opposed to that of the sedentary old. Early left ventricular filling indices in master athletes more closely resembled transmitral inflow patterns of healthy young adults.

Normal diastolic filling in athletes has also been verified using radionuclide angiography. Granger et al.[52] demonstrated no alteration in left ventricular filling in endurance-trained athletes even in the setting of a 43% increase in left ventricular mass over that of control subjects. Hence, while there is a direct relation between the degree of left ventricular hypertrophy and impairment of diastolic filling in patients with pathologic hypertrophy, the physiologic, adaptive left ventricular hypertrophy induced by exercise is not accompanied by alterations in diastolic parameters.

RIGHT VENTRICULAR SIZE AND FUNCTION

The increase in ventricular mass related to athletic training may also include the right ventricle. A small number of studies have evaluated the right ventricular dimension in athletes.[15–19,22,30,31,38,39,53,57] In general, assessment of right ventricular size is more difficult due to the complex shape of the right ventricle and the effect of position on the measurements.[101] The transverse right ventricular cavity dimension is commonly increased as measured by echocardiography. Pooled data reveal an average right ventricular dimension of 22 mm in athletes (maximum 33 mm) compared with an average dimension of 17 mm in control subjects.[58] This represents a difference of 24% between the groups.

ATRIAL ENLARGEMENT

Many athletes have enlargement of the left atrium. Left atrial transverse dimension was significantly greater in athletes than in sedentary control subjects in 11 of 15 studies that compared the two groups.[14,16–19,22,24,26,30,33,38,44,53,57] The mean increase in left atrial dimension in athletes was 16%, but the absolute dimension usually remained within normal limits.[75,102] The cause of left atrial enlargement is unknown, but it is probably due to the increased cardiac output and volume load that cause the increase in left ventricular cavity size. Some authors have suggested that the increase in atrial size is due to impaired left ventricular compliance; however, as discussed earlier, several echocardiographic studies have demonstrated normal left ventricular diastolic function.[51,56,59,95–100]

A significant increase in right atrial dimension was demonstrated in a study by Hauser et al.[53]

VALVULAR REGURGITANT LESIONS

Exercise training is associated with an increased prevalence of mitral and tricuspid regurgitation. Douglas et al.[103] applied pulsed and color flow Doppler techniques to assess the prevalence and severity of valvular regurgitation in athletes versus sedentary control subjects. Regurgitation of at least one of the cardiac valves was found in 91% of the athletes and only 38% of the control subjects. Mitral and tricuspid regurgitation occurred more commonly in athletes than in control subjects (mitral: 69 vs. 27%, tricuspid: 76 vs. 15%). The presence of aortic and pulmonic regurgitation was similar in the two groups. In both groups, the valve regurgitation was no more than mild in severity, and structural valvular lesions were rarely detected. The presence or degree of regurgitant flow was not related to age, heart rate, blood pressure, gender, or the size of the chamber proximal or distal to the measurement being made. A similar increased prevalence of regurgitant flow was noted by Pollak et al.[104] in distance runners as compared to sedentary control subjects.

Regurgitant flow patterns are commonly detected using Doppler echocardiography in normal subjects; however, the true prevalence of "normal" regurgitant flow is unclear.[105] The mechanism of regurgitation in structurally normal valves is unknown. Several characteristics of athlete's heart could be related to the higher prevalence of regurgitation, including slower heart rate, increased chamber or annulus sizes, increased stroke volume, and altered right and left ventricular inflow patterns (high velocities of rapid filling with elevation in the E/A ratio were found in this study). However, none of these variables correlated with the presence or severity of regurgitation. The findings of Douglas and associates[103] confirm the existence of regurgitation in normal valves and also demonstrate an excessive prevalence in athletes, presumably another cardiac adaptation related to athletic training.

CORONARY ARTERIES

Some investigators have looked at the issue of whether coronary circulation undergoes adaptive morphologic changes in the setting of physiologic hypertrophy in order to increase coronary blood flow capacity. Angiographic and histological studies in rats, dogs, and monkeys demonstrate that the proximal coronary arteries increase in size to a degree proportional to the myocardial hypertrophy[106–108] and then decrease in size with deconditioning.[107,108] The early angiographic and pathologic studies in humans[109–113] revealed a relation between the cross-sectional area of the proximal coronary arteries and the myocardial weight, regardless of the etiology of the myocardial hypertrophy. Haskell and associates[113] angiographically studied ultradistance runners and found that the cross-sectional areas of the proximal coronary arteries were no different from inactive men at rest. However, the increase in proximal coronary artery cross-sectional area in response to nitroglycerine was greater for the runners. This dilating capacity was positively correlated with aerobic capacity. Pelliccia et al.[114] echocardiographically assessed coronary size and its relation to physiologic hypertrophy in healthy, trained men. The proximal coronary arteries were viewed and measured in the short axis view just above the aortic valve. They found a significant correlation between coronary artery diameter and left ventricular mass. A separate correlation revealed that the coronary artery diameter correlated with the ventricular wall thickness but not the left ventricular end-diastolic diameter. The morphologic changes in the coronary arteries may contribute in part to increased coronary blood flow.

IMPACT OF THE TYPE, DURATION, AND INTENSITY OF EXERCISE TRAINING ON CARDIAC CHANGES

Several studies suggest that the adaptive cardiac structural changes seen in athletes are related to the type of exercise training.[14,27,36,41,45,47,51] The theory that different patterns of structural change develop in response to different types of athletic training was first suggested by Morganroth and associates[14] who found that athletes participating in isotonic (dynamic) sports show increased left ventricular cavity dimension without significant increase in wall thickness, while athletes participating in isometric (static) sports show increased left ventricular wall thickness with little or no increase in cavity dimension. These patterns of structural adaptation correlated with the predominant volume overload of endurance training and the pressure load of strength training. Several other studies have confirmed these findings.[11,14,36,41,44,47,49,61] However, other investigators have not found significant differences in the cardiac morphologic changes in athletes performing different forms of training.[2,50] In fact, Rost and Hollman[2] found that the greatest increase in left ventricular wall thickness occurred in the hearts with the largest left ventricular cavity dimensions. Spirito et al.[69] assessed the morphologic adaptations of the heart in a large population of elite athletes who represented 27 sports (Table 3.1, Fig. 3.4). They showed that most sports asso-

TABLE 3.1.   CALCULATED EFFECTS OF TYPE OF SPORT ON LEFT VENTRICULAR INTERNAL DIASTOLIC CAVITY DIMENSION (LVIDd) AND WALL THICKNESS IN 947 ATHLETES

Sport	Impact on LVIDd (mm)	Sport	Impact on Wall Thickness (mm)
Endurance cycling	5.91	Rowing	2.13
Cross-country skiing	5.41	Endurance cycling	2.02
Swimming	4.90	Swimming	1.71
Pentathlon	4.35	Canoeing	1.70
Canoeing	4.23	Long-distance track	1.49
Sprint cycling	3.97	Water polo	1.38
Rowing	3.87	Sprint cycling	1.35
Long-distance track	3.47	Weightlifting	1.23
Soccer	3.11	Wrestling/judo	1.21
Team handball	2.87	Tennis	1.00
Tennis	2.69	Pentathlon	0.98
Roller hockey	2.41	Cross-country skiing	0.98
Boxing	2.25	Boxing	0.94
Alpine skiing	2.13	Roller skating	0.88
Fencing	2.09	Soccer	0.76
Taekwondo	2.07	Roller hockey	0.69
Water polo	2.02	Fencing	0.63
Diving	1.70	Sprint track	0.54
Roller skating	1.68	Volleyball	0.39
Volleyball	1.43	Diving	0.38
Bobsledding	1.35	Alpine skiing	0.29
Weightlifting	1.32	Field weight events	0.25
Wrestling/judo	1.25	Taekwondo	0.23
Equestrian	0.43	Team handball	0.19
Field weight events	0.18	Equestrian	0.13
Yachting	0.10	Bobsledding	0.07
Sprint track	0.00	Yachting	0.00

ciated with a larger left ventricular diastolic cavity dimension were also associated with a larger wall thickness. The issue of whether different types of athletic training produce different cardiac structural changes is complicated by a number of factors.[102] Most commonly, a training program does not involve purely isotonic or isometric exercise, but rather includes substantial

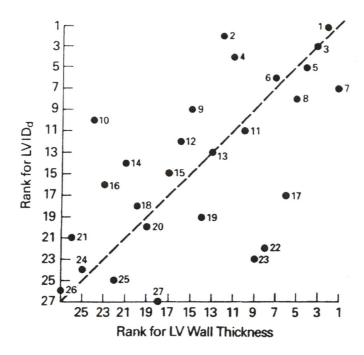

FIGURE 3.4. Twenty-seven sports plotted in rank order on the basis of impact on left ventricular internal diastolic cavity dimension (LVIDd) and LV wall thickness (higher rank indicates larger cardiac dimensions) in elite athletes. Most points are near the 45° line of identity, indicating that these sports have a parallel impact on LVIDd and wall thickness. Individual sports are identified by the number adjacent to each data point. (The 27 sports and their corresponding numbers are listed in the left column in Table 3.1). Although not shown, basketball falls in the middle third for LVIDd.[71] Reprinted from Spirito P, Pelliccia A, Proschan M, et al: Morphology of the "athlete's heart" assessed by echocardiography in 947 elite athletes representing 27 sports. Am J Cardiol 74:804, 1994. Copyright © 1994, with permission from Excerpta Medica. All rights reserved.

overlap of the two disciplines. In addition, the development of left ventricular dilatation in isolation or an increase in wall thickness alone would be nonphysiologic and, in the case of the dilatation, it would lead to an inappropriate, maladaptive increase in wall tension. Although these isolated morphologic changes may occur at the extremes of the spectrum of adaptive cardiac structural changes, most athletes seem to develop a balanced combination of cavity dilatation and increased wall thickness. However, it appears that while both isotonic and isometric athletes have increased left ventricular mass, ventricular dilata-

tion predominates slightly in the endurance athletes and wall thickness predominates in the isometric group.[102]

In addition to the different effects of isotonic and isometric exercise on cardiac dimensions, the specific sport performed within each type of exercise can impact on the cardiac morphologic changes. When Spirito[69] and Pelliccia[71] and associates studied a large group of elite Italian athletes representing 38 different sports, they found that cycling, swimming, rowing, and canoeing were associated with the largest cardiac dimensions (left ventricular end-diastolic cavity dimension and wall thickness), while sports such as sprinting, field weight events, diving, and bobsledding had only a mild impact on cardiac dimensions. Eighty percent of sports had an impact on both left ventricular diastolic cavity dimension and wall thickness. The sports with the largest wall thickness (rowing, cycling, and swimming) also had among the largest left ventricular cavity dimensions. The 185 athletes with left ventricular cavity dimensions of ≥ 60 mm competed in 25 different sporting disciplines with the highest prevalence in road cycling, ice hockey, basketball, rugby, canoeing, and rowing.[71] Spirito et al.[69] found some exceptions to their general finding that athletic training has a balanced impact on both diastolic cavity dimension and wall thickness. Cross-country skiing had the second highest rank for cavity dimension among the sports included, but only a medium rank for wall thickness. In contrast, weightlifting and wrestling, which are primarily isometric sports, had a high rank for wall thickness, but a low rank for cavity dimension. These findings suggest that power sports are associated with a disproportionate increase in wall thickness relative to cavity dimension; however, the wall thickness generally remained close to the normal range (≤ 12 mm).

In addition to the type of athletic training, the duration and intensity of the training have an impact on adaptive cardiac morphologic changes. With increasing intensity of training, a greater degree of left ventricular cavity enlargement and wall thickening may be seen.[50] Several longitudinal echocardiographic studies have been done in previously sedentary adults to evaluate changes in cardiac structure after short-term exercise programs[23,25,28,29,32,34,48,105] A representative study by DeMaria et al.[23] involved echocardiographic evaluation of 24 young adults before and after an 11-week walk-run program in which they exercised for 1 hour per day, 4 days per week. The subjects demonstrated small but statistically significant increases in left ventricular end-diastolic dimension, wall thickness, and left ventricular mass; however, these changes were substantially less than those observed in highly trained athletes

compared to controls suggesting that the intensity and duration of the training affects the degree of structural change. A short-term study of 8 competitive swimmers who had not been involved in any regular training for a period of 2 to 7 months revealed that following 1 week of vigorous training the mean left ventricular diastolic dimension increased by 11% and remained elevated throughout the remainder of the 9-week training period. The left ventricular posterior wall thickness increased by 7% by the end of the training period. Studies in rowers during training[38] have confirmed the rapidity with which cardiac morphologic changes can occur.

Many athletes participate in long-term training programs that span a lifetime. A small number of echocardiographic studies have tried to assess whether there are cumulative effects of this prolonged training on cardiac morphology. Nishimura et al.[26] studied a group of 60 chronically trained professional cyclists of 3 different age groups: 20 to 29 years (average of 5-years training), 30 to 39 years (average of 14-years training), and 40 to 49 years (average of 27-years training). They found that the cyclists who were 20 to 29 and 30 to 39 years of age showed similar increases in left ventricular cavity size, wall thickness, and mass. However, the older cyclists (40 to 49 years) showed greater wall thickness and ventricular mass than the young cyclists. Heath et al.[37] demonstrated that endurance athletes at the master level (average age 59 years) had significantly greater left ventricular end-diastolic volume index and calculated mass than young competitive endurance athletes (average age 22 years), but there was no difference in wall thickness. Other investigators[38] studied 14 senior collegiate rowers who had competed for at least one prior season and 9 freshman rowers beginning their first season. At the beginning of the season, the senior oarsmen had significantly larger cardiac dimensions than the freshman oarsmen and nonathletic controls. By the end of the 7-month season, both the senior and freshman oarsmen demonstrated greater ventricular cavity dimension and wall thickness than did the controls, but the senior oarsmen still had greater cardiac dimensions than the freshmen. These studies suggest many years of athletic training may have a cumulative effect on adaptive morphologic changes of the heart.

EFFECTS OF GENDER, AGE, AND RACE ON EXERCISE-INDUCED CARDIAC CHANGES

While most early echocardiographic studies that investigated the effects of training on cardiac dimensions were limited to male athletes, the increasing participation of women in competitive sports and the increasing interest of the medical community in defining gender-specific differences in the expression of cardiovascular disease has prompted investigations that assess the cardiac structural changes in women in response to athletic training.[2,22,31,39,50,56,70,115–118] Pelliccia et al.[116] assessed the left ventricular end-diastolic cavity dimension and wall thickness in 600 elite female athletes, participating in 27 sports, prospectively from 1986 to 1993. A control group of 65 nonathletic, age-matched women were used, and 738 elite male athletes of similar age, sporting disciplines, and intensity of training were used as a comparison group. The female athletes demonstrated larger left ventricular end-diastolic cavity dimension (49 ± 4 mm) and greater wall thickness (8.2 ± 0.9 mm) than did the controls (46 ± 3 mm, 7.2 ± 0.6 mm). The dimensions were 6 and 14% larger in the athletes than they were in the control group. The left ventricular end-diastolic cavity dimensions ranged from 40 to 66 mm, exceeding the upper limits of normal (> 54 mm) in 47 women (8%) and within the range consistent with dilated cardiomyopathy (≥ 60 mm) in 4 athletes (1%). These 4 athletes included 2 basketball players, a cyclist, and a judo competitor. The left ventricular wall thickness ranged from 6 to 12 mm. Hence, it did not extend into the borderline, overlap zone with hypertrophic cardiomyopathy in any athlete. Compared to the data obtained for the 738 previously studied male athletes, the female athletes demonstrated significantly smaller left ventricular cavity dimension (11% smaller), wall thickness (23% less), and calculated left ventricular mass (31% less). Left ventricular cavity dimension showed a similar broad range of values in female (40–66 mm) and male (44–66 mm) athletes; however, wall thickness demonstrated a more restricted range in women (6–12 mm) than men (7–16 mm) and was within the normal range for all female athletes. In another study,[69] analysis of gender-related differences in cardiac dimensions showed that female athletes had smaller left ventricular cavity dimension (average 2 mm) and smaller wall thickness (average 0.9 mm) than males of the same age and body size who were participating in the same sport. In contrast, Douglas et al.[70] studied 168 male and 67 female triathletes and found that left ventricular hypertrophy is significantly more common among female athletes (36–43%) than it is among male athletes (17–22%) when sex-specific values are used for left ventricular mass.[77,85] In general, the lower prevalence of hypertrophy seen in female athletes may be an artifact of body size—women's hearts should be smaller—and failure to use a gender-specific normal range.

Age has been found to have an effect on the adaptive cardiac morphologic changes due to athletic training. A small number of echocardiographic studies have investigated the effects of training on young athletes.[19,57,117] Allen et al.[19] studied 77 competitive swimmers ages 5 to 17 years and demonstrated that the changes of athlete's heart can be identified early in life. The athletes had increased thickness of the septum and left and right ventricular free walls; however, only 30% of the athletes had a left ventricular end-diastolic cavity dimension greater than that in control subjects. These findings were supported by another study,[117] which found significant increases in wall thickness and calculated mass but no significant increase in left ventricular diastolic dimension in 14-year-old swimmers when compared to age-matched controls. In addition, Geenan et al.[119] showed that 6- and 7-year-old nonathletic children demonstrated increased left ventricular posterior wall thickness and left ventricular mass after an 8-month aerobic exercise program. In contrast, a study of 72 swimmers 8 to 14 years of age found significant increases in left ventricular diastolic dimension when compared to age- and size-matched control subjects.[57] These studies demonstrate that systematic exercise training, as in adults, results in cardiac morphologic changes in children. However, the majority of the studies show left ventricular thickening occurring in the absence of significant left ventricular cavity dilatation, a finding that differs from the majority of studies in adult endurance athletes that demonstrate that left ventricular cavity enlargement is the most consistent structural adaptation to exercise. While this may be due to less vigorous training, the possibility that the cardiovascular effects of training in children may differ from those in adults cannot be excluded.

There have been short-term, often low intensity training studies in subjects with mean ages of 37 and 40 years that did not show any changes in cardiac dimensions after the training period.[25,41,120] The studies imply that the ability of the heart to adapt to the hemodynamic load imposed by exercise decreases with advancing age. However, some of the most dramatic cardiac morphologic changes demonstrated to date have been in elite adult athletes. In fact, in the large study by Spirito et al.,[69] increasing age was associated with larger left ventricular cavity dimension and wall thickness. A 1-year increase in age was associated with an increase of 0.2 mm in cavity dimension and 0.1 mm in wall thickness. These cardiac dimensions may well reflect the duration and intensity of training and not the absolute age of the athletes. Douglas and O'Toole[121] studied 24 young (mean age 23 ± 2 years) and 21 old (58 ± 6 years) triathletes and found higher systolic and diastolic blood pressures, increased wall thickness, and increased relative wall thickness in older compared with younger athletes. Left ventricular mass and mass index both tended to be high, but neither reached statistical significance. In addition, rapid filling velocity was reduced in older compared with younger athletes.

There is limited data evaluating racial differences in the adaptive morphologic response of the heart to exercise; however, there is evidence that suggests that racial differences exist in the response of the heart to certain pathologic loads such as systemic hypertension and that baseline differences may even exist.[122–125] Lewis and associates used echocardiography as a primary screening test to assess 265 collegiate athletes (99% black) for cardiovascular disease. Most athletes had normal left ventricular wall thickness of ≤ 12 mm, but 29 athletes (11%) had ventricular septal thickness ≥ 13 mm. The high prevalence of increased wall thickness may be related to race or perhaps body size and type of sport. Other investigators have confirmed this difference in heart size in normotensive blacks[122] and in the magnitude of the cardiac involvement in black patients with systemic hypertension.[123,124,126] Likewise, it is possible that race could influence the clinical expression of athlete's heart, which reflects the response of the heart to volume and pressure loads. Left ventricular wall thickness that develops in response to systematic training may also be influenced by racial differences in blood pressure response to exercise. Ekelund et al.[127] monitored blood pressure response to treadmill exercise in black and white subjects with similar baseline blood pressures and found that black men had higher systolic blood pressure at each stage of exercise (average 7 mm higher systolic) than did white men. This racial difference in blood pressure response to exercise may impact the cardiac morphologic changes due to exercise but further investigation is necessary.

Bielen et al.[128] studied 15 monozygotic and 9 dizygotic 6- to 8-year-old twin pairs to assess the influence of inheritance on physical exercise capacity and cardiac structure while limiting the effect of environmental factors as much as possible. Their results did not suggest a significant influence of genetic endowment on left ventricular internal diameter or on wall thickness at rest; however, genetic variance was significant for calculated mass. In a follow-up study,[129] Bielen and colleagues performed echocardiograms on 21 pairs of monozygotic and 12 pairs of dizygotic male twins ages 18 to 31 years under resting conditions and during submaximal supine exercise. They found that the capacity to increase end-diastolic left ventricular internal dimension and fractional shortening during submaximal exercise, unlike the findings at rest, has a significant genetic component.

The use of anabolic steroids by athletes has received significant attention. These compounds have been known to have adverse effects on hepatic, reproductive, and emotional function,[130] and some evidence suggests that anabolic steroids may produce abnormalities in left ventricular diastolic function. Thompson et al.[131] performed echocardiographic and Doppler measurements in 23 weight-trained athletes, 12 who were using anabolic steroids and 11 who had never used drugs. They found that left ventricular dimensions were slightly greater in anabolic steroid users, while left ventricular systolic and diastolic function did not differ.

Cocaine use in the United States is widespread, and the effects of cocaine on the heart have been popularized by the sudden deaths of athletes who used the drug. Cocaine has a wide variety of biologic activities that result in a complex spectrum of cardiovascular side effects including accelerated atherosclerosis, coronary thrombosis, coronary vasoconstriction, and increased myocardial oxygen demand, all of which increase the risk of myocardial infarction.[132–134] It has also been shown to cause cardiomyopathy, myocarditis, arrhythmias, aortic rupture, endocarditis, pneumopericardium, and left ventricular hypertrophy.[132–134] The possibility of cocaine use should be considered in young athletes presenting with myocardial infarction, dilated cardiomyopathy, myocarditis, or acute arrhythmias.

LOSS OF CARDIAC ADAPTATIONS AFTER CESSATION OF TRAINING

As discussed earlier, athletic training is associated with adaptive, morphologic cardiac changes that are dynamic and, as demonstrated by short-term longitudinal studies, can occur rapidly.[20,38] What happens to the heart when athletic training is stopped and the hemodynamic load is removed? Several echocardiographic studies have investigated the effect of deconditioning or the cessation of regular training.[135,136] Ehsani et al.[20] demonstrated that a significant decrease in left ventricular diastolic dimension (8%), posterior wall thickness (15%), and left ventricular mass (27%) occurred in competitive runners within 1 week of complete cessation of training. These changes were even more pronounced after two more weeks of deconditioning with decreases of 10, 25, and 39%, respectively. Shapiro and Smith[48] demonstrated similar results in 15 nonathletic subjects studied before and after a 6-week running program. At the end of the 6-week training period, 10 of the subjects stopped running, while 5 continued to train. After 6 weeks of detraining, the cardiac dimensions of the subjects who stopped running had declined to pre-exercise levels, while the subjects who continued to run showed no change in cardiac dimensions from peak exercise. Likewise, Fagard et al.[46] studied 12 competitive cyclists and found decreases in septal and posterior wall thickness during the off season when compared to the competitive season. Similarly, in an effort to look at the effects of deconditioning on left ventricular wall thickness, Maron et al.[137] studied 6 highly trained Olympic athletes. During peak training, all of the athletes had left ventricular wall thickness of 13 to 15 mm. Following reduction of training for 6 to 34 weeks (mean 13 weeks), echocardiographic follow-up was performed. The maximum septal thickness was 13.8 mm (± 0.9 mm) at peak training and 10.5 mm (± 0.5 mm) after deconditioning representing a 15 to 33% change. In addition, Hickson et al.[115] studied normally active subjects before and after a 10-week cycling program. At the end of the training period, all of the subjects demonstrated significant increases in left ventricular end-diastolic dimension, wall thickness, and left ventricular mass. Training was then decreased by two-thirds for 15 weeks and repeat echocardiographic measurements were obtained. There was no significant reduction in the cardiac dimensions demonstrating that training at reduced levels can prevent reversal of training effects on the heart.

CARDIAC FATIGUE

With increasing participation in ultraendurance athletic events, there has been increased interest in determining the effects of extremely exhaustive exercise on cardiac function. It is known that in response to upright submaximal exercise, cardiac output increases due to tachycardia and in stroke volume related to a large end-diastolic volume and a higher ejection fraction.[138,139] When exercise is prolonged, the heart rate continues to rise and the stroke volume falls resulting in either no change or a decrease in the cardiac output.[140] These hemodynamic changes have been referred to as cardiovascular "drift" and are felt to be related to decreases in blood volume, redistribution of blood flow to the skin vasculature to aid in thermoregulation, and cardiac fatigue. Cardiac fatigue refers to reversible alterations in left ventricular performance after prolonged exercise. While studies of recreational and elite athletes have consistently demonstrated adaptive structural cardiac changes (increased left ventricular end-diastolic dimension, increased wall thickness, increased calculated left ventricular mass), which increase the efficiency of the heart in the face of a hemodynamic load, some studies of ultraendurance athletes suggest deleterious effects of extreme exhaustive exercise on left ventricular systolic performance.[138,139,141,143] Niemela and associates[139] studied 13 ultraendurance athletes before and after an uninterrupted competitive 24-hour run. They found that after the race, in the setting of a lower postrace systolic blood pressure (lower afterload), the fractional shortening was decreased by 16% and the mean velocity of circumferential shortening fell by 9% when compared to precompetition values. The end-diastolic dimension was reduced by 7% after the race,

while there was a more variable response in the end-systolic diameter that resulted in a small, but not significant, net increase. The decrease in fractional shortening correlated with increases in end-systolic dimension but not with decreases in end-diastolic dimension, implying a true depression of myocardial contractility. In addition, the changes in left ventricular dimensions and function returned to prerace levels within 2 to 3 days consistent with "fatigue." Douglas and colleagues[142] studied 21 athletes participating in the Hawaii Ironman Triathlon and found similar results. The fractional shortening fell by an average of 10% at race finish. Individual reductions in fractional shortening were correlated with increases in systolic cavity size, but not with decreases in diastolic cavity size. The stress-shortening relation was displaced downward at race finish, while the slope remained unchanged implying that for a given afterload, shortening was reduced. In addition, the stress-shortening regression line returned toward baseline after 1 day of recovery, despite a persistent reduction in left ventricular cavity dimension suggesting that the decreased shortening was due in part to impaired contractility. The fractional shortening returned to the prerace level during recovery (1–2 days). Of interest is that the reduction of fractional shortening tended to be greatest in those athletes with the fastest race times. Likewise in the study by Niemela et al.,[139] increasing impairment was noted throughout the race and a negative correlation was found between the mean velocity of circumferential shortening and the total distance run suggesting that cardiac dysfunction may be related to exercise intensity. Other investigators[141] measured echocardiographic variables in athletes before and after a marathon run of 2.5 to 4.0 h and found no significant change in fractional shortening, implying that the duration of exercise may have been too short to result in depression of myocardial contractility. Similar abnormalities of left ventricular systolic performance have been noted in healthy, young, untrained individuals performing prolonged, exhaustive submaximal exercise. Seals and associates[143] studied 12 men who exercised on a treadmill to exhaustion (170 ± 10 min at 70% maximal oxygen uptake). They found significant reductions in fractional shortening (from 33 to 28%) and mean velocity of circumferential fiber shortening (1.09 ± 0.4 vs 0.97 ± 0.05 circ/s) in the setting of only a small reduction in left ventricular end-diastolic dimension and a lower average end-systolic wall stress. Of note is that the amount of exercise required to impair ventricular function in these healthy, untrained individuals (< 3 h) was substantially less than that needed in highly trained athletes implying that the threshold of cardiac fatigue may vary depending on the baseline level of cardiovascular fitness.

Echocardiographic studies have also assessed the effect of extreme, exhaustive exercise on diastolic ventricular filling.[141,144] Douglas et al.[142] found that following prolonged exhaustive exercise in triathletes, the left ventricular filling pattern showed an increased velocity of atrial or late diastolic inflow, resulting in a reduction in the ratio of early-to-late flow velocities. The changes were readily reversible with return to normal during the 28-h recovery period. Another study by Niemela et al.[144] confirmed the findings of impaired left ventricular diastolic filling in athletes after prolonged strenuous exercise.

The underlying mechanism of cardiac fatigue is unclear. The reversible nature of the lesion is similar to tachycardia- or catecholamine-induced cardiomyopathy, both of which are present during racing as possible substrates. The absence of metabolic alterations including acidosis and electrolyte abnormalities raises the issue of cardiac ischemia and injury. However, the lack of ischemic electrocardiographic changes and significant elevation of the cardiac subfraction of creatinine kinase and lactic dehydrogenase suggest that cardiac injury is insignificant.[142] Troponin T and I levels have been used to assess whether ultraendurance exercise induces cardiomyocyte injury. Laslett et al.[145] studied 5 participants in an ultramarathon race and found that all 5 subjects developed an elevated serum cardiac troponin T level, suggesting myocardial injury. Rifai and associ-

ates[146] assessed whether ultraendurance exercise induced cardiomyocyte injury using plasma troponin T and I measurements and quantitative wall motion analysis and ejection fraction in athletes who participated in the Hawaii Ironman Triathlon. They demonstrated that patients with elevated troponin levels had lower ejection fractions postcompetition.

DISTINGUISHING ATHLETE'S HEART FROM STRUCTURAL HEART DISEASE

The morphologic cardiac changes noted by echocardiography in athlete's heart are generally small in comparison to those seen in patients with primary myocardial disease or significant valvular disease.[2,14,16,20,21,24,26,27,33,36,41,46,48,50,53,56,58,66,68,69] However, not uncommonly, the adaptive cardiac structural changes related to training are substantial enough to raise the question of true structural heart disease. This distinction is crucial as pathologic structural heart disease is associated with an increased risk of sudden death. Identification of cardiovascular disease in an athlete may result in removal of the athlete from competition in an effort to reduce risk.[147] However, incorrect diagnosis may result in unwarranted withdrawal of an athlete from athletic training or competition thereby depriving the athlete of the potential health, emotional, social, and even perhaps financial benefits of sport. Screening of athletes for cardiovascular disease, distinguishing between physiologic changes consistent with athlete's heart and true structural heart disease, and, finally, making recommendations as to whether an athlete is "safe" to continue competing are challenging issues for physicians—issues that are growing in importance to the general population. Not only is an increasing portion of the population participating in athletic training, but the high profile, devastating deaths of several elite basketball players who died suddenly from cardiovascular disease during training or competition have raised everyone's awareness of these issues.[148,149]

Most sudden deaths in young competitive athletes (< 35 years old) occur during training or competition during extreme exertion. Several cardiovascular diseases have been determined to be potential causes of sudden death in young athletes as well as sedentary individuals.[150–152] The most common cause of sudden death in young athletes is hypertrophic cardiomyopathy.[150,151] Other causes that are less common include dilated cardiomyopathy, right ventricular dysplasia, myocarditis, coronary or other congenital anomalies, and the Marfan syndrome.[152] Rare causes of sudden death include aortic valve stenosis, mitral valve prolapse, sarcoid, atherosclerotic coronary disease, and QT prolongation. In the older athlete (> 35 years), sudden death is usually due to atherosclerotic coronary disease.[150]

The differential diagnosis between athlete's heart and pathologic cardiovascular disease most commonly involves hypertrophic cardiomyopathy, the most common cause of sudden death in competitive young athletes.[150] Hypertrophic cardiomyopathy is a term used to describe a hypertrophied, nondilated left ventricle in the absence of other cardiac or systemic disease that could result in hypertrophy of the degree present.[153] In most highly trained athletes, left ventricular wall thickness is within the normal range or only modestly increased (≤ 12 mm;)[2,14,16,20,21,24,26,27,33,36, 41,46,48,50,53,56,58,66,68–71] (Table 3.2). However, in some athletes, the wall thickness may reach 16 mm, thereby raising the question of hypertrophic cardiomyopathy.[68] In hypertrophic cardiomyopathy, the increase in left ventricular wall thickness is usually asymmetric and substantial, with an average reported septal thickness of approximately 20 mm and a peak wall thickness of 50 mm.[154] However, there is a small subset of patients with hypertrophic cardiomyopathy who have relatively modest concentric left ventricular hypertrophy with wall thickness ranging from 13 to 15 mm.[154] These patients fall into an overlap area between adaptive physiological hypertrophy and hypertrophic cardiomyopathy. The differentiation between these two entities can be difficult in some patients, but careful review of echocardiographic findings and clinical features usually allows for the distinction to be made.

In patients with hypertrophic cardiomyopathy, the anterior portion of the ventricular septum is usually the area with the greatest wall thickening; however, the hypertrophy may be heterogeneous and other regions may show the most thickening. Contiguous areas of the left ventricular wall often demonstrate different thickness with abrupt transitions creating significant asymmetry.[155,156] In athletes, there is rarely a discrete area of hypertrophy as the thickness of all regions of the ventricular wall are usually similar, with a septal-to-posterior wall thickness ratio of < 1:3.[72,154] A significant increase in left ventricular wall thickness typically occurs during adolescence in patients with hypertrophic cardiomyopathy.[157] Hence, in young athletes, hypertrophic cardiomyopathy may not be diagnosed because the hypertrophy may not have reached its greatest degree. The distinction from athlete's heart may be difficult at that time, but serial echocardiograms will generally confirm the diagnosis. In addition, female athletes rarely demonstrate left ventricular thickness in the overlap or gray zone between athlete's heart and hypertrophic cardiomyopathy. In a study of 600 elite female athletes,[116] left ventricular thickness ranged from 6 to 12 mm and hence did not substantially exceed the normal limit in any athlete. Due to the decreased absolute value of wall thickness in response to training demonstrated in women, female athletes with modestly elevated left ventricular wall thickness in the set-

TABLE 3.2.   SCREENING ECHOCARDIOGRAPHIC MORPHOLOGIC LIMITS IN ATHLETES

Wall thickness (septal and posterior)	< 1.3 cm
Septal-to-posterior wall thickness ratio	< 1.3
Relative wall thickness	0.30 ≤ and < 0.45
Left ventricular end-diastolic cavity dimension	≤ 6.0 cm
Left ventricular mass	≤ 294 g in men, ≤ 198 g in women

These limits of "normal" for athletes are based on pooled data from several studies involving large numbers of patients. While the morphologic measurements of some athletes may fall outside of these limits, the cutoff points are useful in determining which patients warrant further evaluation and follow-up.

ting of a normal or small cavity size should be suspected of having hypertrophic cardiomyopathy.

While the degree and distribution of left ventricular hypertrophy is usually most helpful in distinguishing athlete's heart from hypertrophic cardiomyopathy, cavity dimension can also be helpful. As discussed earlier, an enlarged end-diastolic cavity dimension typically accompanies increased left ventricular thickness in athletes. In about one-third of highly trained athletes, the left ventricular end-diastolic dimension is > 55 mm.[69] In contrast, the end-diastolic cavity dimension in patients with hypertrophic cardiomyopathy is generally small (< 45 mm).[158] It is only enlarged in patients with hypertrophic cardiomyopathy that has reached its end stage associated with systolic dysfunction and progressive heart failure.[158] Hence, patients with mildly increased wall thickness and small cavity sizes are more likely to have hypertrophic cardiomyopathy than adaptation. This combination (or geometric pattern) is easily recognized and quantified by calculation of relative wall thickness (mean wall thickness ÷ cavity radius), which rarely exceeds 0.45 in normal athletes.[70]

Impairment in left ventricular diastolic filling has been identified in most patients with hypertrophic cardiomyopathy regardless of the degree of hypertrophy or the presence of symptoms or outflow tract obstruction.[159] Typically, there is an inversion of the normal E/A ratio with a decrease in the early peak of transmitral flow velocity, a prolongation of the deceleration time of the early peak, and an increase of the late or atrial flow. In contrast, highly trained athletes have been shown to have normal left ventricular diastolic filling patterns.[51,52,59,68,95,159]

Because of the familial transmission of hypertrophic cardiomyopathy, echocardiographic diagnosis of the disease in a relative of a patient almost definitively establishes the diagnosis in the patient. Screening of family members may therefore be useful.

If distinction of athlete's heart from hypertrophic cardiomyopathy has not been made after

evaluation of wall thickness, cavity size, and diastolic filling, serial echocardiograms can be performed during a period of deconditioning to look for a reduction in wall thickness. Highly trained athletes can show regression of hypertrophy as rapidly as 1 week after cessation of training. Similar changes are not seen with hypertrophic cardiomyopathy.

The degree to which absolute left ventricular cavity dimension is increased by athletic training is modest in most athletes but may be more marked in others, raising the issue of distinguishing physiological structural cardiac change from dilated cardiomyopathy. In Pelliccia et al.'s[71] study of 1309 elite male and female athletes participating in 38 different sports, they demonstrated that 725 (55%) of the athletes had left ventricular diastolic dimensions within the accepted normal range (≤ 54 mm). However, the cavity dimension exceeded the upper limits of normal (≥ 55 mm) in 584 (45%) of the athletes, with marked enlargement (≥ 60 mm) in 185 athletes (14%). Despite the substantial left ventricular enlargement in some of the participants, none of the athletes had evidence of global or segmental systolic dysfunction or impairment in diastolic filling, and wall thickness was also increased in many. In addition, longitudinal follow-up of the 185 athletes with marked left ventricular end-diastolic cavity dimension over 1 to 12 years demonstrated no evidence of global systolic dysfunction or regional wall motion abnormalities.

Right ventricular dysplasia is an idiopathic cardiomyopathy in which there is fibro-fatty replacement of the right ventricular myocardium. There are functional and structural abnormalities of the right ventricle associated with ventricular and supraventricular arrhythmias and an increased risk of sudden death. Most of the deaths related to right ventricular dysplasia have occurred in young athletes (ages 13 to 34 years) during exercise.[160,161] The distinction between athlete's heart and right ventricular dysplasia may be difficult because many highly trained athletes have right ventricular enlargement. Diagnosis of right ventricular dysplasia echocardiographically can be challenging because of the technical difficulty of assessing right ventricular structure and function and because of the common mild morphologic forms of the disease. Magnetic resonance imaging may be helpful in making a noninvasive diagnosis of this disease, not only because of structural abnormalities but also by detection of fatty deposits in the right ventricular free wall.[162] The findings of global or segmental right ventricular dysfunction or marked right ventricular cavity enlargement would favor the diagnosis of right ventricular dysplasia, while the presence of moderate left ventricular cavity enlargement and increased left ventricular wall thickness support the diagnosis of athlete's heart.[2,58,72]

Some series of exercise-related sudden death include cases of myocarditis-induced arrhythmias.[151] Myocarditis is usually infectious in etiology but may occur as a result of drug abuse. Sudden death may occur during the active or healed stages of the disease as a consequence of arrhythmias. Left ventricular enlargement in an athlete suspected of having myocarditis may be due to athletic training or myocarditis. Symptoms such as palpitations or syncope or findings of heart failure, global or segmental systolic dysfunction, or arrhythmias suggest myocarditis.[154]

ECHOCARDIOGRAPHIC SCREENING IN ATHLETES

Cardiovascular preparticipation screening of athletes is an important issue that demands significant attention due to the increasing number of people participating in athletic training and the devastating impact of the sudden death of a healthy athlete.

The potential benefit of screening is based on the fact that athletic training is likely to increase the risk of sudden cardiac death in athletes with significant underlying structural heart disease.[148,151,163,164] While it is not possible to quantify this risk, most young athletes who die suddenly do so during the extreme exertion of competition or training.[151,163,164] Effective detec-

tion of clinically important underlying structural heart disease could allow for therapeutic interventions or avoidance of high-risk activity thereby reducing mortality.

A screening approach must acknowledge that sudden cardiac death is a relatively infrequent event and that only a small subset of the participants in organized sports is at risk.[164] The cardiac abnormalities known to cause sudden death in young athletes occur infrequently in the general population with the most common being hypertrophic cardiomyopathy which occurs at a rate of 1:500.[165] Hence, the combined prevalence of congenital cardiac lesions related to sudden death is on the order of approximately 0.2% in athletic populations. The prevalence of sudden death during training or competition is not accurately known but it appears to be in the range of 1:100,000 to 1:300,000 in high school athletes with a higher prevalence in males.[163] In older athletes (> 30 years), in whom the most common cause of sudden death is coronary artery disease, studies suggest a prevalence of 1:15,000 in joggers[166] and 1:50,000 in marathon runners.[167] Hence, overall, the prevalence of sudden cardiac death in athletes is relatively low. However, the dramatic and devastating effect of sudden death on families, communities, and society as a whole has increased interest in this issue and prompted concern about screening.

Prior to the guidelines proposed by the Sudden Death Committee and Congenital Cardiac Defects Committee of the American Heart Association, there were no generally accepted standards for screening of athletes or any specific certification for health care professionals who perform the screening exams. Currently, the American Heart Association recommends preparticipation cardiovascular screening for all high school and collegiate athletes.[168] They conclude that "a complete and careful personal and family history and physical examination designed to identify (raise the suspicion of) those cardiovascular lesions known to cause sudden death" is the most practical strategy for screening large populations of athletes of all ages.[168] In older athletes, a personal history of coronary risk factors and a family history of premature coronary disease should be obtained before starting competitive exercise. In addition, it may be reasonable to perform exercise stress testing on men older than 40 and women older than 50 who wish to participate in regular athletic training if they are at high risk for coronary disease based on the history obtained.

The addition of echocardiography to the screening process would clearly increase detection of certain cardiovascular abnormalities including hypertrophic cardiomyopathy, valvular heart disease, aortic root dilatation, and left ventricular dysfunction (with dilated cardiomyopathy and myocarditis). However, echocardiography cannot identify all important abnormalities. Many coronary anomalies and even arrhythmogenic right ventricular dysplasia cannot be reliably diagnosed with echocardiography alone. In addition, it is not cost-effective, or even feasible, to echocardiographically screen large populations of athletes. Hence, echocardiographic screening is reserved for those patients in whom cardiovascular abnormalities are identified or suspected after detailed personal and family histories and physical examinations are performed.

Echocardiography can identify several abnormalities including atrial and ventricular septal defects, a patent ductus arteriosus, valvular stenosis and regurgitation, mitral valve prolapse, coarctation of the aorta, some congenital coronary anomalies, aortic dilatation associated with the Marfan syndrome, and hypertrophic cardiomyopathy. Any cardiovascular abnormalities that are definitively identified should be considered in the context of the 26th Bethesda Conference consensus panel guidelines,[147] in order to make the final determination of eligibility for athletic competition.

SUMMARY

Athletic training has become a major component of daily life for a substantial portion of the population. As a result, the cardiovascular adaptations and complications associated with exercise are commanding the attention of physicians and the general population.

Echocardiography has allowed for detailed description of the adaptations of cardiac shape and function that occur with exercise. The typical morphologic changes commonly described as "athlete's heart" include increased left ventricular cavity dimension, wall thickness, and calculated mass. However, other morphologic and functional changes including increased right ventricular cavity size, enlargement of the atria, increased prevalence of mitral and tricuspid regurgitation, large coronary artery diameter, and augmentation of early diastolic filling are often found in athletes. These changes are typically modest and cardiac dimensions often do not exceed the accepted normal range.

The cardiac adaptations to exercise are related to gender, age, and race, and the type, duration, and intensity of the sport performed. They are dynamic and can occur and regress within weeks of onset and cessation of athletic training. The typical cardiac adaptations enhance the heart's ability to meet the aerobic demand of exercise; however, there is a process known as cardiac fatigue in which reversible systolic and diastolic left ventricular dysfunction have been described after prolonged exercise. While the pathophysiological mechanism of this process is unclear, some studies have demonstrated elevated serum tropinin levels in the setting of ventricular dysfunction suggesting myocardial injury.

Distinguishing the physiologic, adaptive morphologic changes of athlete's heart from pathologic structural heart disease that is associated with an increased risk of sudden death is important in order to allow for removal of high-risk athletes from competition, while enabling highly trained athletes with appropriate cardiac adaptations to enjoy participation in sports. This distinction can generally be made with a careful and complete family and personal history and a detailed physical exam, followed by noninvasive testing should any abnormality be found or suspected. Any cardiac abnormality definitively diagnosed should be assessed in the context of the 26th Bethesda Conference consensus panel guidelines in order to make a final recommendation in regard to the safety of participation in athletic competition.

PERSONAL PERSPECTIVE

Athletes and their hearts have long fascinated physicians, scientists, and even athletes themselves; echocardiography provides a marvelous window to discover how the body adapts to exercise training. In the early 1980s, when it became possible to measure diastolic function noninvasively, it became clear that the hypertrophy associated with exercise training was functionally quite different from that of disease states.[56] More detailed studies have since shown that distinctions can also be drawn on a structural basis.[56,68,70] Finally, the utility of echocardiography in distinguishing a healthy athlete's heart from an individual at risk for sudden death is great, but depends on a skilled, experienced observer. Many clinicians accustomed to minor abnormalities in patients with known disease fail to remark on such changes in a healthy individual. Similarly, one not familiar with the pattern and extent of hypertrophy seen in athletes may mistakenly diagnose disease. The literature presents a remarkably consistent picture of the athlete's heart by echocardiography. Careful attention to it will avoid these problems.

While the distinctions between pathologic and physiologic adaptations are obviously important on the playing field and in the doctor's office, physiological hypertrophy is also well worth studying in the laboratory as a model of extreme health and positive adaptation. Having clearly described its phenotype echocardiographically, definition of the underlying biology of this process may provide profound new insights and valuable, novel approaches to treatment of cardiovascular diseases and disease compensation.

Similarly, the entity of cardiac fatigue is well described, but its underlying mechanisms are unknown. It is clear, however, that athletes are "protected" in that they have a much higher threshold of exercise required to produce dysfunction compared to sedentary individuals. Understanding the impact of "overwork" and how the body prevents it is clearly relevant in the clinical arena, where disease is often a gradual process of deterioration. Even as our knowledge of the athlete's heart grows, there remains much to learn.

REFERENCES

1. Henschen S: Skidlauf und Skidwettlauf. Eine medizinische Sportstudie. *Mitt Med Klin Upsala* 2:15, 1899.
2. Rost R, Hollman W: Athlete's Heart—A review of its historical assessment and new aspects. *Int J Sports Med* 4:147, 1983.
3. Marach JH: Physiological and pathological effects of severe exertion, marathon race, on circulatory and renal system. *Arch Intern Med* 5:382, 1910.
4. Gordon B, Levine SA, Welmaers A: A group of marathon runners with special reference to circulation. *Arch Intern Med* 33:425, 1924.
5. Keys A, Friedell HL: Size and stroke of the heart in young men in relation to athletic activity. *Science* 88:456, 1938.
6. Beckner GL, Winsor T: Cardiovascular adaptations to prolonged physical effort. *Circulation* 9:835, 1954.
7. Bevegard S, Holmgren A, Jonsson B: Circulatory studies in well-trained athletes at rest and during heavy exercise with special reference to stroke volume and the influence of body position. *Acta Physiol Scand* 57:26, 1963.
8. Gott PH, Roselle HA, Crampton RS: The athletic heart syndrome. Five-year cardiac evaluation of a champion athlete. *Arch Intern Med* 122:340, 1968.
9. Raskoff WJ, Goldman S, Cohn K: The "athletic heart." Prevalence and physiologic significance of left ventricular enlargement in distance runners. *JAMA* 236:158, 1976.
10. Scheuer J, Tipton CM: Cardiovascular adaptations to physical training. *Annu Rev Physiol* 39: 221, 1977.
11. Longhurst JC, Kelly AR, Gonyea WJ, et al: Cardiovascular responses to static exercise in distance runners and weight lifters. *J Appl Physiol* 49:676, 1980.
12. Blomqvist CG, Saltin B: Cardiovascular adaptations to physical training. *Annu Rev Physiol* 45: 169, 1983.
13. Schaible TF, Scheuer J: Cardiac adaptations to

chronic exercise. *Prog Cardiovasc Dis* 27:297, 1985.

14. Morganroth J, Maron BJ, Henry WL, et al: Comparative left ventricular dimensions in trained athletes. *Ann Intern Med* 82:521, 1975.

15. Roeske WR, O'Rourke RA, Klein A, et al: Non-invasive evaluation of ventricular hypertrophy in professional athletes. *Circulation* 53:286, 1976.

16. Gilbert CA, Nutter DO, Felner JM, et al: Echocardiographic study of cardiac dimensions and function in the endurance-trained athlete. *Am J Cardiol* 40:528, 1977.

17. Underwood RH, Schwade JL: Noninvasive analysis of cardiac function in elite distance runners—echocardiography, vectorcardiography, and cardiac intervals. *Ann N Y Acad Sci* 301:297, 1977.

18. Zoneraich S, Rhee JJ, Zoneraich O, et al: Assessment of cardiac function in marathon runners by graphic noninvasive techniques. *Ann N Y Acad Sci* 301:900, 1977.

19. Allen HD, Goldberg SJ, Sahn DJ, et al: A quantitative echocardiographic study of champion childhood swimmers. *Circulation* 55:142, 1977.

20. Ehsani AA, Hagberg JM, Hickson RC: Rapid changes in left ventricular dimensions and mass in response to physical conditioning and deconditioning. *Am J Cardiol* 42:52, 1978.

21. Parker BM, Londeree BR, Cupp GV, et al: The noninvasive cardiac evaluation of long-distance runners. *Chest* 73:376, 1978.

22. Zeldis SM, Morganroth J, Rubler S: Cardiac hypertrophy in response to dynamic conditioning in female athletes. *J Appl Physiol* 44:849, 1978.

23. DeMaria AN, Neumann A, Lee G, et al: Alterations in ventricular mass and performance induced by exercise training in man evaluated by echocardiography. *Circulation* 57:237, 1978.

24. Ikaheimo MJ, Palatsi IJ, Takkunen JT: Noninvasive evaluation of the athletic heart: Sprinters versus endurance runners. *Am J Cardiol* 44:24, 1979.

25. Wolfe LA, Cunningham DA, Rechnitzer PA, et al: Effects of endurance training on left ventricular dimensions in healthy men. *J Appl Physiol* 47:207, 1979.

26. Nishimura T, Yamada Y, Kawai C: Echocardiographic evaluation of long-term effects of exercise on left ventricular hypertrophy and function in professional bicyclists. *Circulation* 61:832, 1980.

27. Longhurst JC, Kelly AR, Gonyea WJ, et al: Echocardiographic left ventricular masses in distance runners and weight lifters. *J Appl Physiol* 48:154, 1980.

28. Stein RA, Michielli D, Diamond J, et al: The cardiac response to exercise training: Echocardiographic analysis at rest and during exercise. *Am J Cardiol* 46:219, 1980.

29. Kanakis C, Hickson RC: Left ventricular responses to a program of lower-limb strength training. *Chest* 78:618, 1980.

30. Blair NL, Youker JE, McDonald IG, et al: Echocardiographic assessment of cardiac chamber size and left ventricular function in aerobically trained athletes. *Aust N Z J Med* 10:540, 1980.

31. Cohen JL, Gupta PK, Lichstein E, et al: The heart of a dancer: Noninvasive cardiac evaluation of professional ballet dancers. *Am J Cardiol* 45:959, 1980.

32. Peronnet F, Perrault H, Cleroux J, et al: Electro- and echocardiographic study of the left ventricle in man after training. *Eur J Appl Physiol* 45:125, 1980.

33. Bekaert I, Pannier JL, Van De Weghe C, et al: Non-invasive evaluation of cardiac function in professional cyclists. *Br Heart J* 45:213, 1981.

34. Adams TD, Yanowitz FG, Fisher AG, et al: Noninvasive evaluation of exercise training in college-age men. *Circulation* 64:958, 1981.

35. Paulsen W, Boughner DB, Ko P, et al: Left ventricular function in marathon runners: Echocardiographic assessment. *J Appl Physiol* 51:881, 1981.

36. Keul J, Dickhuth HH, Simon G, et al: Effect of static and dynamic exercise on heart volume, contractility, and left ventricular dimensions. *Circ Res* 48(suppl I):I-162, 1981.

37. Heath GW, Hagberg JM, Ehsani AA, et al: A physiological comparison of young and older endurance athletes. *J Appl Physiol* 51:634, 1981.

38. Wieling W, Borghols EA, Hollander AP, et al: Echocardiographic dimensions and maximal oxygen uptake in oarsmen during training. *Br Heart J* 46:190, 1981.

39. Mumford M, Prakash R: Electrocardiographic and echocardiographic characteristics of long distance runners. Comparison of left ventricular function with age- and sex-matched controls. *Am J Sports Med* 9:23, 1981.

40. Rubal BJ, Rosentswieg J, Hamerly B: Echocar-

diographic examination of women collegiate softball champions. *Med Sci Sports Exerc* 13: 176, 1981.

41. Longhurst JC, Kelly AR, Gonyea WJ, et al: Chronic training with static and dynamic exercise: Cardiovascular adaptation and response to exercise. *Circ Res* 48(suppl I):I-171, 1981.

42. Perrault H, Lajoie D, Peronnet F, et al: Left ventricular dimensions following training in young and middle-aged men. *Int J Sports Med* 3:141, 1982.

43. Rost R: The athlete's heart. *Eur Heart J* 3(suppl A):193, 1982.

44. Snoeckx LH, Abeling HF, Lambregts JA, et al: Echocardiographic dimensions in athletes in relation to their training programs. *Med Sci Sports Exerc* 14:428, 1982.

45. Spirito P, Maron BJ, Bonow RO, et al: Prevalence and significance of an abnormal ST segment response to exercise in a young athletic population. *Am J Cardiol* 51:1663, 1983.

46. Fagard R, Aubert A, Lysens R, et al: Noninvasive assessment of seasonal variants in cardiac structure and function in cyclists. *Circulation* 67:896, 1983.

47. Sugishita Y, Koseki S, Matsuda M, et al: Myocardial mechanics of athletic hearts in comparison with diseased hearts. *Am Heart J* 105: 273, 1983.

48. Shapiro LM, Smith RG. Effect of training on left ventricular structure and function. An echocardiographic study. *Br Heart J* 50:534, 1983.

49. Fagard R, Aubert A, Staessen J, et al: Cardiac structure and function in cyclists and runners. Comparative echocardiographic study. *Br Heart J* 52:124, 1984.

50. Shapiro LM: Physiological left ventricular hypertrophy. *Br Heart J* 52:130, 1984.

51. Colan SD, Sanders SP, MacPherson D, et al: Left ventricular diastolic function in elite athletes with physiologic cardiac hypertrophy. *J Am Coll Cardiol* 6:545, 1985.

52. Granger CB, Karimeddini MK, Smith VE, et al: Rapid ventricular filling in left ventricular hypertrophy: I. Physiologic hypertrophy. *J Am Coll Cardiol* 5:862, 1985.

53. Hauser AM, Dressendorfer RH, Vos M, et al: Symmetric cardiac enlargement in highly trained endurance athletes: A two dimensional echocardiographic study. *Am Heart J* 109:1038, 1985.

54. Cohen JL, Segal KR: Left ventricular hypertrophy in athletes: An exercise-echocardiographic study. *Med Sci Sports Exerc* 17:695, 1985.

55. Martin WH III, Coyle EF, Bloomfield SA, et al: Effects of physical deconditioning after intense endurance training on left ventricular dimensions and stroke volume. *J Am Coll Cardiol* 7:982, 1986.

56. Douglas PS, O'Toole ML, Hiller WD, et al: Left ventricular structure and function by echocardiography in ultraendurance athletes. *Am J Cardiol* 58:805, 1986.

57. Medved R, Fabecic-Sabadi V, Medved V: Echocardiographic findings in children participating in swimming training. *Int J Sports Med* 7: 94, 1986.

58. Maron BJ: Structural features of the athlete heart as defined by echocardiography. *J Am Coll Cardiol* 7:190, 1986.

59. Pearson AC, Schiff M, Mrosek D, et al: Left ventricular diastolic function in weight lifters. *Am J Cardiol* 58:1254, 1986.

60. Pavlik G, Bachl N, Wollein W, et al: Resting echocardiographic parameters after cessation of regular endurance training. *Int J Sports Med* 7: 226, 1986.

61. Colan SD, Sanders SP, Borow KM: Physiological hypertrophy: Effects on left ventricular systolic mechanics in athletes. *J Am Coll Cardiol* 9:776, 1987.

62. Cohen CR, Allen HD, Spain J, et al: Cardiac structure and function in elite high school wrestlers. *Am J Dis Child* 141:576, 1987.

63. Maron BJ, Bodison SA, Wesley YE, et al: Results of screening a large group of intercollegiate competitive athletes for cardiovascular disease. *J Am Coll Cardiol* 10:1214, 1987.

64. Lewis JF, Maron BJ, Diggs JA, et al: Preparticipation echocardiographic screening for cardiovascular disease in a large, predominantly black population of collegiate athletes. *Am J Cardiol* 64:1029, 1989.

65. Fagard R, Broeke C, Amery A: Left ventricular dynamics during exercise in elite marathon runners. *J Am Coll Cardiol* 14:112, 1989.

66. Fisher AG, Adams TD, Yanowitz FG, et al: Noninvasive evaluation of world class athletes engaged in different modes of training. *Am J Cardiol* 63:337, 1989.

67. Douglas PS, O'Toole ML, Hiller WD, et al:

Different effects of prolonged exercise on the right and left ventricles. *J Am Coll Cardiol* 15:64, 1990.

68. Pelliccia A, Maron BJ, Spataro A, et al: The upper limit of physiologic cardiac hypertrophy in highly trained elite athletes. *N Engl J Med* 324:295, 1991.

69. Spirito P, Pelliccia A, Proschan MA, et al: Morphology of the "athlete's heart" assessed by echocardiography in 947 elite athletes representing 27 sports. *Am J Cardiol* 74:802, 1994.

70. Douglas PS, O'Toole ML, Katz SE, et al: Left ventricular hypertrophy in athletes. *Am J Cardiol* 80:1384, 1997.

71. Pelliccia A, Culasso F, Di Paolo FM, et al: Physiologic left ventricular cavity dilatation in elite athletes. *Ann Intern Med* 130:23, 1999.

72. Huston TP, Puffer JC, Rodney WM: The athletic heart syndrome. *N Engl J Med* 313:24, 1985.

73. Astrand P, Rodahl K: Mechanical efficiency of muscle contraction, in Van Dalen DB (ed): *Textbook of Work Physiology—Physiological Bases of Exercise.* New York, McGraw-Hill, 1986; p 45.

74. Zepilli S, Sandric S, Cecchetti F, et al: Echocardiographic assessments of cardiac arrangements in different sports activities, in Lubich T, Venerando A (eds): *Sports Cardiology* Bologna, Aulo Gaggi, 1980; p 723.

75. Henry WL, Gardin JM, Ware JH: Echocardiographic measurements in normal subjects from infancy to old age. *Circulation* 62:1054, 1980.

76. Rost R. The athlete's heart: *Eur Heart J* 3(suppl A):193, 1982.

77. Vasan RS, Larson MG, Levy D, et al: Distribution and categorization of echocardiographic measurements in relation to reference limits: The Framingham Heart Study: Formulation of a height- and sex-specific classification and its prospective validation. *Circulation* 96:1863, 1997.

78. Devereux RB, Pickering TG, Harshfield GA, et al: Left ventricular hypertrophy in patients with hypertension: Importance of blood pressure response to regularly recurring stress. *Circulation* 68:470, 1983.

79. Ren JF, Hakki AH, Kotler MN, et al: Exercise systolic blood pressure: A powerful determinant of increased LV mass in patients with hypertension. *J Am Coll Cardiol* 5:1224, 1985.

80. Troy BL, Pombo J, Rackley CE: Measurement of left ventricular wall thickness and mass by echocardiography. *Circulation* 45:602, 1972.

81. Devereux RB, Reichek N: Echocardiographic determination of left ventricular mass in man. Anatomic validation of the method. *Circulation* 55:613, 1977.

82. Devereux RB, Lutas EM, Casale PN, et al: Standardization of M-mode echocardiographic left ventricular anatomic measurements. *J Am Coll Cardiol* 4:1222, 1984.

83. De Simone G, Daniels SR, Devereux RB, et al: Left ventricular mass and body size in normotensive children and adults: Assessment of allometric relations and impact of overweight. *J Am Coll Cardiol* 20:1251, 1992.

84. Levy D, Savage DD, Garrison RJ, et al: Echocardiographic criteria for left ventricular hypertrophy: The Framingham Heart Study. *Am J Cardiol* 59:956, 1987.

85. Lauer MS, Larson MG, Levy D: Gender-specific reference M-mode values in adults: Population-derived values with consideration of the impact of height. *J Am Coll Cardiol* 26:1039, 1995.

86. Popp RL: M-mode echocardiographic assessment of left ventricular function. *Am J Cardiol* 49:1312, 1982.

87. Grossman W, McLaurin LP: Diastolic properties of the left ventricle. *Ann Int Med* 84:316, 1976.

88. Snider AR, Giddings SS, Rocchini AP, et al: Doppler evaluation of left ventricular diastolic filling in children with systemic hypertension. *Am J Cardiol* 56:921, 1985.

89. Phillips RA, Coplan NL, Krakoff LR, et al: Doppler echocardiographic analysis of left ventricular filling in treated hypertensive patients. *J Am Coll Cardiol* 9:317, 1987.

90. Maron BJ, Spirito P, Green KJ, et al: Noninvasive assessment of left ventricular diastolic function by pulsed Doppler echocardiography in patients with hypertrophic cardiomyopathy. *J Am Coll Cardiol* 10:733, 1987.

91. Hanrath P, Mathey DG, Siegert R, et al: Left ventricular relaxation and filling pattern in different forms of left ventricular hypertrophy: An echocardiography study. *Am J Cardiol* 45:15, 1980.

92. Fifer MA, Borow KM, Colan SD, et al: Early diastolic ventricular function in children and adults with aortic stenosis. *J Am Coll Cardiol* 5:1147, 1985.

93. Eichhorn P, Grimm J, Koch R, et al: Left ventric-

ular relaxation in patients with left ventricular hypertrophy secondary to aortic valve disease. *Circulation* 65:1395, 1982.

94. Inouye I, Massie B, Loge D, et al: Abnormal left ventricular filling: An early finding in mild to moderate systemic hypertension. *Am J Cardiol* 53:120, 1984.

95. Fagard R, Van den Broeke C, Bielen E, et al: Assessment of stiffness of the hypertrophied left ventricle of bicyclists using left ventricular inflow Doppler velocimetry. *J Am Coll Cardiol* 9: 1250, 1987.

96. Matsuda M, Sugishita Y, Koseki S, et al: Effect of exercise on left ventricular diastolic filling in athletes and nonathletes. *J Appl Physiol* 55:323, 1983.

97. Shapiro LM, McKenna WJ: Left ventricular hypertrophy: Relation of structure to diastolic function in hypertension. *Br Heart J* 51:637, 1984.

98. Vanoverschelde JJ, Essamri B, Vanbutsele R, et al: Contribution of left ventricular diastolic function to exercise capacity in normal subjects. *J Appl Physiol* 74:2225, 1993.

99. Nixon JV, Wright AR, Porter TR, et al: Effects of exercise on left ventricular diastolic performance in trained athletes. *Am J Cardiol* 68:945, 1991.

100. Forman DE, Manning WJ, Hauser R, et al: Enhanced left ventricular diastolic filling associated with long-term endurance training. *J Gerontol* 47:56, 1992.

101. Sahn DJ, DeMaria A, Kisslo J, et al: Recommendations regarding quantitation in M-mode echocardiography: Results of a survey of echocardiographic measurements. *Circulation* 58:1072, 1978.

102. Presti C, Crawford M: Echocardiographic evaluation of athletes, in Waller B, Harvey WP (eds): *Cardiovascular Evaluation of Athletes.* New Jersey, Laennec, 1993; p 63.

103. Douglas PS, Berman GO, O'Toole ML, et al: Prevalence of multivalvular regurgitation in athletes. *Am J Cardiol* 64:209, 1989.

104. Pollak SJ, McMillan SA, Knopff WD, et al: Cardiac evaluation of women distance runners by echocardiographic color Doppler flow mapping. *J Am Coll Cardiol* 11:89, 1988.

105. Kostucki W, Vandenbossche JL, Friart A, et al: Pulsed Doppler regurgitant flow patterns of normal valves. *Am J Cardiol* 58:309, 1986.

106. Haslam RW, Cobb RB: Frequency of intensive, prolonged exercise as a determinant of relative coronary circumference index. *Int J Sports Med* 3:118, 1982.

107. Leon AS, Bloor CM: Effects of exercise and its cessation on the heart and its blood supply. *J Appl Physiol* 24:485, 1968.

108. Wyatt HL, Mitchell J: Influences of physical conditioning and deconditioning on coronary vasculature of dogs. *J Appl Physiol* 45:619, 1978.

109. Currens JH, White PD: Half a century of running. Clinical, physiologic and autopsy findings in the case of Clarance DeMar ("Mr. Marathon"). *Nord Hyg T* 265:988, 1961.

110. Hutchins GM, Bulkey BH, Miner MM, et al: Correlation of age and heart weight with tortuosity and caliber of normal human coronary arteries. *Am Heart J* 94:196, 1977.

111. Lewis BS, Gotsman MS: Relation between coronary artery size and left ventricular wall mass. *Br Heart J* 35:1150, 1973.

112. O'Keefe JH Jr, Owen RM, Bove AA: Influence of left ventricular mass on coronary artery cross-sectional area. *Am J Cardiol* 59:1395, 1987.

113. Haskell WL, Sims C, Myll J, et al: Coronary artery size and dilating capacity in ultradistance runners. *Circulation* 87:1076, 1993.

114. Pelliccia A, Sparato A, Granata M, et al: Coronary arteries in physiological hypertrophy: Echocardiographic evidence of increased proximal size in athletes. *Int J Sports Med* 11:120, 1990.

115. Hickson RC, Kanakis C Jr, Davis JR, et al: Reduced training duration effects on aerobic power, endurance, and cardiac growth. *J Appl Physiol* 53:225, 1982.

116. Pelliccia A, Maron BJ, Culasso F, et al: Athlete's heart in women: Echocardiographic characterization of highly trained elite female athletes. *JAMA* 276:211, 1996.

117. Lengyel M, Gyarfas I: The importance of echocardiography in the assessment of left ventricular hypertrophy in trained and untrained schoolchildren. *Acta Cardiol* 34:63, 1979.

118. Fagard R, Van den Broeke C, Vanhees L, et al: Noninvasive assessment of systolic and diastolic left ventricular function in female runners. *Eur Heart J* 8:1305, 1987.

119. Geenen DL, Gilliam TB, Crowley D, et al: Echocardiographic measures in 6- to 7-year-old children after an 8 month exercise program. *Am J Cardiol* 49:1090, 1982.

120. Perrault H, Lajoie D, Peronnet F, et al: Left ventricular dimensions following training in young and middle-aged men. *Int J Sports Med* 3:141, 1982.

121. Douglas PS, O'Toole M: Aging and physical activity determine cardiac structure and function in the older athlete. *J Appl Physiol* 72:1969, 1992.

122. Hinderliter AL, Light KC, Willis PW: Racial differences in left ventricular structure in healthy young adults. *Am J Cardiol* 69:1196, 1992.

123. Dunn FG, Oigman W, Sungaard-Riise K, et al: Racial differences in cardiac adaptation to essential hypertension determined by echocardiographic indexes. *J Am Coll Cardiol* 1:1348, 1983.

124. Hypertension Detection and Follow-up Program Cooperative Group: Blood pressure studies in 14 communities. A two stage screen for hypertension. *JAMA* 237:2385, 1997.

125. Lewis JF, Maron BJ, Diggs JA, et al: Preparticipation echocardiographic screening for cardiovascular disease in a large, predominantly black population of collegiate athletes. *Am J Cardiol* 64:1029, 1989.

126. Lewis JF, Maron BJ: Diversity of patterns of hypertrophy in patients with systemic hypertension and marked left ventricular wall thickening. *Am J Cardiol* 65:874, 1990.

127. Ekelund LG, Suchindran CM, Karon JM, et al: Black-white differences in exercise blood pressure. The Lipid Research Clinics Program Prevalence Study. *Circulation* 81:1568, 1990.

128. Bielen E, Fagard R, Amery A: Inheritance of heart structure and physical exercise capacity: A study of left ventricular structure and exercise capacity in 7-year-old twins. *Eur Heart J* 11:7, 1990.

129. Bielen EC, Fagard RH, Amery AK: Inheritance of acute cardiac changes during bicycle exercise: An echocardiographic study in twins. *Med Sci Sports Exerc* 23:1254, 1991.

130. Wilson JD: Androgen abuse in athletes. *Endocr Rev* 9:181, 1988.

131. Thompson PD, Sadaniantz A, Cullinane EM, et al.: Left ventricular function is not impaired in weight-lifters who use anabolic steriods. *J Am Coll Cardiol* 19:278, 1992.

132. Rezkalla SH, Hale S, Kloner RA: Cocaine-induced heart diseases. *Am Heart J* 120:1403, 1990.

133. Kloner RA, Hale S, Alker K, et al: The effects of acute and chronic cocaine use on the heart. *Circulation* 85:407, 1992.

134. Mouhaffel AH, Madu EC, Satmary WA, et al: Cardiovascular complications of cocaine. *Chest* 107:1426, 1995.

135. Coyle EF, Martin WH 3d, Sinacore DR, et al: Time course of loss of adaptations after stopping prolonged intense endurance training. *J Appl Physiol* 57:1857, 1984.

136. Fox EL, Bartels RL, Billings CE, et al: Frequency and duration of interval training programs and changes in aerobic power. *J Appl Physiol* 38:481, 1975.

137. Maron BJ, Pelliccia A, Spataro A, et al. Reduction in left ventricular wall thickness after deconditioning in highly trained Olympic athletes. *Br Heart J* 69:125, 1993.

138. Upton MT, Rerych SK, Roeback JR, et al: Effect of brief and prolonged exercise on left ventricular function. *Am J Cardiol* 45:1154, 1980.

139. Niemela KO, Palatsi IJ, Ikaheimo MJ, et al: Evidence of impaired left ventricular performance after an uninterrupted competitive 24 hour run. *Circulation* 70:350, 1984.

140. Saltin B, Stenberg J: Circulatory response to prolonged severe exercise. *J Appl Physiol* 19:833, 1964.

141. Perrault H, Peronnet F, Lebeau R, et al: Echocardiographic assessment of left ventricular performance before and after marathon running. *Am Heart J* 112:1026, 1986.

142. Douglas PS, O'Toole ML, Hiller WD, et al: Cardiac fatigue after prolonged exercise. *Circulation* 76:1206, 1987.

143. Seals DR, Rogers MA, Hagberg JM, et al: Left ventricular dysfunction after prolonged strenuous exercise in healthy subjects. *Am J Cardiol* 61:875, 1988.

144. Niemela K, Palatsi I, Ikaheimo M, et al: Impaired left ventricular diastolic function in athletes after utterly strenuous prolonged exercise. *Int J Sports Med* 8:61, 1987.

145. Laslett L, Eisenbud E, Lind R: Evidence of myocardial injury during prolonged strenuous exercise. *Am J Cardiol* 78:488, 1996.

146. Rifai N, Douglas PS, O'Toole M, et al: Cardiac troponin T and I, electrocardiographic wall-motion analyses, and ejection fractions in athletes participating in the Hawaii Ironman Triathlon. *Am J Cardiol* 83:1085, 1999.

147. 26th Bethesda Conference: Recommendations for determining eligibility for competition in ath-

letes with cardiovascular abnormalities. *J Am Coll Cardiol* 24:845, 1994.

148. Maron BJ: Sudden death in young athletes. Lessons from the Hank Gathers affair. *N Engl J Med* 329:55, 1993.

149. The death of Reggie Lewis: A search for answers. *Boston Globe,* September 12, 1993.

150. Maron BJ, Epstein SE, Roberts WC: Causes of sudden death in the competitive athletes. *J Am Coll Cardiol* 7:204, 1986.

151. Burke AP, Farb A, Virmani R, et al: Sports-related and non-sports-related sudden cardiac death in young adults. *Am Heart J* 121:568, 1991.

152. Corrado D, Thiene G, Nava A, et al: Sudden death in young competitive athletes: Clinicopathologic correlations in 22 cases. *Am J Med* 89:588, 1990.

153. Maron BJ, Epstein SE: Hypertrophic cardiomyopathy: A discussion of nomenclature. *Am J Cardiol* 43:1242, 1979.

154. Maron BJ, Pelliccia A, Spirito P: Cardiac disease in young trained athletes. Insights into methods for distinguishing athlete's heart from structural heart disease, with particular emphasis on hypertrophic cardiomyopathy. *Circulation* 91:1596, 1995.

155. Maron BJ, Gottdiener JS, Epstein SE: Patterns and significance of the distribution of left ventricular hypertrophy in hypertrophic cardiomyopathy. A wide-angle, two-dimensional echocardiographic study of 125 patients. *Am J Cardiol* 48:418, 1981.

156. Maron BJ, Bonow RO, Cannon RO, et al: Hypertrophic cardiomyopathy. Interrelations of clinical manifestations, pathophysiology, and therapy. *N Engl J Med* 316:780, 1987.

157. Maron BJ, Spirito P, Wesley Y, et al: Development and progression of left ventricular hypertrophy in children with hypertrophic cardiomyopathy. *N Engl J Med* 315:610, 1986.

158. Spirito P, Maron BJ, Bonow RO, et al: Occurrence and significance of progressive left ventricular wall thinning and relative cavity dilatation in patients with hypertrophic cardiomyopathy. *Am J Cardiol* 69:123, 1987.

159. Lewis JF, Spirito P, Pelliccia A, et al: Usefulness of Doppler echocardiographic assessment of diastolic filling in distinguishing "athlete's heart" from hypertrophic cardiomyopathy. *Br Heart J* 68:296, 1992.

160. Goodin JC, Farb A, Smialek JE, et al: Right ventricular dysplasia associated with sudden death in young adults. *Mod Pathol* 4:702, 1991.

161. Nava A, Thiene G, Canciani B, et al: Familial occurrence of right ventricular dysplasia: A study involving nine families. *J Am Coll Cardiol* 12:1222, 1988.

162. Ricci C, Longo R, Pagnan L, et al: Magnetic resonance imaging in right ventricular dysplasia. *Am J Cardiol* 70:1589, 1992.

163. Maron BJ, Shirani J, Poliac LC, et al: Sudden death in young competitive athletes. Clinical, demographic, and pathological profiles. *JAMA* 276:199, 1996.

164. Maron BJ, Roberts WC, McAllister HA, et al: Sudden death in young athletes. *Circulation* 62:218, 1980.

165. Maron BJ, Gardin JM, Flack JM, et al: Prevalence of hypertrophic cardiomyopathy in a general population of young adults: Echocardiographic analysis of 4111 subjects in the CARDIA Study—Coronary Artery Risk Development in (Young) Adults. *Circulation* 92:785, 1995.

166. Thompson PD, Funk EJ, Carleton RA, et al: Incidence of death during jogging in Rhode Island from 1975 though 1980. *JAMA* 247:2535, 1982.

167. Maron BJ, Poliac LC, Roberts WO: Risk for sudden cardiac death associated with marathon running. *J Am Coll Cardiol* 28:428, 1996.

168. Maron BJ, Thompson PD, Puffer JC, et al: Cardiovascular preparticipation screening of competitive athletes. A statement for health professionals from the Sudden Death Committee (Clinical Cardiology) and the Congenital Cardiac Defects Committee (Cardiovascular Disease in the Young) American Heart Association. *Circulation* 94:850, 1996.

Chapter 4

OVERVIEW
OF EXERCISE TESTING

Cynthia M. Ferguson, B.S.   *Jonathan Myers, Ph.D.*   *Victor F. Froelicher, M.D.*

The exercise test continues to have an integral place in cardiovascular medicine because of its high yield of diagnostic, prognostic, and functional information.[1] Exercise testing can also be an important tool for the evaluation of the competitive and noncompetitive athlete. When conducting an exercise test the method and analysis of the data should be determined by the objective of the test. The objective or goal of the exercise test differs when used in athletes as compared to routine clinical use. In the clinical setting the major indications for exercise testing are the diagnosis and prognostication of heart disease. While determination of functional capacity, as measured by gas analysis, is helpful in quantifying exercise capacity and monitoring the disease state of patients with chronic obstructive pulmonary disease, chronic heart disease, and known coronary heart disease, the major emphasis is on the analysis of the electrocardiogram (ECG) in the majority of clinical tests. Also, careful monitoring for reproduction of symptoms such as angina or presyncope is vital in the clinical setting.

   In athletes exercise testing is commonly used

71

for evaluation of response to training, decline in performance, or exercise-induced symptoms. The measurement of exercise capacity, particularly by analysis of expired gases, becomes more important than the ECG in athletes. Exceptions to this generalization are in the older (over 40-year-old) or master athlete in whom coronary artery disease is the most common cause of sudden death during exercise or in athletes complaining of palpitations or exercise-induced syncope.

In order to address the specific goals of testing in the athlete the order of presentation of material in this chapter will vary from the usual exercise-testing chapter. It will begin with methodology of exercise testing, the hemodynamic responses to exercise, and the evaluation of functional capacity. It will then provide a brief review of the exercise ECG, outline the use to the exercise test for screening and diagnosis, and finish with a summary.

METHODS

Excellent guidelines have been updated by organizations such as the American Heart Association, the American Association of Cardiovascular and Pulmonary Rehabilitation, and the American College of Sports Medicine that are based on a multitude of research studies over the last 20 years, and have led to greater uniformity in methods.[2] These should be followed as closely as possible. General concerns prior to performing an exercise test include safety precautions and equipment needs, patient preparation, choosing a test type, choosing a test protocol, patient monitoring, reasons to terminate a test, and posttest monitoring.

SAFETY PRECAUTIONS AND EQUIPMENT

The safety precautions outlined by the American Heart Association are explicit in regard to the requirements for exercise testing. Everything necessary for cardiopulmonary resuscitation must be available, and regular drills should be performed to ascertain that both personnel and equipment

are ready for a cardiac emergency. The first survey of clinical exercise facilities[3] showed exercise testing to be a safe procedure, with approximately 1 death and 5 nonfatal complications per 10,000 tests. Perhaps due to an expanded knowledge concerning indications, contraindications, and endpoints, maximal exercise testing appears safer today than 20 years ago. Gibbons et al.[4] reported the safety of exercise testing in 71,914 tests conducted over a 16-year period. The complication rate was 0.8 per 10,000 tests. The authors suggested that the low complication rate might be due to a cool-down walk, but present authors have observed a low complication rate despite laying even high-risk patients supine immediately after the test.[5]

Besides emergency equipment, the safety and accuracy of the testing equipment should be considered. The treadmill should have front and side rails for subjects to steady themselves. It should be calibrated monthly. Some models can be greatly affected by the weight of the subject and will not deliver the appropriate workload to heavy individuals. An emergency stop button should be readily available to the staff only. A small platform or stepping area at the level of the belt is advisable so that the subject can start the test by "pedaling" the belt with one foot prior to stepping on.

Though numerous clever devices have been developed to automate blood pressure measurement during exercise, none can be recommended. The time-proven method of holding the subject's arm with a stethoscope placed over the brachial artery remains most reliable. The subject's arm should be free of the handrails so that noise is not transmitted up the arm. It is sometimes helpful to mark the brachial artery. An anesthesiologist's auscultatory piece or an electronic microphone can be fastened to the arm. A device that inflates and deflates the cuff on the push of a button can be helpful also.

EXERCISE TESTING

PRETEST PREPARATIONS
Detection of disease in the athlete may depend on this initial screening more than it would in the

typical patient, as the former frequently does not have symptoms commonly associated with heart disease. During the evaluation, the physician should establish an understanding of any patterns of cardiopulmonary compromise associated with exercise. The physician should note the type, length, and intensity of the athlete's workout, document any reasons why the athlete has had to interrupt or stop an exercise program, and discuss any problems associated with exertion (i.e., syncope, palpitations, or dyspnea).[6] The athlete should be asked whether he or she has ever become light-headed or has fainted while exercising and whether anyone in the family has died suddenly during exercise. The physician should also ask about family history and general medical history, making note of any conditions that may increase the risk of sudden death (i.e., smoking, drug use, diabetes mellitus, and hyperlipidemia).

A brief physical examination should always be performed prior to testing to rule out significant obstructive aortic valvular disease. Cardiac evaluation of a healthy athlete may reveal changes that are considered abnormal in the untrained person. Upon auscultation, ventricular gallops and soft systolic murmurs frequently are heard. If a significant systolic murmur is heard, an echocardiogram should be obtained before exercise testing. Additionally, palpation of the heart may reveal cardiomegaly, which is due to physiological rather than pathologic hypertrophy.[7]

In some instances, such as when asymptomatic, apparently healthy subjects are tested for functional capacity, or a repeat treadmill test is performed on a patient whose condition is stable and established, a physician need not be present, but should be in close proximity and prepared to respond promptly. The response to signs or symptoms should be moderated by the information the patient gives regarding his or her usual activity. If abnormal findings occur at levels of exercise that the patient usually performs, then it may not be necessary to stop the test for them. Also, the patient's activity history should help determine appropriate work rates for testing.

Table 4.1 lists the absolute and relative con-

TABLE 4.1. CONTRAINDICATIONS TO EXERCISE TESTING

Absolute

Acute myocardial infarction (within 2 days)
Unstable angina not previously stabilized by medical therapy[a]
Uncontrolled cardiac arrhythmias causing symptoms or hemodynamic compromise
Symptomatic severe aortic stenosis
Uncontrolled symptomatic heart failure
Acute pulmonary embolus or pulmonary infarction
Acute myocarditis or pericarditis
Acute aortic dissection

Relative[b]

Left main coronary stenosis
Moderate stenotic valvular heart disease
Electrolyte abnormalities
Severe arterial hypertension[c]
Tachyarrhythmias or bradyarrhythmias
Hypertrophic cardiomyopathy and other forms of outflow tract obstruction
Mental or physical impairment leading to inability to exercise adequately
High-degree atrioventricular block

[a] Appropriate timing of testing depends on level of risk of unstable angina, as defined by the Agency for Health Care Policy and Research Unstable Angina Guidelines.

[b] Relative contraindications can be superseded if the benefits of exercise outweigh the risks.

[c] In the absence of definitive evidence, the committee suggests a systolic blood pressure > 200 mmHg and/or diastolic blood pressure > 110 mmHg.

Adapted with permission from Fletcher GF, Balady G, Froelicher VF, et al: Exercise standards: A statement for healthcare professionals from the American Heart Association. Special report. *Circulation* 91:580–615, 1995.

traindications to performing an exercise test, as well as the factors to consider in assessing the degree of exercise. The contraindications to exercise testing in the athlete are the same as those applied to the general population.

Preparations for exercise testing include the following:

1. The subject should be instructed not to eat or smoke at least 2 h prior to the test and to come dressed for exercise.
2. A brief history and physical examination (particularly noting systolic murmurs) should be

accomplished to rule out any contraindications to testing (Table 4.1).

3. Specific questioning should determine which drugs are being taken, and potential electrolyte abnormalities should be considered. The labeled medication bottles should be brought along so that they can be identified and recorded. Because of a greater potential for cardiac events with the sudden cessation of beta blockers, they should not be automatically stopped prior to testing, but done so gradually under physician guidance only after consideration of the purpose of the test.

4. Pretest standard 12-lead ECGs are necessary in both the supine and standing positions. Good skin preparation must cause some discomfort, but it is necessary for good conductance and avoidance of artifact. The changes caused by exercise electrode placement can be kept to a minimum by keeping the arm electrodes off the chest, placing them on the shoulders, and by recording the baseline ECG supine. In this situation, the modified exercise limb lead placement of Mason and Likar can serve well as the reference resting ECG prior to an exercise test.[7a]

5. Hyperventilation is not necessary prior to testing. Subjects both with and without disease may or may not exhibit ST-segment changes with hyperventilation; the value of this procedure in lessening the number of false-positive responders is no longer considered useful by most researchers.[7a]

DURING THE TEST

Most problems can be avoided by having an experienced physician, nurse, or exercise physiologist standing next to the subject, measuring blood pressure, and assessing appearance during the test. The exercise technician should operate the recorder and treadmill, take the appropriate tracings, enter data on a form, and alert the physician to any abnormalities that may appear on the monitor scope.

Subjects should be reminded to not grasp the front or side rails as this decreases the work performed and thus decreases oxygen uptake. The result of which is an increase in exercise time, and therefore an overestimation of exercise capacity.

Target heart rates based on age should not be used because the relation between maximal heart rate and age is poor, and a wide scatter exists around the many different recommended regression lines. Such heart rate targets result in a submaximal test for some individuals, a maximal test for some, and an unrealistic goal for others. The Borg scales are an excellent means of quantifying a person's effort. At 1 to 2 min intervals, subjects should be monitored for perceived effort level by using the 6 to 20 Borg scale or the nonlinear 1 to 10 scale of perceived exertion.[8,9]

INDICATIONS FOR TEST TERMINATION

The absolute and relative indications for termination of an exercise test listed in Table 4.2 have been derived from clinical experience. Absolute indications are clear-cut, whereas relative indications can sometimes be disregarded if good clinical judgment is used. Absolute indications include a drop in systolic blood pressure despite an increase in workload, a more than usual anginal chest pain, central nervous system symptoms, signs of poor perfusion (such as pallor, cyanosis, and cold skin), serious dysrhythmias, technical problems with monitoring the patient, patient's request to stop, and marked electrocardiographic changes (e.g., more than 0.3 mV of horizontal or downsloping ST-segment depression, and 0.2 mV of ST-segment elevation). Relative indications for termination include other worrisome ST or QRS changes such as excessive junctional depression; increasing chest pain; fatigue, shortness of breath, wheezing, leg cramps, or intermittent claudication, worrisome appearance, hypertensive response (systolic pressure greater than 260 mmHg, diastolic pressure greater than 115 mmHg), and less serious dysrhythmias including supraventricular tachycardias. If more information is required, the test can be repeated later after symptoms have stabilized.

TABLE 4.2. INDICATIONS FOR TERMINATING EXERCISE TESTING

Absolute Indications

Drop in systolic blood pressure of > 10 mmHg from baseline blood pressure despite an increase in workload, when accompanied by other evidence of ischemia

Moderate to severe angina

Increasing nervous system symptoms (e.g., ataxia, dizziness, or near-syncope)

Signs of poor perfusion (cyanosis or pallor)

Technical difficulties in monitoring ECG or systolic blood pressure

Subject's desire to stop

Sustained ventricular tachycardia

ST elevation ($\geq$ 1.0 mm) in leads without diagnostic Q waves (other than V_1 or a V_R)

Relative Indications

Drop in systolic blood pressure of $\geq$ 10 mmHg from baseline blood pressure despite an increase in workload, in the absence of other evidence of ischemia

ST or QRS changes such as excessive ST depression (> 2 mm of horizontal or downsloping ST-segment depression) or marked axis shift

Arrhythmias other than sustained ventricular tachycardia, including multifocal PVCs, triplets of PVCs, supraventricular tachycardia, heart block, or bradyarrhythmias

Fatigue, shortness of breath, wheezing, leg cramps, or claudication

Development of bundle branch block or IVCD that cannot be distinguished from ventricular tachycardia

Increasing chest pain

Hypertensive response[a]

[a] In the absence of definitive evidence, the committee suggests systolic blood pressure of > 250 mmHg and/or a diastolic blood pressure of > 115 mmHg. ECG indicates electrocardiogram; PVCs, premature ventricular contractions; IVCD, intraventricular conduction delay.

Adapted with permission from Fletcher GF, Froelicher VF, Hartley LH, et al: Exercise standards: A statement for health professionals from the American Heart Association. *Circulation* 82:2286–2322, 1990.

POSTEXERCISE

If maximal sensitivity for ischemic markers is to be achieved with an exercise test, patients should be supine during the postexercise period. It is advisable to record about 10 s of electrocardiographic data while the patient is standing motionless, but still experiencing near maximal heart rate, and then have the patient lay down. Having the patient perform a cool-down walk after the test can delay or eliminate the appearance of ST-segment depression.[10] According to the law of LaPlace, the increase in venous return and thus ventricular volume in the supine position increases myocardial oxygen demand. Data from our laboratory[11] suggest that having patients lie down may enhance ST-segment abnormalities in recovery. However, this is usually not an issue in young athletes, and a cool down makes the test more comfortable for them.

Monitoring should continue for at least 5 min after exercise or until changes stabilize. An abnormal response occurring only in the recovery period is not unusual. All such responses are not false positives, as has been suggested. Experiments confirm mechanical dysfunction and electrophysiological abnormalities in the ischemic ventricle following exercise. A cool-down walk can be helpful when performing tests on patients with established diagnoses who are undergoing testing for other than diagnostic reasons, when testing athletes, or when testing patients with dangerous dysrhythmias. When this is the case, it may be preferable to walk slowly (1.0 to 1.5 mi/h) or continue cycling against 0 or minimal resistance (0 to 25 W when testing with a cycle ergometer) for several minutes following the test.

EXERCISE TEST MODALITIES

Three types of exercise can be used to stress the cardiovascular system: isometric, dynamic, and a combination of the two. Isometric exercise, defined as constant muscular contraction without movement (such as handgrip), imposes a disproportionate pressure load on the left ventricle relative to the body's ability to supply oxygen. Dynamic exercise is defined as rhythmic muscular activity resulting in movement and initiates a more appropriate increase in cardiac output and oxygen exchange. Since a delivered workload can be accurately calibrated and the physiological response easily measured, dynamic exercise is preferred for clinical testing.

Numerous modalities have been used to provide dynamic exercise for exercise testing, including steps, escalators, and ladder mills. Today, however, the bicycle ergometer and the treadmill are the most commonly used dynamic exercise devices. In cases of spinal cord injury, peripheral neuropathy, or orthopedic disorders, arm ergometry is also performed for exercise testing. A wheelchair ergometer has been developed for spinal-cord-injured patients who compete as wheelchair athletes.

Whenever possible, the testing of an athlete should be done as to maximize the congruence between mode of ergometer exercise and the sport activity.[12,13] In order to accurately measure functional capacity and determine anaerobic threshold, the runner should be tested on a treadmill and the cyclists on a bicycle ergometer. However, this is not as important when the exercise test is performed for screening and diagnostic purposes.

SUPINE VERSUS UPRIGHT EXERCISE TESTING

A great deal of the information available on hemodynamic responses to exercise has come from supine exercise, mostly because cardiac catheterization is required to obtain much of this information. However, there are marked differences between the body's responses to acute exercise in the supine versus upright positions. During supine bicycle exercise, stroke volume and end-diastolic volume do not change much from values obtained at rest, whereas in the upright position, these values increase during mild work and then plateau. Naturally, exercise capac-

ity is markedly lower in the supine position than when it is compared to upright cycling. As with upright exercise, a linear relation between cardiac output and oxygen uptake during supine bicycle exercise has been observed and has been used to separate heart disease patients from healthy people. Exercise factor, or the increase in cardiac output for a given increase in oxygen uptake, is based on studies of normal persons. For every 100 ml increase in oxygen consumption, cardiac output should increase by 500 ml. Left ventricular filling pressure does not increase in proportion to work in normal persons, but often increases in patients with heart disease. Radionuclide imaging has shown that the ejection fraction usually increases in normal subjects, but can decrease during exercise in patients with ischemia or left ventricular dysfunction, or in the elderly.

BICYCLE ERGOMETER VERSUS TREADMILL

The bicycle ergometer is usually cheaper, takes up less space, and makes less noise. Although bicycling is a dynamic exercise, most individuals perform more work on a treadmill because a greater muscle mass is involved and most subjects are more familiar with walking than cycling. However, this is not the case for cyclists. Upper body motion is usually reduced, but care must be taken so that the arms do not perform isometric exercise. The workload administered by the simple bicycle ergometers is not well calibrated and is dependent upon pedaling speed. It is too easy for a subject to slow pedaling speed during exercise testing and decrease the administered workload. More expensive electronically braked bicycle ergometers keep the workload at a specified level over a wide range of pedaling speeds. These are particularly needed for supine exercise testing.

In most studies comparing the upright cycle ergometer with treadmill exercise, maximal heart rate values have been demonstrated to be roughly similar, whereas maximal oxygen uptake has been shown to be 6 to 25% greater during treadmill exercise.[14,15] Early hemodynamic studies[16] concluded that bicycle exercise constitutes a greater stress on the cardiovascular system for any given oxygen uptake than does treadmill exercise. The clinical importance of these findings in relation to patients with cardiovascular disease undergoing exercise testing is that slightly higher maximal oxygen uptakes are achieved with slightly less hemodynamic stress when treadmill exercise is used.

ARM ERGOMETRY

For a given submaximal workload, arm exercise requires a greater myocardial oxygen demand than leg exercise. At maximal effort, however, physiological responses are generally greater in leg exercise than they are in arm exercise. At a given power output (expressed as kilopond meters per minute [kpm/min] or watts [W]), heart rate, systolic and diastolic blood pressure, the product of heart rate multiplied by systolic blood pressure, minute ventilation (V_E), and blood lactate concentration are higher during arm exercise than they are in leg exercise. In contrast, stroke volume and the ventilatory threshold (the latter expressed as a percentage of aerobic capacity) are lower during arm exercise than when compared with leg exercise.[17,18] Since cardiac output is nearly the same in arm and leg exercise at a given oxygen uptake,[19] the elevated blood pressure during arm exercise is due to increased peripheral vascular resistance.

This difference in cardiopulmonary and hemodynamic responses to arm exercise as compared to leg exercise at identical workloads appears to be due to several factors. Mechanical efficiency is lower during arm exercise than it is during leg exercise. This may reflect the involvement of smaller muscle groups and the static effort by the torso muscles to stabilize the shoulder girdle required for arm work.[20] Both could increase oxygen requirements but not affect the external work output performed by the arms. The higher rate-pressure product and estimated myocardial oxygen demand at a given external workload for arm work as compared with leg work may be due to a number of factors. These include increased sym-

pathetic tone during arm exercise (due to reduced stroke volume with compensatory tachycardia), isometric contraction of torso muscles, and vasoconstriction in the nonexercising leg muscles.[21,22]

Maximal oxygen uptake (V_{O_2} max) during arm ergometry in men generally varies between 64 and 80% of leg ergometry V_{O_2} max. Similarly, maximal cardiac output is lower during arm exercise than when compared with leg exercise, whereas maximal heart rate, systolic blood pressure, and rate-pressure product are comparable[23] or slightly lower[24] during arm exercise. Although women have a lower arm V_{O_2} max than men, it appears that their aerobic capacity for arm work is not disproportionately inferior to that of men's. Vander et al.[25] found that the relation between arm and leg ergometry in women, expressed as arm V_{O_2} max/leg V_{O_2} max, was 79%, comparable to the mean value of 72% derived from 7 separate studies on men (Table 4.3).

Several investigators have examined the ability of leg or arm exercise testing to predict performance capacity of the other extremities in able-

TABLE 4.3. COMPARISON OF THE MAXIMAL OXYGEN CONSUMPTION (V_{O_2} max) IN RESPONSE TO ARM AND LEG ERGOMETRY IN MEN AND WOMEN

Reference	V_{O_2} max (L/min) Arms	V_{O_2} max (L/min) Legs	$\dfrac{V_{O_2}\text{ max (arms)}}{V_{O_2}\text{ max (legs)}}$ %
Men			
Åstrand and Saltin (1961)[a]	3.27	4.66	70
Stenberg et al. (1967)	2.55	3.87	66
Vokac et al. (1975)	NA[b]	NA[b]	78
Bergh et al. (1976)	3.01	4.12	73
Davis et al. (1976)	2.34	3.68	64
Fardy et al. (1977)	2.23	3.20	70
Franklin et al. (1983)	2.54	3.17	80
Mean	2.66	3.78	72
Women			
Vander et al. (1984a)	1.60	2.02	79

[a] See Ref. 1 for complete list of references.
[b] NA = data not available

bodied subjects. Asmussen and Hemmingsen[26] showed that it was not possible to estimate leg V_{O_2} max from experiments with arm work and vice versa. Franklin et al. found weak correlations between maximal power output and V_{O_2} max for arm and leg exercise.[27]

EXERCISE PROTOCOLS

The many different exercise protocols in use has led to some confusion regarding how physicians compare tests between patients and serial tests in the same patient. The most common protocols, their stages, and the predicted oxygen cost of each stage are illustrated in Figure 4.1. When treadmill and cycle ergometer testing were first introduced into clinical practice, practitioners adopted protocols used by major researchers.[28,29] The large and uneven work increments in some of these protocols have been shown to result in a tendency to overestimate exercise capacity.[30] Investigators have since recommended protocols with smaller and more equal increments.[31,32] Guidelines suggest that protocols should be individualized for each subject such that test duration is approximately 8 to 12 min.

RAMP TESTING

An approach to exercise testing that has gained interest is the ramp protocol, in which work increases constantly and continuously (Fig. 4.2). The call for "optimizing" exercise testing would appear to be facilitated by the ramp approach, since work increments are small, and, since it allows for increases in work to be individualized, a given test duration can be targeted.

To investigate this, the authors compared ramp treadmill and bicycle tests to protocols which are more commonly used clinically.[33] Ten patients

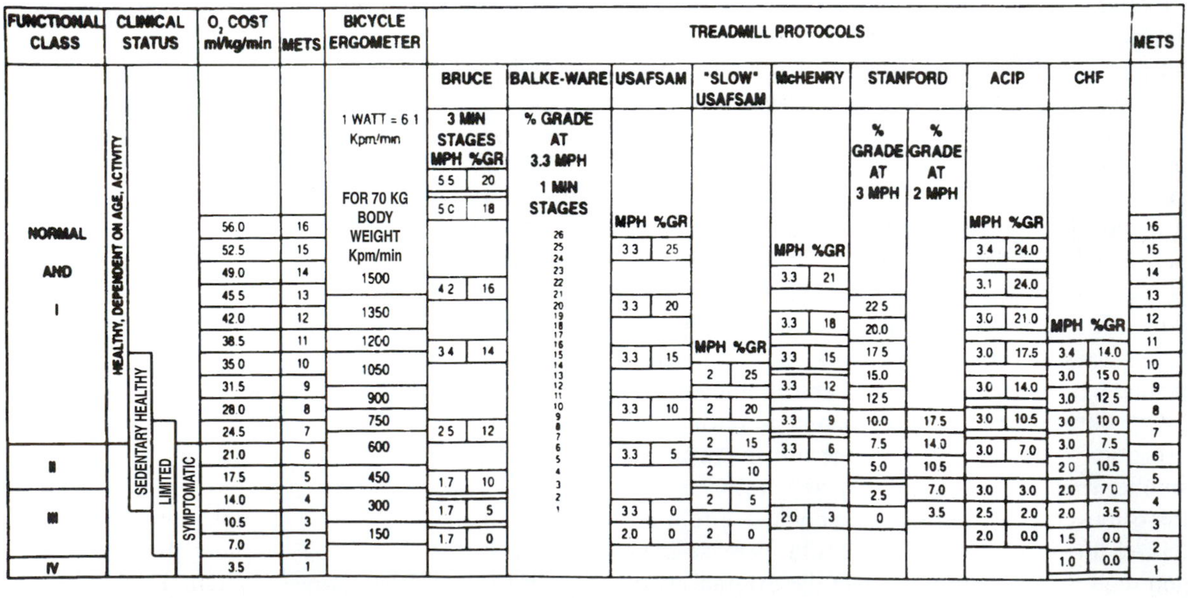

FUNCTIONAL CLASS	CLINICAL STATUS	O₂ COST ml/kg/min	METS	BICYCLE ERGOMETER	BRUCE 3 MIN STAGES MPH / %GR	BALKE-WARE % GRADE AT 3.3 MPH 1 MIN STAGES	USAFSAM MPH / %GR	"SLOW" USAFSAM MPH / %GR	McHENRY MPH / %GR	STANFORD % GRADE AT 3 MPH	STANFORD % GRADE AT 2 MPH	ACIP MPH / %GR	CHF MPH / %GR	METS
NORMAL AND I	HEALTHY, DEPENDENT ON AGE, ACTIVITY	56.0	16		5.5 20 / 5.0 18	26								16
		52.5	15			25	3.3 25					3.4 24.0		15
		49.0	14			24 / 23			3.3 21					14
		45.5	13		4.2 16	22 / 21				22.5		3.1 24.0		13
		42.0	12	1500 / 1350		20 / 19 / 18	3.3 20		3.3 18	20.0		3.0 21.0		12
	SEDENTARY HEALTHY	38.5	11	1200	3.4 14	17 / 16		2 25	3.3 15	17.5		3.0 17.5		11
		35.0	10	1050		15 / 14	3.3 15		3.3 12	15.0		3.0 14.0	3.4 14.0	10
		31.5	9	900		13 / 12				12.5		3.0 15.0	3.0 15.0	9
		28.0	8	750		11 / 10	3.3 10	2 20	3.3 9	10.0	17.5	3.0 12.5	3.0 12.5	8
	LIMITED	24.5	7		2.5 12	9 / 8				7.5	14.0	3.0 10.5	3.0 10.0	7
II		21.0	6	600		7 / 6	3.3 5	2 15	3.3 6	5.0	10.5	3.0 7.0	2.0 10.5	6
		17.5	5	450	1.7 10	5		2 10		2.5	7.0	3.0 3.0	2.0 7.0	5
III	SYMPTOMATIC	14.0	4	300	1.7 5	4 / 3		2 5			3.0	2.5 2.0	2.0 3.5	4
		10.5	3	150	1.7 0	2	3.3 0	2 0	2.0 3	0	3.5	2.0 0.0	1.5 0.0	3
		7.0	2			1	2.0 0		2.0 0			1.0 0.0	2.0 3.5	2
IV		3.5	1										1.0 0.0	1

FIGURE 4.1. The most common protocols, their stages, and the predicted oxygen cost of each stage. Key: USAFSAM, United States Air Force School of Aerospace Medicine; ACIP, asymptomatic cardiac ischemia pilot; CHF, congestive heart failure (modified Naughton); Kpm/min, kilopond meters per minute; METS, metabolic equivalents; MPH, miles per hour; %GR, percent grade.

Note: Bicycle ergometer: 1 WATT = 6.1 Kpm/min; for 70 kg body weight, Kpm/min values (1500, 1350, 1200, 1050, 900, 750, 600, 450, 300, 150).

EXERCISE PROTOCOLS

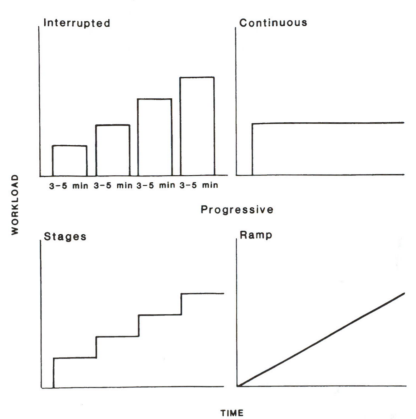

FIGURE 4.2. An approach to exercise testing that has gained interest is the ramp protocol, in which work increases constantly and continuously as shown in this illustration.

with chronic heart failure, 10 with coronary artery disease who were limited by angina during exercise, 10 with coronary artery disease who were asymptomatic during exercise, and 10 age-matched normal subjects performed 3 bicycle tests (25 W per 2-min stage, 50 W per 2-min stage, and ramp) and 3 treadmill tests (Bruce, Balke, and ramp) in randomized order on different days. For the ramp tests, ramp rates on the bicycle and treadmill were individualized to yield a test duration of approximately 10 min for each subject. Maximal oxygen uptake was significantly higher (18%) on the treadmill protocols versus the bicycle protocols collectively, confirming previous observations. Only minor differences in maximal oxygen uptake, however, were observed among the treadmill protocols themselves or among the cycle ergometer protocols themselves.

The relations between oxygen uptake and work rate (predicted oxygen uptake), which reflect the degree of change in oxygen uptake for a given increase in work (a slope of unity would suggest that the cardiopulmonary system is adapting in direct accordance with the demands of the work), were highest for the ramp tests and lowest for the protocols containing the greatest increments in work. Further, the variance about the slope (standard error estimate (SEE) in oxygen uptake, milliliters per kilogram per minute) was largest for the tests with the largest increments between stages (Bruce treadmill and 50 W per stage bicycle) and smallest for the ramp tests. These observations suggest that: (a) oxygen uptake is overestimated from tests that contain large increments in work; and (b) the variability in estimating oxygen uptake from work rate is markedly greater on these tests than it is on individualized ramp treadmill tests.

Because this approach appears to offer several advantages, at present we perform all our clinical, athletic, and research testing using the ramp. A number of equipment manufacturers have developed treadmill controllers that can automatically ramp to reach an input metabolic equivalent level in a specified time; however, it is easy to implement a ramp manually.

HEMODYNAMIC RESPONSES

Monitoring hemodynamic responses while conducting a treadmill test is vital to assessing patient's response to exercise. Measurements are used for diagnosis and prognosis and can necessitate test termination. In the trained athlete, initial evaluation may reveal values that are considered abnormal in the untrained person. The heart rate will commonly be bradycardic, and the patient may exhibit hypotension. It is not uncommon for diastolic blood pressures to be 0 mmHg (the fifth Korotkov sound) in well-conditioned athletes during exercise. However, basic hemodynamic trends should be the same for both populations.

MAXIMAL HEART RATE

METHODS OF RECORDING

Although measuring a patient's maximal heart rate should be a simple matter, the different ways of recording rate and differences in the type of exercise used may affect its measurement. The best way to measure maximal heart rate is to use a standard ECG recorder and from the R-R intervals calculate the instantaneous heart rate. Methods using the arterial pulse or capillary blush technique are much more affected by artifact than electrocardiographic techniques. Some investigators have used an average over the last minute of exercise or in immediate recovery; both of these methods are inaccurate. Heart rate drops quickly in recovery and can climb steeply even in the last seconds of exercise. Premature beats can affect averaging and must be eliminated in order to obtain the actual heart rate. Cardiotachometers are available but may fail to trigger or may trigger inappropriately on T waves, artifact, or aberrant beats thus yielding inaccurate results. Not all cardiotachometers have the accuracy of the ECG paper technique.

FACTORS LIMITING MAXIMAL HEART RATE

Several factors may affect the maximal heart rate during dynamic exercise.[1] Maximal heart rate declines with advancing years and is affected by gender. Height, weight, and even lean body weight apparently do not greatly affect maximal heart rate. The physiological limits on maximal heart rate in normal man are determined by rapidity of sinus node recovery, cardiac dimensions, left ventricular filling, and contractile state. Systole has a relatively fixed-time interval; in contrast, relatively less time of the cardiac cycle is spent in diastole when heart rate increases. It seems logical that a limit would be approached where an increase in heart rate would not effectively increase cardiac output due to decreased diastolic filling; not only would the heart receive less blood to pump thereby imposing mechanical limitations, but the degree of coronary artery perfusion would decrease, imposing metabolic constraints. Although this theoretical limitation is reasonable, there is little experimental work to support it. Many studies have reported maximal heart rate during treadmill testing in a variety of patients. Regressions with age have varied depending on the population studied and other factors. Table 4.4 and Figure 4.3 summarize these studies of maximal heart rate; some of the major studies will be discussed.

TABLE 4.4.   SUMMARY OF STUDIES ASSESSING MAXIMAL HEART RATE

Study	Number	Population Studied	Mean Age ±SD (Range)	Mean HR MAX (SD)	Regression Line (y; age)	Correlation Coefficient	Standard Error of the Estimate (beats/min)
Astrand[a]	100	Asymptomatic men	50 (20–69)	166 ± 22	211 –0.922	NA	NA
Bruce	2091	Asymptomatic men	44 ± 8	181 ± 12	210–0.662	−0.44	14
Cooper	2535	Asymptomatic men	43 (11–79)	181 ± 16	217–0.845	NA	NA
Ellestad[b]	2583	Asymptomatic men	42 ± 7 (10–60)	173 ± 11	197–0.556	NA	NA
Froelicher	1317	Asymptomatic men	38 ± 8 (28–54)	183	207–0.64	−0.43	10
Lester	148	Asymptomatic men	43 (15–75)	187	205–0.411	−0.58	NA
Robinson	92	Asymptomatic men	30 (6–76)	189	212–0.775	NA	NA
Sheffield	95	Men with CHD	39 (19–69)	176 ± 14	±216–0.88	−0.58	11[c]
Bruce	1295	Men with CHD	52 ± 8	148 ± 23	204–1.07	−0.36	25[c]
Hammond	156	Men with CHD	53 ± 9	157 ± 20	209–1.0	−0.30	19
Morris	244	Asymptomatic men	45 (20–72)	167 ± 19	200–0.72	−0.55	15
Graettinger	114	Asymptomatic men	46 ± 13 (19–73)	168 ± 18	199–0.63	−0.47	NA
Morris	1388	Men referred for evaluation for CHD	57 (21–89)	144 ± 20	196–0.9	−0.43	21

[a] Astrand used bicycle ergometry; all other studies performed on treadmill. See Ref.1 for complete list of references.

[b] Data compiled from graphs in reference cited.

[c] Calculated from available data.

CHD, coronary heart disease; HR max, maximal heart rate; NA, not able to calculate from available data.

Bruce and colleagues attempted to separate the effects of aging from the effects of cardiovascular disease on maximal heart rate by analyzing data on over 2000 healthy middle-aged men and subgroups of over 2000 ambulatory male patients with hypertension, coronary heart disease, or both.[34] All men were given maximal treadmill tests, and the data from each subgroup was regressed on age and compared. Any substantial difference in slope would imply that disease, independently from age, influenced maximal heart rates. Bruce found an age-related decline in all groups with correlation coefficients ranging from −.3 to −.5.

Cooper and associates examined the maximal heart rate response to treadmill testing in over 2500 men ranging in age from 10 to 80 years with a mean of 43.[35] Patients with abnormal resting ECGs and those unable to give a maximal effort were eliminated from the study. Levels of cardiovascular fitness were determined by age-adjusted treadmill times using the Balke-Ware protocol. Their data demonstrated that those subjects with low fitness achieved lower maximal heart rates and that these differences were more divergent at advanced ages. In additon, with the cardiovascularly fit population there was a less rapid decline of maximal heart rates with aging when compared with the cardiovascularly unfit population.

In an effort to clarify the relation between maximal heart rate and age, Londeree and Moeschberger performed a comprehensive review of the literature compiling over 23,000 subjects aged 5 to 81 years.[36] A stepwise multiple regression revealed that age alone accounted for 75% of the variability; other factors added only about 5% and included mode of exercise, level of fitness, and continent of origin but not sex. The 95% confidence interval, even when accounting for these factors, was 45 beats per minute (Fig. 4.4). Heart rates at maximal exercise were lower on bicycle ergometry than they were on the treadmill and were still lower with swimming. Their analysis revealed that trained individuals had significantly lowered maximal heart rates.

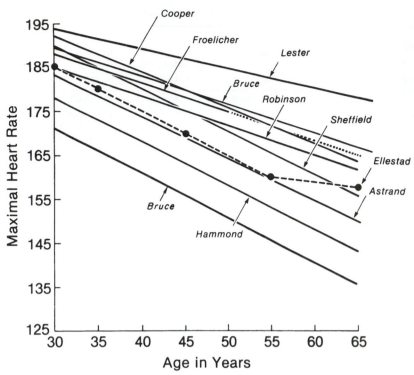

FIGURE 4.3. Many studies as shown in this illustration have reported maximal heart rate during treadmill testing in a variety of patients. Regressions with age have varied depending on the population studied and other factors.

At the United States Airforce School of Aerospace Medicine, Froelicher et al. compared the cardiovascular responses to maximal treadmill testing using 3 different popular treadmill protocols to evaluate reproducibility among tests.[37] The Bruce, Balke, and Taylor protocols were used in the evaluation of 15 healthy men; each man performed 1 test per week for 9 weeks repeating each protocol 3 times in randomized order. The maximal heart rates achieved were reproducible within each protocol, and there were no significant differences in heart rate achieved among the three protocols. Also, large numbers of normal persons were studied as shown in Figure 4.5, which also shows the wide scatter. Graettinger et al. looked at clinical, echocardiographic, and functional determinants of maximal heart rate in preliminary form.[38] Despite controlling for age, activity status, sex, and hyperten-

sion, measures of cardiac size and function added little to the prediction of maximal heart rate. Most of the variance in maximal heart rate was accounted for simply by age. Given the large degree of individual variability in cardiac variables as well as the maximal heart rate per age relation, maximal heart rate may always be a difficult variable to explain.

Bedrest. Another factor that affects maximal heart rate and that is important to clinical medicine is bedrest. Convertino and colleagues examined the cardiovascular responses to maximal exercise in normal men following 10 days of bedrest.[39] A significant increase in maximal heart rate was found following bedrest when compared to prebedrest tests. It was suggested that lack of gravitational forces on baroreceptor mechanisms played a role in this accentuated heart rate re-

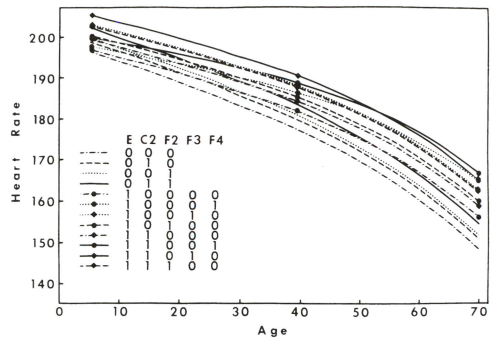

FIGURE 4.4. In an effort to clarify the relation between maximal heart rate and age, Londeree and Moeschberger performed a comprehensive review of the literature compiling over 23,000 subjects aged 5 to 81 years. These were their results. Under ergometer (E), 0 = bicycle, 1 = tread-mill; under C2, 1 = European study, 0 = non-European; Under F2, 1 = sedentary, 0 = not seden-tary; Under F3, 1 = active, 0 = not active; Under F4, 1 = endurance trained, 0 = not endurance trained. Adapted with permission from Londeree BR, Moeschberger ML: Influence of age and other factors on maximal heart rate. J Cardiac Rehab 4:44–49, 1984.

sponse. Measurements of Vo_2 max in both the supine and upright positions revealed low values with upright exercise. Since maximal heart rates increased significantly but Vo_2 max decreased, changes in heart volume are likely involved and may reflect changes in plasma volume during prolonged bedrest.

Altitude. Altitude may affect the heart rate response to exercise. Hartley and coworkers examined maximal heart rate before and after the administration of atropine in 5 normal untrained men who lived at sea level all of their lives.[40] The subjects were studied with bicycle ergometry at sea level and at 15,000 feet altitude. The maximal heart rates decreased a mean of 24 beats per minute, and the maximal oxygen uptake decreased 26% at this altitude. Atropine administration did not affect maximal heart rate at sea level but significantly increased maximal heart rate at high altitude (165 to 176 beats per minute). At high altitude there is an increased parasympathetic tone at maximal exercise. This may be secondary to increased sympathetic tone and the baroreceptor reflex. Mean maximal heart rate did not increase with the administration of supplemental oxygen so the impaired heart rate response was not due to hypoxia alone.

State of Training. Some investigators report substantially low maximal heart rates in well-trained athletes. Perhaps blood volume changes and cardiac hypertrophy can explain this. However, this has not been a consistent finding. While

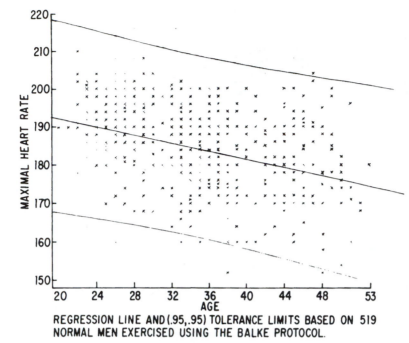

REGRESSION LINE AND (.95,.95) TOLERANCE LIMITS BASED ON 519
NORMAL MEN EXERCISED USING THE BALKE PROTOCOL.

FIGURE 4.5. The results of a large number of normal persons who underwent a progressive treadmill test show the wide scatter of maximal heart rate.

this point remains unsettled, it is possible that training in early life may result in cardiac hypertrophy and/or dilation. Perhaps cardiac dimensions determine the maximal heart rate in individuals with a healthy sinus node.

Motivation. A final factor determining maximal exercise heart rate is motivation to exert oneself maximally. Older patients may be restrained by poor muscle tone, pulmonary disease, claudication, orthopedic problems, and other noncardiac causes of limitation. The usual decline in maximal heart rate with age is not as steep in people who are free from myocardial disease and stay active, but it still occurs.

BLOOD PRESSURE RESPONSE

Systolic blood pressure should rise with increasing treadmill workload while diastolic blood pressure usually remains about the same. A rising diastolic blood pressure can be associated with coronary heart disease; however, it is more likely a marker for labile hypertension, which leads to coronary disease. A drop in systolic blood pressure below preexercise values is the most ominous criterion, whereas a drop of 20 mmHg or more without a fall below preexercise values appears to have less predictive value. Exercise-induced hypotension (EIH) can be due to either left ventricular dysfunction or ischemia or outflow obstruction. When EIH occurs without association with either of these two factors, EIH appears to be benign. Though speculative, other potential mechanisms of EIH that deserve further investigation include exercise-induced mitral regurgitation and a (noncardiac) peripheral vasodilatory mechanism.

The highest systolic blood pressure should be achieved at maximal workload. When exercise is stopped, approximately 10% of people tested will abruptly drop their systolic blood pressure owing to peripheral pooling. To avoid fainting, patients should not be left standing on the treadmill. The systolic blood pressure usually normalizes upon resuming the supine position during recovery but may remain below normal for several hours after the test. In spite of studies showing discrepancies between noninvasively and invasively measured blood pressure, the product of heart rate and systolic blood pressure, determined by cuff and auscultation, correlates with measured myocardial oxygen consumption during exercise. Usually, an individual patient's angina pectoris will be precipitated at the same double product (systolic blood pressure multiplied by heart rate). This product is also an estimate of the maximal workload that the left ventricle can perform.

Irving and colleagues examined variations in clinical noninvasive systolic pressure at the point of symptom-limited exercise on a treadmill in 6 groups of subjects: 5459 men and 749 women classified into three categories each.[41] Among the men, 2532 were asymptomatic healthy, 592 were hypertensive, and 1586 had clinical manifestations of coronary heart disease. Among the women, 244, 158, and 347 were in these respective clinical categories. Retesting of 156 persons from 1 to 32 months later showed that pressure values agreed within 10% in two-thirds, the overall mean difference was only 8.6 mmHg, and the correlation at maximal exercise was superior to that of the resting observations just before exercise. Among men, the lowest maximal systolic pressure was observed in the group with coronary heart disease; among women, the lowest mean pressure was found in the healthy group. Maximal systolic pressures correlated fairly well ($r = 0.46 - 0.68$ for the various groups) with resting systolic pressure, and this relation was independent of the diagnosis of cardiovascular disease in both men and women. Relations between pressure and the number of stenotic coronary arteries and impaired ejection fraction at rest were examined in 22 men without and 182 men with coronary artery disease. Low maximal systolic pressures were often associated with disease involving two or three vessels or reduced ejection fraction, or both. The annual rate of sudden cardiac death decreased from 97.9 per 1000 men to 25.3 and 6.6 per 1000 men as the range of maximal systolic pressure increased from less than 140, to 140 to 199, and to 200 mmHg or more, respectively. In addition, men with systolic pressures < 140 were more likely of have cardiomegaly, Q waves in the resting ECG, and persistent postexertional ST depression than men with higher maximal systolic pressures.

The 3-min systolic blood pressure ratio is a useful and readily obtainable measure that can be applied in all patients who are undergoing exercise testing for the evaluation of known or suspected ischemic heart disease.[42] The ratio is calculated by dividing the systolic blood pressure 3 min into the recovery phase of a treadmill exercise test by the systolic blood pressure at peak exercise. A 3-min systolic blood pressure ratio greater than 0.90 is considered abnormal and has a diagnostic accuracy of approximately 75% for the detection of coronary artery disease (i.e., an accuracy comparable to that of ST-segment depression). High values for the ratio are associated with more extensive coronary artery disease, as well as an adverse prognosis after myocardial infarction.

FUNCTIONAL CAPACITY

Maximal ventilatory oxygen uptake (VO_2 max) is the greatest amount of oxygen that a person can extract from inspired air while performing dynamic exercise involving a large part of the total body muscle mass.[1] Since maximal ventilatory oxygen uptake is equal to the product of cardiac output and arterial venous oxygen (aVO_2) difference, it is a measure of the functional limits of the cardiovascular system. Maximal aVO_2 difference is physiologically limited to roughly 15 to 17 vol%. Thus, maximal aVO_2 difference behaves more or less as a constant, making maximal oxygen uptake an indirect estimate of maximal cardiac output.

Maximal oxygen uptake is dependent on many factors, including natural physical endowment, activity status, age, and sex, but it is the best index of exercise capacity and maximal cardiovascular function. As a rough reference, the maximal oxygen uptake of the normal sedentary adult is often considered approximately 30 ml O_2 per kilogram per minute and the minimal level for physical fitness is often considered roughly 40 ml O_2 per kilogram per minute. In general, aerobic training can increase maximal oxygen uptake by up to 25%. This increase is dependent on the initial level of fitness and age as well as the intensity, frequency, and length of training sessions. Individuals performing aerobic training such as distance running can have maximal oxygen uptakes as high as 60 to 90 ml per O_2 per kilogram per minute. For convenience, oxygen consumption is often expressed in multiples of basal resting requirements (metabolic equivalents). The metabolic equivalent is a unit of basal oxygen consumption, equal to approximately 3.5 ml O_2

per kilogram per minute. This value is the oxygen required to sustain life in the resting state.

Figure 4.6 illustrates the relation between maximal oxygen uptake to exercise habits and age.[43] Though the 3 activity levels have regression lines that fit the data, as one would expect, there is much scatter around the lines and the correlation coefficients are poor. This finding demonstrates the inaccuracy involved with trying to predict maximal oxygen uptake from age and habitual physical activity. It is preferable to estimate an individual's maximal oxygen uptake from the workload reached while performing an exercise test. Maximal oxygen uptake is of course most precisely determined by direct measurement using ventilatory gas exchange techniques. Thus, if quantifying work with precision is an important objective, such as in athletics, research studies,

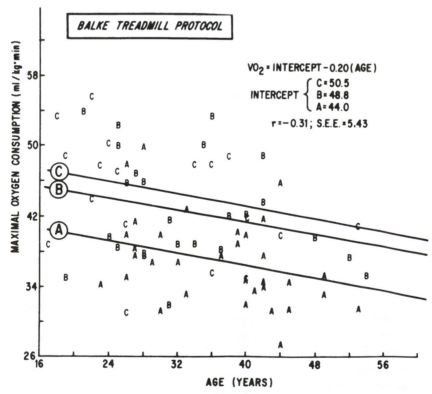

FIGURE 4.6. This illustrates the relation between maximal oxygen uptake to exercise habits and age.

and patients considered for cardiac transplantation, a direct measurement is essential.

MEASUREMENT OF EXPIRED GASES

Oxygen uptake can be predicted from treadmill or cycle ergometer workload, but it can be very misleading (Table 4.5). Although measured and estimated metabolic equivalents are directly related, with correlation coefficients ranging between 0.8 and 0.9, there is a wide scatter around the regression line. Figure 4.7 illustrates that the 95% confidence limits for predicting oxygen uptake based on treadmill time range more than 20 ml/kg/min (nearly 6 METs). An important consideration, particularly when serially testing athletes, is the reliability and reproducibility of the data. This has been one of the most important arguments in favor of the use of gas exchange techniques. The tendency to increase treadmill time with serial testing without an increase in Vo_2 max is well documented.

The measurement of oxygen uptake can be roughly described as simply the product of ventilation (Ve) in a given interval and the fraction of oxygen in that ventilation which has been consumed by the working muscle:

$$Vo_2 \text{ ml/min (STPD)} = Ve \times (Fio_2 - Feo_2)$$

TABLE 4.5. FACTORS AFFECTING THE RELATIONSHIP BETWEEN MEASURED AND PREDICTED OXYGEN UPTAKE

Factor	Affect
Habituation	Oxygen uptake and variability decrease, reproducibility increases with treadmill experience
Fitness	Oxygen uptake, variability decreases with increased fitness
Heart disease	Oxygen uptake is overpredicted in patients with heart disease
Handrail holding	Oxygen uptake reduced by holding handrails
Exercise protocol	Oxygen uptake overpredicted, variability increases with rapidly incremented, demanding protocols

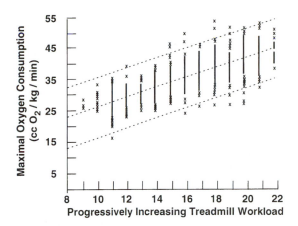

FIGURE 4.7. The 95% confidence limits for predicting oxygen uptake based on treadmill time.

where Fio_2 is the fraction of inspired oxygen and Feo_2 is the fraction of expired oxygen. Fio_2 is equal to 20.93% at sea level and 0% humidity, and Ve is converted to standard temperature and pressure, dry (STPD). Thus, $Fio_2 - Feo_2$ represents the amount of oxygen consumed by the working muscle for a given sample, sometimes called "true O_2."

The preceding equation is oversimplified, as it assumes that expired air is dry and that inspired and expired volumes are not different. Because this is generally not the case (unless the respiratory exchange ratio equals 1), several additional calculations are necessary to accurately determine oxygen uptake. First, the sample of air that is analyzed for O_2 and CO_2 content must be dried. Second, because oxygen uptake is the difference between the fraction of oxygen in the inspired and expired ventilation, both inspired and expired ventilation must be known precisely. Ventilatory volume is frequently measured only from the expired air. Inspired volume, however, can be determined from the expired volume and the fractions of oxygen and carbon dioxide. This is possible because nitrogen (N_2) and other inert gasses do not affect the body's gas exchange processes.

Thus, given that the concentrations of N_2, CO_2, and O_2 of the inspired air are known to be .7904, 0, and .2093, respectively, the fraction of inert gasses (N_2) in the expired air (F_{EN_2}) becomes:

$$F_{EN_2} = 1 - F_{EO_2} - F_{ECO_2}$$

Thus, inspiratory volume (V_I) can be expressed as the difference between the fraction of inert gasses in the expired air and the fraction of inert gasses in the atmosphere:

$$V_I = \frac{[V_E \times (1 - F_{EO_2} - F_{ECO_2})]}{0.7904}$$

And the equation for oxygen uptake becomes:

$$V_{O_2} \text{ L/min STPD} = \frac{(1 - F_{EO_2} - F_{ECO_2})}{0.7904} \times (F_{IO_2} - F_{EO_2}) \times V_E \text{ STPD}$$

COLLECTION OF EXPIRED VENTILATION

The measurement of gas exchange variables during exercise requires that the patient have a mouthpiece in place that seals tightly and a clip to seal the nose. Facemasks that cover the nose and mouth are also commonly used. While these make speaking possible, caution must be used to ascertain that no leaking of ventilation occurs, which can sometimes be a problem at high ventilation rates. According to the earlier equation, the measurement of oxygen uptake requires that the gases be analyzed for total volume as well as oxygen and carbon dioxide content. This requires that the water content of the inspired air be accounted for by adjusting for standard pressure and temperature (thus, the correction for STPD). As originally performed, expired gases were collected in a container requiring a great deal of technician time and limited precision. Today, gas analysis is performed "on-line"; various types of flow meters are used including mass transducers, Fleisch pneumotacometers, hot-wire devices, small propellers or turbines, or dry gas meters. A mixing chamber from which expired gases are sampled is frequently required. The Fleisch device measures the pressure drop due to the Venturi effect caused by airflow through a tube; the "hot wires" drop in temperature when cooled by air, and the propellers are spun by airflow. One of the problems with these devices is the difficulty in measuring ventilatory gas volume directly from a rapidly breathing individual. The phasic nature of breathing affects these devices.

Most modern metabolic systems today measure ventilation directly at the mouth using a lightweight, disposable flow meter. These clever devices obviate the need for headgear, valve apparatus, and collection tubes, which can often be cumbersome. Flow is determined by a difference in pressure between the front and back of a strut or between 2 screens positioned in the center of the pneumotacometer. The relation between the volume of airflow and the change in pressure is stated by Bernoulli's law (flow is proportional to the square root of the pressure difference), permitting the quantification of ventilation.

The availability of these rapidly responding gas analyzers, while facilitating precision and convenience, has led to confusion regarding data sampling. For example, differences in sampling (i.e., breath by breath, 30 s, 60 s, or "running" breath averaging) can greatly affect precision and variability in measuring oxygen uptake. Shorter sampling intervals increase precision, but also increase the variability.[44]

Data derived from small sampling intervals should be interpreted with caution, and one should resist the tendency to use breath-by-breath data simply because the technology is available. Breath-by-breath sampling can be invaluable for certain research applications, such as oxygen kinetics, but it is inappropriate for general clinical applications. The literature has commonly reported 30-s samples for treatment effects and when applying peak V_{O_2} in a prognostic context. Because 30-s samples can also limit precision (e.g., few patients complete the test precisely at a 30-s interval), the use of a "rolling" or "moving" average of 30-s data, printed more frequently, is useful. Regardless of the sample chosen, investigators should report the sampling interval used, and the intervals should be consistent throughout a given trial when studying interventions.

INFORMATION FROM VENTILATORY GAS EXCHANGE DATA DURING EXERCISE

Maximal Oxygen Uptake. V_{O_2} max is an objective measurement of exercise capacity: It defines the upper limits of the cardiopulmonary system. It is determined by the capacity to increase heart rate, augment stroke volume, and direct blood flow to the active muscles. It is often the most important variable measured, although this depends on the setting and the context of the particular patient being tested. Initially, V_{O_2} max should be considered in terms of what is normal for a given individual if he or she were healthy. The observation that V_{O_2} max falls within the normal range for a given gender and age makes a strong statement that the individual has no significant impairment in the cardiopulmonary system. Implicit with this statement, of course, is that the patient has no major limitations to cardiac output, its redistribution, or skeletal muscle metabolism or function. Changes in V_{O_2} max following training or detraining or those caused by disease closely parallel changes in cardiac size and maximal cardiac output.[45,46] Clearly, V_{O_2} max is directly related to the integrated function of several systems.

Minute Ventilation (VE).   Minute ventilation is the volume of air moving into and out of the lungs expressed as liters per minute (BTPS). It is determined by the product of respiratory rate and the volume of air exhaled with each breath (the tidal volume). *True O_2* or the difference between inspired and expired oxygen content varies little between individuals regardless of fitness level. Thus, ventilation rate is the major component of oxygen uptake during exercise. Fit individuals with high maximal ventilations and thus high maximal oxygen uptakes in addition must also have cardiac outputs that match ventilation in the lung. The ratio of alveolar ventilation to alveolar capillary blood flow, termed the *ventilation-perfu-*

sion ratio, is roughly 0.80 at rest. With exercise, ventilation and alveolar blood flow increase such that this ratio may approach 5.0. Abnormal ventilation is an important characteristic of both patients with chronic heart failure and with pulmonary disease, due in part to a mismatching of the ratio of ventilation to perfusion.

Carbon Dioxide Production (VCO₂).   Carbon dioxide produced by the body during exercise is expressed in liters per minutes, STPD. V_{CO_2} is generated from two sources during exercise. One source, the metabolic CO_2, is produced by oxidative metabolism. Roughly 75% of the O_2 consumed by the body is converted to CO_2, which is returned to the right heart by the venous blood, enters the lungs, and is exhaled as V_{CO_2}. A second source of CO_2 is often called *nonmetabolic* and results from the buffering of lactate at high levels of exercise. An elevation in CO_2 in the blood can quickly result in respiratory acidosis. Fortunately, the major determinants of ventilation during exercise are these two sources of CO_2 in the blood, which are reflected in the expired air as V_{CO_2}. Thus, V_{CO_2} closely matches V_E during exercise, and the body maintains a relatively normal pH under most conditions. V_{CO_2} and V_E also parallel increases in V_{O_2}, or work rate, during exercise levels up to roughly 50% to 70% of V_{O_2} max. At exercise levels beyond this, V_E increases disproportionately to V_{O_2}. This is because as exercise increases in intensity, lactate is produced at a greater rate than it is removed from the blood. The lactate must be buffered, and this process yields an additional source CO_2 that stimulates ventilation.

Respiratory Exchange Ratio.   The respiratory exchange ratio (RER) represents the amount of CO_2 produced divided by the amount of O_2 consumed. Normally, roughly 75% of the O_2 consumed is converted to CO_2. Thus, RER at rest generally ranges from 0.70 to 0.85. Because RER depends on the type of fuel used by the cells, it can provide an index of carbohydrate or fat metabolism. If carbohydrates were the predominant fuel, RER would equal one given the formula:

$$C_6H_{12}O_6 \text{ (glucose)} + 6\,O_2 \leftrightarrow 6\,CO_2 + 6\,H_2O$$
$$RER = V_{CO_2} \div V_{O_2} = 6\,CO_2 \div 6\,O_2 = 1.0$$

Because relatively more oxygen is required to burn fat, the respiratory exchange ratio for fat metabolism is lower than it is for carbohydrates, roughly 0.70. At high levels of exercise, CO_2 production exceeds O_2 uptake; thus, an RER exceeding 1.0 to 1.2 is often used to indicate the maximal effort of the subject. However, peak RER values vary greatly and generally are not a precise cutpoint for "maximal" exercise.

Oxygen Pulse (O_2 Pulse).   Oxygen pulse is an indirect index of combined cardiopulmonary oxygen transport. It is calculated by dividing O_2 uptake (ml/min) by heart rate. In effect, O_2 pulse is equal to the product of stroke volume and aV_{O_2} difference. Thus, circulatory adjustments that occur during exercise (i.e., widening aV_{O_2} difference, increased cardiac output, and redistribution of blood flow to the working muscle), will increase O_2 pulse. Maximal O_2 pulse is high in fit subjects, low in the presence of heart disease, and more importantly, is high at any given workload in the fit or healthy individual. Conversely, O_2 pulse will be reduced in any condition which reduces stroke volume (left ventricular dysfunction secondary to ischemia or infarction) or reduces arterial O_2 content (anemia, hypoxemia).

Ventilatory Equivalents for Oxygen and Carbon Dioxide. V_E/V_{O_2} and V_E/V_{CO_2} are calculated by dividing ventilation (L/min, BTPS) by V_{O_2} or V_{CO_2} (L/min, STPD). A great deal of ventilation (25 to 40 L) is required to consume a single liter of oxygen; thus, V_E/V_{O_2} is often in the 30s at rest. A decrease in V_E/V_{O_2} is frequently observed from rest to submaximal exercise, followed by a rapid increase at high levels of exercise when V_E increases in response to the need to buffer lactate. V_E/V_{O_2} reflects the ventilatory requirement for any given oxygen uptake; thus, it is an index of ventilatory efficiency. High V_E/V_{O_2} values during exercise occur in patients with lung disease and/or chronic heart failure. V_E/V_{CO_2} represents

the ventilatory requirement to eliminate a given amount of CO_2 produced by the metabolizing tissues. Since metabolic CO_2 is a strong stimulus for ventilation during exercise, V_E and V_{CO_2} closely mirror one another, and after a drop in early exercise, V_E/V_{CO_2} normally does not increase significantly throughout submaximal exercise.

Breathing Reserve.   The breathing reserve is calculated as the ratio of maximal voluntary ventilation at rest (MVV) to maximal exercise ventilation. Most healthy subjects achieve maximal ventilation of only 60 to 80% of MVV at peak exercise. One characteristic of chronic pulmonary disease is maximal ventilation that approximates or equals the individual's MVV. These patients reach a "ventilatory" limit during exercise, while normal subjects generally have a substantial ventilatory reserve (20 to 40%) at peak exercise and are limited by other factors.

Ventilatory Threshold.   A sudden rise in the blood lactate level during exercise has been associated with muscle anaerobiosis and has therefore been termed the anaerobic *threshold*.[47] Historically, the anaerobic threshold has been defined as the highest oxygen uptake during exercise above which a sustained lactic acidosis occurs. When this level of exercise is reached, excess H^+ ions of lactate must be buffered to maintain physiological pH. Because bicarbonate buffering yields an additional source of CO_2, ventilation is further stimulated. This point of nonlinear increase in ventilation has been used to detect the anaerobic threshold noninvasively and is often termed the *gas exchange anaerobic threshold* or the *ventilatory threshold (VT)*.

Changes in oxygen uptake at the VT have been used clinically during pharmacological and other investigations to imply that a change in oxygen supply to the working muscle has occurred. Many studies now suggest that lactate production occurs at all times, even in resting conditions. Further, the turnover rate of lactate (the ratio of appearance and disappearance) is linearly related to oxygen uptake during exercise.[48,49] This relation is possible because studies have shown that lactate is "shuttled" from fibers where it is produced (presumably fast twitch muscle) to those where it is used as an energy source (such as the heart and slow twitch fibers). The "lactate shuttle" has engendered the concept that production, transport, and use of lactate represents an important source of energy from carbohydrates during exercise.[50]

It is argued whether lactate during exercise in fact increases in a pattern which is mathematically "continuous" rather than as a threshold.[51,52] The cumulative effect of these studies has led to the conclusion that the anaerobic threshold is not strictly related to muscle anaerobiosis but instead reflects an imbalance between lactate appearance and disappearance. The term *ventilatory* threshold has been suggested as preferable to anaerobic as it does not imply the onset of anaerobiosis. No matter what causes the VT, lactate does accumulate in the blood during exercise, ventilation must respond to maintain physiological pH, a breakpoint in ventilation appears to occur reproducibly, and this point is related to various measures of cardiopulmonary performance in normal persons and patients with heart disease.[53,54] A common argument in favor of the use of the VT is that, as a submaximal parameter, it is better associated with patient's everyday activities than is maximal exercise, and using the VT avoids the increased risk and discomfort of maximal exercise. We make the following suggestions concerning the use of the VT during exercise testing:

1. Regardless of the mechanism, ventilatory changes appear strongly correlated with a lactate threshold.
2. An alteration in the VT reflects a change in the balance between lactate production and removal.
3. References to muscle anaerobiosis should be avoided.

Because lactate is strongly associated with muscle fatigue, a change in this relation that can be attributed to an intervention may add important information concerning the intervention. An additional consideration concerns the method of choosing the VT. VT can vary markedly depending on both the observer and the method of determination.[55]

Oxygen Kinetics. Although the measurement of oxygen kinetics often requires a specialized exercise test, is defined differently by various laboratories, and requires mathematical computations not familiar to most clinicians, this measurement is probably underutilized as an index of cardiopulmonary function clinically. Put simply, oxygen kinetics quantify the ability of the cardiopulmonary system to respond to the demands of a given amount of work; it is usually defined as the rate at which oxygen uptake reaches a steady state value. However, measures such as the oxygen uptake/work rate relation, oxygen debt, steepness of the slope of the relation between work rate and oxygen uptake, and various other measures of the difference between predicted and measured oxygen uptake generally describe oxygen kinetics. Oxygen kinetics are greater below versus above the ventilatory threshold and greater after a program of physical conditioning.[56]

Plateau in Oxygen Uptake. Maximal oxygen uptake is considered the best index of aerobic capacity and maximal cardiorespiratory function. By defining the limits of the cardiopulmonary system, it has been an invaluable measurement clinically for assessing the efficacy of drugs, exercise training, or invasive procedures. No other measure of work is as accurate, reliable, or reproducible as ventilatory maximal oxygen uptake. The collection and analysis of an expired gas sample taken during the last minute of an exercise test has generally been used to determine maximal oxygen uptake. From early studies using interrupted protocols, a test was only considered "maximal" when there was no further increase in oxygen uptake despite further increases in workload. Conversely, oxygen uptake has been considered "peak" when the subject reaches a point of fatigue, while no plateau in oxygen uptake was observed. Unfortunately, the many problems associated with the determination and criteria for the "plateau" in oxygen uptake makes these definitions more semantic that physiological. A brief history of this concept and its inherent problems are outlined later.

In 1955, Taylor and associates[57] established the criteria of plateauing as a failure to increase oxygen uptake more than 150 ml/min, or 2.1 ml/kg/min with an increase in workload. Their original research was done using interrupted progressive treadmill protocols. With interrupted protocols, stages of exercise could be separated by rest periods ranging from minutes to days. Taylor and coworkers found that 75% of his subjects fulfilled these criteria. Using continuous treadmill protocols, Pollock et al.[58] found that 69% of subjects plateaued when tested using the Balke, 69% with Bruce, 59% with Ellestad, and 80% with the Astrand protocols. Froelicher and coworkers[59] found that only 33% of healthy subjects met these criteria during testing with the Taylor, 17% with Balke, and 7% with the Bruce protocols, despite that there were no significant differences between the protocols in maximal heart rate, VO_2 max, or blood pressure. Taylor and coworkers later reported that plateauing did not occur when using continuous treadmill protocols.

The plateau concept is long ingrained in exercise physiology. Intuitively, the body's respiratory and metabolic systems must reach some finite limit beyond which oxygen uptake can no longer increase, and some subjects who are highly motivated may exhibit a plateau. However, the occurrence of a plateau depends as much on the criteria applied, the sampling interval, and methodology as the subject's health, fitness, and motivation. We contend that the plateau concept has limitations for general application during standard exercise testing.

NORMAL VALUES FOR EXERCISE CAPACITY

Maximal oxygen uptake declines with increasing age, and high values are observed among men

as compared with women. Thus, when measuring or estimating maximal oxygen uptake, it is useful to have reference values for comparison. Many clever attempts have been made to improve the prediction of what represents a "normal" exercise capacity by including height, weight, body composition, activity status, exercise mode, and such clinical and demographic factors as smoking history, heart disease, and medications. It is important to note that a normal value is only a number that has been inferred from some population. A predicted normal value usually refers to age and gender, but many other factors affect one's exercise capacity. In addition to those mentioned earlier, these include some that are not so easily measured, such as genetics and the type and extent of disease (Table 4.6).

Regression Equations.   The following are commonly used generalized equations based on data published in North America and Europe in the 1950s, 60s, and 70s:[60–63]

Males

$$VO_2 \text{ max (L/min)} = 4.2 - 0.032 \text{ (age) (SD} \pm 0.4)$$
$$VO_2 \text{ max (ml/kg/min)} = 60 - .55 \text{ (age) (SD} \pm 7.5)$$

Females

$$VO_2 \text{ max (L/min)} = 2.6 - 0.014 \text{ (age) (SD} \pm 0.4)$$
$$VO_2 \text{ max (ml/kg/min)} = 48 - 0.37 \text{ (age) (SD} \pm 7.0)$$

TABLE 4.6.   FACTORS TO CONSIDER IN REFERENCE POPULATION WHEN APPLYING FORMULAS FOR EXERCISE CAPACITY

Population tested:
  Age
  Gender
  Anthropometric characteristics
  Health and fitness
  Heart disease
  Pulmonary disease
Exercise mode and protocol
Reason tested:
  Clinical referral
  Screening apparently healthy volunteers
Exercise capacity estimated versus measured directly
Units of measurement
Variability of predicted values (usually 10–30%)

Efforts have been made to improve the precision of predictive equations by considering specific populations, body size, and other demographic factors, in addition to gender. Hansen et al. and Wasserman and associates[64] have published predicted values for maximal oxygen uptake that consider sex, age, height, weight, and whether testing was performed on a treadmill or a cycle ergometer:

	Mode	Overweight	Predicted $\dot{V}O_2$ max (ml/min)
Males			
	Cycle*	No	$W \times (50.72 - 0.372 \times A)$
		Yes	$(0.79 \times H - 60.7) \times (50.72 - 0.372 \times A)$
	Treadmill[†]	No	$W \times (56.36 - 0.413 \times A)$
		Yes	$(0.79 \times H - 60.7) \times (56.36 - 0.413 \times A)$
Females			
	Cycle*	No	$(42.8 \times W) \times (22.78 - 0.17 \times A)$
		Yes	$H \times (14.81 - 0.11 \times A)$
	Treadmill[§]	No	$W \times (44.37 - 0.413 \times A)$
		Yes	$(0.79 \times H - 68.2) \times (44.37 - 0.413 \times A)$

W = weight in kg; H = height in cm; A = age in years
*Overweight is $W > (0.79 \times H - 60.7)$.
[†]Overweight is $W > (0.65 \times H - 42.8)$.
[§]Overweight is $W > (0.79 \times H - 68.2)$.

Jones et al.[65] studied healthy adults on a cycle ergometer and reported the following regression equation (H = height in cm, and gender is coded 0 for males, 1 for females):

$$\dot{V}O_2 \text{ max (L/min)} = 0.046(H) - 0.021(age) - 0.62(gender) - 4.31$$
$$(r = 0.87, \text{SEE} = 0.46)$$

Cooper and Weiler-Ravell[66] developed regression equations from California school children (ages 6 to 17) that considered height rather than age (H = height in cm):

$$\text{Boys: } \dot{V}O_2 \text{ (ml/min)} = 43.6(H) - 4547$$
$$\text{Girls: } \dot{V}O_2 \text{ (ml/min)} = 22.5(H) - 1837$$

Application of Nomograms. Morris and associates[67] developed a nomogram from 1388 veteran patients (Fig. 4.8). The regression equations derived from the group were as follows:

$$\text{All Subjects: METs} = 18.0 - .15 \text{ (age)},$$
$$\text{SEE} = 3.3, r = -0.46, p < .001$$

$$\text{Active Subjects: METs} = 18.7 - 0.15 \text{ (age)},$$
$$\text{SEE} = 3.0, r = -0.49, p < .001$$

$$\text{Sedentary Subjects: METs} = 16.6 - 0.16 \text{ (age)},$$
$$\text{SEE} = 3.2, r = -0.43, p < .001$$

When using regression equations or nomograms for reference purposes, it is important to consider several points. First, as mentioned, the relation between exercise capacity and age is rather poor ($r = -0.30$ to -0.60). Second, nearly all equations are derived from different populations using different protocols. Thus, to some extent, they are both population- and protocol-specific. Moreover, since treadmill time or workload tends to overpredict maximal METs, it is important to consider whether gas exchange techniques were used in developing the equations. For example, the equations developed by Morris et al. were derived from a large group of veterans referred for testing for clinical reasons.[67] Thus, they had a greater prevalence of heart disease than the other studies, and it is not surprising that a steeper slope was present with a faster decline in $\dot{V}O_2$ max with age.

To account for the differences in measured versus predicted oxygen uptake, a nomogram was also developed using measured oxygen uptake among 244 active or sedentary apparently healthy males. The metabolic equivalent values are shifted downward roughly 1.0 to 1.5 METs for any given age, reflecting the lower but more precise measures of exercise capacity:

$$\text{All Subjects: METs} = 14.7 - .11 \text{ (age)}$$
$$\text{Active Subjects: METs} = 16.4 - .13 \text{ (age)}$$
$$\text{Sedentary Subjects: METs} = 11.9 - .07 \text{ (age)}$$

Thus, such scales are specific to both the population tested and to whether oxygen uptake was measured directly or predicted. Within these limitations, these equations and the nomograms derived from them can provide reasonable references for normal values and can facilitate communication with patients and between physicians regarding their level of exercise capacity in relation to their peers.

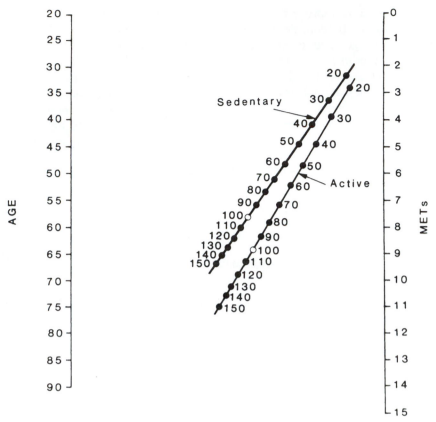

FIGURE 4.8. The functional capacity nomogram for estimating aerobic impairment. Exercise capacity (% of normal in referral males).

ECG INTERPRETATION

ST ANALYSIS

ST-segment depression is a representation of global subendocardial ischemia, with a direction determined largely by the placement of the heart in the chest. ST depression does not localize coronary artery lesions. V_5 is the lead predominating in significant ST depression. Depression isolated to other leads is usually due to Q-wave distortion of the resting ECG. ST depression in the inferior leads (II, aV_F) is most often due to the atrial repolarization wave, which begins in the PR segment and can extend to the beginning of the ST segment. When ST depression is isolated to these leads and there are no diagnostic Q waves,

it is usually a false positive. ST-segment depression limited to the recovery period does not generally represent a false positive response. Inclusion of analysis during this time period increases the diagnostic yield of the exercise test.

When the resting ECG shows Q waves of an old myocardial infarction, ST elevation is due to wall motion abnormalities. Accompanying ST depression can be due to a second area of ischemia or reciprocal changes. When the resting ECG is normal, exercise-induced ST elevation is due to severe ischemia (spasm or a critical lesion), though accompanying ST depression is reciprocal. Such ST elevation is uncommon, very arrhythmogenic, and localizes the involved coronary artery. Exercise-induced ST elevation (not over diagnostic Q waves) and ST depression both represent ischemia, but they are quite distinctive: Elevation is due to transmural ischemia, is arrythmogenic, has a 0.1% prevalence, and localizes the artery where there is spasm or a tight lesion. *Depression* is due to subendocardial ischemia, is not arrythmogenic, has a 5 to 50% prevalence, is rarely due to spasm, and does not localize. Figure 4.9 illustrates the various patterns. The standard criterion for abnormal is 1 ml of horizontal or downsloping ST depression below the PR isoelectric line or 1 ml further depression if there is

baseline depression. Most information is available in lead V_5 with maximal exercise and 3 min recovery being the most important times to look for ST depression.[68] ECG recordings should continue for 5 min in recovery or until any new changes from the baseline stabilize.

Athletes commonly have abnormal resting ECGs with left ventricular hypertrophy, right ventricular hypertrophy, and IVCDs predominating. It is antedotally reported that they more likely have false-positive ST responses, or ST changes suggesting ischemia. However, the prevalence of

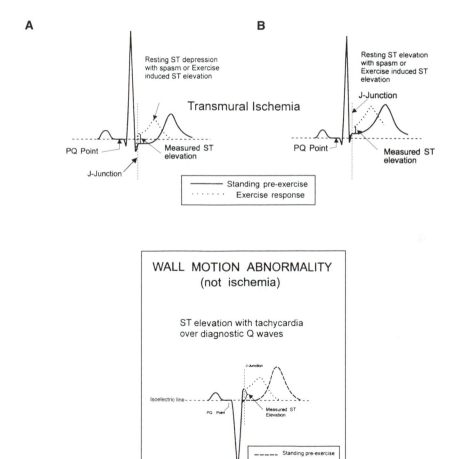

FIGURE 4.9. This illustrates the various patterns of ST shift. The standard criterion for abnormal is 1 ml of horizontal or downsloping ST depression below the PR isoelectric line or 1 ml further depression if there is baseline depression.

abnormal responses is low and most would be false positives because of the low prevalence of coronary disease in this population.

Nonsustained ventricular tachycardia is uncommon during routine clinical treadmill testing (prevalence less than 2%), is well tolerated, and its prognosis is determined by the accompanying ischemia and left ventricular damage.[69]

THE AMERICAN COLLEGE OF CARDIOLOGY AND THE AMERICAN HEART ASSOCIATION GUIDELINES FOR THE USE OF THE STANDARD EXERCISE TEST

In 1986 and 1997 a task force established guidelines for the use of exercise testing.[70] The 1997 publication had some dramatic changes, including the recommendation that the standard exercise test be the first diagnostic procedure in women and in most patients with resting ECG abnormalities rather than that of imaging studies. The following classifications were used to summarize the indications for exercise testing:

Class I: Conditions for which there is evidence and/or general agreement that the exercise test is useful and effective (appropriate).

Class II: Conditions for which there is conflicting evidence and/or a divergence of opinion about the usefulness/efficacy of the exercise test.

IIa: Weight of evidence/opinion is in favor of usefulness/efficacy (probably appropriate).

IIb: Usefulness/efficacy is less well established by evidence/opinion (may be appropriate).

Class III: Conditions for which there is evidence and/or general agreement that the exercise test is not useful or effective and in some cases may be harmful (not appropriate).

Patients who are candidates for exercise testing may have stable symptoms of chest pain, may be stabilized by medical therapy following symptoms of unstable chest pain, or may be postmyocardial infarction or postrevascularization patients. The indications provided in the guidelines are subsequently summarized.

FOR DIAGNOSIS OF CORONARY DISEASE

Exercise testing for the diagnosis of obstructive coronary artery disease is one of the most common uses of exercise testing. Most relative evidence for this use has been gathered in patients presenting with chest pain, though it has been logically extended to those with other symptomatology or ECG changes possibly due to coronary disease. Appropriate evidence-based use of the test for this application (Class I) is in adult patients (including those with complete right bundle branch block or less than 1 mm of resting ST depression) with an intermediate pretest probability of coronary artery disease based on gender, age, and symptoms (Table 4.7). A probable diagnostic use of the test (less evidence) is in patients with vasospastic angina (Class IIa). The efficacy is less well established by evidence and opinion (Class IIb) in patients with a low or high pretest probability of coronary artery disease by age, symptoms, and gender and in patients with less than 1 mm of baseline ST depression and taking digoxin or with left ventricular hypertrophy. The exercise ST analysis should not be used for diagnosis (Class III) in patients with Wolff-Parkinson-White syndrome, left bundle branch block, electronic pacemakers, or with greater than 1 mm of resting ST depression. Patients with a documented myocardial infarction or prior coronary angiography or intervention demonstrating significant disease should not be tested for diagnosis since they have an established diagnosis of coronary artery disease; however, ischemia and risk can be determined by testing.

Diagnostic testing is most valuable in patients with an intermediate pretest probability. Exercise testing for the diagnosis of coronary artery disease is most commonly expressed by sensitivity and specificity. Results of correlative studies have

TABLE 4.7. PRETEST PROBABILITY OF CORONARY DISEASE BY SYMPTOMS, GENDER, AND AGE

Age	Gender	Typical/Definite Angina Pectoris	Atypical/Probable Angina Pectoris	Non-anginal Chest Pain	Asymptomatic
30–39	Males	Intermediate	Intermediate	Low (< 10%)	Very low (< 5%)
	Females	Intermediate	Very Low (< 5%)	Very low	Very low
40–49	Males	High	Intermediate	Intermediate	Low
	Females	Intermediate	Low	Very low	Very low
50–59	Males	High (> 90%)	Intermediate	Intermediate	Low
	Females	Intermediate	Intermediate	Low	Very low
60–69	Males	High	Intermediate	Intermediate	Low
	Females	High	Intermediate	Intermediate	Low

High = > 90%; intermediate = 10–90%; low = < 10%; very low = < 5%.

There is no data for patients or athletes younger than 30 or older than 69, but it can be assumed that coronary artery disease prevalence increases with age.

been divided over the use of 50 or 70% luminal diameter occlusion. Meta-analysis of 58 consecutively published reports involving 11,691 patients without prior myocardial infarction who underwent coronary angiography and exercise testing revealed a wide variability in sensitivity and specificity.[71] Mean sensitivity was 67%, and mean specificity was 72%. In the studies where workup bias was avoided by having the patients agree to undergo both procedures, the approximate sensitivity and specificity of 1 mm of horizontal or downsloping ST depression for diagnosis of coronary artery disease were 50 and 90%, respectively.[72] The true diagnostic value of the exercise ECG lays in its relatively high specificity but the sensitivity can be enhanced by the consideration of clinical and hemodynamic variables in scores.

SCREENING

A diagnostic test such as the exercise ECG can be used to screen asymptomatic individuals for cardiac disease. As previously reviewed, there are

12 studies using the exercise test to do such.[73] Patients were screened for silent heart disease using the exercise test and have been followed for 5 to 10 years for cardiac events. Considerably different results have been obtained in these studies according to the endpoints considered. When angina is included as an endpoint, nonspecific symptoms in a subject with an abnormal test are more likely to be called coronary disease during the follow-up period. Hard endpoints, such as death or myocardial infarction, eliminate this misclassification and are more appropriate. The first screening studies included angina as an endpoint; the last 4 have used only hard endpoints. In Table 4.8, you can see that the first studies tested 5000 subjects and ranged in size from 113 to 1390 individuals. Sensitivity was 50%, specificity was 90%, risk ratio was 9 times, and the predictive value of a positive response was 25%. That means that 1 out of 4 patients with abnormal tests went on to have a cardiac event. Remember that some of these events will be angina, which was probably not truly due to cardiac disease or truly angina. The last 4 studies have been larger in size

TABLE 4.8. THE TWELVE SCREENING STUDIES

Study	Patients	Sensitivity (%)	Specificity (%)	Risk Ratio	Predictive Value + (%)
First 8 (soft endpoints)	5526 (100–1390)	50	90	9 ×	25
Last 4 (hard endpoints)	12,212	25	90	4 ×	5

and have included only hard endpoints. The sensitivity of the test has been about 25%, specificity about 90%, risk ratio 4 times, and the predictive value of a positive response has only 5%. That means that only 1 out of 20 people with an abnormal test went on to a cardiac event. Because of this limited predicted value, in any asymptomatic population, screening has not been recommended. It can cause more harm than good and can lead to unnecessary tests. Several studies have even tried to raise the pretest probability by considering risk factors and have not been able to do so to a level that limits the false positives and improves the predicted value. However, theoretically this should be possible by using a risk-factor score.

The argument could be made that a prediction should be able to be made as to which patients will have milder forms of coronary disease and which will die or have myocardial infarction (i.e., angina). Certainly this is the objective; however, the endpoints created by the test result present difficulties. For example, using soft endpoints exaggerates the sensitivity and predictive value of the test. This could be avoided by blinding all parties to the test result, but this has been considered unethical. Since some of the asymptomatic individuals developing chest pain really have angina due to coronary disease, the sensitivity probably lies between the 25 and 50% obtained in the studies that used respectively hard and hard plus soft endpoints. While soft endpoints are appropriate for intervention studies, they can result in important prediction errors in studies of diagnostic procedures.

Screening studies have other population selection considerations than do diagnostic studies. First, the population should truly be asymptomatic and should represent a random sample of the target population. Volunteers are not appropriate since they usually represent the extremes of the population: the healthiest and those who are concerned for personal reasons regarding their health (i.e., family history, symptoms they chose to deny, etc.). Volunteers represent a subtle form of limited challenge.

COMPARISON WITH OTHER DIAGNOSTIC TESTS

While the studies of the standard exercise test have been helpful in illustrating the problems in demonstrating test characteristics, new technologies have often been evaluated by studies with the same limitations. Nonetheless, it is appropriate to compare the newer diagnostic modalities with the standard exercise test since it is a mature, established technology. The equipment and personnel for performing it are readily available. Exercise testing equipment is relatively inexpensive so that replacement or updating is not a major limitation. The exercise test can be performed in the doctor's office and does not require injections or exposure to radiation. It can be an extension of the medical history and physical exam, providing more than simply diagnostic information. Furthermore, it can determine the degree of disability and impairment to quality of life as well as be the first step in rehabilitation and altering a major risk factor (physical inactivity).

Some of the add-ons or substitutes for the exercise test have the advantage of being able to localize ischemia as well as diagnose coronary disease when the baseline ECG negates ST analysis (more than 1 ml ST depression, left bundle branch block, Wolff-Parkinson-White syndrome). The substitutes for exercise also have the advantage of not requiring the patient to exercise, which is particularly valuable clinically for those who cannot walk. However, while these technologies appear to have better diagnostic characteristics, this is not always the case particularly when more than the ST segments from the exercise test are used in scores.

The evaluation of diagnostic tests has been advanced by the writings of Philbrick et al.,[74] Reid et al.,[75] and Guyatt,[76] creating a better guidline method of reviewing research concerning test characteristics. A number of researchers have applied these guidelines along with meta-analysis to come to consensus on the diagnostic characteristics of the available tests for angiographic coronary artery disease.[77,78] Table 4.9 presents some of the results from meta-analysis and from multi-

TABLE 4.9. COMPARISON OF EXERCISE TESTING AND ADD-ONS OR OTHER TEST MODALITIES

Grouping	Studies	Total Patients	Sensitivity (%)	Specificity (%)	Predictive Accuracy (%)
Meta-analysis of standard exercise ECG	147	24,047	68	77	73
Excluding MI patients	58	11,691	67	72	69
Limiting workup bias	2	> 1000	50	90	69
Meta-analysis of exercise test scores	24	11,788			80
Thallium scintigraphy	59	6038	85	85	85
SPECT without MI	27	2136	86	62	74
Exercise echocardiography	58	5000	84	75	80
Exercise echocardiography excluding MI patients	24	2109	87	84	85
Nonexercise stress tests					
Persantine thallium	11	< 1000	85	91	87
Dobutamine echocardiography	5	< 1000	88	84	86
Electron beam computed tomography	5	2373	90	45	61

ECG, electrocardiogram; MI, myocardial infarction; SPECT, single-photon-emitted computed tomography.

center studies. Techniques listed include electron-beam computed tomography (EBCT), a fast radiographic technique that can make a quantitative measurement of coronary artery calcification.[79,80] Nuclear perfusion imaging includes both the early studies mainly using thallium radiographic images and the more modern use of single-photon-emitted computed tomography (SPECT), which requires computer enhancement of the emissions of thallium and other agents.

Since sensitivity and specificity are inversely related and altered by the chosen cutpoint for normal and abnormal, the predictive accuracy (percentage of patients correctly classified as normal and abnormal) is a convenient way to compare tests. For instance, while the sensitivity and specificity for exercise testing and EBCT are nearly opposite, the predictive accuracy of the tests are similar. This means that by altering their cutpoints (i.e., lowering the amount of ST-segment depression or raising the calcium score) similar sensitivities and specificities would result. Since predictive accuracy can be thought of as the number of individuals correctly classified out of 100 tested, simply subtracting predictive accuracy provides an estimate of how many more patients are classified by substituting one test for another. However, this does assume a disease prevalence of 50% that is the intermediate probability for ap-propriate use of diagnostic tests (i.e., predictive accuracy is affected by disease prevalence).

While the nonexercise stress tests are useful, the results shown in Table 4.9 are probably an overestimation of their predictive accuracy because of patient selection. For studies of diagnostic characteristics, patients with a prior myocardial infarction should be excluded since diagnosis of coronary disease is not an issue for them.

EXERCISE TEST SCORES

The exercise testing studies that have considered additional information in addition to the ST response have been reviewed and demonstrate the improved test characteristics obtained using this approach.[81] The Duke prognostic score has been extended to diagnosis,[82] and a consensus approach that uses a number of equations appears to make the scores more portable to other populations.[83]

EXERCISE NUCLEAR PERFUSION AND ECHOCARDIOGRAPHY

Investigators from the University of California San Francisco reviewed the contemporary literature to compare the diagnostic performance of exercise echocardiography and exercise nuclear perfusion scanning in the diagnosis of coronary artery disease.[84] Studies published between January

1990 and October 1997 were identified from MEDLINE search; bibliographies of reviews and original articles; and suggestions from experts in each area. Articles were included if they discussed exercise echocardiography and/or exercise perfusion imaging for detection and/or evaluation of coronary artery disease; if data on coronary angiography were presented as the reference test; and if the absolute numbers of true-positive, false-negative, true-negative, and false-positive observations were available or derivable from the data presented. Studies performed exclusively in patients after myocardial infarction, with coronary interventions, or with recent unstable coronary syndromes were excluded. Two reviewers used a standardized spreadsheet to independently extract data and discrepancies were resolved by consensus. There were 51 articles that met inclusion criteria: 24 reported exercise echocardiography results in 2637 patients with a weighted mean age of 59 years, 69% were men, 66% had angiographic coronary disease, and 20% had prior myocardial infarction; 27 reported exercise SPECT in 3237 patients, 70% were men, 78% had angiographic coronary disease, and 33% had prior myocardial infarction. In pooled data weighted by the sample size of each study, exercise echocardiography had a sensitivity of 85% (95% confidence interval (CI), 83–87%) with a specificity of 77% (95% CI, 74–80%). Exercise perfusion yielded a similar sensitivity of 87% (95% CI, 86–88%), but a lower specificity of 64% (95% CI, 60–68%).

ELECTRON BEAM COMPUTED TOMOGRAPHY

Of the angiographic correlative studies of EBCT, there were 5 with more than 200 subjects without overlapping populations. There were 160 men and women with coronary disease (45–62 years), of whom 138 had obstructive coronary artery disease and 22 had normal coronary arteries. In addition, 56 age-matched healthy control subjects underwent double-helix CT.[85] Sensitivity in detecting obstructive coronary artery disease was high (91%); however, specificity was low (52%)

because of calcification in nonobstructive lesions. A multicenter study evaluated patients referred for angiography.[86] Between 1989 and 1993, 491 symptomatic patients underwent coronary angiography and EBCT at 5 different centers. The area under the range of characteristics (ROC) curve was 0.75 for the coronary calcium score. In this group, sensitivity of any detectable calcification by EBCT as an indicator of significant stenosis (greater than 50% narrowing) was 92% and specificity 43%. When these CT images were reinterpreted in a blinded and standardized manner, however, specificity was only 31%. In another multicenter study[87] of 710 enrolled patients, 427 had significant angiographic disease, and coronary calcification was detected in 404, yielding a sensitivity of 95%. Of the 283 patients without angiographically significant disease, 124 had negative EBCT studies for a specificity of 44%. Ultrafast CT was used to detect and quantify coronary artery calcium levels in 584 subjects (mean age 48), 19% of whom had clinical coronary artery disease.[88] Sensitivity, specificity, and predictive values for clinical coronary artery disease were calculated for several total calcium scores in each decade. For age groups 40 to 49 and 50 to 59 years, a total score of 50 resulted in a sensitivity of 71% and 74% and a specificity of 91% and 70%, respectively. For the age group 60 to 69 years, a total score of 300 gave a sensitivity of 74% and a specificity of 81%. Between April 1989 and December 1993, 368 symptomatic patients underwent coronary angiography and EBCT at 4 different centers.[89] There were 158 patients (43%) who had angiographically obstructive coronary artery disease (> 50%), and 297 (81%) had coronary calcification. It appears that even the best studies of EBCT suffer from limited challenge and workup bias so that the true characteristics of this procedure are not known. However, averages of the 5 studies in Table 4.9 demonstrated a high sensitivity and a low specificity with a predictive accuracy of about 61%. While adjustment of the cutpoint for calcium density can alter the sensitivity and specificity, the EBCT is not more diagnostic for angiographic coronary artery disease than is the standard exercise test.

Risk assessment (prognostication) and post-myocardial infarction are the next two applications of the standard exercise ECG. The test should not be performed in these situations in patients with severe comorbidity likely to limit life expectancy and/or candidacy for revascularization (Class III).

FOR RISK ASSESSMENT AND PROGNOSIS

The second major application of the exercise ECG is for assessment of risk and prognosis in patients with symptoms or a prior history of coronary artery disease. Appropriate evidence-based use of the test for this application (Class I) is in patients undergoing initial evaluation or in patients with significant change in clinical status with suspected or known coronary artery disease.

Exercise testing may be useful for prognostic assessment of patients on digoxin or with abnormal resting ECGs, but its usefulness is less well established in this setting (Class IIb). Also, the exercise test may still provide prognostic information (particularly exercise capacity) in patients with preexcitation, ventricular paced rhythm, more than 1 mm ST depression, and left bundle branch block. It cannot, however, be used to identify ischemia. The test may also be used in patients with a stable clinical course who undergo periodic monitoring to guide treatment. The Duke treadmill score (see nomogram in Fig. 4.10) incorporates two of the major prognostic markers (exercise capacity and exercise-induced ischemia) and was strongly recommended.[90]

AFTER MYOCARDIAL INFARCTION

The third major application of the exercise ECG is for patients within 2 months of a myocardial infarction. Appropriate evidence-based uses of the test for prognostic assessment, activity prescription, evaluation of medical therapy, and cardiac rehabilitation of these patients (Class I) are (a) before discharge for prognostic assessment, activity prescription, or evaluation of medical therapy (submaximal at about 4 to 7 days); (b) early after discharge if the predischarge exercise test was not done (symptom-limited, about 14 to 21 days); and (c) late after discharge if the early exercise test was submaximal (symptom-limited, about 3 to 6 weeks). A probable postmyocardial infarction use of the test (less evidence) is for activity counseling and/or exercise training as part of cardiac rehabilitation in patients who have undergone coronary revascularization (Class IIa). The efficacy is less well established by evidence or opinion (Class IIb) before discharge in patients who have undergone cardiac catheterization to identify ischemia in the distribution of a coronary lesion of borderline severity or in those with the previously mentioned ECG abnormalities that interfere with the recognition of ischemia or for periodic monitoring in patients who continue to participate in exercise training or cardiac rehabilitation.

A meta-analysis of 28 studies involving 15,613 patients found that markers of ventricular dysfunction were more accurate predictors of adverse cardiac events after myocardial infarction than they were measures of exercise-induced ischemia.[91]

EXERCISE TESTING USING VENTILATORY GAS ANALYSIS

Evidence supports the addition of ventilatory gas analysis to the exercise test (Class I) for the evaluation of exercise capacity and response to therapy in patients with heart failure who are considered for heart transplantation and when assistance is needed in differentiating cardiac versus pulmonary limitations as a cause of exercise-induced dyspnea or impaired exercise capacity.

A probable reason to add gas analysis to the exercise test (less evidence, Class IIa) is for the evaluation of exercise capacity when indicated for medical reasons in patients in whom subjective assessment of maximal exercise is unreliable.

The efficacy of adding gas analysis is less well established by evidence or opinion (Class IIb) for

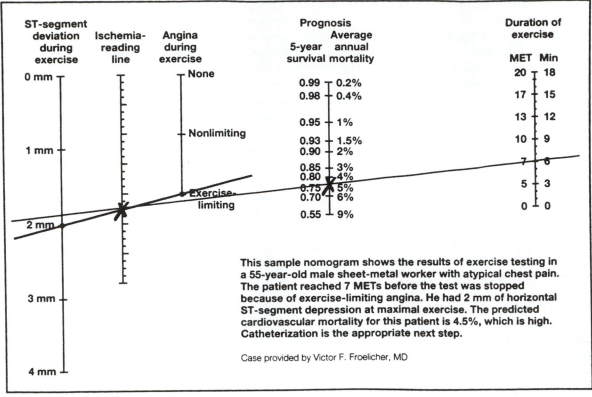

FIGURE 4.10. The Duke treadmill score nomogram for predicting CV mortality from treadmill testing.

evaluation of the patient's response to specific therapeutic interventions in which improvement of exercise tolerance is an important goal or endpoint or for the determination of the intensity for exercise training as part of comprehensive cardiac rehabilitation.

Expired gas analysis is not indicated (Class III) routinely to evaluate exercise capacity.

SCREENING FOR SILENT CORONARY DISEASE IN ASYMPTOMATIC INDIVIDUALS

There is no Class I indication for the use of the exercise test in asymptomatic persons without known coronary artery disease since the available evidence demonstrates a large number of false positives in low prevalence populations.

The efficacy of using the exercise test in evaluation of persons with multiple risk factors or of asymptomatic men older than 40 years and women older than 50 years who plan to start vigorous exercise (especially if sedentary) or who are involved in occupations in which impairment might impact public safety or who are at high risk for coronary artery disease due to other diseases (e.g., chronic renal failure) is possibly but not definitely supported by evidence (Class IIb).

The test should not be used for routine screening (Class III) of asymptomatic men or women.

VALVULAR HEART DISEASE

There is no evidence-based Class I indication for testing patients with valvular heart disease. The test can possibly be used though there is no convincing data to evaluate exercise capacity in patients with valvular heart disease (Class IIb). The exercise ECG should not be used to diagnose coronary artery disease in patients with valvular heart disease (Class III).

BEFORE AND AFTER REVASCULARIZATION

The evidence supports the use of the exercise ECG test to demonstrate ischemia before revascularization and to evaluate patients with recurrent symptoms suggesting ischemia after revascularization (Class I)

A probable use of the test (less evidence) is after discharge for activity counseling and/or exercise training as part of cardiac rehabilitation in patients who have undergone coronary revascularization (Class IIa). The efficacy is less well established by evidence or opinion (Class IIb) for detection of restenosis in selected, high-risk asymptomatic patients within the first months after angioplasty or for periodic monitoring of selected, high-risk asymptomatic patients for restenosis, graft occlusion, or disease progression.

The test should not be used to localize ischemia for determining the site of intervention or for routine, periodic monitoring of asymptomatic patients after percutaneous transluminal coronary angioplasty (PTCA) or coronary artery bypass grafting without specific indications (Class III).

INVESTIGATION OF HEART RHYTHM DISORDERS

The exercise test should be used to identify the appropriate settings in patients with rate-adaptive pacemakers (Class I).

A probable use of the test (less evidence) is for evaluation of patients with known or suspected exercise-induced arrhythmias or for evaluation of medical, surgical, or ablative therapy in patients with exercise-induced arrhythmias (including atrial fibrillation) (Class IIa). The efficacy is less well established by evidence or opinion for inves-

tigation of isolated ventricular ectopic beats in middle-aged patients without other evidence of coronary artery disease (Class IIb).

The test should not be used to investigate isolated ectopic beats in young patients (Class III).

PEDIATRIC TESTING: EXERCISE TESTING IN CHILDREN AND ADOLESCENTS

Evidence supports the exercise test for evaluation of exercise capacity in the following:

1. Children or adolescents with congenital heart disease
2. Those who have had surgery for congenital heart disease
3. Children who have acquired valvular or myocardial disease
4. The rare child with anginal chest pain
5. Young athletes to assess the response of an artificial pacing system to exertion and to evaluate exercise-related symptoms
6. Children with tachyarrhythmias that were found during exercise testing before therapy to evaluate the adequacy of the response to medical, surgical, or radio frequency ablation treatment
7. Those with congenital or acquired valvular lesions, especially aortic valve stenosis, as an adjunct in assessment of its severity
8. Patients with known or suspected exercise-induced arrhythmia to evaluate their rhythm during exercise (Class I)

The efficacy is less well established by evidence or opinion (Class IIb) as a component of the evaluation of children or adolescents who have a family history of unexplained sudden death related to exercise in young persons or who have follow-up of cardiac abnormalities with possible late coronary involvement such as Kawasaki disease and systemic lupus erythematosus. It is also less well established in the assessment of ventricular rate response and development of ventricular arrhythmia in children and adolescents with congenital complete atrioventricular block, quantitation of the heart-rate response to exercise in children and adolescents treated with beta-blocker therapy to estimate the adequacy of blockade, and in the measurement of response of shortening or prolongation of the corrected QT interval to exercise as an adjunct in the diagnosis of hereditary syndromes of prolongation of the QT interval. In addition, there is less evidence for evaluation of blood pressure response or arm-to-leg gradient after the repair of coarctation of the aorta or in the assessment of degree of desaturation with exercise in patients with relatively well-balanced or palliated cyanotic congenital cardiac defects.

The exercise test should not be used (Class III) to screen healthy children and adolescents before athletic participation, for routine use of exercise testing for evaluating noncardiac chest pain, or for evaluation of premature atrial and ventricular contractions in otherwise healthy children and adolescents.

SUMMARY

Utilization of proper methodology is critical to safety and to obtain accurate and comparable results. The use of specific criteria for exclusion and termination, interaction with the subject, and appropriate emergency equipment are essential. The exercise protocol should be progressive with even increments in speed and grade whenever possible. Rather than using the same protocol for every patient or athlete, it is important to individualize the exercise protocol.

In all individuals tested, athletes included, a pretest physical exam and medical history should be performed. The treadmill protocol should be adjusted to the subject, and one protocol is not appropriate for all. The optimal test duration is from 8 to 12 min and so the protocol workloads should be adjusted to permit this duration. Exercise capacity should be reported in metabolic equivalents, not minutes of exercise, in order to permit comparison of the results of many different exercise testing protocols. Hyperventilation

prior to testing is not indicated. Effort level should be recorded by using the Borg scale, and test termination should be determined by established clinical criteria. Age-predicted heart rate targets are only a part of the assessment of effort because of the wide scatter for any age. While patients should immediately be placed supine in order for the test to have its greatest diagnostic value, a cool-down walk is more appropriate when testing athletes.

The use of gas exchange techniques can greatly supplement exercise testing by adding precision and reproducibility and increasing the yield of information concerning cardiopulmonary function. Quantifying work from treadmill or cycle ergometer workload introduces a great deal of error and variability. The limitations of quantifying work in terms of exercise time or workload make gas exchange techniques essential when using exercise to quantify aerobic capacity and the effects of training.

Maximal oxygen uptake is considered the best index of aerobic capacity and maximal cardiorespiratory function. By defining the limits of the cardiopulmonary system, it has been an invaluable measurement clinically for assessing the efficacy of drugs, exercise training, or invasive procedures. No other measurement of work is as accurate, reliable, or reproducible as maximal ventilatory oxygen uptake. Oxygen uptake is quantified by measuring the volume of expired ventilation and determining the difference in the oxygen content of inspired and expired air. Hemodynamically, oxygen uptake is equal to the product of cardiac output and arteriovenous oxygen difference. Historically, the maximal cardiopulmonary limit was considered achieved when oxygen uptake does not increase further with an increase in work (plateau). However, the many criteria and definitions used to describe this point and differences in data sampling limit its utility. Determining what a given athlete's maximal oxygen uptake is relative to "normal" can be imprecise, because this determination is dependent not only upon age and gender, but also many clinical and demographic variables. An effort should be made to apply the most population-specific reference equation for normality.

The American College of Cardiology and the American Heart Association guidelines for exercise testing clearly indicate the correct uses of exercise testing. Since the last guidelines, the application of the standard exercise test has been extended to include the first diagnostic test in women and in individuals with right bundle branch block and resting ST depression. The Duke prognostic nomogram and scores based on additional data to the ECG increase the value of the exercise test. In fact, this method results in test characteristics that approach the nuclear and echogardiographic add-ons to the exercise test.

PERSONAL PERSPECTIVE

Technology continues to drive up the cost of health care. The public and health care providers need to realize that every new test is not better than the older tests. Consider EBCT. This was the latest high technology diagnostic test. Each unit costs $2 million and requires $200,000 yearly maintenance only to become obsolete in 5 years. In spite of this price tag, meta-analysis demonstrates that its diagnostic characteristics are no better than the standard exercise test. Most cardiologists are no longer interested in the standard exercise test because other tests provide greater reimbursement. While it seems reasonable that many internists and general practitioners are beginning to perform exercise testing, they are not well trained and are only comfortable testing low-risk patients who need testing the least. One solution to this problem is the development of specialized services that come to the clinic or hospital with standardization and overreading via centralization. Such services could help to train internists and/or do the tests for them. They will also make electrocardiography, in general, more cost-effective. Also decreasing cost but improving services, ECG technology utilizing personal-computer-based systems can bring high-quality ECGs to the doctors' offices and provide overreading and serial comparison services over the Internet. No matter what the future brings, the exercise test will remain essential to medicine because exercise capacity is the most universal and consistent predictor of prognosis and means of assessing disability.

REFERENCES

1. Froelicher VF, Myers J: *Exercise and the Heart,* 4th ed. Philadelphia, WB Saunders, 1999.
2. American Association of Cardiovascular and Pulmonary Rehabilitation: *Guidelines for Cardiac Rehabilitation Programs.* Champaign, Illinois, Human Kinetics, 1991.
3. Rochmis P, Blackburn H: Exercise tests: A survey of procedures, safety, and litigation experience in approximately 170,000 tests. *JAMA* 217:1061–1066, 1971.
4. Gibbons L, Blair SN, Kohl HW, et al: The safety of maximal exercise testing. *Circulation* 80:846–852, 1989.
5. Yang JC, Wesley RC, Froelicher VF: Ventricular tachycardia during routine treadmill testing. *Arch Intern Med* 151:349–353, 1991.
6. Hizon J, Rodney WM: *The Team Physician's Handbook.* Philadelphia, Hanley & Belfus, 1990.
7. Grumet J, Hizon J, Froelicher VF: Special considerations in exercise testing. *Prim Care* 21(3):459–474, 1994.
7a. Mason RE, Likar I: A new system of multiple-lead exercise electrocardiography. *AM Heart J* 41:196–205, 1966.
8. Borg G: Perceived exertion as an indicator of somatic stress. *Scand J Rehab Med* 23:92–93, 1970.
9. Borg G, Holmgren A, Lindblad I: Quantitative evaluation of chest pain. *Acta Med Scand* 644:43–45, 1981.
10. Gutman RA, Alexander ER, Li YB, et al: Delay of ST depression after maximal exercise by walking for two minutes. *Circulation* 42:229–233, 1970.
11. Lachterman B, Lehmann KG, Abrahamson D, et al: "Recovery only" ST segment depression and the predictive accuracy of the exercise test. *Ann Int Med* 112:11–16, 1990.
12. Verstappen FT, Huppertz RM, Snoeckx LH: Effect of training on specificity on maximal treadmill and bicycle ergometer exercise. *Int J Sports Med* 3:43–46, 1982.
13. Pannier JL, Vrijens J, Van Cauter C: Cardiorespiratory response to treadmill and bicycle exercise in runners. *Eur J Appl Physiol* 43:243–251, 1980.
14. Myers J, Froelicher VF: Optimizing the exercise test for pharmacological investigations. *Circulation* 82:1839–1846, 1990.
15. Buchfuhrer MJ, Hansen JE, Robinson TE, et al:

Optimizing the exercise protocol for cardiopulmonary assessment. *J Appl Physiol* 55:1558–1564, 1983.

16. Niederberger M, Bruce RA, Kusumi F, et al: Disparities in ventilatory and circulatory responses to bicycle and treadmill exercise. *Br Heart J* 36:377, 1974.

17. Astrand P, Ekblom B, Messin R, et al: Intra-arterial blood pressure during exercise with different muscle groups. *J Appl Physiol* 20:253–256, 1965.

18. Davis JA, Vodak P, Wilmore JH, et al: Anaerobic threshold and maximal aerobic power for three modes of exercise. *J Appl Physiol* 41:544–550, 1976.

19. Asmussen E, Nielsen M: Regulation of body temperature during work performed with arms and legs. *Acta Physiol Scand* 14:373–382, 1947.

20. Klefbeck B, Mattsson E, Weinberg J: The effect of trunk support on performance during arm ergometry in patients with cervical cord injuries. *Paraplegia* 34:167–172, 1996.

21. Astrand I, Guharay A, Wahren J: Circulatory responses to arm exercise with different arm positions. *J Appl Physiol* 25:528–532, 1968.

22. Wahren J, Bygdeman S: Onset of angina pectoris in relation to circulatory adaptation during arm and leg exercise. *Circulation* 44:432–441, 1971.

23. Shaw DJ, Crawford MH, Karliner JS, et al: Arm crank ergometry: A new method for the evaluation of coronary artery disease. *Am J Cardiol* 33:801–805, 1974.

24. DeBusk RF, Valdez R, Houston N, et al: Cardiovascular responses to dynamic and static effort soon after myocardial infarction: Application to occupational work assessment. *Circulation* 58:368–375, 1978.

25. Vander LB, Franklin BA, Wrisley D, et al: Cardiorespiratory responses to arm and leg ergometry in women. *Phys Sports Med* 12:101–106, 1984.

26. Asmussen E, Hemmingsen I: Determination of maximum working capacity at different ages in work with the legs or with the arms. *Scand J Clin Lab Invest* 10:67–71, 1958.

27. Franklin BA, Vander L, Wrisley D, et al: Aerobic requirements of arm ergometry: Implications for exercise testing and training. *Phys Sports Med* 11:81–90, 1983.

28. Balke B, Ware R: An experimental study of physical fitness of air force personnel. *US Armed Forces Med J* 10:675–688, 1959.

29. Ellestad MH, Allen W, Wan MCK, et al: Maximal treadmill stress testing for cardiovascular evaluation. *Circulation* 39:517–522, 1969.

30. Sullivan M, McKirnan MD: Errors in predicting functional capacity for postmyocardial infarction patients using a modified Bruce protocol. *Am Heart J* 107:486–491, 1984.

31. Webster MWI, Sharpe DN: Exercise testing in angina pectoris: The importance of protocol design in clinical trials. *Am Heart J* 117:505–508, 1989.

32. Panza JA, Quyyumi AA, Diodati JG, et al: Prediction of the frequency and duration of ambulatory myocardial ischemia in patients with stable coronary artery disease by determination of the ischemic threshold from exercise testing: Importance of the exercise protocol. *J Am Coll Cardiol* 17:657–663, 1991.

33. Myers J, Buchanan N, Walsh D, et al: Comparison of the ramp versus standard exercise protocols. *J Am Coll Cardiol* 17:1334–1342, 1991.

34. Bruce RA, Gey GO Jr, Cooper MN, et al: Seattle Heart Watch: Initial clinical, circulatory and electrocardiographic response to maximal exercise. *Am J Cardiol* 33:459, 1974.

35. Cooper KH, Purdy JG, White SR, et al: Age-fitness adjusted maximal heart rates. *Med Sport* 10:78–88, 1977.

36. Londeree BR, Moeschberger ML: Influence of age and other factors on maximal heart rate. *J Cardiac Rehab* 4:44–49, 1984.

37. Froelicher VF, Brammel H, Davis G, et al: A comparison of three maximal treadmill exercise protocols. *J Appl Physiol* 36:720–725, 1974.

38. Graettinger W, Smith D, Neupel J, et al: Influence of LV chamber size on maximal heart rate. *Circulation* 84:II-187, 1991.

39. Convertino V, Hung J, Goldwater D, et al: Cardiovascular responses to exercise in middle-aged man after 10 days of bedrest. *Circulation* 65:134-140, 1982.

40. Hartley LH, Vogel JA, Cruz JC: Reduction of maximal exercise heart rate at altitude and its reversal with atropine. *J Appl Physiol* 36:362–365, 1974.

41. Irving JB, Bruce RA, DeRouen TA: Variations in

and significance of systolic pressure during maximal exercise (treadmill) testing. *Am J Cardiol* 39:841–848, 1977.

42. Taylor AJ, Beller GA: Postexercise systolic blood pressure response: Clinical application to the assessment of ischemic heart disease. *Am Fam Phys* 58:1126–1130, 1998.

43. Froelicher VF, Thompson AJ, Noquero I, et al: Prediction of maximal oxygen consumption. Comparison of the Bruce and Balke treadmill protocols. *Chest* 68:331–336, 1975.

44. Myers J, Walsh D, Sullivan M, et al: Effect of sampling on variability and plateau in oxygen uptake. *J Appl Physiol* 68:404–410, 1990.

45. Ehsani AA, Hagberg JM, Hickson RC: Rapid changes in left ventricular dimensions and mass in response to physical conditioning and deconditioning. *Am J Cardiol* 42:52–56, 1978.

46. Blomqvist CG, Saltin B: Cardiovascular adaptations to physical training. *Ann Rev Physiol* 45:169–189, 1983.

47. Wasserman K, McElroy MB: Detecting the threshold of anaerobic metabolism in cardiac patients during exercise. *Am J Cardiol* 14:844–852, 1964.

48. Issekutz B, Shaw WAS, Issekutz AC: Lactate metabolism in resting and exercising dogs. *J Appl Physiol* 40:312–319, 1976.

49. Stanley WC, Neese RA, Wisneski JA, et al: Lactate kinetics during submaximal exercise in humans: Studies with isotopic tracers. *J Cardiopul Rehabil* 8:331–340, 1988.

50. Brooks GA: Mammalian fuel utilization during sustained exercise. *Comp Biochem Physiol B Biochem Mol Biol* 120:89–107, 1998.

51. Campbell ME, Hughson RL, Green HJ: Continuous increase in blood lactate concentration during different ramp exercise protocols. *J Appl Physiol* 66:1104–1107, 1989.

52. Dennis SC, Noakes TD, Bosch AN: Ventilation and blood lactate increase exponentially during incremental exercise. *J Sport Sci* 10:437–449, 1992.

53. Tanaka K, Matsuura Y, Matsuyaka A, et al: A longitudinal assessment of anaerobic threshold and distance running performance. *Med Sci Sports Exerc* 16:278–282, 1986.

54. Sullivan MJ, Cobb FR: The anaerobic threshold in chronic heart failure. Relationship to blood lactate, ventilatory basis, reproducibility, and response to exercise training. *Circulation* 81:1147–1158, 1990.

55. Shimizu M, Myers J, Buchanan N, et al: The ventilatory threshold: Method, protocol, and evaluator agreement. *Am Heart J* 122:509–516, 1991.

56. Hickson RC, Bomze HA, Holloszy JO: Faster adjustment of O_2 uptake to the energy requirement of exercise in the trained state. *J Appl Physiol* 44:877–881, 1978.

57. Taylor HL, Buskirk E, Heuschel A: Maximal oxygen intake as an objective measurement of cardiorespiratory performance. *J Appl Physiol* 8:73–80, 1955.

58. Pollock ML, Bohannon RL, Cooper KH, et al: A comparative analysis of four protocols for maximal treadmill stress testing. *Am Heart J* 92:39–46, 1976.

59. Froelicher VF, Brammell H, Davis G, et al: A comparison of the reproducibility and physiologic response to three maximal treadmill exercise protocols. *Chest* 65:512–517, 1974.

60. Shephard RJ: *Endurance Fitness.* Toronto, University of Toronto Press, 1969.

61. Astrand P: Human physical fitness, with special reference to sex and age. *Physiol Rev* 36(suppl 2):307–335, 1956.

62. Astrand I: Aerobic work capacity in men and women with special reference to age. *Acta Physiol Scand* 49(suppl 196):1–92, 1960.

63. Lange-Anderson K, Shephard RJ, Denolin H, et al: *Fundamentals of Exercise Testing.* World Health Organization, Geneva, 1971.

64. Wasserman K, Hansen JE, Sue DY, et al: *Principles of Exercise Testing and Interpretation.* Philadelphia, Lea and Febiger, 1987, pp. 72–86.

65. Jones NL, Markrides L, Hitchcock C, et al: Normal standards for an incremental progressive cycle ergometer test. *Am Rev Respir Dis* 131:700–708, 1985.

66. Cooper CM, Weiler-Ravell D: Gas exchange response to exercise in children. *Am Rev Respir Dis* 129(suppl):547–548, 1984.

67. Morris CK, Myers J, Kawaguchi T, et al: Based on metabolic equivalents and age for aerobic exercise capacity in men. *J Amer Coll Cardiol* 22:175–182, 1993.

68. Lachterman B, Lehmann KG, Abrahamson D, et al: "Recovery only" ST-segment depression and the predictive accuracy of the exercise test. *Ann Intern Med* 112:11–16, 1990.

69. Yang JC, Wesley RC, Froelicher VF: Ventricular

tachycardia during routine treadmill testing. Risk and prognosis. *Arch Intern Med* 151:349–353, 1991.

70. Gibbons RJ, Balady GJ, Beasley JW, et al: ACC/AHA Guidelines for Exercise Testing. A report of the American College of Cardiology/ American Heart Association Task Force on Practice Guidelines (Committee on Exercise Testing). *J Am Coll Cardiol.* 30:260–311, 1997.

71. Gianrossi R, Detrano R, Lehmann K, et al: Exercise-induced ST depression in the diagnosis of coronary artery disease. A meta-analysis. *Circulation* 80:87–98, 1989.

72. Froelicher VF, Lehmann KG, Thomas R, et al: The electrocardiographic exercise test in a population with reduced workup bias: Diagnostic performance, computerized interpretation, and multivariable prediction. Veterans Affairs Cooperative Study in Health Services #016 (QUEXTA) Study Group. Quantitative Exercise Testing and Angiography. *Ann Intern Med* 128: 965–974, 1998.

73. Froelicher VF, Quaglietti S: *Handbook Exercise Testing.* Boston, Little Brown Publishers, 1995.

74. Philbrick JT, Horowitz RI, Feinstein AR: Methodological problems of exercise testing for coronary artery disease: Groups, analysis and bias. *Am J Cardiol* 64:1117–1122, 1989.

75. Reid M, Lachs M, Feinstein A: Use of methodological standards in diagnostic test research. *JAMA* 274:645–651, 1995.

76. Guyatt GH: Readers' guide for articles evaluating diagnostic tests: What ACP Journal Club does for you and what you must do yourself. *ACP J Club* 115:A-16, 1991.

77. Gianrossi R, Detrano R, Columbo A, et al: Cardiac fluoroscopy for the diagnosis of coronary artery disease: A meta-analytic review. *Am Heart J* 120:1179–1188, 1990.

78. Detrano R, Janosi A, Marcondes G, et al: Factors affecting sensitivity and specificity of a diagnostic test: The exercise thallium scintigram. *Am J Med* 84:699–710, 1988.

79. Wexler L, Brundage B, Crouse J, et al: Coronary artery calcification: Pathophysiology, epidemiology, imaging methods, and clinical implications. A statement for health professionals from the American Heart Association. Writing Group. *Circulation* 94:1175–1192, 1996.

80. Fiorino AS: Electron-beam computed tomography, coronary artery calcium, and evaluation of patients with coronary artery disease. *Ann Intern Med* 128:839–847, 1998.

81. Yamada H, Do D, Morise A, et al: Review of studies utilizing multi-variable analysis of clinical and exercise test data to predict angiographic coronary artery disease. *Prog CV Dis* 39:457–481, 1997.

82. Shaw LJ, Peterson ED, Shaw LK, et al: Use of a prognostic treadmill score in identifying diagnostic coronary disease subgroups. *Circulation* 98: 1622–1630, 1998.

83. Do D, West JA, Morise A, et al: A consensus approach to diagnosing coronary artery disease based on clinical and exercise test data. *Chest* 111: 1742–1749, 1997.

84. Fleischmann KE, Hunink MG, Kuntz KM, et al: Exercise echocardiography or exercise SPECT imaging? A meta-analysis of diagnostic test performance. *JAMA* 280:913–920, 1998.

85. Shemesh J, Apter S, Rozenman J, et al: Calcification of coronary arteries: Detection and quantification with double-helix CT. *Radiology* 197:779–783, 1995.

86. Detrano R, Hsiai T, Wang S, et al: Prognostic value of coronary calcification and angiographic stenoses in patients undergoing coronary angiography. *J Am Coll Cardiol* 27:285–290, 1996.

87. Budhoff MJ, Georgiou D, Brody A, et al: Ultrafast computed tomography as a diagnostic modality in the detection of coronary artery disease: A multicenter study. *Circulation* 93:898–904, 1996.

88. Agatston AS, Janowitz WR, Hildner FJ, et al: Quantification of coronary artery calcium using ultrafast computed tomography. *J Am Coll Cardiol* 15:827–832, 1990.

89. Kennedy J, Shavelle R, Wang S, et al: Coronary calcium and standard risk factors in symptomatic patients referred for coronary angiography. *Am Heart J* 135:696–702, 1998.

90. Mark DB, Hlatky MA, Harrell FE, et al: Exercise treadmill score for predicting prognosis in coronary artery disease. *Ann Int Med* 106:793–800, 1987.

91. Froelicher VF, Perdue S, Pewen W, et al: Application of meta-analysis using an electronic spread sheet to exercise testing in patients after myocardial infarction. *Am Jour Med* 83:1045–1054, 1987.

Chapter 5

PRINCIPLES OF EXERCISE TRAINING FOR PHYSICIANS

Niall M. Moyna, Ph.D.

The primary purpose of any training program is to optimize performance during competition. To accomplish this goal, the coach needs to design and implement a comprehensive conditioning program that is appropriate to the needs and abilities of each athlete and the level of competition. In many team sports the coach is faced with the additional problem of integrating conditioning with technique and skill development.

A high level of physical fitness, although important, does not guarantee superior performance during competition. In team sports the ability to execute skills and make split-second decisions, coupled with a thorough knowledge of individual and team tactics is equally important. Inadequate attention to mental preparation may also negate superior fitness. An excellent example is that of a world record holder in the 10,000 meters race who, unable to cope with the stress and expectations of top-level competition, ran off the track during the final of a major championship.

There is large interindividual variation in physiological response and performance levels to exercise training programs.[1–3] Successful athletes tend to be superiorly endowed with the physiological attributes necessary for success in their sport.[4-6] They also tend to demonstrate the greatest response to exercise training (i.e., they are high responders).[1,2] Some of the physiological attributes such as gender are determined at birth. Others are acquired through growth, maturation, and training, and some result from the interaction of genetic and environmental factors. The degree and nature of these interactive effects remains largely unknown.

There is no ideal training blueprint that is appropriate for all sports. A training program for wrestling would be inappropriate for basketball or football. Likewise it would be unwise for a high school middle distance runner to replicate the training program of an Olympic champion. Cellular, organ, and systemic alterations occur in a relatively predictable and uniform manner when conditioning programs adhere to four basic training principles—overload, progression, specificity, and reversal. These training principles have evolved largely as a result of the trial and error observations of innovative coaches and the outstanding performance of their athletes and teams.[7] They provide a framework on which to base training recommendations which can be applied to any sport, at any level of competition, and to the development of any performance attribute.

The purpose of this review is to summarize these training principles and their application to individual and team sports. This should permit clinicians to better understand current training regimens, and the special needs of coaches and athletes. The review will focus on competitive sports, although the principles can also be applied to recreational activities.

OVERLOAD

Overload refers to a training stimulus that disturbs the stability of the internal environment and produces physiological adaptations called *training effects*. Collectively, the adaptive responses increase fitness levels, which helps to diminish the magnitude of the disruptions to the internal environment from future exercise at the same absolute intensity.

The mechanism by which an overload stimulus improves fitness is illustrated in Figure 5.1. Exercise that demands more than the normal capability of the body produces acute changes that temporarily lower the power-generating capacity of muscle resulting in fatigue. The mechanisms responsible for fatigue depend on such factors as the intensity, type, and duration of the exercise, the contractile activity, the fiber composition of the contracting muscle, and the individual's level of fitness.[8]

Cells, tissue, and organs that are disturbed during exercise are restored to their pretraining levels in the hours and days following each workout (the restoration phase). The restoration rate depends on a number of factors including the physiological systems stressed, individual fitness level, the intensity, type, and duration of the contractile activity, nutritional status, and other lifestyle habits such as sleeping patterns, alcohol consumption, and tobacco use.

Typically, heart rate, respiration, body temperature, enzymatic activity, and neuroendocrine function return to resting levels within minutes to hours following an acute bout of exercise.[9] In contrast, it may take 2 or more days to replenish carbohydrate stores,[10,11] and repair damaged muscle tissue.[12]

Following the restoration phase, the various cells, tissue, and organ systems disturbed during the workout undergo changes in their structure and function. This is referred to as the adaptation phase. This in turn permits an athlete to exercise subsequently for a longer duration at the same absolute work rate before the onset of fatigue. These physiological adaptations include increases in the size,[13] strength,[14] mitochondrial density,[15] enzymatic activity,[16] capillary number,[17] and fuel storage capacity[10] of the exercised muscle, as well as systemic changes such as increased blood volume,[18] heart size,[19] maximal stroke volume,[20] and maximal cardiac output.[20] The pattern of over-

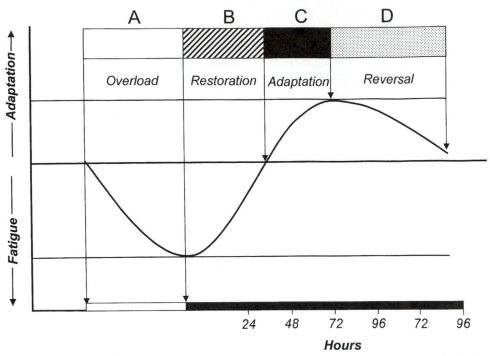

FIGURE 5.1. Supercompensation cycle. (A) Training that overloads one or more physiological systems results in temporary fatigue; (B) cells, tissues, and organs are restored to pretraining levels in the hours and days following each workout; (C) fitness improves due to structural changes and adaptations; and (D) fitness gains are lost if training is stopped.

load, restoration, and adaptation is called a *supercompensation cycle*. Each cycle produces a new fitness level that benefits future training and performance.

Physiological adaptations and the magnitude of improvements in exercise performance vary depending on age,[13,21] intensity, duration, and frequency of exercise,[22,23] genetic factors,[1–3,5] and initial fitness level.[24] Adaptive changes in the cardiovascular system[20] and skeletal muscle[17] begin almost immediately after initiation of endurance exercise training in previously sedentary individuals. For example, changes in mitochondrial and nonmitochondrial enzymes occur within 2 to 7 days after the onset of training and are associated with a low blood lactate response and altered substrate utilization at the same absolute exercise intensity.[21,25]

Absolute and relative increases in fitness for the same increases in training effort decrease as the individual's fitness improves. This means that additional intense training is required to increase fitness as the individual becomes increasingly fit. Indeed, improvements in performance may become so insignificant that training time may be better spent on developing technique and team tactics for sports requiring a combination of fitness and skill. In contrast, small changes in fitness may be the difference between finishing first and second in sports such as speed skating and middle-distance running where fitness is paramount.

Overload is achieved by manipulating the intensity, duration, and frequency of exercise. For endurance events such as long-distance running, swimming, rowing, and cycling, intensity can be defined as the percentage of maximal speed, maximal oxygen uptake (VO_2 max), or maximal heart rate achieved. In resistance training programs, intensity is normally described as a percentage of the maximal possible weight that can be lifted for one (1 rep/max) or more (X rep/max) repetitions. Intensity and duration are generally inversely related. The failure to reduce training volume when intensity is increased is a common mistake, particularly among novice coaches.

Adaptation occurs only with repetitive application of an optimal training load and recovery interval. Ideally, physically demanding workouts should occur at the peak of the adaptation phase (Fig. 5.2A). This will help to ensure that the effects of training are both positive and cumulative. It is not necessary to wait for complete recovery

if subsequent training sessions have different objectives, such as improving tactics or skill.

The recovery rate following strenuous exercise is slower in sedentary individuals as compared to highly trained athletes. The different recovery rates have important implications when planning high intensity workouts. In the example in Figure 5.3, it would be unwise to schedule a vigorous workout for the previously sedentary individual until 3 days after the training session. Ideally, the next strenuous workout should be undertaken on day 6 when peak adaptation has occurred. In contrast, the highly trained athlete has fully recovered within 24 h of the workout and could undertake a strenuous workout 24 h later.

If the recovery interval between successive hard training sessions is prolonged, the adaptations may

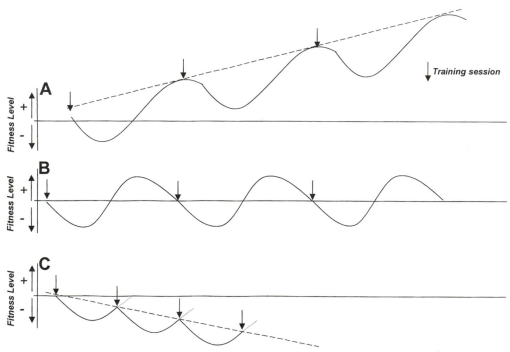

FIGURE 5.2. Effect of recovery interval on functional capacity. (A) Fitness improvements are maximized when strenuous workouts are planned to occur at the peak of the adaptation phase; (B) fitness improvements are minimal if the interval between successive workouts is prolonged; (C) fatigue and/or overtraining occurs when the recovery interval between strenuous workouts is too short.

fade, leading to reversal of gains (Fig. 5.3B). High intensity or high volume days should generally be followed by days of complete rest or low-to-medium intensity and volume. Failure to allow adequate time between stressful training sessions will slow the rate of recovery and result in fatigue (Fig. 5.3C). Over time this may result in injury, overtraining, or a chronically fatigued state.

Inadequate recovery may suppress the immune system and increase susceptibility to upper respiratory tract infections.[26] Acute exercise transiently alters the number and function of immune cells.[27–29] The magnitude of the changes is related to the intensity and duration of exercise.[27,29] Moderate physical activity enhances immune responses.[29,30] In contrast, vigorous exercise decreases innate[31] and adaptive[32,33] immune mechanisms for several hours to a week or longer. Vulnerability to opportunistic infections is increased during this temporary period of immune suppression.[34] There is accumulating anecdotal evidence that athletes who undertake multiple daily workouts with inadequate recovery or who undertake successive days of high intensity training are at higher risk for immune suppression and infection.

Failure to replenish muscle glycogen stores may also delay restoration and adversely affect future workouts and performance.[35] Adequate dietary intake of carbohydrate is particularly important for athletes who undertake more than 1 workout per day or who train vigorously on consecutive days. The timing of carbohydrate ingestion should take into account the fact that muscle glycogen synthesis rate is highest immediately following exercise.[36] Athletes who train daily should ingest 0.70 g of glucose per kilogram of body weight, or approximately 200 calories for a 70-kg individual, every 2 h during the first 4 to 6 h following a workout.[11]

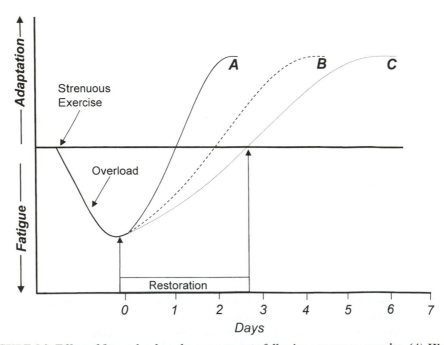

FIGURE 5.3. Effect of fitness level on the recovery rate following strenuous exercise. (A) Highly trained athlete, (B) moderately trained athlete, (C) sedentary individual.

PROGRESSION

Progression refers to a planned, systematic increase in the training load. Training loads that optimally stimulate adaptation early in a conditioning program no longer provide an adequate stimulus once fitness levels have improved. For example, strength gains are minimal or nonexistent if the weight or number of repetitions is not increased during a resistance training program. Systematic application of the progressive overload principle with adequate provision for recovery also adds variety to training, reduces injuries, and helps avoid overtraining.

The rate of progression is important. Training programs that progress too rapidly often fail. It is not possible to change prolonged periods of inactivity and negative lifestyle habits in a relatively short period of time. Application of the progressive overload principle is best achieved by systematically planning quantitative and qualitative changes in the volume and intensity of training. Systematic variations in the yearly, monthly, and weekly training volume and intensity are called *periodization*.

Classic periodization divides the training year into phases of varying duration (Fig. 5.4A). The major training phases are the (a) pre-season, (b) competitive season, and (c) off-season. The length of each training phase and the type of training undertaken will vary depending on the nature of the sport and the competition schedule.

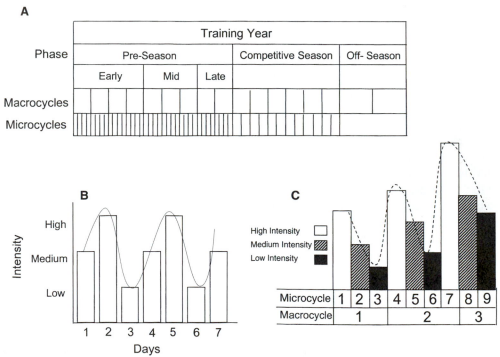

FIGURE 5.4. (A) Classic periodization of the training year into phases, macrocycles, and microcycles; (B) individual microcycle consisting of 2 high intensity workouts followed by low and moderate intensity recovery days; (C) three successive macrocycles. Each macrocycle consists of 3 weekly microcycles. There is a progressive, cyclic increase in exercise intensity from week 1 to week 9.

The aim of the pre-season is to prepare for the upcoming season. The pre-season is usually divided into early, middle, and late phases. The focus during the early pre-season is on developing basic physical conditioning. This is achieved by undertaking high volume-low intensity training. By middle pre-season, there is a transition to more sport-specific training involving a decrease in volume and an increase in intensity. Immediately prior to competition, the volume continues to decrease and intensity increases. Competition-specific training is emphasized during the late pre-season.

Training during the competitive season is designed to maintain conditioning in order to optimize performance during competition. Training intensity and skill development is emphasized, and training volume is low. The number of competitions will vary among different sports. Sports such as track and field are usually focused on a single championship competition. In contrast, team sports may involve participating in one or more games per week for up to 6 months.

The off-season begins after the final competition of the season. This period should be used to allow recovery from the mental and physical strains of competition. The length of the off-season varies among sports and is determined by the duration of the competitive season. Light-to-moderate levels of physical activity should be undertaken 3 to 5 times per week.

Microcycles are the smallest training unit within the periodization framework and are normally 7 days in duration. The dynamics of each microcycle will depend on the nature of the sport, the training phase, and the training objective. Each microcycle should be planned around 1 or more days of moderate-to-high intensity training (Fig. 5.4B). Depending on the sport, the other training days should be used to recover and to develop technical, tactical, and psychological capabilities.

The combination of 2 or more microcycles is called a *macrocycle* (Fig. 5.4C). Each macrocycle has a specific objective and is associated with a specific training phase. Individual microcycles are classified as high, medium, or low intensity. The number of high, medium, and low intensity microcycles and their order within a macrocycle will depend on the athlete's fitness level and the specific fitness objective of the macrocycle. One or more high intensity microcycles should be followed by a low intensity recovery and adaptation week. This is particularly important when peaking for a major game or competition.

Continuous training over a number of years is necessary for success using periodization. Long periods of inactivity eliminate the physiological gains of training, produce a detraining effect, and eliminate the athlete's ability to build on prior fitness. The effects of detraining become more dramatic with age. The yearly, monthly, and weekly periodization process is complex and requires some trial and error on the part of the coach. However, when applied correctly it can take much of the guess work out of coaching and maximize an athlete's performance during competition.

SPECIFICITY

The physiological adaptations to exercise training are highly specific to the type of activity performed,[37,38] the motor units recruited and their recruitment pattern,[9] and the volume and intensity of exercise.[39] A conditioning program designed to improve strength will have little or no impact on cardiorespiratory endurance.[40] According to the principle of specificity, the greatest physiological adaptations occur in the muscle groups that are stressed during exercise. For example, swim training results in a significant increase in maximal aerobic capacity (Vo_2 max) during swimming, and no change during treadmill running.[41] Similarly, the increase in Vo_2 max is significantly greater during arm exercise than when compared to treadmill running following 10 weeks of arm training.[42]

Conditioning programs should focus on developing the fitness attributes that are critical for optimal performance in a given sport. These attributes are determined by the characteristics and specific physical demands of each sport. For example, many coaches involved in team sports view speed simply as the ability to cover a specified distance in the shortest possible time. An athlete who can sprint 40 m in 4.6 s is considered to be faster than another athlete who can cover the same distance in 4.9 s. However, this rather narrow view fails to recognize the unique speed requirements of many different sports.

Sports such a tennis, volleyball, basketball, football, and soccer are characterized by frequent quick starts and sudden stops, interspersed with constant changes of speed and direction. In these and other sports the ability to accelerate, decelerate, and change direction is more important than maximal running speed. In fact, the development of maximal linear sprinting speed represents a poor use of time considering that athletes in many sports seldom reach maximal speed during the course of a game.

Cardiovascular endurance, strength, speed, and flexibility compose the basic fitness components required for performance in most sports (Fig. 5.5A). The time devoted to each fitness component will depend on the nature of the sport and the training phase. Training for predominantly endurance events such as marathon running and distance swimming require high levels of cardiovascular endurance. In contrast, the development of strength and speed should be emphasized for weightlifters and sprinters, respectively.

Many sports require fitness attributes that combine one or more of the basic fitness components (Fig. 5.5B). Power is the product of strength and speed. It is an important fitness attribute for sports such as football, basketball, and sprinting. The combination of speed and endurance or speed endurance is important for success in middle-distance running. Muscular or strength endurance, the combination of strength and endurance, is important for sports such as wrestling and football that require sustained or repeat contractions involving a high percentage of an athlete's maximal strength.

Cross-training is a nonspecific form of training that has grown in popularity.[43] It involves the si-

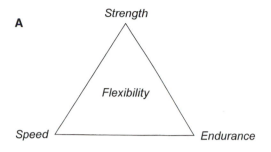

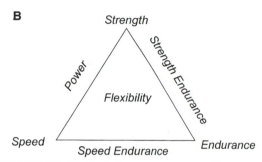

FIGURE 5.5. *(A) Basic fitness components that are required for the majority of sports; (B) some sport-specific fitness attributes.*

multaneous use of more than one mode of exercise training. Advocates of this form of training contend that despite the principle of specificity of training, performance in one mode of exercise can be improved by training using another mode. Cross-training has become popular because it adds variety to the training regimen and allows the athlete to train at a high intensity with less risk of overuse injury.

Evidence linking cross-training to successful performance in competitive sports is based primarily on cross-sectional comparisons among various athletes during treadmill running, cycling, and swimming.[43] Treadmill running increases maximal aerobic power[44,45] and work rate corresponding to the lactate threshold[46] during running and cycling. In contrast, Vo_2 max during treadmill running has been found to increase[45,46] or remain unchanged[44] following training on a cycle ergometer. The failure to find an improvement in Vo_2 max during treadmill running may be related to differences in muscle mass involved, motor unit recruitment pattern, different training regimens, and whether training intensity is equated based on maximal heart rate or as a percentage of Vo_2 max.[43] Swim training has little or no effect on maximal oxygen uptake during running.[41] This is probably because swimming and running use primarily upper and lower body muscles, respectively.

Relatively few studies have examined the effects of cross-training on endurance exercise performance. Foster et al.[47] found a decrease in 5 km run time in well-trained men and women following 10 weeks of running only or a combination of running and swimming. The decrease in run time in the cross-trained groups was 13.2 s as compared to 26.4 s in the running only group. The treadmill speed associated with a blood lactate concentration of 4 mmol·L^{-1} increased in the run but not in the cross-trained group. These findings suggest that while cross-training occasionally might show some transfer effects, the size of the effects will be less than for those which could be attained by increasing specific training by a similar amount. It appears that cross-training may be appropriate for moderately fit recreational athletes who wish to maintain or increase general aerobic fitness. In athletes who are well-trained, exercise needs to be specific and should simulate the exercise motions in order to enhance performance.[44]

Athletes routinely undergo various forms of testing to monitor training adaptations, prescribe training intensities, develop race strategies, and predict performance in competition. Some of the tests, such as time trials over a specific distance, are easy to administer, while others require specialized equipment to assess various physiological parameters.

Adaptations to endurance exercise training are commonly assessed by measuring changes in Vo_2 max. However, Vo_2 max provides little information regarding physiological and metabolic changes during submaximal exercise. Furthermore, significant improvements in endurance exercise performance can occur despite no change in Vo_2 max. Submaximal responses to exercise training in endurance athletes can be assessed by measuring heart rate and/or Vo_2 and blood lactate levels during 3 to 5 submaximal workloads of 3- to 4-min duration.

The relation between heart rate and Vo_2 during incremental exercise is linear. This relation can be expressed as a simple regression equation, $y = mx + c$, where y is the heart rate, x is the Vo_2 demand, c is the intercept, and m is the slope of the line of best fit for the data. The equation can be generated using a calculator with the appropriate function or a simple spreadsheet program such as Excel. A unique feature of individual regression equations is that they can be used to determine the heart rate or workload corresponding to a percentage of Vo_2 max. This information can be used by coaches to accurately prescribe training intensities.

The regression lines in Figures 5.6A and B were generated from data collected during 4 submaximal workloads of 3-min duration. The athlete had a Vo_2 max of 44.36 ml/kg/min. How can the coach use the information to determine the heart rate and speed corresponding to 75% Vo_2 max? When the x or Vo_2 value is known, the corresponding heart rate can be determined by solving for y. The Vo_2 corresponding to 75% Vo_2 max is 33.27 ml/kg/min, and solving the equation for $y = (3.5)(33.27) + 26.7$ results in a heart rate of 143 beats per minute. The speed corresponding to a heart rate of 141 beats per minute can subsequently be determined from the running speed–heart rate regression equation (Fig. 5.6B). Since the heart rate or y variable is known, the equation is solved for the speed or x variable and the result is 7.3 mi/h. In situations where athletes do not have access to a laboratory that can measure Vo_2, the heart rate–speed relation can be determined on a running track using a heart rate monitor.

Alterations in blood lactate levels during submaximal exercise may be a better indication of training-induced improvements in endurance performance than are changes in Vo_2 max.[48] Indeed, the Vo_2 or workload at which blood lactate exhibits an abrupt nonlinear increase above resting

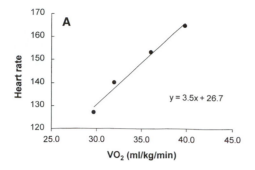

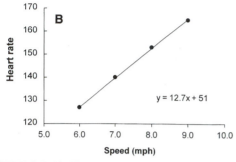

FIGURE 5.6. (A) Heart rate–Vo_2 regression equation can be used to predict heart rate when Vo_2 is known and vice versa; (B) heart rate–running speed regression equation can be used to predict running speed when heart rate is known and vice versa.

levels, called the *lactate threshold (LT),* has been found to be a better predictor of endurance performance than is Vo_2 max.[49,50] The point at which expired ventilation demonstrates a nonlinear increase in relation to Vo_2 is thought to reflect the LT. This inflection point is defined as the *ventilatory threshold* and can also be used as a sensitive noninvasive method to assess changes in endurance fitness and to predict running performance over varying distances.[51]

Laboratory tests should replicate the movement patterns of training in order to objectively evaluate maximal and submaximal performance parameters. Maximal oxgyen uptake values are higher, and lactate and ventilatory threshold occur at a greater relative percent of Vo_2 when athletes are tested on the exercise modality which is specific to their training.[52,53]

REVERSIBILITY

When exercise training is stopped, the physiological systems readjust to the diminished physiological stimuli.[54] This readjustment is simply a reversal of the physiological changes which produced the trained state. The rate of readjustment is dependent in part on the level of fitness[54,55] and the nature of the activity.[56]

Improvements in maximal aerobic power in previously sedentary individuals who undertake 6 to 10 weeks of low-to-moderate intensity and duration exercise are totally reversed following 3 months of inactivity.[55] In contrast, among highly trained endurance athletes, a number of physiological adaptations persist following 12 weeks of detraining.[54] These adaptations maintain Vo_2 max values higher than those of habitually sedentary individuals.

The decline in Vo_2 max results from alterations of both central and peripheral components of the oxygen delivery system. The decline is biphasic and is characterized by an initial rapid reduction in the first 3 weeks followed by a slower decline during weeks 4 to 12 of detraining. The initial decrease is due primarily to changes in the central component of the oxygen delivery system. Cardiac output at maximal exercise decreases 8% during the first 21 days of detraining and returns to pretraining levels by 12 weeks even in highly trained endurance athletes.[54]

The decline in Vo_2 max following the initial 4 weeks of detraining is associated with changes in the peripheral component of the oxygen delivery system. Unlike the cardiovascular system, the effect of detraining on the peripheral component of the oxygen delivery system is dependent on training history. Complete reversal of training induced peripheral adaptations occurs within 6 to 8 weeks following cessation of moderate exercise training.[55,57] In contrast, mitochondrial enzyme activity and muscle capillary density remain significantly elevated following 12 weeks of detraining in previously highly trained athletes.[54] The persistent increase in peripheral adaptations contribute to the relatively high atrioventricular O_2

difference and maximal oxygen uptake observed in highly trained endurance athletes following 12 weeks of detraining.[58]

Even with the best intentions athletes will from time to time lapse from their normal training routine. Missing 1 or 2 weeks of training or even a month of training does not always result in large losses of fitness. Since peripheral adaptations remain elevated for up to 12 weeks after training is stopped, highly trained athletes who become injured during the season should undertake cross-training to minimize the decrements in the central component of the oxygen delivery system. This should help to ensure a more expeditious return to competition.

Deep water running is an attractive sport-specific alternative to on-land running for runners with musculoskeletal injuries. In one study, competitive distance runners were able to maintain running performance, submaximal VO_2, running velocity corresponding to the LT, and VO_2 max following 4 weeks of deep water running.[59]

In many sports the training time allotted to conditioning is decreased in favor of skill and technique during the competitive season. Coaches need to focus on optimizing the limited time available for physical training. Understanding the interaction between exercise frequency, duration, and intensity during reduced training will help the coach decide how best to use the limited time.

Exercise intensity plays a principal role in regulating the maintenance of endurance training adaptations during periods of reduced training. Improvements in short-term endurance performance in response to 10 weeks of training can be maintained for 15 weeks when training intensity is reduced by one-third and training frequency and volume are maintained at training levels.[60] In contrast, short-term cycling and running endurance performance decreases significantly after 10 and 15 weeks, respectively, when intensity is reduced by two-thirds and duration and frequency are maintained for an identical 15-week period.[41] In the same 15-week study paradigm, endurance time to exhaustion at 80% VO_2 max decreased by 30 and 21% when intensity was reduced by two-

thirds and one-third, respectively. Despite these decrements, long-term endurance time remained more than 100% greater than that of pretraining levels. Running and cycling VO_2 max are maintained at training levels when duration and frequency are reduced by two-thirds for 15 weeks and intensity is kept constant.[61,62]

Advances in sports science have allowed coaches to become more scientific and individualized in the preparation of their athletes. Application of exercise training principles has improved the ability of coaches to design programs that optimally blend optimal training loads and recuperation. Clinicians are becoming an integral part of the support system for competitive athletics. Depending on the circumstances, the clinician may be the primary source of information to young athletes or may act as a bridge between the coach and athlete. Understanding the training principles and their application to individual and team sports will permit the clinician to better serve the athletes under his or her care.

PERSONAL PERSPECTIVE

There have been remarkable improvements in the performance of athletes in virtually all sports in the past decade. Athletes are bigger, faster, and stronger than their predecessors. World records have been set in the men's 100, 400, 1500, 5000, and 10,000 m, mile, and marathon in the past 24 months. The world record in the 10,000 m has improved more in the past 5 years than it has in the previous 30 years. For the first time in history an athlete has run 2 miles in less than 8 min. Prior to 1994, Said Aouita of Morocco was the only athlete ever to run under 13 min for 5000 m. Nine different athletes ran the 5000 m in less than 13 min on 19 different occasions in 1999.

Many factors have contributed to the dramatic improvements in sports performance in the past decade. Surprisingly, improvements in endurance performance have occurred even though VO_2 max values among elite endurance athletes have remained stagnant during the past 30 years. I believe that athletes are currently training at intensities that would have been unthinkable only 10 years ago. These training programs are preparing athletes to exercise at or close to VO_2 max for long periods of time. Khalid Khannouchi of Morocco ran a 26.2 marathon at an average speed of 4.47 min per mile. This is equivalent to running 104 consecutive laps of a 400-m track at an average speed of 71.43 s per lap.

I believe that diagnosis and treatment of overtraining is a major issue of concern among athletes and coaches. Overtraining is considered to be a syndrome that is associated with chronic fatigue, underperformance, and an increased susceptibility to injury and infection. The main feature of the syndrome is a sudden unexpected drop in performance during training or competition. There is currently no diagnostic test available to detect overtraining. The diagnosis is complicated by the fact that the syndrome has no single etiology. Psychological, neuroendocrine, physiological, biochemical, and immunological factors have all been implicated as putative mechanisms. Future studies need to identify the principal markers of overtraining and develop an algorithm that can be used by clinicians to identify the stage and severity of functional impairment.

Clinicians and coaches need to recognize that there are large interindividual variations in the physiological responses to an exercise training program. This is important because coaches are constantly faced with the problem of how to handle a large number of athletes and still cater to individual needs and differences. I believe that advances in molecular genetics will in the future enable clinicians and coaches to identify responders and nonresponders and to tailor the training programs more effectively to the individual.

REFERENCES

1. Lortie G, Simoneau JA, Hamel P, et al: Responses of maximal aerobic power and capacity to aerobic training. *Int J Sports Med* 5:232, 1984.
2. Prud'homme D, Bouchard C, Leblanc C, et al: E Sensitivity of maximal aerobic power to training is genotype-dependent. *Med Sci Sports Exerc* 16:489, 1984.
3. Hamel P, Simoneau JA, Lortie G, et al: Heredity and muscle adaptation to endurance training. *Med Sci Sports Exerc* 18:690, 1986.
4. Fagard R, Bielen E, Amery A: Heritability of aerobic power and anaerobic energy generation during exercise. *J Appl Physiol* 70:357, 1992.
5. Park JH, Brown RL, Park CR, et al: Energy metabolism of the untrained muscle of elite runners as observed by 31P magnetic resonance spectroscopy: Evidence suggesting a genetic endowment for endurance exercise. *Proc Natl Acad Sci U S A* 85:8780, 1988.
6. Bouchard C, An P, Rice T, et al: Familial aggregation of VO(2max) response to exercise training: Results from the HERITAGE Family Study. *J Appl Physiol* 87:1003, 1999.
7. Newsholme E, Leech T, Duester D: *Keep on running: The Science of Training and Performance.* Chichester, England, John Wiley & Sons Ltd, 1994.
8. Fitts RH: Cellular mechanisms of muscle fatigue. Department of Biology, Marquette University, Milwaukee, Wisconsin. *Physiol Rev* 74:49, 1994.
9. Brooks GA, Fahey TD, White TP: *Exercise Physiology: Human Biogenergetics and Its Application.* Mountain View, CA, Mayfield, 1996.
10. Greiwe JS, Hickner RC, Hansen P, et al: Effects of endurance exercise training on muscle glycogen accumulation in humans. *J Appl Physiol* 87:222, 1999.
11. Ivy JL: Role of carbohydrate in physical activity. *Clin Sports Med* 18:469, 1999.
12. Clarkson PM, Sayers SP: Etiology of exercise-induced muscle damage. *Can J Appl Physiol* 24:234, 1999.
13. Hakkinen K, Newton RU, Gordon SE, et al: Changes in muscle morphology, electromyographic activity, and force production characteristics during progressive strength training in young and older men. *J Gerontol A Biol Sci Med Sci* 53:B415, 1998.
14. Kraemer WJ, Patton JF, Gordon SE, et al: Compatibility of high-intensity strength and endurance training on hormonal and skeletal muscle adaptations. *J Appl Physiol* 78:976, 1995.
15. Holloszy JO, Coyle EF: Adaptations of skeletal muscle to endurance exercise and their metabolic consequences. *J Appl Physiol* 56:831, 1984.
16. Wibom R, Hultman E, Johansson M, et al: Adaptation of mitochondrial ATP production in human skeletal muscle to endurance training and detraining. *J Appl Physiol* 73:2004, 1992.
17. Brodal P, Ingjer F, Hermansen L: Capillary supply of skeletal muscle fibers in untrained and endurance-trained men. *Am J Physiol* 232:H705, 1977.
18. Convertino VA: Blood volume: Its adaptation to

endurance training. *Med Sci Sports Exerc* 23:1338, 1991.

19. Fagard RH: Impact of different sports and training on cardiac structure and function. *Cardiol Clin* 15:397, 1997.

20. Mier CM, Turner MJ, Ehsani AA, et al: Cardiovascular adaptations to 10 days of cycle exercise. *J Appl Physiol* 83:1900, 1997.

21. Chesley A, Heigenhauser GJ, Spriet LL: Regulation of muscle glycogen phosphorylase activity following short-term endurance training. *Am J Physiol* 270:E328, 1996.

22. Mujika I: The influence of training characteristics and tapering on the adaptation in highly trained individuals: A review. *Int J Sports Med* 19:439, 1998.

23. Wenger HA, Bell GJ: The interactions of intensity, frequency and duration of exercise training in altering cardiorespiratory fitness. *Sports Med* 1986 3:346, 1986.

24. Mujika I, Chatard JC, Busso T, et al: Effects of training on performance in competitive swimming. *Can J Appl Physiol* 20:395, 1995.

25. Spina RJ, Chi MM, Hopkins MG, et al: Mitochondrial enzymes increase in muscle in response to 7-10 days of cycle exercise. *J Appl Physiol* 80:2250, 1996.

26. Peters EM: Exercise, immunology and upper respiratory tract infections. *Int J Sports Med Suppl* 1:S69, 1997.

27. Moyna NM, Acker GR, Weber KM, et al: The effects of incremental submaximal exercise on circulating leukocytes in physically active and sedentary males and females. *Eur J Appl Physiol* 74:211, 1996.

28. Moyna NM, Acker GR, Fulton JR, et al: Lymphocyte function and cytokine production during incremental exercise in active and sedentary males and females. *Int J Sports Med* 17:585, 1996.

29. Moyna NM, Acker GR, Weber KM, et al: Exercise-induced alterations in natural killer cell number and function. *Eur J Appl Physiol* 74:227, 1996.

30. Huupponen MR, Makinen LH, Hyvonen PM, et al: The effect of N-acetylcysteine on exercise-induced priming of human neutrophils. A chemilluminescence study. *Int J Sports Med* 16:399, 1995.

31. Gabriel H, Muller HJ, Urhausen A, et al:

Suppressed PMA-induced oxidative burst and unimpaired phagocytosis of circulating granulocytes one week after a long endurance exercise. *Int J Sports Med* 15:441, 1994.

32. Fry RW, Morton AR, Crawford GP, et al: Cell numbers and in vitro responses of leucocytes and lymphocyte subpopulations following maximal exercise and interval training sessions of different intensities. *Eur J Appl Physiol* 64:218, 1992.

33. Tharp GD, Barnes MW: Reduction of saliva immunoglobulin levels by swim training. *Eur J Appl Physiol* 60:61, 1990.

34. Shephard RJ: *Physical Activity, Training and the Immune Response.* Carmel, IN, Cooper Publishing Group, 1997.

35. Costill DL, Bowers R, Branam G: Muscle glycogen utilization during prolonged exercise on successive days. *J Appl Physiol* 31:834, 1971.

36. Friedman JE, Neufer PD, Dohm GL: Regulation of glycogen resynthesis following exercise. Dietary considerations. *Sports Med* 11:232, 1991.

37. Magel JR, Foglia GF, McArdle WD, et al: Specificity of swim training on maximum oxygen uptake. *J Appl Physiol* 38:151, 1975.

38. McArdle WD, Margel JR, Delio DJ, et al: Specificity of run training on Vo_2 max and heart rate changes during running and swimming. *Med Sci Sports* 10:16, 1978.

39. Mujika I, Chatard JC, Busso T, et al: Effects of training on performance in competitive swimming. *Can J Appl Physiol* 20:395, 1995.

40. Hurley BF, Seals DR, Ehsani AA, et al: Effects of high-intensity strength training on cardiovascular function. *Med Sci Sports Exerc* 16:483, 1984.

41. Gergley TJ, McArdle WD, DeJesus P, et al: Specificity of arm training on aerobic power during swimming and running. *Med Sci Sports Exerc* 16:349, 1984.

42. Magel JR, McArdle WD, Toner M, et al: Metabolic and cardiovascular adjustment to arm training. *J Appl Physiol* 45:75, 1978.

43. Tanaka H: Effects of cross-training. Transfer of training effects on Vo_2max between cycling, running and swimming. *Sports Med* 18:330, 1994.

44. Roberts JA, Alspaugh JW: Specificity of training effects resulting from programs of treadmill running and bicycle ergometer riding. *Med Sci Sports* 4:6, 1972.

45. Pechar GS, McArdle WD, Katch FI, et al:

Specificity of cardiorespiratory adaptation to bicycle and treadmill training. *J Appl Physiol* 36:753, 1974.

46. Pierce EF, Weltman A, Seip RL, et al: Effects of training specificity on the lactate threshold and Vo$_2$ peak. *Int J Sports Med* 11:267, 1990.

47. Foster C, Hector LL, Welsh R, et al: Effects of specific versus cross-training on running performance. *Eur J Appl Physiol* 70:367, 1995.

48. Brooks GA, Anaerobic Threshold: Review of the concept and directions for future research. *Med Sci Sports Exerc* 17:22, 1985.

49. Tanaka KY, Matsuura A, Matsuzaka K, et al: A longitudinal assessment of anaerobic threshold and distance-running performance. *Med Sci Sports Exerc* 16:278, 1984.

50. Tanaka KH, Watanabe Y, Konishi R, et al: Longitudinal associations between anaerobic threshold and distance running performance. *Eur J Appl Physiol* 55:248, 1986.

51. Cunningham LN: Relationship of running economy, ventilatory threshold, and maximal oxygen consumption to running performance in high school females. *Res Quart Exerc Sport* 61:369, 1990.

52. Mazzeo RS, Marshall P: Influence of plasma catecholamines on the lactate threshold during graded exercise. *J Appl Physiol* 67:1319, 1989.

53. Davis JA, Vodak P, Wilmore JH, et al: Anaerobic threshold and maximal aerobic power for three modes of exercise. *J Appl Physiol* 41:544, 1976.

54. Coyle EF, Martin WH, Sinacore DR, et al: Time course of loss of adaptations after stopping prolonged intense endurance training. *J Appl Physiol* 57:1857, 1984.

55. Klausen K, Andersen LB, Pelle I: Adaptive changes in work capacity, skeletal muscle capillarization and enzyme levels during training and detraining. *Acta Physiol Scand* 113:9, 1981.

56. Linossier MT, Dormois D, Perier C, et al: Enzyme adaptations of human skeletal muscle during bicycle short-sprint training and detraining. *Acta Physiol Scand* 161:439, 1997.

57. Henriksson J, Reitman JS: Time course of changes in human skeletal muscle succinate dehydrogenase and cytochrome oxidase activities and maximal oxygen uptake with physical activity and inactivity. *Acta Physiol Scand* 99:91, 1977.

58. Chi MM, Hintz CS, Coyle EF, et al: Effects of detraining on enzymes of energy metabolism in individual human muscle fibers. *Am J Physiol* 244:C276, 1983.

59. Bushman BA, Flynn MG, Andres FF, et al: Effect of 4 wk of deep water run training on running performance. *Med Sci Sports Exerc* 29:694, 1997.

60. Hickson RC, Foster C, Pollock ML, et al: Reduced training intensities and loss of aerobic power, endurance, and cardiac growth. *J Appl Physiol* 58:492, 1985.

61. Hickson R, Kanakis CJ, Davis J, et al: Reduced training duration effects on aerobic power, endurance, and cardiac growth. *J Appl Physiol* 53:225, 1982

62. Hickson RC, Rosenkoetter MA: Reduced training frequencies and maintenance of increased aerobic power. *Med Sci Sports Exerc* 13:13, 1981.

PART II

CARDIAC
RISKS OF
EXERCISE

Chapter 6

THE CARDIOVASCULAR RISKS OF EXERCISE

Paul D. Thompson

Sudden cardiac death and acute myocardial infarction (MI) are the most important cardiovascular complications of exercise based on both frequency and seriousness. Other serious but rare complications include exercise-related aortic dissection and cerebrovascular accidents.[1] Exercise can also induce nonfatal cardiac arrhythmias including ventricular tachycardia, paroxysmal atrial tachycardia, and atrial fibrillation. Postexercise vasovagal syncope is a common cardiac problem especially in well-trained endurance athletes predisposed to this because of enhanced parasympathetic nervous system tone. Various peripheral vascular complications can also be induced by exercise. So-called effort thrombosis, most frequently of the subclavian vein in association with repetitive arm movements such as baseball pitching, is well-known. Exercise has also been associated with other unusual vascular problems such as mesenteric infarction[2] and even subclavian artery aneurysm as experienced by the Yankees' baseball pitcher, David Cone.

The acute cardiovascular adjustments to exercise provide a plausible link between exercise and these cardiovascular complications. Increases in heart rate and systolic blood pressure increase myocardial oxygen demand, which induces cardiac ischemia and the likelihood of malignant ventricular arrhythmia in patients with flow-limiting coronary artery lesions. Increases in left ventricular end-diastolic diameter and decreases in end-systolic diameter require greater excursion of the epicardial coronary arteries during cardiac contraction. This increases the possibility of plaque rupture in the less flexible atherosclerotic segments. Increased cathecholamines augment platelet adhesion, especially in habitually sedentary subjects[3,4] and could contribute to coronary or other vessel thrombosis. Postexercise vascular dilation in exercised muscle increases the likelihood of postexertion syncope in subjects who remain upright and stationary after leg exercise. In addition to such plausibility relationships, exercise has also been statistically linked to the most serious cardiovascular events—sudden cardiac death and MI.[5–9]

This chapter will examine the risk of exercise using data for the most serious cardiovascular complications of exercise—sudden cardiac death and acute MI.

PATHOLOGY OF EXERCISE-RELATED CARDIAC EVENTS IN ADULTS

Atherosclerotic vascular disease is the primary cause of almost all exercise-related deaths in adults. An adult may die occasionally during exertion from other causes such as hypertrophic cardiomyopathy, cardiac amyloidosis,[10] and intramyocardial coronary arteries.[11] The term *adult* in these studies has been variously defined as an age > 29 or > 39 years. Ragosta and associates examined the causes of death in 80 men and 1 woman who died during or immediately after recreational exercise.[1] Seventy-five of these deaths occurred in individuals over age 29, and all of these deaths were related to atherosclerotic vascular disease, including atherosclerotic coro-

nary artery disease in 71 people, hypertensive heart disease diagnosed by history alone in 2, and dissecting aortic aneurysm and cerebrovascular accident in 1 each. In addition to being the primary cause of exercise-related death, atherosclerotic coronary artery disease causes virtually all exercise-related MIs.

Sudden coronary death and acute MI in *previously healthy adults* in the general population are generally produced by atherosclerotic plaque rupture with acute coronary thrombosis.[12] Long before the concept of the ruptured atherosclerotic plaque was widely known, Black et al. reported clinical, autopsy, and angiographic evidence of acute plaque rupture in 13 individuals who died or suffered an MI during vigorous exertion.[13] This mechanism was labeled "Black's Crack in the Plaque." Black believed the plaque produced coronary spasm with subsequent infarction (A. Black, personal communication, 12/16/1985), although recent evidence[12] supports the concept of plaque rupture induced thrombosis.

Black's observation of plaque disruption during exertion has subsequently been confirmed by others who have also demonstrated a high prevalence of intracoronary thrombosis in the victims of exercise-related coronary events. Ciampricotti et al. performed coronary angiography within 4 h of the onset of symptoms in 36 well-trained athletes and 36 comparison subjects.[14] All of the athletes had the onset of symptoms during or within 1 h of sports participation, whereas the comparison group had symptoms occurring at rest. The athletes had unstable angina ($n = 4$), acute MI ($n = 23$), or sudden cardiac death ($n = 9$). When angiography was performed, 65% of both patient groups showed eccentric coronary lesions suggestive of plaque rupture and 45% of both groups had residual thrombus. The latter value underestimates the presence of thrombus in this situation, however, because some of these patients received intravenous streptokinase before angiography.

Hammoudeh and Haft[15] reported angiographic findings on 15 individuals who developed acute coronary syndromes during snow shoveling. Evidence of plaque disruption and coronary thrombosis was found in all subjects.[15] Giri and associates compared coronary angiographic findings in 640 subjects who did ($n = 64$) or did not ($n = 576$) suffer an acute MI during or within 1 h of vigorous exertion.[9] All subjects were referred for primary angioplasty treatment of their MI. None received thrombolytics, and all angiograms were obtained within 12 h of the onset of symptoms. A coronary clot of more than 2 mm was present in 64% of the exercise MI patients, but was present in only 35% of the comparison subjects. This difference between the exercise MI and sedentary MI group suggests differences in the mechanism causing rest and exercise MIs.

Alan Burke in Renu Virmani's group at the Armed Forces Institute of Pathology compared the coronary artery anatomy of 141 men who died suddenly either during exertion ($n = 25$) or at rest ($n = 116$).[16] Of the 25 exertion-related deaths, 14 occurred during unaccustomed exertion, 4 during habitual exercise training regimens, and 7 during emotional stress. Atherosclerotic plaque rupture was found at necropsy in 68% of the exertion-related deaths, but in only 23% of the nonexertion group. Healing ruptured plaque (0 vs. 4%), stable plaques (24 vs. 53%), and plaque erosion (8 vs. 21%) accounted for the remaining coronary findings in the exertion and nonexertion groups, respectively. Coronary plaque rupture is presumably more frequent at the site of "vulnerable plaques," which are characterized by a thin, fibrous cap, macrophage infiltration of the cap, and a large lipid-laden, necrotic core.[16] Men dying during exertion were not only more likely to die of plaque rupture, but they also had a larger total number of vulnerable plaques throughout the coronary tree, 1.6 ± 1.5 versus 0.9 ± 1.2. In the general population approximately 63% of plaque ruptures occur at the shoulder of the atherosclerotic lesion where the fibrous cap intersects with the more normal arterial wall.[17] Rupture through the center of the cap is responsible for the remaining 37% of events.[17] In only 16 of the 25 exertion-related deaths and only 20 of 116 nonexertion rest victims could the site of rupture be determined.[16] Nevertheless, exertion-relate deaths

had rupture of the shoulder region in only 25% of the events, as compared to 65% of the victims who died at rest. The minimum thickness of the ruptured fibrous caps was less in the exertion group than it was in the nonexertion subjects. Furthermore, the number of intraplaque vasa vasorum at the site of plaque rupture was higher in the exertion group, and hemorrhage into the plaque occurred in 72% of the exertion-related deaths and 41% of the nonexertion group.

The significance of these pathologic differences is uncertain. One would expect the fibrous cap to be thicker in the exercise group, if exercise was required to provoke the event, but the caps were thinner in the exercise subjects. The role of increased vasa vasorum in the plaques of the exertion-related subjects is also unclear, although bleeding from the vasa vasorum has been suggested as a possible cause of coronary plaque hemorrhage and rupture. These findings will require confirmation, but they do suggest that the pathology of exertion-related cardiac events may differ from the pathology of sudden cardiac death occurring at rest.

How could exercise induce plaque disruption and thrombosis, leading to an acute MI or cardiac death? Exercise could induce arterial injury, worsen an existing injury, or increase the risk of thrombosis in a damaged arterial segment. Black et al. postulated that the increased "twisting and bending" of coronary arteries during vigorous exertion increased the frequency of plaque rupture.[13] These authors noted that the coronary arteries were subjected to 5 "stress motions," including a ballooning action from the pulsation of blood, an accordion motion associated with lengthening and contracting during the cardiac cycle, a twisting motion, acute bending during contraction, and flow currents.[13] These motions are exacerbated by the increases in heart rate and contractility produced by exercise. Exercise also increases the excursion of the epicardial coronary arteries because of increased end-diastolic and reduced end-systolic cardiac dimensions during exertion. Also, exercise dilates normal coronary arteries, but can produce vasoconstriction in atherosclerotic segments.[18] Such spasm over a thickened, noncompliant atherosclerotic plaque could itself induce plaque rupture.

Exercise could also facilitate plaque disruption by chemical mechanisms. A 25-min progressive exercise session to exhaustion in healthy young men not only increases platelet aggregability, but also increases platelet-to-leukocyte aggregation and plasma elastase levels.[4] Increased platelet-to-leukocyte aggregation could increase leukocyte adherence to the arterial wall. This in turn could facilitate leukocyte migration into the vessel wall where the leukocytes could contribute to disruption of the fibrous cap.[4] Elastase is secreted by activated neutrophils and can attack elastic fibers in the extracellular matrix. This could further facilitate plaque disruption.

Exercise also has multiple prothrombotic effects that could increase the risk of thrombosis over an injured arterial segment. Progressive exercise to maximal exertion on a cycle ergometer increases platelet P-selectin expression and platelet-to-platelet aggregation.[4] Both changes contribute to the development of platelet thrombi. Exercise-induced platelet aggregation is greater in sedentary than in active subjects,[3] possibly because exercise training reduces the catecholamine response to any absolute workload. Lower catecholamine levels reduce the chance of catecholamine-induced platelet aggregation.

Exercise might also induce acute events by deepening existing coronary fissures. Physical exertion increases systolic blood pressure, thereby increasing shear forces in the coronaries and possibly increasing coronary fissuring. Plaque rupture without coronary thrombosis is common. Coronary plaque fissuring without thrombosis was found in 17% of people who died of noncoronary atherosclerosis and in 9% of subjects dying in motor vehicle accidents and suicides.[19] Consequently, it could be that vigorous exercise induces coronary thrombosis by worsening previously damaged coronary plaques that were only mildly fissured.

It must be emphasized that the preceding discussion of plaque rupture and thrombosis as a cause of exercise-related cardiac death applies primarily to previously *asymptomatic* subjects. Patients with known coronary heart disease who die during exertion may, but often do not, demonstrate evidence of an acute coronary lesion or recent myocardial injury.[20] Patients without evidence of an acute coronary lesion often demonstrate evidence of previous infarction. The absence of any acute lesions in the coronary arteries of these patients suggests that such subjects probably die of ventricular fibrillation originating from areas of myocardial scarring.

PATHOLOGY OF EXERCISE-RELATED CARDIAC EVENTS IN CHILDREN AND YOUNG ADULTS

In contrast to the findings in adults, coronary artery disease is a rare cause of exercise-related deaths in young subjects. In the Rhode Island report, none of the sudden deaths during recreational physical activity in young subjects could be attributed to atherosclerotic coronary artery disease.[1] Similarly, among high school and college athletes, only 3 of 100 exercise-related cardiovascular deaths were caused by coronary artery disease.[21] When young athletes do die of atherosclerotic coronary artery disease, it is often associated with primary hypercholesterolemia and genetic abnormalities in the low density lipoprotein receptor.[22] Indeed, if atherosclerotic coronary artery disease is documented as a cause of exercise-related deaths in young subjects, family members should be examined for primary hypercholesterolemia.

Congenital cardiac abnormalities and nonatherosclerotic acquired cardiac diseases are the primary cause of nontraumatic, exercise-related cardiac deaths in young subjects.[21–23] Van Camp et al examined 136 deaths that occurred during or within 1 h of sports participation over 10 years.[21] The cases were collected by the National Center for Catastrophic Sports Injury Research. Cardiac conditions were responsible for 100 deaths.

Definite or probable hypertrophic cardiomyopathy (HCM; 56% of the cases), coronary artery anomalies (13%), myocarditis (7%), aortic stenosis (6%), and dilated cardiomyopathy (6%) were the most frequent causes of death (Table 6.1) The coronary artery anomalies included anomalous origin, intramyocardial course, and an ostial ridge at the coronary origin. Some coronary anomalies such as an acute take-off of the artery from the aorta[24] may be overlooked or unappreciated during autopsy. Interestingly, only 1 case was attributed to right ventricular dysplasia, a condition in which there is fibrosis and fatty tissue replacement of the right ventricular myocardium. The dominance of HCM as a cause of exercise-related death and the rarity of right ventricular dysplasia in this report[21] is similar to other reports from American researchers.[22–23] In contrast, right ventricular cardiomyopathy, also known as right ventricular dysplasia, is the most frequent cause of exercise-related deaths in young Italians in the Veneto region of Italy,[25] and HCM is a rare cause of exertion-related deaths in this population. Among 60 Italians aged < 35 years, 12 died from right ventricular cardiomyopathy and only 3 died from HCM.[25] Ten of the right ventricular cardiomyopathy deaths occurred during exercise. Consequently, the causes of exercise-related sudden death vary not only by age, but also by nationality.

There are several clinically important observations from these pathological studies of exercise-related sudden cardiac death. First, deaths among women are extremely rare. This does not appear to be related to participation rates. Absolute incidence rates in women of exercise-related sudden cardiac death are also lower than in men.[21] One cannot exclude differences in the intensity of training or competition, but this is an unlikely explanation and indeed studies in the general population have also noted low rates of sudden cardiac death among women.[26] The low death rates may be related to cardiac size, since women have smaller hearts than men and heart size appears to be a risk factor for sudden death.[27,28] Second, deaths related to mitral valve prolapse (MVP) are rare. MVP is a frequently overdiagnosed,[29] cardiac condition that has been assumed to affect as many as 10% of the general population.[29] The rarity of this diagnosis among victims of exercise-related deaths is reassuring to the many patients who have been appropriately or inappropriately diagnosed with MVP. Third, anomalous atrioventricular (AV) cardiac conduction, such as the Wolff-Parkinson-White (WPW) syndrome, is also a rare cause of exercise-related cardiac events. WPW pattern conduction is present in approximately 1% of ECGs obtained from healthy subjects.[30] The WPW pattern is probably even more prevalent in endurance athletes who are more likely to conduct down the accessory pathway than through the AV node because of enhanced vagal tone.[31] The rarity of exercise-related deaths among athletes with WPW syndrome is im-

TABLE 6.1. CARDIAC CAUSES OF DEATH IN HIGH SCHOOL AND COLLEGE ATHLETES (*n* = 100)

	Men	Women
Hypertrophic cardiomyopathy[a]	50	1
Probable hypertrophic cardiomyopathy	5	0
Coronary artery anomalies[b]	11	2
Myocarditis	7	—
Aortic stenosis	6	—
Cardiomyopathy	6	—
Atherosclerotic coronary disease	2	1
Aortic rupture	2	—
Subaortic stenosis	2	—
Coronary aneurysm	—	1
Mitral prolapse	1	—
Right ventricular dysplasia	—	1
Cerebral arteriovenous malformation	—	1
Subarachnoid hemorrhage	—	1

[a] 3 also had coronary anomalies, 1 had Wolff-Parkinson-White syndrome.

[b] Includes: anomalous left coronary artery from right sinus of Valsalva (*n* = 4); intramural left anterior descending (*n* = 4); anomalous left coronary artery from pulmonary artery (*n* = 2); anomalous right coronary artery from left sinus (*n* = 2); hypoplastic right coronary artery (*n* = 2); and ostial ridge of the left coronary artery (*n* = 2). Three subjects with coronary anomalies also had hypertrophic cardiomyopathy and are tabulated with that group.

Adapted with permission from Van Camp SP, Bloor CM, Mueller FO, et al: Nontraumatic sports death in high school and college athletes. *Med Sci Sports Exerc* 27:641–647, 1995.

portant, however, because of a growing tendency among cardiologists to recommend ablative therapy for such athletes even when the athletes are asymptomatic. Finally, some exercise-related deaths remain unexplained and may represent subtle abnormalities of the cardiac conduction system that are not detectable by routine autopsy.

It is also important to remember that these reports do not provide any information on how many individuals with cardiac conditions were prohibited from participating in sports and thereby escaped an exercise-related complication. It seems unlikely to have markedly affected the results, however. Maron et al. also using the National Center for Catastrophic Sports Injury Research database plus other sources, identified 134 athletes dying of cardiovascular disease, 90% or 121 of whom suffered sudden cardiac death during or immediately after training or competition.[32] Eighty-six percent or 115 of the victims had undergone a standard preparticipation examination, but cardiac disease was suspected in only 3% ($n = 4$) and the fatal cardiac malformation (Marfan syndrome) was correctly diagnosed in only one athlete. Fifteen additional athletes underwent evaluations in addition to the standard school preparticipation physical. These athletes were evaluated further because of signs or symptoms of cardiac disease, but it is unclear how many of these workups were prompted by findings on the school screening exam. Even among this more extensively evaluated group, the correct clinical diagnosis was made in only 7 athletes and only 2 were disqualified from competition. Such results *suggest* that few athletes are denied participation on the basis of health issues. Nevertheless, it remains undefined how many potential victims were saved because they were excluded from sport.

RISK OF SUDDEN DEATH DURING EXERCISE IN ADULTS

The risk of exercise varies by population depending on the prevalence of cardiac abnormalities associated with exercise-related deaths. Since the most common cardiac abnormality, and the most common cause of exercise cardiac complications, is atherosclerotic coronary artery disease, deaths are more frequent in older populations and among subjects with known atherosclerosis. Nevertheless, even in the adult population, exercise complications are rare and the rarity of exercise-related events limits the number of cases available for estimating incidence.

Two of the most frequently cited studies on the incidence of exercise-related deaths in Rhode Island[5] and cardiac arrests in Seattle[6] were based on only 10 and 9 deaths, respectively. Small changes in such a small numerator can greatly affect the estimated incidence. Also, few studies are based on well-defined, unselected populations. Selected populations, such as military recruits, may undergo cardiovascular screening or be otherwise selected so that their results are not applicable to the general population.

Despite such problems, these studies do provide useful estimates on the incidence of exercise-related sudden death in adults. In cooperation with William Sturner, the state medical examiner, Thompson and associates collected data on all deaths during jogging from 1975 through 1980 in Rhode Island.[5] The number of joggers was calculated using the percentage of joggers determined by a random digit dial telephone survey and state population estimates. There was 1 death per year for every 7620 male joggers aged 30 through 65. Half of the victims had known coronary artery disease by history or electrocardiogram (ECG) criteria. If these men are eliminated and the assumption made that no other joggers had known coronary artery disease, the annual incidence of sudden death can be estimated as 1 per every 15,240 previously healthy joggers.

There are a number of problems with this study. The prevalence of joggers was based on self-report from the random digit telephone survey. Self-report may overestimate the number of joggers and underestimate the rate of jogging deaths. Alternatively, the study design may have underestimated the number of joggers and thereby overestimated exercise risks. Telephone calls were placed between 5 and 8 pm. The first person over age 15 years to answer the phone was interviewed. If joggers were running during this time period, the prevalence of joggers would have been underestimated and their death rate overestimated. An additional problem in estimating the risk for previously asymptomatic men is the assumption that other men with known heart disease did not jog. Despite these problems, the incidence figure for healthy subjects agrees with the annual incidence of exercise-related cardiac arrests determined among previously healthy adults in Seattle where there was an estimated 1 death for every 18,000 physically active men.[6] Both the Rhode Island and Seattle estimates also have wide confidence limits because they are based on only 10 and 9 subjects, respectively, and the Rhode Island study had only 5 previously healthy sudden death victims. The 95% confidence limits for the Rhode Island study suggest that 1 death during jogging will occur per year for every 4000 to 26,000 asymptomatic men.[5] These studies were also published over 15 years ago, but this author is unaware of later studies of exercise-related deaths in the general population.

This author is also unaware of published incidence figures for exercise-related sudden cardiac deaths in adult women. This probably reflects the delayed development of coronary artery disease in women, lower rates of vigorous physical activity among older women and men, and the lower incidence of sudden cardiac death in women in general.

Although the absolute death rate appears low, the death rate per hour of exercise in both the Rhode Island and Seattle studies was increased over the resting rate.[5,6] The relative risk of sudden death was sevenfold higher during jogging than during more sedentary activities in Rhode Island.[5] The Seattle study calculated the incidence of cardiac arrest based on the individual's habitual activity level. In men who spent < 20 min per week in activities requiring ≥ 6 kcal/min of energy expenditure, the relative risk of an exercise-related cardiac arrest was 56 times greater than it was at rest whereas the relative risk was increased only fivefold in men who spent ≥ 140 min per week in such activities.[6] This study demonstrates that regular exercise reduces the chance of sudden death during exercise, but that exercise transiently increases the risk of cardiac arrest even among habitually active individuals.

It is possible that this protective effect is overestimated when evaluated as the absolute hourly risk for an individual. The lower risk among the active subjects is based on risk per personhours of exercise. The more active men exercise more hours and therefore have a lower risk per hour of exercise than sedentary men. It is difficult to put much faith in calculating annual death rates for men of various physical activity levels because the number of subjects in each group ranges from 2 to 4.[6] Nevertheless, when such a calculation is made, the annualized risk of sudden death during exertion is 1 death per 17,000; 23,000; and 13,000 individuals for men expending 1 to 19, 20 to 139, or ≥ 140 min per week in activity requiring ≥ 6 kcal/min of exertion, respectively. This variation with activity level is considerably less than the 56- to fivefold decrease when the risk is expressed as the relative risk of exercise and rest.

If exercise does indeed reduce the absolute annual incidence of exercise-related sudden death, the annualized death rate should be considerably lower in middle-aged athletes. Unfortunately, few studies have estimated the incidence of sudden death among such subjects. Maron et al. calculated the frequency of cardiac arrest among 215,413 participants in the Marine Corps and Twin Cities Marathons from 1976 to 1994.[33] There were 4 deaths or 1 death per 50,000 participants over this time span. If a marathon time of 4 h was used, the death rate was 1 per every 215,000 h of competition. This number exceeds the incidence of sudden death among joggers in the Rhode Island population (1 per 396,000 exercise h),[5] as well as the incidence of cardiac arrest among the most active group in the Seattle study (1 arrest per 4,800,000 exercise h).[6] The number of marathoners who died is far too few to make firm conclusions, but the results do suggest that prolonged competitive tasks may increase the exercise risk.

Interestingly, in both the Rhode Island and Seattle studies, the relative risk of an exercise-related sudden death versus other activities was greatest in the youngest adults. In Rhode Island, the relative risk of jogging versus more sedentary activities was 99 times greater than at rest in men aged 30 to 39, 13 times greater for those 40 to 49, and 5 times greater for those 50 to 59 years. The number of deaths per hour of jogging varied from 1 per 482,600 h for the youngest group to 1 per 309,400 h for the oldest group, suggesting approximately equivalent hourly event rates. In Seattle, 6 of the 9 cases of cardiac arrest occurred in men under age 45 years. The younger men spent more time exercising, however, so that the cardiac arrest incidence figures were actually similar in the older and younger men.[6,34] Consequently, it appears that in young men, the high relative risk of death during vigorous exercise is due in part to the low risk of sudden death in this age group during sedentary activities. This supports the concept that vigorous exercise is indeed a provocateur of sudden cardiac death from coronary artery disease, especially among young subjects.

RISK OF MYOCARDIAL INFARCTION DURING EXERCISE

The risk of myocardial infarction is also related to the habitual fitness level of the subject. Mittleman et al. examined the relative risk of suffering a myocardial infarction during or within 1 h of exercise requiring ≥ 6 (metabolic equivalents) METs.[7] A MET refers to a multiple of resting energy expenditure which is approximately 3.5 ml of oxygen per minute per kilogram of body weight. For a 70-kg individual, 6 METs would be approximately 21 ml of oxygen per minute. The study population was derived from 22 community and 23 tertiary care hospitals in the United States. Of 1228 MI patients qualifying for inclusion, only 54 or 4.4% of the patients experienced initial

symptoms of their MI during or within 1 h of exercise. Three comparisons were performed: (a) within the MI patients between their habitual level of activity and their activity within 1 h of their MI; (b) within the patients between the day of their MI and the same time period 1 day earlier; and (c) between patients and community controls. In each of these comparisons the relative risk of an MI during or soon after exercise was at least 5.6-fold greater than the risk during less vigorous activity. Common activities associated with MI included lifting or pushing (18%), isotonic activities such as jogging (30%), and yard work such as gardening and chopping wood (52%). In patients who were usually sedentary, the relative risk of suffering an MI was 107-fold higher during exercise than it was at rest. Among those who habitually exercised at least 5 times weekly, the relative risk was only 2.7-fold higher than it was at rest. Diabetics had a relative risk of an exercise-related MI that was 18.9 times higher than their risk at rest.

Willich et al. compared the frequency of MIs during or within 1 h of exercise requiring ≥ 6 METs with that during less vigorous activity in Berlin and Augsburg, Germany.[34] Two comparisons were performed: (a) a within-patient comparison using the patients' usual frequency of exertion to calculate the expected chance of an MI occurring with exertion compared to that of the actual frequency; and (b) a comparison between patients and a telephone control group. The control group was asked to describe their activity at the time the MI victims suffered their MI. Over a 2-year period there were 1194 patients who agreed to participate. Of these, 69 patients (5.8%) had an exercise-associated MI. The patient group was not restricted to patients with first-time MI and consequently the MI patients had more prior MIs, more cardiac risk factors, and used more cardiac medications than the telephoned controls. Nevertheless, after adjustment for these differences, the relative risk of an MI during exercise was 2.1 higher than it was for those at rest. The same increase in relative risk was also found for the within-subject comparison.

Giri et al. stratified the relative risk of exercise-related MI by the subjects' habitual activity level in 640 patients who underwent primary angioplasty as treatment for their MI.[35] Of the 640 patients, 10% or 64 suffered their MI during or within 1 h of exertion requiring ≥ 6 METs. The overall risk of suffering an MI during exertion was 10.1 greater than it was for those at rest (95% confidence interval [CI] = 1.6–65.6), but the risk varied with the patients' habitual activity level. Among the least active patients, the relative risk of an MI was 30.5 higher during exercise than it was at rest (CI = 4.4–209.9), whereas the exercise risk was not significantly higher than it was at rest among the most active men (RR = 1.2; CI = 0.3–5.2). These results confirm that exercise increases the risk of MI, but suggest that such events occur primarily among habitually inactive individuals performing unaccustomed physical activity.

All of these studies[7–9] on the relative risk of exercise MI are not readily applicable to athletes or to the healthy population because they all included patients with known heart disease. To obviate this problem, this author analyzed the relative risk of exercise versus rest MI in 547 previously healthy patients with MI who were treated by primary angioplasty.[35] Of these patients, 12% or 66 had suffered their MI during or within 1 h after exertion requiring ≥ 6 METs. This population included some of the same patients studied previously.[9] The risk of MI during exertion was 12-fold higher than it was at rest. The risk was again greatest among the least active (RR = 55.1, CI = 8–391) and lowest among the most active men (RR = 2.9, CI = 0.7–2.9).

This author is unaware of studies providing an absolute incidence of MI during vigorous exercise in previously healthy individuals, but has estimated the incidence from other data.[36] In the Lipid Clinics Primary Prevention Trial of previously healthy hypercholesterolemic men, the incidence of exercise-related MI was 7 times higher than the incidence of sudden cardiac death.[37] This relative rate of MI and sudden death contrasts with the relative rate of these two events among patients with known coronary disease participating in cardiac rehabilitation programs. In the latter situation, the ratio of exercise MIs to sudden death is reversed with sudden death 2.6[38] to 7[39] times more frequent. Since these studies originate from the pre-angioplasty era, many of the patients had suffered an MI and sustained myocardial injury, so the increased relative risk of ventricular fibrillation is probably due to the presence of myocardial scar.[39] Nevertheless, assuming an absolute risk of sudden death during exercise as 1 per 15,000[5] to 18,000[6] healthy men and the risk of MI as 7 times more frequent, there is an absolute annual incidence of 1 MI during exertion for every 2142 to 2571 exercising men. The annual rate of exercise MI could range from 1 per 571 to 3714 men per year if the 95% CI for sudden death during exercise from the Rhode Island study (1 death per 4000 to 26,000 men per year)[5] are used to calculate the incidence.

This estimated risk is not trivial, but may be overestimated. In the Giri et al study of exercise-related MIs, patients who suffered exercise-related infarcts were more likely to present with ventricular fibrillation than were subjects experiencing a nonexertion MI.[9] This suggests that more exercise-related MIs present as sudden death, thereby increasing the incidence of exercise-related sudden death. If the sudden death incidence is subsequently used to estimate the incidence of exercise-related MI, the latter will almost certainly be overestimated.

RISK OF SUDDEN DEATH DURING EXERCISE IN YOUNG SUBJECTS

In contrast to the prevalence of coronary artery disease in adults, the prevalence of cardiac abnormalities among younger individuals is extremely low. Consequently, the incidence of sudden death during exercise is low and the incidence of exercise-related MI among young subjects is almost nonexistent. Indeed, when MIs do occur among young individuals, nonatherosclerotic causes including arteritis, intramural coronary arteries, and anomalous coronary origin and course, as well as cocaine use[40,41] should be considered unless the individual has marked hypercholesterolemia.

Van Camp et al. have estimated an absolute rate of exercise-related death among high school and college athletes as 1 per 133,000 men and 769,000 women.[21] These estimates include all sports-related nontraumatic deaths and are not restricted to cardiac events. The death rate is higher among college men than high school men (1.45 vs. 0.66 per 100,000) for unclear reasons. This author has speculated that this may be related to cardiac size, since evidence in hypertensive patients suggests that cardiac size itself is a risk factor for cardiac death[27,28] and more mature athletes should have larger hearts.

RISK OF EXERCISE FOR SPECIAL POPULATIONS

CARDIAC EVENT RATES IN PATIENTS WITH KNOWN CORONARY ARTERY DISEASE

The best estimates on the risk of exercise among patients with known cardiac disease are from studies of cardiac rehabilitation programs. Unfortunately, the two primary studies were published in the mid 1970s[39] and 1980s[38] and might not be directly applicable to present day patients who are more likely to receive aggressive medical and interventional therapy for their disease. Haskell queried 30 rehabilitation centers and reported 1 cardiac arrest, MI, and death for every 33,000; 223,000; and 116,000 patient-hours of participation, respectively.[39] Van Camp and Peterson[38] surveyed 167 rehabilitation programs and reported 1 cardiac arrest, MI, and death every 112,000; 294,000; and 784,000 hours of participation.[38] The lower exercise event rates in the later study may be due to improved patient selection and supervision, as well as to better treatment of underlying coronary artery disease. Both studies suggest that cardiac arrest is more frequent than MI in this patient group. These studies also demonstrate that prompt treatment of cardiac arrest contributes to the low mortality of cardiac rehabilitation programs.

RISKS OF EXERCISE STRESS TESTING

The risks of exercise stress testing, similar to the risks of exercise itself, vary by the prevalence of disease in the population being tested. Exercise testing among healthy athletes has extremely low risk with no complications reported for exercise tests performed on 353,638 sportsmen.[42] In contrast, among 263 patients with known ventricular arrhythmias who underwent 1377 maximal exercise tests, 24 or 9.1% of the patients developed ventricular fibrillation, ventricular tachycardia, or bradycardia requiring cardioversion, intravenous medication, or closed-chest cardiac compression.[43] The complication rate from 7 reports in usual clinical settings over the last 30 years suggests that there are approximately 1 MI, 2 episodes of ventricular fibrillation or major arrhythmia, 0.3 deaths, and less than 3 hospitalizations for every 10,000 exercise tests or approximately 6 major complications per 10,000 exercise tests (Table 6.2).[44-50] This low rate has prompted some clinicians to use physician extenders to administer the exercise stress tests,[50] but as of January 1, 1998, the physician is required to be physically present in the room when exercise testing is performed.[51]

INDIVIDUALS WITH SICKLE CELL TRAIT

In their study of nontraumatic sudden death among high school and college athletes, Van Camp et al. reported that 7 of 160 sports-related deaths were due to rhabdomyolysis in individuals with sickle cell trait.[21] Kark et al. examined deaths during basic training in 2 million U.S. Military recruits between 1977 and 1981.[52] All of the sudden deaths, "unexplained" by prior disease, were related to physical exertion and were caused by cardiac events, heat illness, or exertional rhabdomyolysis. Unfortunately, it is not possible from this report to decipher exactly how many of these exercise-related deaths were due to cardiac causes. Nevertheless, the relative risk of sudden unexplained death among African-Americans with sickle cell trait was 27 times higher than it was in African-Americans without

TABLE 6.2.   CARDIAC COMPLICATIONS OF EXERCISE TESTING

Reference	Year	Site	No. of Tests	MI	VF	Death	Hospitalization	Comment
44	1971	73 U.S. Centers	170,000	NA	NA	1	3	34% of tests were symptom limited; 50% of deaths in 8 h, 50% over next 4 days
45	1977	15 Seattle Facilities	10,700	NA	4.67	0	NR	
46	1977	Hospital	12,000	0	0	0	0	
47	1979	20 Swedish Centers	50,000	0.8	0.8	6.4	5.2	
48	1980	1,375 U.S. Centers	518,448	3.58	4.78	0.5	NR	VF includes other arrhythmias requiring treatment
49	1989	Cooper Clinic	71,914	0.56	0.29	0	NR	Only 4% of men and 2% of women had CAD
50	1995	Geisinger Cardiology Service	20,133	1.42	1.77	0	NR	25% were inpatients' tests supervised by non-MDs
SUM				1.06	2.05	0.27	2.73	

MI, myocardial infarction; VF, ventricular fibrillation; NA, not available; NR, not recorded; CAD, coronary artery disease.

sickle cell trait, and 40 times higher than in other races. The risk appeared higher in older recruits. This author estimates that the absolute annual death rate in African-Americans with sickle cell trait during 8 to 11 weeks of basic training was approximately 1 death for every 3000 recruits. This is a remarkably high rate given that the absolute annual death rate among high school athletes is only 1 per 133,000 men and women and among college athletes 769,000.[51] The explanation for the excess mortality rate among individuals with sickle cell trait deserves additional investigation.

REDUCING THE CARDIOVASCULAR RISKS OF EXERCISE

YOUNG SUBJECTS

The death of an athlete during training or competition or the death of any previously healthy individual during vigorous exertion is a shock and a tragedy for the individual's family and community. Such deaths often prompt a community call for more extensive screening of athletes and have also prompted some entrepreneurial physicians to initiate screening programs as a means of stimulating testing income. This author has been skep-

tical about the effectiveness of the more extensive screening programs and has advocated routine medical screening as a prudent approach,[53] along with the aggressive evaluation of symptomatic athletes. Also suggested is that all coaches be required to know basic life-support techniques. Despite position stands by such prominent groups as the American Heart Association, there remains a lack of consensus on this issue and some experts strongly advocate more extensive screening of athletes.

The argument in favor of screening received considerable support after publication of the Italian experience evaluating competitive athletes.[54] Italy has had a national law since 1971 requiring that athletes undergo an extensive examination before being allowed to compete. The physician issuing the clearance is legally responsible for the health of the athlete and can be prosecuted in both civil and criminal actions if something happens to the athlete.[55] The basic exam includes a medical history, physical examination, ECG, and step test. Those with abnormalities can subsequently be referred for a 24-h ECG recording, an echocardiogram, and a formal exercise test. This program has screened 33,735 athletes and referred 3016 for echocardiography.[54] Of these, 621 athletes were disqualified from competition,

58.7% because of cardiac issues including 22 athletes with HCM. Four disqualified athletes died over 8.2 ± 5 years (mean ± standard deviation) of follow-up. None of the 22 athletes with HCM died. A total of 49 nondisqualified athletes died yielding an annual death rate of 1 per 62,500 athletes. The authors compared the frequency of HCM as a cause of exercise deaths in the United States and in Italy and concluded that the low prevalence of HCM among their athletes who died was most likely a result of the screening program.

There are several major problems with this conclusion. First, the prevalence of HCM in this population is low. Only 0.06% of the athletes had this diagnosis, whereas the expected prevalence, at least in a sample of healthy young Americans, is 0.2%.[56] Second, few excluded athletes died. Only 4 athletes died out of the 365 athletes who were denied participation because of a cardiac condition. It is not known how these excluded athletes were medically managed, but the death rate is extremely low, raising the possibility that screening prohibited individuals who were not at great risk. Third, the annual death rate of 1 per 62,500 athletes is similar to, if not higher than, the death rate of 1 per 133,000 male athletes reported for American athletes who presumably underwent far less screening.[21] Consequently, instead of supporting extensive screening, these results[54] actually raise questions about its effectiveness.

At least 5 American studies,[57–61] including 5458 high school and collegiate athletes, have examined the utility of screening echocardiography, but no cases of definite HCM were detected (Table 6.3). This is surprising since approximately 11 cases would be expected given the 0.2% prevalence of HCM in the general population.[56] The paucity of athletes found to have HCM in such studies raises the possibility that individuals with this abnormality self-select themselves away from athletic participation and that those who do die during athletic activity represent an undefined subset of the disease. A variety of cardiac abnormalities were detected in these screening studies, but most of the findings were inconsequential or could have been detected by simpler techniques (Table 6.3).

One of these studies performed only selective echocardiography.[57] Out of 501 college athletes, 90 were selected for echocardiography because of abnormalities detected by medical history, physical examination, or resting ECG. Three athletes had increased left ventricular septal thickness, but none were diagnosed as having HCM or excluded from competition.

Other authors have suggested an ECG should be routinely included in the screening of young athletes. Fuller et al. obtained a medical history, had a cardiologist perform cardiac auscultation, and recorded a resting ECG on 5615 athletes from 30 schools in the Reno, Nevada, area.[62] Cardiovascular abnormalities were detected in 582 or 10.4% of the athletes. These included an abnormal cardiac history in 2% of the athletes, abnormal auscultatory findings in 3%, hypertension in 0.3%, and an abnormal ECG in 2.6%. After further evaluation, only 22 athletes were denied participation for severe aortic insufficiency (AI; $n = 1$), severe hypertension ($n = 5$), WPW ECG pattern ($n = 6$), premature ventricular contractions (PVCs; $n = 5$), right bundle branch block ($n = 4$), and supraventricular tachycardia (SVT; $n = 1$). The reasons for excluding the athletes with WPW, PVCs, and right bundle branch block were not provided. Among the 22 excluded athletes, the patient with severe AI underwent valve replacement, the hypertensive patients were treated, and the patient with SVT underwent therapeutic ablation. Unfortunately, 15 of the excluded subjects were lost to follow-up. Over the 3 years of the study, there was 1 cardiac arrest in an athlete. This occurred in an athlete with an anomalous right coronary artery who had successfully passed screening. The authors reason that including ECG in the evaluation of high school athletes increases the detection of cardiac abnormalities. An alternative interpretation is that most important abnormalities could have been detected by sphygmomanometry and auscultation alone and that the ECG only increases the detection of

TABLE 6.3. RESULTS OF SCREENING ATHLETES

Reference #	*n*	Techniques	Group	Results
57	501	History, Physical, ECG (*n* = 501) Selective 2D echo (*n* = 90)	Collegiate 357 men 144 women	MVP (*n* = 14) Septal thickening (*n* = 3)
58	265	2D echo	Collegiate 220 men 45 women	MVP (*n* = 11) ASD (*n* = 1)
59	125	"Limited" 2D echo	Collegiate 83 men 42 women	MVP (*n* = 13) Bicuspid AoV (*n* = 2)
60	1570	2D echo	High school 1570 men	Dextrocardia (*n* = 1)
61	2997	"Screening" 2D echo	High school	MVP (*n* = 40) Bicuspid AoV (*n* = 10) Dilated Ao root (*n* = 4) VSD (*n* = 2) Dilated coronary sinus (*n* = 2) ASD (*n* = 1) RV mass (*n* = 1) Septal hypertrophy (*n* = 1)

ECG, electrocardiogram; 2D, two dimensional; echo, echocardiogram; MVP, mitral valve prolapse; ASD, atrial septal defect; AoV, aortic valve, VSD, ventricular septal defect; RV, right ventricular.

asymptomatic abnormalities unlikely to be of major significance to the athlete.

The American Heart Association has issued a medical and scientific statement on the cardiovascular preparticipation screening of competitive athletes.[53] This document recommends a personal and family history as well as a physical examination before high school participation, with the examination repeated at least every 4 years. The examination should be done by someone who is knowledgeable about the risks of exercise and qualified to perform the cardiac examination. Extensive testing is warranted in certain instances and a careful evaluation should be performed in all symptomatic athletes whose symptoms are potentially cardiac in origin. For athletes with known cardiovascular disease and for those in whom abnormalities have been detected, recommendations on eligibility for competitive athletics have been presented as part of the 26th Bethesda Conference.[63] Finally, it makes excellent sense to ensure that coaches and other personnel who attend athletic training and competition possess basic resuscitation skills.

ADULTS

Preventing cardiac-related events in adults ultimately requires preventing atherosclerotic cardiovascular disease. Clearly, individuals with the most risk factors are at the greatest risk of developing cardiac problems in the general population. The same principle applies to preventing exercise-related cardiac events in adults. Exercise-related MIs are frequent in patients who smoke[9] and in those who are hyperlipidemic,[9] obese,[9] diabetic,[7] and physically least active.[7,9] Surprisingly, the risk-factor profile of athletes who develop exercise-related atherosclerotic coronary events appears different from the profile of individuals in the general population who experience a cardiac event at rest. Ciampricotti et al. compared the clinical characteristics of 36 well-conditioned athletes who suffered sudden cardiac death, MI, or unstable angina within 1 h of exertion with those of 36 other men who developed the same syndromes at rest.[64] Risk factors for heart disease including hypertension (19 vs. 33%), hypercholesterolemia (14 vs. 56%), and cigarette smoking (58 vs. 94%) were less frequent in the athletes. Ages for the two groups were similar. Thus, it appears that athletes who suffer exercise-related coronary artery disease events, in contrast to nonathletes who suffer exercise-related cardiac events,[9] have fewer risk factors than individuals in the general population with coronary artery disease. This makes it more difficult to identify adult athletes at risk for exercise-related cardiac events by risk factors alone. This does not, of course, obviate the need to treat aggressively risk factors in both athletes and nonathletes because aggressive reduction of risk factors probably stabilizes coronary plaques thereby reducing the chance that exercise will induce a cardiac event.

This author has championed the importance of informing exercising adults of the nature of cardiac prodromal symptoms so that they can seek appropriate attention and avoid exertion if such symptoms appear. Among 13 individuals who died during or immediately after exercise from coronary artery disease, 6 had prodromal symptoms before the event.[65] Noakes summarized the clinical history of 36 marathoners who suffered sudden cardiac death or acute MI.[66] Prodromal symptoms were present in 71% of the 28 cases where information was available. In contrast, Ciampricotti and associates noted prodromal symptoms in 47% of sedentary men who developed acute coronary syndromes at rest, but in only 8% of athletes suffering the same events during exercise.[64] Consequently, although prodromal symptoms can help identify individuals at risk for exercise-related events, they are variable and may be less frequent among athletes possibly because such events in habitually active subjects are due to the rapid progression of previously noncritical coronary lesions.

The issue of exercise stress testing before embarking on an exercise program is also controversial. The American College of Sports Medicine recommends that high-risk individuals undergo exercise stress testing prior to vigorous exercise.[67] The high-risk classification includes men over 40 and women over 50 years of age, individuals with more than 1 coronary disease risk factor, and

those with known coronary disease. The American College of Cardiology and the Ameri-can Heart Association considered the evidence for using screening exercise tests in formulating Guidelines for Exercise Testing.[68] A minority of the writing committee, the present author included, favored classifying the use of exercise testing prior to starting an exercise program as not useful. The overall committee classified such testing as not well-established by evidence or opinion, but stopped short of calling such testing unjustified.

The committee's reluctance to give a more enthusiastic endorsement of exercise testing in asymptomatic adults is that exercise testing is a poor predictor of the major cardiac complications during exercise, MI, and sudden cardiac death. A true positive exercise test requires a hemodynamically significant coronary obstruction, whereas acute coronary events often involve plaque rupture and thrombosis at the site of previously nonobstructive atherosclerotic plaque.[69]

Studies evaluating the utility of exercise testing in ostensibly healthy populations support this hypothesis. McHenry et al. studied 916 Indiana State Troopers who underwent maximal exercise tests, had repeat testing at intervals of 1 to 5 years, and were followed for a mean of 12.7 years.[70] Only 61 men (6.6%) ever demonstrated a positive ECG response to exercise. Of these, 21 (34%) developed clinical signs of coronary disease including angina pectoris in 18, an acute MI in 1, and sudden cardiac death in 1. An additional asymptomatic man underwent coronary bypass surgery. Among the 833 men with normal ECG responses, only 44 (5%) subsequently developed clinical coronary disease: 25 developed MI, 7 died suddenly, and 12 developed angina. These data demonstrate that ostensibly healthy individuals with a positive exercise test have a sixfold higher chance of developing coronary artery disease (32 vs. 5%), but that the predominant presentation in these men is angina and not sudden cardiac death or MI. This is probably because positive tests identify individuals with hemodynamically significant coronary lesions that are often tolerated until the appearance of angina.

Screening only individuals at high risk produces similar results. Exercise testing was used to screen for heart disease in 3617 men participating in the Lipid Research Clinics Primary Prevention Trial.[37] All men had prerandomization low-density lipoprotein cholesterol values above 4.91 (190) mmol/L (mg/dl). Exercise tests to 90% of age-predicted maximal heart rate were performed at baseline and annually thereafter. Sixty-two men developed an exercise-related event: 54 acute myocardial infarctions and 8 sudden deaths. Only 11 of the 62 events occurred in men with a positive exercise test. The predictive value of a positive exercise test for an acute exercise event was only 4%, in part because such events are rare. The authors concluded that routine exercise testing is not effective in preventing exercise-related acute cardiac events even in high-risk populations.

Such results suggest that routine exercise testing is not justified to identify asymptomatic individuals at risk for exercise-related cardiac events. This conclusion ignores the high rate of false-positive tests in an asymptomatic active population. Given that exercise-induced ischemia requires a hemodynamically restrictive coronary lesion, it is unlikely that radionuclide or echocardiographic imaging would greatly alter this conclusion although such techniques should reduce the incidence of falsely positive ECG responses.

RECOMMENDATIONS

Reducing the risk of exercise-related cardiac events is extremely difficult because of the rarity of such events and the poor predictive value of most screening procedures. There are, however, prudent measures that should be followed even if they are of unproven effectiveness. These include the medical examination of young athletes prior to vigorous sports by an examiner who is knowledgeable about conditions associated with exercise-related cardiac events. Schools should provide a competent examiner for athletes who cannot otherwise afford this service. Many of the conditions associated with sudden death during exercise can often be detected by simple inspection and cardiac auscultation. Adults should be cautioned to reduce coronary artery disease risk factors and not to assume that exercise is a coronary artery disease prevention panacea. Active adults should also know the nature of cardiac prodromal symptoms and their need for prompt medical attention. Any active person or athlete, young or old, who develops possible cardiac symptoms during exercise should undergo a careful cardiac evaluation prior to returning to training or competition. It should be emphasized that cardiac discomfort is often not perceived as "pain," but as discomfort, tightness, or heartburn. Indeed, "gastrointestinal" symptoms are such a common precedent of cardiac disease that the present author cautions internists to begin all gastrointestinal evaluations with a stress test. Exercise stress testing is especially useful in evaluating nonspecific discomforts in active people. Excluding important cardiac disease in *symptomatic* athletes is probably the most efficient way to prevent exercise-related complications, since many athletes have premonitory symptoms before their final event. The present author is repeatedly impressed with the number of athletes who die during exercise after having exercise symptoms that were ignored or inadequately evaluated. The most threatening symptom is often exercise-induced syncope, which nearly always portends ill.

The present author also strongly recommends that individuals who officiate at sporting events learn and update yearly their cardiopulmonary resuscitation skills. Coaches are most frequently present when athletes collapse. If properlytrained, coaches may be able to prevent some of these exercise-related deaths. Competency in cardiac resuscitation should be a prerequisite for a coaching certificate. Finally, athletes with known heart disease and their physicians should follow the recommendations of the 26th Bethesda Conference[63] on determining eligibility for competitive athletics. These guidelines are conservative, but are designed to reduce the incidence of exercise-related cardiac events.

PERSONAL PERSPECTIVE

My personal perspective on the risks of exercise have been forged by over 20 years of interest in this topic.[65] The cardiovascular complications of exercise are often ignored by public health officials. This is appropriate given the benefits of habitual physical activity, but between 4 and 10% of MIs are associated with exercise,[7,9] for example, and the cardiac risks of exertion remain a major concern for practitioners who often fear legal liability for failing to detect cardiac abnormalities. More research is needed to determine who is at risk and in which patient groups the risks of vigorous exertion outweigh its benefits.

More careful research is needed into how much and what intensity of exercise is required to reduce coronary artery disease. It is likely that risk rises with intensity. If coronary artery disease prevention benefits occur at moderate intensity, more patients could benefit with less risk.

The risks of exercise are both over- and underestimated. The risk is overestimated in healthy young individuals. I suspect that too much money and effort are expended on formal screening programs for young athletes. This service probably could be done best by a competent family physician who knows the individual and the family. The risk of exercise is underestimated, however, in patients with known disease. The public health emphasis on the benefits of exercise encourages some coronary artery disease patients to believe that they can cure their coronary artery disease by vigorous exercise. Such patients often ignore the aggressive management of other risk factors and even ignore the risk of vigorous exercise. This can have fatal consequences. All coronary artery disease patients should pursue an exercise training regimen, but most patients should be prohibited from vigorous exertion and competition.

REFERENCES

1. Ragosta M, Crabtree J, Sturner WQ, et al: Death during recreational exercise in the state of Rhode Island. *Med Sci Sports Exerc* 16:339–342, 1984.
2. Kam LW, Pease WE, Thompson PD: Exercise-related mesenteric infarction. *Am J Gastroenterol* 89:1899–1900, 1994.
3. Kestin AS, Ellis PA, Barnard MR, et al: Effect of strenuous exercise on platelet activation state and reactivity. *Circulation* 88:1502–1511, 1993.
4. Li N, Wallen H, Hjemdahl P: Evidence of prothrombotic effects of exercise and limited protection by aspirin. *Circulation* 100:1374–1379, 1999.
5. Thompson PD, Funk EJ, Carleton RA, et al: Incidence of death during jogging in Rhode Island from 1975 through 1980. *JAMA* 247:2535–2538, 1982.
6. Siscovick DS, Weiss NS, Fletcher RH, et al: The incidence of primary cardiac arrest during vigorous exercise. *N Engl J Med* 311:874–877, 1984.
7. Mittleman MA, Maclure M, Tofler GH, et al: Triggering of acute myocardial infarction by heavy exertion: Protection against triggering by regular exercise. *N Engl J Med* 329:1677–1683, 1993.
8. Willich SN, Lewis M, Lowell H, et al: Physical exertion as a trigger of acute myocardial infarction. *N Engl J Med* 329:1684–1690, 1993.
9. Giri S, Thompson PD, Kiernan FJ, et al: Clinical and angiographic characteristics of exertion-related acute myocardial infarction. *JAMA* 282:1731–1736, 1999.
10. Siegel RJ, French WJ, Roberts WC: Spontaneous exercise testing: Running as an early unmasker of underlying cardiac amyloidosis. *Arch Int Med* 142:345, 1982.
11. Thompson PD, Klocke FJ, Levine BD, et al: 26th Bethesda conference: Recommendations for determining eligibility for competition in athletes with cardiovascular abnormalities. Task Force 5: Coronary artery disease. *J Am Coll Cardiol* 24:888–892, 1994.
12. Davies MJ, Thomas AC: Plaque fissuring—the cause of acute myocardial infarction, sudden ischaemic death, and crescendo angina. *Br Heart J* 53:363–373, 1985.
13. Black A, Black MM, Gensini G: Exertion and acute coronary artery injury. *Angiology* 26:759–783, 1975.
14. Ciampricotti R, Deckers JW, Taverne R, et al: Characteristics of conditioned and sedentary men with acute coronary syndromes. *Am J Cardiol* 73:219–222, 1994.
15. Hammoudeh AJ, Haft JI: Coronary-plaque rupture in acute coronary syndromes triggered by snow shoveling. *N Engl J Med* 335:2001, 1996.
16. Burke AP, Farb A, Malcom GT, et al: Plaque rup-

ture and sudden death related to exertion in men with coronary artery disease. *JAMA* 281:921–926, 1999.

17. Richardson PD, Davies MJ, Born GVR: Influence of plaque configuration and stress distribution on fissuring of coronary atherosclerotic plaques. *Lancet* 2:941–944, 1989.

18. Gordon JB, Ganz J, Nabel EG, et al: Atherosclerosis influences the vasomotor response of epicardial coronary arteries to exercise. *J Clin Invest* 83:1946–1952, 1989.

19. Davies MJ, Bland JM, Hangartner JR, et al: Factors influencing the presence or absence of acute coronary artery thrombi in sudden ischaemic death. *Eur Heart J* 10:203–208, 1989.

20. Cobb LA, Weaver WD: Exercise: A risk for sudden death in patients with coronary heart disease. *J Am Coll Cardiol* 7:215–219, 1986.

21. Van Camp SP, Bloor CM, Mueller FO, et al: Nontraumatic sports death in high school and college athletes. *Med Sci Sports Exerc* 27:641–647, 1995.

22. Maron BJ, Roberts WC, McAllister HA, et al: Sudden death in young athletes. *Circulation* 62:218–229, 1980.

23. Burke AP, Farb A, Virmani R, et al: Sports-related and non-sports-related sudden cardiac death in young adults. *Am Heart J* 121:568–575, 1991.

24. Virmani R, Chun PK, Goldstein RE, et al: Acute takeoffs of the coronary arteries along the aortic wall and congenital coronary ostial valve-like ridges: Association with sudden death. *J Am Coll Cardiol* 3:766–771, 1984.

25. Thiene G, Nava A, Corrado D, et al: Right ventricular cardiomyopathy and sudden death in young people. *N Engl J Med* 318:129–133, 1988.

26. Kannel WB, Thomas E Jr: Sudden coronary death: The Framingham study. *Ann N Y Acad Sci* 3–21, 1982.

27. Cooper RS, Simmons BE, Castaner A, et al: Left ventricular hypertrophy is associated with worse survival independent of ventricular function and number of coronary arteries severely narrowed. *Am J Cardiol* 65:441–445, 1990.

28. Kragel AH, Roberts WC: Sudden death and cardiomegaly unassociated with coronary, valvular, congenital or specific myocardial disease. *Am J Cardiol* 61:659, 1988.

29. Freed LA, Levy D, Levine RA, et al: Prevalence and clinical outcome of mitral-valve prolapse. *N Engl J Med* 341:1–7, 1999.

30. Bigger JT Jr: Mechanisms and diagnosis of arrhythmias, in Braunwald E (ed): *Heart Disease: A Textbook of Cardiovascular Medicine.* Philadelphia: WB Saunders Company, 1980: p. 687.

31. Huston TP, Puffer JC, Rodney WMN: The athletic heart syndrome. *N Engl J Med* 313:24–32, 1985.

32. Maron BJ, Shirani J, Poliac LC, et al: Sudden death in young competitive athletes. Clinical, demographic, and pathological profiles. *JAMA* 276(3):199–204, 1996.

33. Maron BJ, Poliac LC, Roberts WO: Risk for sudden cardiac death associated with marathon running. *J Am Coll Cardiol* 28:428–431, 1996.

34. Siscovick DS: Risks of exercising: Sudden cardiac death and injuries, in Bouchard C, Shephard RJ, Stephens T, et al. (ed): *Exercise, Fitness, and Health: A Consensus of Current Knowledge.* Champaign: Human Kinetics Books, 1990: pp. 707–713.

35. Giri S, Waters DD, Kiernan FJ, et al: Risk of exertion-related acute myocardial infarction in subjects with no history of coronary artery disease. *Circulation* 100:I–523,1999.

36. Thompson PD: The relative risk of myocardial infarction during exercise, in Fletcher G, ed. *Cardiovasculr Response to Exercise.* Mount Kisco, NY: Futura Publishing, 1994: pp. 291–300.

37. Siscovick DS, Ekelund LG, Johnson JL, et al: Sensitivity of exercise electrocardiography for acute cardiac events during moderate and strenuous physical activity: The lipid research clinics coronary primary prevention trial. *Arch Int Med* 151:325–330, 1991.

38. Van Camp SP, Peterson RA: Cardiovascular complications of outpatient cardiac rehabilitation programs. *JAMA* 256:1160–1163, 1986.

39. Haskell WL: Cardiovascular complications during exercise training of cardiac patients. *Circulation* 57:920–924, 1978.

40. Isner JM, Estes NAM, Thompson PD, et al: Acute cardiac events temporally related to cocaine abuse. *N Engl J Med* 315:1438–1443, 1986.

41. Kolodgie FD, Virmani R, Cornhill JF, et al: Increase in atherosclerosis and adventitial mast cells in cocaine abusers: An alternative mechanism of cocaine-associated coronary vasospasm and thrombosis. *J Am Coll Cardiol* 17:1553–1560, 1991.

42. Scherer D, Kaltenbach M: Häufigkeit lebensbedrohlicher Komplikationen bei ergometrischen Belastungsuntersuchungen. *Dtsch Med Wochenschr* 104:1161–1165, 1979.

43. Young DZ, Lampert S, Graboys TB, et al: Safety of maximal exercise testing in patients at high risk for ventricular arrhythmia. *Circulation* 70:184–191, 1984.

44. Rochmis P, Blackburn H: Exercise Tests: A survey of procedures, safety, and litigation experience in approximately 170,000 tests. *JAMA* 217:1061–1066, 1971.

45. Irving JB, Bruce RA: Exertional hypotension and postexertional ventricular fibrillation in stress testing. *Am J Cardiol* 39:849–851, 1977.

46. McHenry PL: Risks of graded exercise testing. *Am J Cardiol* 39:935–937, 1977.

47. Atterhög JH, Jonsson B, Samuelsson R: Exercise testing: A prospective study of complication rates. *Am Heart J* 98(5):572–579, 1979.

48. Stuart RJ Jr, Ellestad MH: National survey of exercise stress testing facilities. *Chest* 77:94–97, 1980.

49. Gibbons L, Blair SN, Kohl HW, et al: The safety of maximal exercise testing. *Circulation* 80:846–852, 1989.

50. Knight JA, Laubach CA Jr, Butcher RJ, et al: Supervision of clinical exercise testing by exercise physiologists. *Am J Cardiol* 75:390–391,1995.

51. Federal Register V62#211:59059–59062, October 31, 1997.

52. Kark JA, Posey DM, Schumacher HR, et al: Sickle-cell trait as a risk factor for sudden death in physical training. *N Engl J Med* 317:781–787, 1987.

53. Maron BJ, Thompson PD, Puffer JC, et al: Cardiovascular preparticipating screening of competitive athletes. *Circulation* 94:850–856, 1996.

54. Corrado D, Basso C, Schiavon M, et al: Screening for hypertrophic cardiomyopathy in young athletes. *N Engl J Med* 339:364–369, 1998.

55. Pelliccia A, Maron BJ: Preparticipation cardiovascular evaluation of the competitive athlete: Perspectives from the 30-year Italian experience. *Am J Cardiol* 75:827–829, 1995.

56. Maron BJ, Gardin JM, Gidding SS, et al: Prevalence of hypertrophic cardiomyopathy in a general population of young adults: Echocardiographic analysis of 4111 subjects in the CARDIA study. *Circulation* 92:785–789, 1995.

57. Maron BJ, Bodison SA, Wesley YE, et al: Results of screening a large group of intercollegiate athletes for cardiovascular disease. *J Am Coll Cardiol* 10:1214–1221, 1987.

58. Lewis JF, Maron BJ, Diggs JA, et al: Preparticipation echocardiographic screening for cardiovascular disease in a large, predominantly black population of collegiate athletes. *Am J Cardiol* 64:1029–1033, 1989.

59. Murray PM, Cantwell JD, Heath DL, et al: The role of limited echocardiography in screening athletes. *Am J Cardiol* 76:849–850, 1995.

60. Feinstein RA, Colvin E, Oh KM: Echocardiographic screening as part of a preparticipation examination. *Clin J Sports Med* 3:149–152, 1993.

61. Weidenbener EJ, Krauss MD, Waller BF, et al: Incorporation of screening echocardiography in the preparticipation exam. *Clin J Sports Med* 5:86–89, 1995.

62. Fuller CM, McNulty CM, Spring DA, et al: Prospective screening of 5,615 high school athletes for risk of sudden cardiac death. *Med Sci Sports Exerc* 29:1131–1138, 1997.

63. 26th Bethesda conference: Recommendations for determining eligibility for competition in athletes with cardiovascular abnormalities. *J Am Coll Cardiol* 24:846–899, 1994.

64. Ciampricotti R, Deckers JW, Taverne R, et al: Characteristics of conditioned and sedentary men with acute coronary syndromes. *Am J Cardiol* 73:219–222, 1994.

65. Thompson PD, Stern MP, Williams P, et al: Death during jogging or running: A study of 18 cases. *JAMA* 242:1265–1267, 1979.

66. Noakes TD: Heart disease in marathon runners: A Review. *Med Sci Sports Exerc* 19:187–194, 1987.

67. Mahler DA, Froelicher VF, Miller NH, York TD: Health screening and risk satisfaction, in Kenney WL, Humphrey RH, Bryant CX (eds.): *ACSM's Guidelines for Exercise Testing and Prescription.* 5th ed. Philadelphia, PA: A. Waverly Company, 1995: pp. 12–26.

68. Gibbons RJ, Balady GJ, Beasley JW, et al: ACC/AHA Guidelines for Exercise Testing. *J Am Coll Cardiol* 30:260–311, 1997.

69. Little WC, Constantinescu M, Applegate RJ, et al: Can coronary angiography predict the site of a subsequent myocardial infarction in patients with mild-to-moderate coronary artery disease? *Circulation* 78:1157–1166, 1988.

70. McHenry PL, O'Donnell J, Morris SN, et al: The abnormal exercise electrocardiogram in apparently healthy men: A predictor of angina pectoris as an initial coronary event during long-term follow-up. *Circulation* 70:547–551, 1984.

Chapter 7

CORONARY ARTERY DISEASE

Joseph R. Libonati, Ph.D.   Helene L. Glassberg, M.D.   Gary J. Balady, M.D.

There exists compelling data summarized in the Surgeon General's report on Physical Activity and Health[1] that physical activity reduces mortality related to coronary heart disease, hypertension, diabetes, and some cancers. Despite the benefits associated with physical activity, there are also risks. The absolute incidence of cardiovascular complications during physical activity in healthy individuals is low, but there are reports of sudden death and myocardial infarction (MI) during physical exertion in asymptomatic, presumably "fit" individuals. These cases are widely publicized and leave the lay public concerned with the cardiovascular risks of exercise. The cardiovascular risks of exercise are also a major concern for practicing physicians as they often evaluate patients prior to participation in regular exercise. Physicians must evaluate exercise-induced symptoms and may be held legally responsible for their activity recommendations.[2] The purpose of this chapter is to review the pathophysiology, risks, and incidence of exercise-related coronary artery events.

ATHEROSCLEROTIC CORONARY ARTERY DISEASE AND EXERCISE

SUPPLY–DEMAND IMBALANCE

During acute aerobic exercise, the total body oxygen needs are met by increases in cardiac output and the arteriovenous oxygen difference (AVo_2 difference). The increase in cardiac output is achieved in part by an increased heart rate, which increases the myocardial oxygen demand (MVo_2). The major factors that determine the MVo_2 during exercise are: heart rate, systolic blood pressure, myocardial inotropy, and left ventricular wall stress. Typically, the rate-pressure product, an index of the MVo_2, is used to quantify myocardial work during exercise.[3] During exercise, when MVo_2 is increased, the coronary flow must rise to supply myocardial demand because the myocardial AVo_2 difference is nearly maximal at rest.

Myocardial ischemia is the result of a mismatch between coronary blood flow (supply) and myocardial oxygen demand. The coronary artery area and the velocity of flow are critical determinants of flow, with the vessel radius (raised to the fourth power) being the primary determinant. The development of coronary atherosclerotic plaque, resulting in a decrease in vascular luminal area, can greatly compromise coronary flow and result in myocardial ischemia during exercise. Coronary artery vasoconstriction also contributes to exercise-induced ischemia in coronary artery disease patients.

FACTORS CONTRIBUTING TO ACUTE CARDIAC EVENTS

Factors such as the extent of luminal stenosis, the length of the atherosclerotic plaque, the development of coronary collaterals, the amount of muscle mass, the degree of vascular autoregulatory function, and the shape and stability of the atheroma are important determinants of how coronary atherosclerosis affects coronary flow.[4,5] Although the increased heart rate and consequent increased myocardial oxygen demand produced by exercise can generate myocardial ischemia and angina, increased MVo_2 alone is an unlikely cause of exercise-related acute cardiac events. The shape and stability of atherosclerotic plaque is important in understanding how physical exertion may trigger coronary events. Little et al have shown that the coronary lesions associated with subsequent acute MI are often only minimal-to-moderate stenoses and are generally less than 70% of the angiographic coronary diameter.[6] These data suggest that plaque rupture and coronary thrombosis, and not critically tight coronary lesions, produce most myocardial infarcts. Plaque rupture is also important in the pathogenesis of exercise-induced MI.[7] Atherosclerotic plaque typically has a lipid core encased by a fibrous cap. The inherent strength of the fibrous cap determines the vulnerability of the plaque to rupture. Typically vulnerable plaques have a thin fibrous cap that is sensitive to physical or chemical changes. The stability of the atherosclerotic fibrous cap is greatly influenced by cytokines and inflammatory processes. Pathologic studies demonstrate that plaque disruption is frequently localized to an area in the luminal wall where normal endothelium and atherosclerotic surfaces join.[4]

There are several mechanisms by which exercise may induce plaque rupture. The first possibility involves exercise-induced vasomotion of the coronary arteries. In individuals with healthy coronary arteries, exercise induces coronary vasodilation. However, in patients with coronary artery disease, exercise paradoxically produces coronary artery vasoconstriction.[8] The mechanical forces associated with coronary vasoconstriction may disrupt the fibrous cap of the coronary atheroma with subsequent thrombosis. In addition to the mechanical forces on the artery wall produced by vasomotion, vasoconstriction could also increase intracoronary pressure and turbulent flow and thereby increase the shear forces exerted on the fibrous cap and thereby contribute to plaque fissure and rupture.

The second possibility involves the stress placed on vulnerable plaque by the acute hemodynamic responses to exercise. The epicardial coronary arteries are forced to track the myocardium during contraction. Exercise increases heart rate,[9] which makes the coronary arteries experience more frequent bending and twisting with myocardial contraction. Furthermore, exercise decreases end-systolic volume and increases end-diastolic volume. This magnifies the excursion of the epicardial arteries and may contribute to cracking and rupture of the inflexible coronary plaque much as twisting a dried rubber hose contributes to its rupture. Exercise also increases systolic blood pressure, which would add to the shear stress placed on the plaque surface.[10]

Exercise could also contribute to thrombosis and an acute cardiac event once plaque disruption has occurred. During acute exercise, plasma catecholamine concentrations increase proportionally to the work rate. Catecholamines stimulate platelet aggregation[11] and could contribute to coronary thrombosis. Interestingly, platelet aggregation with exercise is most apt to occur in sedentary subjects since exercise elicits a more pronounced catecholamine release in these subjects.[11] Consequently, although there are several mechanisms by which exercise may initiate coronary events (see Fig. 7.1), all are mediated via the derangements in vascular endothelial function. Coronary vascular endothelium regulates coronary vasodilation, platelet activity, leukocyte adhesion, and intimal proliferation. The vascular endothelium dictates the balance between thrombosis and fibrinolysis. Through the synthesis and local release of several paracrine substances such as nitric oxide and prostaglandins, the vascular endothelium regulates vascular function. The pathophysiology of several vascular diseases is associated with disturbances of these regulatory functions or direct injury to the vascular endothelium. When considering vascular endothelial function, the nitric oxide system is unequivocally the most important factor in the pathophysiology of coronary events. Cardiac complications are less frequent in habitual exercisers and are perhaps due to the upregulation of the nitric oxide system as discussed later.

NITRIC OXIDE

One of the most potent endothelial-derived vasodilators is nitric oxide (NO). Initial studies showed that acetylcholine induces vasodilation in isolated rabbit aorta, as long as the vascular endothelium was present. However, when the vascular endothelium was denuded, acetylcholine-induced relaxation was attenuated.[12] These studies clearly showed the importance of vascular endothelium in vasoregulation. Nitric oxide induces vasodilation by activating soluble guanylyl cyclase and increasing intracellular cyclic 3′,5′-guanosine monophosphate (cyclic GMP) in smooth muscle cells. Beyond its role as a vasodilator, there appears to be several other impor-

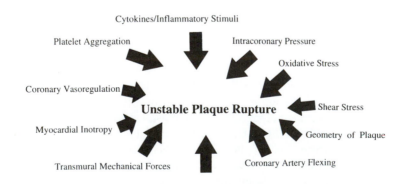

FIGURE 7.1. Potential mechanisms related to the rupture of unstable plaque.

tant actions of NO, such as inhibition of platelet activation and thrombosis[13–15] and limitation of leukocyte adhesion.[16]

Nitric oxide is synthesized from L-arginine in endothelial cells and undergoes oxidation to form citrulline and the free radical NO–.[17] This reaction is regulated by the enzyme nitric oxide synthase (NOS). There are 2 primary isoforms of NOS: the constitutive class (cNOS) and the inducible class (iNOS). The constitutive class (cNOS), consists of an endothelial form (eNOS) and the neuronal form (nNOS). Agonists such as acetylcholine and bradykinin activate the phosphoinositol second messenger system in the endothelium, thereby activating endoplasmic reticulum calcium release.[18] The increase in intracellular calcium activates cNOS, which produces NO until calcium levels return to resting concentrations.[19] Vascular tone is, in part, maintained by the basal, intermittent production of NO through the activation of cNOS.[20]

Endothelial cells produce NO in response to several physiological stimuli including platelet products, thrombin, changes in oxygen tension, and shear stress. Endothelial cells are sensitive to changes in shear stress and stretch forces produced by blood flow and pressure. An increase in blood flow appears to activate shear-sensitive calcium-dependent potassium channels that act as mechanochemical receptors, thereby inducing NO release.[21] Under normal physiological conditions, shear stress and stretch are likely responsible for tonic, basal release of NO. Inhibitors of NO synthesis, such as N-monomethyl-L-arginine (LNMMA), are known to cause vasoconstriction and hypertension,[22] suggesting that continuous endothelial production of NO is involved in the maintenance of blood pressure. Nitric oxide activity appears to be highest in large-diameter arteries, which are subject to the greatest changes in flow and shear stress.[21] Furthermore, Awolesi et al showed that cultured bovine aortic endothelial cells subjected to cyclic strain increase eNOS gene expression, protein synthesis, and activity.[23] This suggests that, in addition to the contribution of shear stress and stretch on the tonic release of NO, strain-induced increases in eNOS may, in part, explain the beneficial effects of exercise on cardiovascular disease. Sessa and coworkers showed that exercise training in dogs increases the production of coronary vascular NO, which was associated with an increase in the aortic endothelial cell expression of eNOS, suggesting that exercise-related elevations in aortic flow rates might upregulate the production of eNOS.[24] By increasing NO release, shear stress enhances endothelium-dependent vasodilation.

Nitric oxide also inhibits the aggregation of platelets in response to serotonin, ADP, and/or coagulation factors, such as thrombin.[25] Platelet inhibition occurs when NO diffuses across the vessel lumen and activates guanylyl cyclase and cyclic GMP.[20] Nitric oxide also appears to inhibit endothelial neutrophil aggregation and leukocyte adhesion.[26] The effects of NO on neutrophils are related to its action on the reactive superoxide oxygen anion. Mast cells are activated by the superoxide anion, resulting in degranulation and leukocyte adhesion to vascular endothelium.[27] By inhibiting the superoxide anion, NO reduces degranulation and leukocyte adhesion.

Impaired NO reactivity associated with atherosclerosis appears to be related to increased oxidative stress.[28] Reactive oxygen species and subsequent oxidation of low-density lipoprotein may suppress the action of NO through several mechanisms. Particularly, the superoxide anion attenuates the biological activity of NO.[29] The deleterious effects of superoxide anion have been demonstrated by studies documenting improved endothelial mediated vasoreactivity when superoxide anion is removed by free radical scavengers.[28]

Smooth-muscle proliferation is also important in the pathogenesis of atherosclerosis. The vascular endothelium is involved in cell growth as the release of several endothelial factors is linked to the proliferation of smooth-muscle cells. Mechanical removal of the endothelium is followed by proliferation of the intima,[30,31] and balloon-induced endothelial injury is inversely related to acetylcholine-induced vasodilation.[32]

These former findings[30,31] suggest that endothelium-dependent factors may suppress intimal growth, whereas the latter documents the key role of the endothelium in vasodilation.

FIBRINOLYSIS

Fibrinolysis is also regulated by the endothelium via the release of several factors, including tissue-type plasminogen activator (*t*-PA) and plasminogen activator inhibitor (PAI-1). *t*-PA is a serine protease that binds to fibrin, converting plasminogen to plasmin, which activates clot lysis. Thrombin, histamine, cytokines, and shear stress stimulate *t*-PA release. Endothelial cells have *t*-PA receptors that localize plasminogen activation.[33] PAI-1 acts to inhibit *t*-PA in plasma, which enhances thrombosis.[34] The endothelium also regulates thrombosis through synthesis of von Willebrand factor, a glycoprotein that mediates platelet adhesion to injured vascular surfaces.[33] Evidence suggests that exercise training favorably affects the fibrinolytic system. In healthy, older (60–82 years) patients who participated in 6 months of strenuous endurance exercise, there was a significant improvement in hemostatic parameters, with an increase in *t*-PA, and a reduction in fibrinogen and PAI-1.[35]

VASOACTIVE SUBSTANCES

In addition to NO, other vasorelaxing factors, such as prostacyclin and endothelium-derived hyperpolarizing factor, are secreted from the vascular endothelium. Prostaglandins are produced when arachidonic acid is generated from calcium-activated phospholipase A_2. Arachidonic acid leads to the formation of prostaglandins after it is metabolized to prostaglandin G_2 and H_2 by cyclooxygenase. The most abundantly produced prostaglandin, prostacyclin, relaxes smooth muscle and inhibits platelet aggregation by adenyl cyclase activation. All of the prostanoids, including prostacyclin, have the potential to induce vasoconstriction, although the most potent vasoconstrictors are thromboxane A_2 and the endoperoxide intermediates, PGG_2 and PGH_2.

Nitric oxide and prostacyclin indirectly oppose vasoconstriction associated with thromboxane A_2 by attenuating platelet activation and adhesion. Endothelium-derived hyperpolarizing factor is another endothelially released vasoregulator. Endothelium-derived hyperpolarizing factor hyperpolarizes vascular smooth-muscle cells by stimulating potassium efflux, thereby causing vasodilation by inhibiting calcium entry into the smooth-muscle cells.[36,37] Endothelial cells also secrete potent vasoconstrictors, substances which include endothelin and angiotensin II.

EFFECT OF HABITUAL EXERCISE ON ENDOTHELIAL FUNCTION

As discussed earlier, the majority of exercise-related acute cardiac events are likely due to endothelial dysfunction and atherosclerotic plaque rupture.[7] Multiple studies have documented that such exercise-related events are more frequent in habitually sedentary individuals and less frequent in physically active people. Sudden death during exercise, for example, is more frequent among inactive subjects as is exercise-related acute MI. Consequently, it is possible that physical activity reduces the frequency of exercise-related events by improving endothelial function. Wang and coworkers showed an improvement in endothelium-dependent epicardial vasodilation after 7 days of treadmill exercise in dogs.[38] Others have shown that exercise training enhances acetylcholine-stimulated nitrite production in dogs, reflecting an increase in NO synthesis and in messenger ribonucleic acid (mRNA) levels for eNOS.[24]

Libonati and associates[39] also documented improved endothelial function in physically active subjects suggesting that NOS production is increased following exercise training. High-resolution brachial artery ultrasound was used to assess peripheral arterial flow-mediated dilation as a measure of endothelial function, and it was observed that physical fitness was highly correlated with postocclusion hyperemia in both men and women.[39]

Exercise training or habitual physical activity

may also improve platelet function, although available studies have examined the effect of exercise on platelets directly and not the effect of exercise on the endothelial-platelet interaction. Kestin and coworkers[40] demonstrated that strenuous exercise acutely increases platelet activation and hyperreactivity in sedentary subjects, but has no effect on these parameters in physically fit subjects. Furthermore, Rauramaa and colleagues[41] showed that 12 weeks of regular moderate-intensity activity in middle-aged, overweight, and mildly hypertensive men resulted in decreased platelet aggregation.

To summarize, there is a large body of evidence that indicates that endothelial dysfunction is an important mechanism in the development of atherosclerotic diseases. Alteration in any of the activities of the endothelium and fibrinolytic system may accelerate the pathophysiology of atherosclerosis. A reduction in NO activity may result in unopposed vasoconstriction, platelet aggregation, intravascular thrombosis, and smooth-muscle proliferation. Moreover, an increased production of oxygen-derived free radicals further enhances vascular pathogenicity. A growing body of literature suggests that exercise training confers beneficial effects on endothelial function, platelet aggregation, and thrombosis. However, the role of endothelial dysfunction as it relates to plaque rupture during an acute bout of exercise is a mechanism that needs further elucidation.

EPIDEMIOLOGY OF ADVERSE CARDIOVASCULAR EVENTS DURING EXERCISE

There are two major cardiac problems during exercise due to coronary artery disease: sudden cardiac death and acute MI. Both events are primarily due to atherosclerosis and consequently confined to adults. Exercise-related coronary events in younger subjects are extremely rare and most frequently are due to congenital abnormalities in coronary artery origin and course.

SUDDEN CARDIAC DEATH

In apparently healthy subjects, the absolute risk of sudden death during exercise is quite low. Thompson et al[42] reported that the incidence of death during jogging in Rhode Island men aged 30 to 65 during the years 1975 through 1980 was only 1 death per 7620 joggers per year. However, if men with known heart disease were excluded, the annual death rate was estimated to be only 1 death per 15,000 joggers.[42] All deaths in these middle-aged men were due to coronary artery disease. Similarly, a case-controlled study of cardiac arrest during vigorous exercise documented only 1 episode of cardiac arrest occurred per every 18,000 healthy male exercisers per year.[43] Thus, on the basis of these and other studies, the exertional-related sudden death rate in previously healthy, middle-aged men is approximately 6 to 7 per 100,000 exercisers per year.[42,43]

The risk of sudden death during exercise in young individuals is much lower than it is for middle-aged adults because of the absence of advanced coronary artery disease in this group and the rarity of congenital cardiovascular problems. Van Camp et al estimated the incidence of sudden death in high school and college athletes within 1 h of competition as only 1 death per 133,333 men and 769,230 women, respectively.[44] Also, in contrast to adults where coronary artery disease predominates, only 20% of the deaths were related to coronary artery problems including anomalous coronary artery origin or course (16%), atherosclerotic disease (3%), and coronary artery aneurysm (1%), the latter possibly related to Kawasaki disease.

In both the young and old subject groups, sudden death related to exercise is more common in men. Studies in high school and college athletes suggest that the event rate is almost sixfold higher in male than in female athletes.[44] Sudden death during exercise among adult women is also rare. The explanation for these differences is not clear, but may be related to the later onset of coronary artery disease in women and the relative paucity of vigorous exercise among postmenopausal women.[45]

Despite the low absolute risk of sudden cardiac death, the rate of sudden death is considerably greater during exercise than it is at rest. Thompson et al reported a sevenfold increase in sudden death rate while jogging as compared to other activities.[42] Siscovick et al showed that inactive Seattle men were 56 times more likely to experience cardiac arrest during vigorous activity than at rest.[43] In comparison, regular exercisers were only 5 times more likely to experience cardiac arrest during vigorous exercise than they were at rest.[43] These data emphasize both the transient increase risk of sudden death during exercise and the stronger inverse relation between physical activity and all cause mortality.[46,47] (See Fig. 7.2.)

MYOCARDIAL INFARCTION

Exercise is also a potent trigger of myocardial infarction. Between 4 to 20% of MIs occur during or soon after exertion,[48–50] and the incidence of MI during exertion is 2 to 6 times greater than the incidence of MI at rest.[48,49] The symptoms of MI may manifest during the exertion, but most studies of this problem have included infarctions oc-

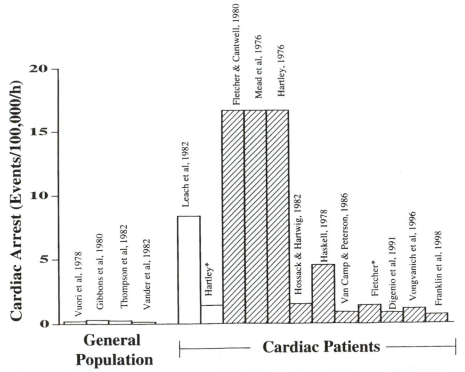

FIGURE 7.2. Cardiac arrest rate in the general population and in cardiac patients. Unsupervised exercise programs are represented by open bars and supervised exercise programs are represented by hatched bars. * Indicates unpublished data. *Adapted and modified with permission from Fletcher GF, Balady G, Froelicher VF, et al: Exercise Standards: A statement for healthcare professionals from the American Heart Association.* Circulation *91(2):580–615, 1995; and Franklin BA, Bonzheim K, Gordon S, Timmis GC: Safety of medically supervised outpatient cardiac rehabilitation exercise therapy.* Chest *114:902–906,1998.*

curring within one h of previous exercise. The incidence of MI during exercise in previously healthy, hypercholesterolemic men is 7 times greater than that of sudden cardiac death.[51] If this is true and if the annual risk of sudden death during exercise in healthy men is 1 in 15,000 to 18,000 individuals,[51,52] the risk of MI during exertion could be estimated as 1 per 2142 to 2571 asymptomatic men per year.[52]

The relative risk is greater in people who do not exercise regularly.[48,49] In sedentary people the relative risk of MI during vigorous exercise was 107 times that during less strenuous activity. Among individuals who exercised 5 times per week, the relative risk of infarction during exercise was only 2.4 times greater than at other times.[48] Such observations suggest that the potentially beneficial effects of exercise training on endothelial function and platelet activation may have direct effects on the cardiac risks of exercise.

PRODROMAL SYMPTOMS OF EXERCISE-RELATED CARDIAC EVENTS

Many "healthy" victims of cardiac-related events have prior symptoms that were ignored. Noakes reported that cardiovascular symptoms such as nausea, dizziness, and even chest discomfort had preceded sudden death in 20 of 28 marathon runners.[53] However, despite the importance of these cautionary symptoms, the runners continued running, subsequently leading to a fatal outcome.[53] It is imperative that the public recognizes prodromal cardiovascular symptoms and that clinicians advise their patients of the nature of these complaints.

CARDIOVASCULAR RISKS OF EXERCISE TESTING

The risks of exercise testing depend primarily on what group is undergoing the test. Rochmis and Blackburn in 1969 reported 8 deaths occurring within 1 h of exercise in 170,000 exercise tests.[54] In a study of 50,000 exercise tests among predominantly patient subjects, Atterhög et al re-

ported 0.4 deaths per 10,000 tests and 1.4 MIs per 10,000 tests.[55] Both of these studies examined exercise tests done in the usual clinical setting and would have included patients with known or suspected heart disease. In contrast, Wendt et al noted only 0.11 MIs and 0.02 fatal MIs per 10,000 tests in a review of 1,741,106 exercise tests that included both patients and young, healthy individuals.[56] Most of the subjects who experienced cardiovascular complications had suspected or known coronary vascular disease.[56] Among the young athletic subjects presumably without heart disease, there were no events reported in 380,000 exercise tests[56] and only 1 test complication in 71,914 persons. Based on these and other data, the estimated composite risk of death is 1 per 10,000 tests, MI is 4 per 10,000, and/or hospital admission is 5 per 10,000. These event rates can be applied to exercise testing when performed in the usual clinical setting and include both known cardiac patients and healthy individuals.[57] The absolute figures for any facility will depend primarily on the patient mix.

EXERCISE-RELATED CARDIAC EVENTS IN PATIENTS WITH DIAGNOSED CORONARY ARTERY DISEASE

The discussion to date has focused on the risks of exercise in healthy, previously asymptomatic subjects. Similar risk-benefit data exist for exercise training in patients with diagnosed coronary artery disease. A meta-analysis has documented that participation in cardiac rehabilitation exercise programs is associated with reductions in total mortality, cardiovascular mortality, and fatal reinfarctions of 20, 22, and 25%, respectively, over 3 years, but no significant difference in the 1 year rate of recurrent nonfatal infarctions.[58] Such data suggest that exercise training in such patients increases survival after a cardiac event, but does not reduce the frequency of reinfarction. Exercise training reduces the incidence of ventricular fibrillation in an animal model of cardiac ischemia.[59] Exercise training has also been shown to increase the ischemic tolerance of the myocardium.[60] Both factors could increase survival after a cardiac event in patients with preexisting disease.

Nevertheless, there are risks associated with vigorous exercise in coronary artery disease patients. Haskell[60a] compiled questionnaire data from the experience of 30 rehabilitation programs during the 1970s. One cardiac arrest, MI, and death occurred for every 33,000, 233,000, and 116,000 patient h of participation, respectively. Van Camp and Peterson evaluated statistics from 167 programs in 1985.[61] There was 1 cardiac arrest, for every 112,000, 1 MI for every 294,000, and 1 death for every 784,000 patient-h of participation.[61]

Both studies suggest that cardiac arrest is 2 to 7 times more frequent than MI in patients with known disease. This contrasts with the results in previously healthy subjects who experience exercise-related events where the ratio of sudden death to MI is approximately 1:7.[51] This may reflect the presence of myocardial scarring in the cardiac patients, which increases the risk of ventricular fibrillation.

RISK OF DELETERIOUS VENTRICULAR REMODELING AFTER MYOCARDIAL INFARCTION

Cardiac rehabilitation is standard care for patients with coronary artery disease as stated by the American Heart Association.[62] However, despite the many beneficial effects of exercise on work capacity and metabolism, the influence of exercise on left ventricular remodeling remains controversial.[63–65] Since left ventricular dilatation is inversely related to patient survival,[66] much concern has been raised whether exercise training contributed to potentially deleterious left ventricular dilatation in cardiac patients. Jugdutt et al demonstrated an increase in left ventricular dilatation and a decrease in regional and global function in a subset of patients with extensive anterior wall MI who participated in exercise training.[63] Two other studies found a similar degree of dilatation in patients after an anterior MI whether or not these patients participated in an exercise

training program. In other words, there was no worsening of this remodeling process by exercise.[64,65]

The dynamic process of left ventricular remodeling can profoundly alter the size and shape of the left ventricle. Initially, this process involves the infarcted area but may lead to subsequent geometrical alterations in noninfarcted areas. In some cases, these changes can serve as precursors to progressive left ventricular enlargement and regional shape distortion. An increase in left ventricular size[63,66] and the development of a more spherical geometry[67] tend to worsen post-MI outcome. There are several factors that have been shown to influence the extent of left ventricular remodeling after infarction. Particularly, large anterior wall infarctions involving the apex appear most susceptible to severe changes in left ventricular size and adverse myocardial function over time.

The effect of exercise on the process of left ventricular remodeling remains an important area of research since exercise training after MI is widely encouraged[62] Experimental studies on rats with surgical occlusion of the left anterior descending artery and subsequent transmural MI, who are exposed to repeated swimming exercise, have shown scar thinning and increased left ventricular dilatation when compared to sedentary rats.[68–70] However, rats with experimental infarctions who are subjected to treadmill training do not show adverse differences in cardiac function when compared to sedentary controls.[71,72]

The initial published study in humans by Jugdutt et al found that patients after the first anterior Q-wave infarction with >18% left ventricular asynergy, experienced a further increase in asynergy and a decrease in ejection fraction after 12 weeks of exercise training when compared to nonexercising controls.[63] These control patients were matched to the exercise patients by time after infarction. This study, however, is limited by small sample size, a poorly standardized exercise program, and the use of only echocardiographic short-axis views for the determination of left ventricular asynergy. In the larger multicenter

Exercise in Anterior MI (EAMI) trial, exercise training in patients after a first anterior Q-wave infarction did not result in any significant changes in global or regional left ventricular size for the group as a whole. Among patients with an ejection fraction < 40%, spontaneous global and regional left ventricular dilatation was seen similarly in both the exercise and control groups, but was not influenced by exercise training.[64] Dubach et al conducted a controlled trial of 25 patients with reduced left ventricular function (mean ejection fraction 32%) using serial left ventricular measurements obtained from magnetic resonance imaging (MRI).[65] No detrimental effects from 2 months of moderate intensity cycle exercise training on left ventricular volume or ejection fraction were noted, or was any change in these indices noted over time in the control group.[65] Cannistra et al[73] also found no overall adverse effects of exercise on various parameters of left ventricular geometry and remodeling in a controlled study of exercise in patients entered into cardiac rehabilitation early after their first MI. No index of left ventricular geometry changed significantly after 12 weeks of exercise training.[73]

Collectively, there appears to be a greater body of evidence to suggest that exercise training in patients after a first MI does not adversely affect left ventricular remodeling. To date, there is no definitive justification for withholding moderate intensity exercise training in patients who are at least 3 weeks post MI. The effects of exercise training earlier than this have yet to be studied. Thus, from the majority of the available data, moderate-to-high intensity exercise initiated 3 weeks after MI appears safe and beneficial.

NONATHEROSCLEROTIC CORONARY ARTERY DISEASE

Atherosclerotic coronary artery disease is the predominant cause of exercise-related MI and sudden cardiac death in adults. Coronary artery disease in general and atherosclerotic disease in particular are uncommon causes of exercise-

related deaths in young subjects. As noted earlier,[61] only 20% of the cardiovascular deaths in young athletes are related to coronary artery abnormalities such as anomalous coronary artery origin or course (16%), atherosclerotic disease (3%), or coronary artery aneurysm (1%). Atherosclerosis is also an unusual cause of MI in young subjects. Of all patients with acute MI, 4 to 7% do not have atherosclerotic coronary artery disease. According to necropsy data[74–76] from patients with fatal acute MI, 95% have at least 1 major epicardial coronary artery with severe luminal narrowing or total occlusion, and 5% have normal coronary arteries. Of the 95% of patients with luminal narrowing, 95% of these have typical atherosclerotic plaque. The other 5% with significant luminal narrowing have a variety of etiologies including coronary arteritis, metabolic disorders, and intimal proliferation. Of the 5% with normal coronary arteries, slightly more than one-half have coronary spasm, and the other half involves spontaneous recanalization, disproportionate myocardial oxygen supply–demand, and congenital coronary artery anomalies[74] (Fig. 7.3).

ANOMALOUS CORONARY ARTERY ORIGIN AND COURSE

Coronary artery anomalies are second only to hypertrophic cardiomyopathy as the most common cause of exercise-related deaths in young athletes.[77] Anomalous coronary arteries arise from an atypical location or follow an atypical course to the myocardium. Examples of coronary anomalies include the left coronary artery arising from the anterior sinus of Valsalva,[78] a single coronary artery, the origin of left coronary artery from the pulmonary artery, and hypoplastic coronaries. Without overt symptoms, these anomalies are difficult to identify. Symptoms when they do occur include syncope and exertional angina or patients may have resting electrocardiogram (ECG) abnormalities.[78]

Congenital coronary anomalies are found in 1 to 2% of the general population.[74,79–81] Certain anomalies are more prone to produce myocardial

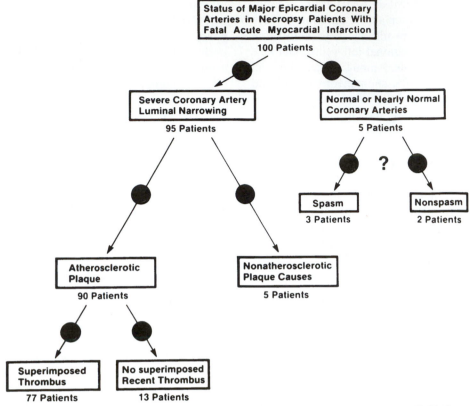

FIGURE 7.3. Coronary artery findings in necropsy patients with fatal acute myocardial infarction. *Adapted with permission from Waller BF: Atherosclerotic and nonatherosclerotic coronary artery factors in acute myocardial infarction, in Pepine CJ (ed.):* Acute Myocardial Infarction Cardiovascular Clinics. *Philadelphia, FA Davis Co. 1989, p. 20.*

ischemia/infarction, such as myocardial bridges, ostial obstruction, or passage between the pulmonary artery and the aorta. One necropsy study of 150 cases of sudden death in subjects younger than 35 years reported that 48 cases were attributed to coronary artery disease, of which 16 (33%) were nonatherosclerotic. Twelve subjects had congenital anomalies: a deep intramyocardial course in 6, origin from the wrong sinus in 3, and ostial obstruction in 3. In 6 of the 150 cases, sudden death was related to physical exertion.[82]

Taylor and colleagues[83] reported 142 cardiac deaths among 242 patients with coronary artery anomalies; 32% had sudden death, nearly one-half of which occurred during exercise. The most common coronary anomalies associated with sudden death and exercise-related death were: left main coronary artery originating for the right coronary sinus, right coronary artery originating from the left coronary sinus, and when either artery coursed between the pulmonary artery and aorta. Younger patients (< 30 years) with these conditions were more likely to die suddenly (62 vs. 12%) or during exercise (40 vs. 2%) than older patients (≥ 30 years), but this could simply reflect a survival bias in that older patients had survived their anomaly. The mechanism of sudden death, ischemia, and infarction produced by the anomalous origin of the right coronary artery from the left coronary sinus, or the left coronary artery from the right coronary sinus, is likely the altered shape of the ostium. With exercise, the pulmonary artery and the aorta dilate, and the already narrowed ostium becomes compressed and more severely narrowed. (See Figs. 7.4 and 7.5.)

MYOCARDIAL BRIDGING

Myocardial bridging, or "tunneled" epicardial coronary arteries refer to the coursing of these vessels into the subepicardial myocardium, then reappearing on the epicardial surface. The functional consequences of this anomaly remain controversial. However, the implication is that contraction of the perivascular myocardium, particularly at increased heart rates, leads to increases in systolic narrowing of the tunneled segment's luminal diameter and ultimately causes myocardial ischemia (Fig. 7.6). Yetman et al, examined the clinical significance and prognostic implications of myocardial bridging of the left anterior descending artery in children with hypertrophic cardiomyopathy.[84] Angiograms of 36 children demonstrated myocardial bridging in 28% of those studied. Compared with patients without bridging, there was a greater incidence of chest pain (60 vs. 19%), cardiac arrest (50% vs. 4%), and ventricular tachycardia (80 vs. 8%). The patients with bridging also demonstrated a reduction in blood pressure, greater ST-segment depression, and greater QT-interval dispersion with exercise, and had a shorter duration of exercise.

The diagnosis of coronary artery anomalies requires a high index of suspicion when obtaining the medical history and examination. Physical examination, ECG, and chest x-ray are usually normal. Screening exercise tests have low sensitivity, and normal results do not exclude significant anomalies. Echocardiography may be useful if specific attention is focused on coronary arteries. Although coronary angiography is the gold standard, noninvasive techniques such as MRI and nuclear imaging may become important diagnostic tools.[85]

CORONARY ARTERY VASCULITIS (ARTERITIS)

Coronary artery vasculitis can lead to myocardial ischemia/infarction and may or may not be associated with arterial thrombosis. Polyarteritis nodosa, likely the most common cause of coronary arteritis, is a necrotizing vasculitis that affects medium and small-sized vessels. Holsinger and coworkers[86] reported involvement of epicardial coronary arteries in 41 (62%) of 66 cases of polyarteritis nodosa studied, and 41 cases had MIs. Coronary arteritis has been reported at autopsy in up to 20% of patients with rheumatoid arthritis, but it rarely has clinical manifestations.[87] Cardiac involvement is a common complication in systemic lupus erythematosus (SLE), and the incidence of coronary artery disease is greater in women with SLE than it is in healthy subjects.[88] Coronary artery disease in patients with SLE has been attributed to vasculitis, immune-complex mediated endothelial injury, coronary artery thrombosis associated with the presence of antiphospholipid antibodies, and premature accelerated atherosclerosis, particularly in those treated with glucocorticosteroids.[88–90]

Various infectious diseases have been associated with coronary arteritis, including infective endocarditis,[91,92] salmonellosis,[76,92] and syphilis.[92,93] These may result in myocardial ischemia and infarction. Kawasaki disease is an acute vasculitis of unknown etiology that predominantly affects the coronary arteries of children after acute, self-limited febrile illness. In approximately 20% of patients, coronary vasculitis leads to the formation of coronary aneurysms, thrombosis, and MI. Burns and colleagues[93] reported that the mean age at presentation with cardiac sequelae was 24.7 years, and symptoms at presentation included chest pain/MI (60.8%), arrhythmia (10.8%), and sudden death (16.2%). Interestingly, these symptoms were precipitated by exercise in 82% of patients.

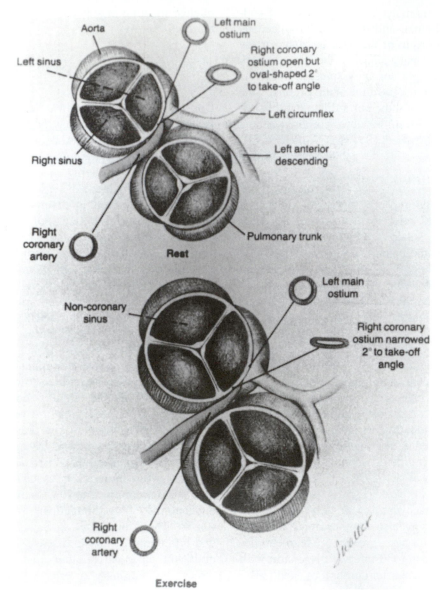

FIGURE 7.4. Illustration of the proposed mechanism of ischemia associated with anomalous origin of the right coronary artery from the left sinus of Valsalva. Exercise causes the aorta and pulmonary trunk to dilate, thereby reducing the already narrowed coronary ostium of the anomalous right coronary artery. *Adapted with permission from Waller BF: Atherosclerotic and nonatherosclerotic coronary artery factors in acute myocardial infarction, in Pepine CJ (ed.):* Acute Myocardial Infarction Cardiovascular Clinics. *Philadelphia, FA Davis Co. 1989, p. 20.*

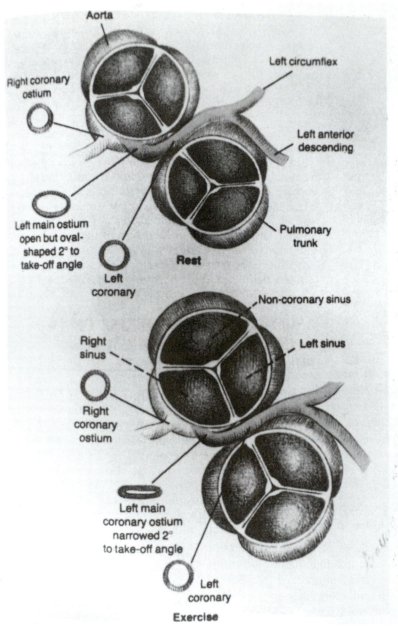

FIGURE 7.5. Illustration of the proposed mechanism of ischemia associated with anomalous origin of the left coronary artery from the right sinus of Valsalva. Exercise causes the aorta and pulmonary trunk to dilate, thereby reducing the already narrowed coronary ostium of the anomalous left coronary artery. *Adapted with permission from Waller BF: Atherosclerotic and nonatherosclerotic coronary artery factors in acute myocardial infarction, in Pepine CJ (ed.):* Acute Myocardial Infarction Cardiovascular Clinics. *Philadelphia, FA Davis Co. 1989, p. 20.*

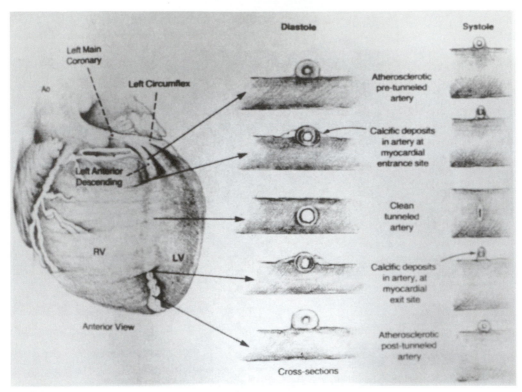

FIGURE 7.6. Illustration of tunneled and untunneled segments of coronary artery with changes during systole and diastole. Ao, aorta; LV, left ventricle; RV, right ventricle. *Adapted with permission from Waller BF: Atherosclerotic and nonatherosclerotic coronary artery factors in acute myocardial infarction, in Pepine CJ (ed.):* Acute Myocardial Infarction Cardiovascular Clinics. *Philadelphia, FA Davis Co. 1989, p. 20.*

OTHER CAUSES OF NONATHEROSCLEROTIC CORONARY DISEASE

Other less common causes of nonatherosclerotic coronary artery disease that may manifest during exercise include radiation-induced coronary stenosis following radiation therapy; cardiac transplant-associated coronary arteriopathy, presumably caused by chronic immune injury; coronary artery aneurysm, and metabolic disorders, such as homocystinuria and amyloidosis.

CORONARY ARTERY SPASM

Exertion can induce coronary artery vasospasm.[94] Vasospasm most often occurs at or near a vascu-lar segment that has been damaged by atherosclerosis, but can occur in arteries without atherosclerosis.[94] Coronary vasospasm may be suspected when myocardial ischemia occurs without significant coronary obstruction, or when great variations in the ischemic threshold occur during exercise.[95] Some of the mechanisms that induce coronary vasospasm are: atherosclerosis-induced hypercontractility of the arterial wall, elevated plasma concentrations of vasoconstrictive agents, and dysfunction of the coronary endothelium. The overall risk of exercise in patients with coronary vasospasm is unknown.

Prinzmetal's angina is also an important vasospastic syndrome. Prinzmetal's angina is defined as an atypical form of angina pectoris that is thought to be secondary to the vasospasm of otherwise normal coronary arteries. It is described as a chest discomfort that occurs most often at rest and is not usually precipitated by physical exertion. Patients tend to be young and without coronary risk factors, except that they are often cigarette smokers. Often there are frequent episodes of angina and cardiac events for 6 months following initial presentation with Prinzmetal's angina. The 5-year survival ranges from 89 to 97%, although nonfatal MI can occur in up to 20% of patients.[94,96] Moreover, vasospastic angina can result in the development of serious arrhythmias, such as ventricular tachycardia or atrioventricular block.[94] Because of the potential complications that can occur secondary to coronary vasospasm, a cautious approach to exercise in such patients is recommended where this condition is well documented.[97] Athletes with mild degrees of atherosclerosis and known vasospasm should be advised similarly to athletes with significant coronary atherosclerosis.[97] Athletes with vasospasm and angiographically normal coronary arteries should be limited to low-intensity competitive activities. For greater detail see Recommendations from the 26th Bethesda Conference.[97]

PREEXERCISE SCREENING AND EVALUATION FOR CORONARY ARTERY DISEASE

SCREENING MECHANISMS AND TOOLS

Preexercise screening is important in identifying individuals who are at risk for a cardiovascular event during exercise. The major purpose of preparticipation cardiovascular screening is to identify persons with known cardiovascular disease, symptoms of cardiovascular disease, and/or risk factors for disease development.[98] Screening also identifies persons with known cardiovascular disease who should not participate in an exercise program or who should participate at least initially in a medically supervised program, as well as persons with other special needs.[99,100] Even

simple screening instruments such as the Physical Activity Readiness Questionnaire (PAR-Q), are capable of identifying persons at risk and may increase the safety of exercise participation.[101] Even though the risk of MI and sudden death related to exertion is low, it is reasonable to assume that cardiovascular screening, particularly in old individuals, will diminish adverse cardiovascular events during exercise.

The extent and practicality of preparticipation screening is an important consideration. For instance, the wide use of exercise testing as a screening tool for all asymptomatic persons may lead to a high rate of false-positive findings.[102] Such tests are characteristically followed-up with further diagnostic procedures. This process would be both costly and inefficient. Moreover, given our understanding of the triggering factors for MI and sudden death during exercise (e.g., unstable plaque rupture), exercise testing alone may not be capable of detecting individuals at risk for an acute adverse event. An extremely thorough and mandatory screening process may also prohibit individuals from participating in an exercise program and may be counterproductive in encouraging exercise and physical activity.

Preparticipation screening should identify persons at high risk and should be simple and easy to perform. Public health efforts should focus on increasing the use of preparticipation screening at a wide variety of sites: at office visits with health care providers; at health/fitness facilities upon enrollment or registration; upon registration for athletic competition or team sports; or self-administered by an individual who wishes to begin an exercise program. The American Heart Association and the American College of Sports Medicine recommend 2 practical tools for preparticipation screening.[98] The PAR-Q is a simple, self-administered questionnaire that addresses questions concerning symptoms that possibly suggest angina pectoris. Based upon answering "yes" to one or more of the questions, individuals are encouraged to contact their physician prior to exercise. Musculoskeletal status is also addressed in the PAR-Q.

The American Heart Association and the American College of Sports Medicine Preexercise Screening Questionnaire is slightly more complex than PAR-Q.[98] It uses history, symptoms, and risk factors (including age) to assess one's risk of exercise. Individuals that are at risk for a cardiovascular event are then encouraged to contact their physician (or appropriate health care provider) before participation. High-risk individuals who wish to begin a moderate-to-vigorous exercise program are encouraged initially to exercise in health/fitness facilities with appropriate staff supervision.

Cardiovascular screening of all new members should be a sound policy for all health/fitness facilities offering exercise equipment. Currently, preexercise screening is performed only on a sporadic basis.[103] All exercise facilities must incorporate prescreening exercise health appraisals into their policies of operation. Widespread use of prescreening is important in educating new members about the signs and symptoms suggestive of cardiovascular disease during exercise. By increasing the public awareness of cardiovascular signs and symptoms during exercise, individuals would probably be more apt to appropriately terminate exercise. Without preexercise screening, it is impossible to determine whether a person may be at significant risk of injury or even death by participating in an exercise program or activity.[98]

Part of the responsibility of preparticipation health screening also falls on the prospective participant. Individuals who undergo a health appraisal and are identified as having symptoms of or known cardiovascular disease, yet neglect to obtain the recommended medical evaluation, or those who fail to complete the health appraisal questionnaire, may be excluded from participation in exercise at a health/fitness facility or athletic competition to the extent as permitted by the law.

RISK STRATIFICATION

Following the initial health appraisal and medical consultation (when indicated), individuals can be classified for exercise training using data modified from existing AHA[99] and ACSM guidelines. The following is a brief overview of the classifications developed in the AHA/ACSM Scientific Statement for Recommendations for Cardiovascular Screening, Staff, and Emergency Policies at Health Fitness Facilities. For a more detailed description, see Balady et al.[98]

Class A: Apparently healthy. There is no evidence of increased cardiovascular risk for exercise. This classification includes (a) "apparently healthy" young persons (Class A-1) and (b) old persons (Class A-2) and those with ≥ 2 cardiovascular risk factors (Class A-3) who have a normal diagnostic maximal exercise test.

Class B: Presence of known, stable cardiovascular disease with low risk for vigorous exercise but slightly greater than that for apparently healthy persons. This classification includes clinically stable persons with (a) coronary artery disease, (b) valvular heart disease, (c) congenital heart disease, (d) cardiomyopathy, (e) and exercise test abnormalities that do not meet the criteria outlined in Class C following.

Class C: Those at moderate to high risk for cardiac complications during exercise and/or who are unable to self-regulate activity or understand the recommended activity level. This classification includes persons with (a) coronary artery disease; (b) acquired valvular disease; (c) congenital heart disease; (d) cardiomyopathy; (e) exercise test abnormalities not directly related to ischema; (f) a previous episode of ventricular fibrillation or cardiac arrest that did not occur in the presence of an acute ischemic event or cardiac procedure; (g) complex ventricular arrhythmia's that are uncontrolled at mild-to-moderate work intensity with medication; (h) 3-vessel or left main coronary artery disease; and (i) ejection fraction < 30%.

Class D: Unstable conditions with activity restriction. This classification includes those with (a) unstable ischemia; (b) heart failure that is not compensated; (c) uncontrolled arrhythmias; (d) severe and symptomatic aortic stenosis; (e) hypertrophic cardiomyopathy or cardiomyopathy from recent myocarditis; (f) severe pulmonary hypertension; or (g) other conditions that could be aggravated by exercise (e.g., resting systolic blood pressure >200 mmHg or resting diastolic blood pressure > 110 mmHg; active or suspected myocarditis or pericarditis; suspected or known dissecting aneurysm; thrombophlebitis and recent systemic or pulmonary embolus). In this population, no physical activity is recommended for conditioning purposes.

On the basis of these strata it is recommended that Classes A-1 through A-3 may participate in activity of moderate intensity (but not vigorous intensity) without prior medical examination or symptom-limited exercise test. Apparently healthy young persons (Class A-1) can partake in vigorous activity without previous medical examination and/or exercise test. Classes B and C should undergo a medical examination and perform a maximal exercise test before participation in moderate or vigorous exercise unless exercise is contraindicated (i.e., Class D). Data from a medical evaluation performed within 1 year are acceptable unless clinical status has changed.

Other issues also need to be considered. Comorbidities such as insulin-dependent diabetes mellitus, morbid obesity, severe pulmonary disease, complicated pregnancy, or debilitating neurological or orthopedic conditions may constitute contraindication to exercise and/or warrant closer supervision.

Although there is an overall increased risk of cardiac events during physical exertion, the risk is small. However, this does warrant serious consideration by both the physician and patient when initiating an exercise program, as the risk may be high for an individual patient. In order to appropriately advise individuals on the risks and benefits of exercise, physicians, health care professionals, health fitness facility staff, and athletic trainers or directors should understand the risks of exercise, have a strategy for identifying those at risk, and know the proper exercise modalities to minimize such risk. In turn, all persons who participate in exercise or athletic activities should be familiar with their exercise tolerance, self-monitoring during exercise, and with their warning symptoms.

RECOMMENDATIONS FOR EXERCISE TRAINING IN PATIENTS WITH ISCHEMIC HEART DISEASE

Exercise training in patients with ischemic heart disease is an important form of therapy. However, as with other types of treatment, the efficacy of exercise must outweigh the involved risks. Exercise programs should be individualized and suited to meet the needs of the patient. Any patient with ischemic heart disease who is considering or being considered for an exercise program should undergo medical evaluation by a qualified health care provider. A complete medical history and cardiovascular status must be assessed. The training prescription is optimized when exercise is performed 3 to 5 times per week for 30 to 40 min duration at a specified intensity (range: 50-85% of VO_2 peak achieved on the exercise test).[104,105] Exercise intensity is easily monitored with the heart rate. In addition, if angina or ischemic ST depression occur, then the exercise intensity should be adjusted to an intensity that is at least 10 beats below the heart rate at which the ischemic threshold occurs.

The mode of exercise should focus on movements that require large muscle groups used in a repetitive fashion (e.g., walking or cycling). The physiological responses to exercise vary with the type of work being performed (isometric vs. dynamic) and the volume of muscle mass executing the work. At a given absolute level of external work, arm ergometry is known to yield a greater rate-pressure product than does leg ergometry or treadmill work. Yet it appears that during arm ergometry, the ischemic threshold as measured by the rate-pressure product is higher than that detected during treadmill testing.[106] Resistance training is also an important adjunct to aerobic exercise. Skeletal muscle strength and endurance have been shown to improve in cardiac patients following a program of circuit weight training[107] and, with correct supervision, can be performed safely.

PERSONAL PERSPECTIVE

WHY EXERCISE?

Despite the risks of exercise in patients with coronary artery disease as detailed in this chapter, the scientific evidence regarding the benefits of exercise argues heavily in favor of a physically active lifestyle and a program of regular exercise in most patients. Data compiled in 2 major publications from the National Institutes of Health (the Surgeon General's Report on Physical Activity and Health[1] and the AHCPR Clinical Practice Guideline on Cardiac Rehabilitation[108]) provide the most current and comprehensive overviews regarding the benefits of physical activity among persons of all ages and those with cardiovascular disease.

The specific mechanisms by which physical activity and physical fitness decrease mortality have not been well elucidated. Physical activity has been associated with favorable modifications of cardiovascular disease risk through a reduction in obesity, improved distribution of body fat, and lower incidence of non-insulin-dependent diabetes.[1] Regular exercise also yields a modest but beneficial effect on blood pressure and lipoprotein profiles.[109,110] However, the beneficial effect of physical activity cannot be accounted for solely by means of risk factor reduction, since the association with reduced mortality is independent of other coronary risk factors.[111] Emerging evidence suggests that exercise training favorably alters the fibrinolytic system,[112] autonomic nervous system,[113] and endothelial function,[114] yielding changes that may modify cardiovascular function and, thereby, reduce subsequent cardiovascular risk. Furthermore, exercise training among those with known coronary artery disease has been shown to reduce progression of atherosclerosis, reduce levels of myocardial ischemia at a given level of effort, and improve myocardial perfusion. Data suggest that these latter effects on perfusion appear to yield benefits in clinical outcome, including a significant reduction in adverse cardiac events.[115,116]

UNANSWERED QUESTIONS FOR FUTURE RESEARCH

Estimates of cardiovascular risk during exercise are drawn primarily from case reports, small regional series, and surveys that rely upon self-reporting. Indeed it is fair to state, that the absolute risk of an adverse event during exercise for a given individual remains unknown. Numerous confounding variables exist, including the modality, intensity, and duration of exercise; presence and extent of atherosclerosis and vulnerable plaque; degree of left ventricular dysfunction; cardioactive medications that work to reduce ischemia, but may induce postexercise hypotension; and comorbidities such as diabetes and chronic lung disease. As exercise and physical activity are now recognized in the broad scope of cardiovascular therapies, physicians and health care providers must become adept in prescribing safe and effective exercise programs for their patients. How can such information be integrated into the curriculum of our primary care providers and cardiologists? What resources are present to assist them in this effort? What are the most efficient methods of evaluating, risk stratifying and instructing patients regarding exercise?

Although exercise testing has important diagnostic and prognostic power, its utility in predicting events during an acute bout of exercise has not been studied. It has been assumed that exercise test variables that predict an adverse long-term outcome (e.g., ischemia at a low work rate) also predict risk of adverse events during exercise. Yet, the latter has not been demonstrated. What is the most cost-effective use of exercise testing in establishing the exercise prescription? Perhaps a risk classification scheme that incorporates both clinical and exercise test variables can be developed to provide an accurate measure of relative risk for an adverse event during a given mode and intensity of exercise.

The American Heart Association and the American College of Sports Medicine have published recommendations regarding screening, staffing, and emergency policies and procedures at the more than 15,000 health/fitness facilities in the United States. To what extent are these recommendations being followed? What is the cardiovascular emergency event rate at health/fitness facilities? Is there a reduction in cardiovascular emergency events, or at least a reduction in morbidity and mortality following such events when the AHA/ACSM recommendations are applied? Are there other screening questionnaires or simple techniques that can effectively and efficiently identify high-risk persons of any age prior to engaging in an exercise program?

REFERENCES

1. U.S. Department of Health and Human Services. Physical Activity and Health: A Report of the Surgeon General. Atlanta, GA: U.S. Department of Health and Human Services, Centers for Disease Control and Prevention, National Center for Chronic Disease Prevention and Health Promotion, 1996.
2. Thompson PD: The cardiovascular complications of vigorous physical activity. *Arch Intern Med* 156:2297–2302, 1996.
3. Kitamura K, Jorgensen CR, Gobel FL, et al: Hemodynamic correlates of myocardial oxygen consumption during upright exercise. *J Appl Physiol* 32:516–522, 1972.
4. Fuster V, Lewis A: Conner Memorial Lecture. Mechanisms leading to myocardial infarction: Insight from studies of vascular biology. *Circulation* 90:2126–2146, 1994.
5. Herzel HO, Leutwyler R, Krayenbuehl HP: Silent myocardial ischemia: Hemodynamic changes during exercise in patients with proven coronary artery disease despite absence of angina pectoris. *J Am Coll Cardiol* 6:275–284, 1985.
6. Little WC, Constantinescu M, Applegate RJ, et al: Can coronary angiography predict the site of a subsequent myocardial infarction in patients with mild-to-moderate coronary artery disease? *Circulation* 78:1157–1166, 1988.
7. Burke AP, Farb A, Malcom GT, et al: Plaque rupture and sudden death related to exertion in men with coronary artery disease. *JAMA* 281:921–926, 1999.
8. Gordon JB, Nabel EG, Fish RD, et al: Atherosclerosis influences the vasomotor response of epicardial coronary arteries to exercise. *J Clin Invest* 83:1946–1952, 1989.
9. Libonati JR, Colby AM, Caldwell TM, et al: Systolic and diastolic cardiac function time intervals and exercise capacity in women. *Med Sci Sports Exerc* 31:258–263, 1999.
10. Black BM, Gensini G: Exertion and acute coronary artery injury. *Angiology* 26:759–783, 1975.
11. Kestin AS, Kellis PA, Barnard MR, et al: Effect of strenuous exercise on platelet activation state and reactivity. *Circulation.* 88:1502–1511, 1993.

12. Furchgott RF, Zawadzki JV: The obligatory role of endothelial cells in the relaxation of arterial smooth muscle by acetylcholine. *Nature* 288:373–376, 1980.
13. Ignarro LJ, Buga GM, Wood KS, et al: Endothelium-derived relaxing factor produced and released from artery and vein is nitric oxide. *Proc Natl Acad Sci USA* 84:9265–9269, 1987.
14. Stamler JS, Singel DJ, Loscalzo J: Biochemistry of nitric oxide and its redox-activated forms. *Science* 258:1898–1902, 1992.
15. Radomski MW, Palmer RM, Moncada S: Modulation of platelet aggregation by an L-arginine-nitric oxide pathway. *Trends Pharmacol Sci* 12:87–88, 1991.
16. Kubes P, Suzuki M, Granger DN: Nitric oxide: An endogenous modulator of leukocyte adhesion. *Proc Natl Acad Sci USA* 88:4651–4655, 1991.
17. Nathan C: NO as a secretory product of mammalian cells. *FASEB J* 6:3051–3064, 1992.
18. Dinerman JL, Lowenstein CJ, Snyder SH: Molecular mechanisms and nitric oxide regulation. *Circ Res* 73:217–222, 1993.
19. Bredt DS, Ferris CD, Snyder SH: NOS regulatory sites. *J Biol Chem* 267:10976–10981, 1992.
20. Ignarro LJ, Burke TM, Wood KS, et al: Association between cyclic GMP accumulation and acetylcholine-elicited relaxation of bovine intrapulmonary artery. *J Pharmacol Exp Ther* 228:682–690, 1984.
21. Rubanyi GM, Romero JC, Vanhoutte PM: Flow-induced release of endothelium derived relaxing factor. *Am J Physiol* 250:1145–1149, 1986.
22. Vallance P, Collier JG, Moncada S: Effect of endothelium-derived nitric oxide on peripheral arteriolar tone in man. *Lancet* 28:997–1000, 1989.
23. Awolesi MA, Widmann MD, Sessa WC, et al: Cyclic strain increases endothelial nitric oxide synthase activity. *Surgery* 116:439–444, 1994.
24. Sessa W, Pritchard K, Seyedi N, et al: Chronic exercise in dogs increases coronary vascular nitric oxide production and endothelial cell nitric oxide synthase gene expression. *Circ Res* 74:349–353, 1994.
25. Lusher TF, Diederich D, Siebenbaum R, et al: Difference between endothelium-dependent relaxation in arterial and in venous coronary bypass graft. *N Engl J Med* 319:462–467, 1988.

26. Ohara Y, Peterson TE, Harrison DG: Hypercholesterolemia increases endothelial superoxide anion production. *J Clin Invest* 91:2546–2551, 1993.
27. Wei EP, Kontos HA, Christman CW, et al: Superoxide generation and reversal of acetylcholine-induced cerebral arteriolar dilatation after acute hypertension. *Circ Res* 57:781–787, 1985.
28. Anderson TJ, Merideth IT, Yeung AC, et al: The effect of cholesterol-lowering therapy and antioxidant therapy on endothelium dependent coronary vasomotion. *N Engl J Med* 332:488–493, 1995.
29. Rubanyi GM, Vanhoutte PM: Superoxide anions and hypoxia inactivate endothelium-derived relaxing factor. *Am J Physiol* 250:H822–H827, 1986.
30. Clowes AW, Reidy MA, Clowes MM: Kinetics of cellular proliferation after arterial injury. Smooth muscle growth in the absence of endothelium. *Lab Invest* 49:327–333, 1983.
31. Reidy MA: Biology of disease. A reassessment of endothelial injury and arterial lesion formation. *Lab Invest* 53:513–520, 1985.
32. Weidinger FF, McLenachan JM, Cybulski MI, et al: Persistent dysfunction of regenerated endothelium after balloon angioplasty of rabbit iliac artery. *Circulation* 81:1667–1679, 1990.
33. Meyer DE, Baumgartner HR: Role of von Willebrand factor in platelet adhesion to the subendothelium. *Br J Haematol* 54:1–9, 1983.
34. Sprengers ED, Kluft C: Plasminogen activator inhibitors. *Blood* 69:381–387, 1987.
35. Stratton JR, Chandler WL, Schwartz RS, et al: Effects of physical conditioning on fibrinolytic variables and fibrinogen in young and old healthy adults. *Circulation* 83:1692–1697, 1991.
36. Taylor SG, Weston AH: Endothelium-derived hyperpolarizing factor. A new endogenous inhibitor from the vascular endothelium. *Trends Pharmacol Sci* 9:272–274, 1988.
37. Weston AH, Edwards G: Recent progress in potassium channel opener pharmacology. *Biochem Pharmacol* 43:47–54, 1992.
38. Wang J, Wolin MS, Hintze TH: Chronic exercise enhances endothelium-mediated dilation of epicardial coronary artery in conscious dogs. *Circulation Res* 73:829–838, 1992.
39. Libonati JR, Glassberg HL, Caldwell C, et al: Brachial artery post-occlusion hyperemia

strongly predicts exercise capacity. *Circulation* 98(Suppl):I–156, 1998.
40. Kestin AS, Ellis PA, Barnard MR, et al: Effect of strenuous exercise on platelet activation state and reactivity. *Circulation* 88:1502–1511, 1993.
41. Rauramaa R, Salonen JT, Seppanen K, et al: Inhibition of platelet aggregability by moderate-intensity physical exercise: A randomized clinical trial in overweight men. *Circulation* 74:939–944, 1986.
42. Thompson PD, Funk EJ, Carleton RA, et al: Incidence of death during jogging in Rhode Island from 1975 through 1980. *JAMA* 247:2535, 1982.
43. Siscovick DS, Weiss NS, Fletcher RH, et al: The incidence of primary cardiac arrest during vigorous exercise. *N Engl J Med* 311:874–877, 1984.
44. Van Camp SP, Bloor CM, Mueller FU, et al: Nontraumatic sports deaths in high school and college athletes. *Med Sci Sports Exerc* 27:641–647, 1995.
45. Glassberg HL, Balady GJ: Exercise, women, and heart disease. *Cardiol in Rev* 7:301–308, 1999.
46. Blair SN, Kampert JB, Kuhl HW, et al: Influences of cardiorespiratory fitness and other precursors on cardiovascular disease and all-cause mortality in men and women. *JAMA* 276:205–210, 1996.
47. Powell KE, Thompson PD, Caspersen CJ, et al: Physical activity and the incidence of coronary heart disease. *Ann Rev Pub Health* 8:253–287, 1987.
48. Mittleman MA, MaClure M, Tofler GH, et al: Triggering of acute myocardial infarction by heavy physical exertion. *N Engl J Med* 329:1677–1683, 1993.
49. Willich SN, Lewis M, Lowel H, et al: Physical exertion as a trigger of acute myocardial infarction. *N Engl J Med* 329:1684–1690, 1993.
50. Tofler GH, Muller JE, Stone PH, et al: Modifiers of timing and possible triggers of acute myocardial infarction in the thrombolysis on myocardial infarction phase II (TIMI II) study group. *J Am Coll Cardiol* 20:1049–1055, 1992.
51. Siscovick DS, Ekelund LG, Johnson JL, et al: Sensitivity of exercise electrocardiography for acute cardiac events during moderate and strenous physical activity: The Lipid Research Clinics Coronary Primary Prevention Trial. *Arch Intern Med* 151:325–330, 1991.

52. Thompson PD: The cardiovascular complications of vigorous physical activity. *Arch Intern Med* 156:2297–2302, 1996.

53. Noakes TD: Heart disease in marathon runners: A review. *Med Sci Sports Exerc* 19:187–194, 1987.

54. Rochmis P, Blackburn H: Exercise tests: A survey of procedures, safety, and litigation experience in approximately 170,000 tests. *JAMA* 217:1061, 1971.

55. Atterhög JH, Bjorn J, Samuelsson R: Exercise testing: A prospective study of complication rates. *Am Heart J* 98:572–579, 1979.

56. Wendt TH, Scherer D, Kaltenbach M: Life-threatening complications in 1,741,106 ergometries. *Dtsch Med Wochenschr* 109:123–127, 1984.

57. Thompson PD: The Safety of Exercise Testing and Participation, in ACSM Resource Manual for Guidelines for Exercise Testing and Prescription, 2nd ed. Durstine L (ed). Media, PA: Williams & Wilkins, 1993, pp. 359–363.

58. O'Connor GT, Burling JE, Yusef S, et al: An overview of randomized trials of rehabilitation with exercise after myocardial infarction. *Circulation* 80:234–244, 1989.

59. Noakes TD, Higginson L, Opie LH: Physical training increases ventricular fibrillation thresholds of isolated rat hearts during normoxia, hypoxia and regional ischemia. *Circulation* 67:24–30, 1983.

60. Libonati JR, Gaughan JP, Hefner CA, et al: Reduced ischemia and reperfusion injury following exercise training. *Med Sci Sports Exerc* 29:509–516, 1997.

60a. Haskell WL: Cardiovascular complications during exercise training of cardiac patients. *Circulation* 57:920–924, 1978.

61. VanCamp SP, Peterson RA: Cardiovascular complications of outpatient cardiac rehabilitation programs. *JAMA* 256:1160–1163, 1986.

62. Balady GJ, Fletcher BJ, Froelicher ES, et al: Cardiac rehabilitation programs: A statement for healthcare professionals from the American Heart Association. *Circulation* 90:1602–1610, 1994.

63. Jugdutt BI, Michorowski BL, Kappagoda CT: Exercise training after anterior Q wave myocardial infarction: Importance of regional left ventricular function and topography. *J Am Coll Cardiol* 12:362–372, 1988.

64. Giannuzzi P, Tavazzi L, Temporelli PL, et al: Long-term physical training and left ventricular remodeling after myocardial infarction: Results of the exercise in anterior myocardial infarction (EAMI) trial. *J Am Coll Cardiol* 22:1821–1829, 1993.

65. Dubach P, Meyers J, Dziekan G, et al: Effect of exercise training on myocardial remodeling in patients with reduced left ventricular function after myocardial infarction; application of magnetic resonance imaging. *Circulation* 95:2060–2067, 1997.

66. Braunwald E, Pfeffer MA: Ventricular enlargement and remodeling following acute myocardial infarction: Mechanisms and management. *Am J Cardiol* 68:1D–6D, 1991.

67. Lamas GA, Vaughan DE, Parisi AF, et al: Effects of left ventricular shape and captopril therapy on exercise capacity after anterior wall acute myocardial infarction. *Am J Cardiol* 63:1167–1173, 1989.

68. Kloner RA, Kloner JA: The effect of early exercise in myocardial infarct scar formation. *Am Heart J* 5:1009–1013, 1983.

69. Hammerman H, Schoen FJ, Kloner RA: Short-term exercise has a prolonged effect on scar formation after experimental acute infarction. *J Am Coll Cardiol* 2:979–982, 1983.

70. Gaudron P, Kai H, Schamberger R, et al: Effect of endurance training early or late after coronary artery occlusion on left ventricular remodeling, hemodynamics, and survival in rats with chronic transmural myocardial infarction. *Circulation* 89:402–412, 1994.

71. Libonati JR, Apstein CS, Ngoy S, et al: Moderate intensity exercise training and ventricular remodeling following infarction: Echocardiographic and isolated heart studies. *Circulation* 92(8, Suppl):I–398, 1995.

72. Orenstein TL, Parker TG, Butany JW, et al: Favorable left ventricular remodeling following large myocardial infarction by exercise training. *J Clin Invest* 96:858–866, 1995.

73. Cannistra LB, Davidoff R, Picard MH, et al: Effect of exercise training after myocardial infarction on left ventricular remodeling relative to infarct size. *J Cardiopul Rehab* 19:373–380, 1999.

74. Waller BF: Atherosclerotic and nonatherosclerotic coronary artery factors in acute myocardial infarction, in Pepine CJ (ed): *Acute Myocardial Infarction*. Philadelphia, PA: FA Davis, 1989, pp. 29–104.

75. Eliot RS, Baroldi G: Necropsy studies in myocardial infarction with minimal or no coronary luminal reduction due to atherosclerosis. *Circulation* 49:1127–1131, 1974.

76. Cheitlin MD, McAllister HA, deCastro CM: Myocardial infarction without atherosclerosis. *JAMA* 231:951–959, 1975.

77. Maron BJ, Shirani J, Poliac LC, et al: Sudden death in young competitive athletes: Clinical, demographic and pathological profiles. *JAMA* 276:199–204,1996

78. Barth CW, Roberts WC: Left main coronary artery originating from the right sinus of Valsalva and coursing between the aorta and pulmonary trunk. *J Am Coll Cardiol* 7:366–373, 1986.

79. Roberts WC: Major anomalies of coronary arterial origin seen in adulthood. *Am Heart J* 111:941–963, 1986.

80. Levin DC, Fellows KE, Abrams HL: Hemodynamically significant primary anomalies of the coronary arteries. Angiographic aspects. *Circulation* 58:25–34, 1978.

81. Virmani R, Chun PKC, Goldstein RE, et al: Acute takeoffs of the coronary arteries along the aortic wall and congenital coronary ostial valve-like ridges. Association with sudden death. *J Am Coll Cardiol* 3:766–771, 1984.

82. Corrado D, Thiene G, Cocco P, et al: Nonatherosclerotic coronary artery disease and sudden death in the young. *Br Heart J* 68:601–607, 1992.

83. Taylor AJ, Rogan KM, Virmani R: Sudden death associated with isolated congenital coronary artery anomalies. *J Am Coll Cardiol* 20:640–647, 1992.

84. Yetman AT, McCrindle BW, MacDonald C, et al: Myocardial bridging in children with hypertrophic cardiomyopathy: A risk factor for sudden death. *N Engl J Med* 339:1201–1209, 1998.

85. Chu E, Cheitlin MD: Diagnostic considerations in patients with suspected coronary artery anomalies. *Am Heart J* 1427–1438, 1993.

86. Holsinger DR, Osmundson PJ, Edwards JE: The heart in periarteritis nodosa. *Circulation* 25:610–618, 1962.

87. Morris PB, Imber MJ, Heinsimer JA, et al: Rheumatoid arthritis and coronary arteritis. *Am J Cardiol* 57:689, 1986.

88. Bidani AK, Roberts JL, Schwartz M, et al: Immunopathology of cardiac lesions in fatal systemic lupus erythematosus. *Am J Med* 69:849, 1980.

89. Korbet SM, Schwartz MM, Lewis EJ: Immune complex deposition and coronary vasculitis in systemic lupus erythematosus: Report of two cases. *Am J Med* 77:141, 1984.

90. Leung WH, Wong KL, Lau CP, et al: Association between antiphospholipid antibodies and cardiac abnormalities in patients with systemic lupus erythematosus. *Am J Med* 89:411, 1990.

91. Saphir O, Katz LN, Gore I: The myocardium in subacute bacterial endocarditis. *Circulation* 1:1155–1167, 1950.

92. Waller BF: Nonatherosclerotic coronary heart disease, in Hurst JW, Schlant RC, Alexander RW, O'Rourke RA, Roberts R, Sonnenblick EH (eds): *The Heart,* 8th ed. New York, McGraw-Hill, 1994, pp. 1255.

93. Burns JC, Shike H, Gordon JB, et al. Sequelae of Kawasaki disease in adolescents and young adults. *J Am Coll Cardiol* 28:253–257, 1996.

94. Yasue H, Takizawa D, Nagao M, et al: Long term prognosis of patients with variant angina and influential factors. *Circulation* 78:1, 1988.

95. Ciampricotti R, El Gamal MIH, Bonnier JJ, et al: Myocardial infarction and sudden death after sport: Acute coronary angiographic findings. *Cathet Cardiovasc Diagn* 17:193–197, 1989.

96. Gersh BJ, Braunwald E, Rutherford JD: Chronic coronary artery disease, in Braunwald E (ed.): *Heart Disease: A Textbook of Cardiovascular Medicine,* 5th ed. Philadelphia: WB Saunders, 1997.

97. Thompson PD, Klocke FJ, Levine BD, et al: Task Force 5: Coronary artery disease. 26th Bethesda Conference. Recommendations for determining eligibility for competition in athletes with cardiovascular abnormalities. *J Am Coll Cardiol* 24:845–899, 1994.

98. Balady GJ, Chaitman B, Driscoll D, et al: Recommendations for cardiovascular screening, staffing, and emergency policies at health/fitness facilities. *Circulation* 97:2283–2293, 1998.

99. Fletcher GF, Balady G, Froelicher VF, et al: Exercise standards: A statement for healthcare professionals from the American Heart Association. *Circulation* 91:580–615, 1995.

100. Fletcher GF, Balady G, Blair SN, et al: Statement on exercise: Benefits and recommendations for

physical activity programs for all Americans. A statement for health professionals by the Committee on Exercise and Cardiac Rehabilitation of the Council in Clinical Cardiology, American Heart Association. *Circulation* 94:857, 1996.

101. Shephard RJ, Thomas S, Weller I: The Canadian home fitness test: 1991 update. *Sports Med* 11:358–366, 1991.

102. Gibbons RJ, Balady GJ, Beasley JW, et al: ACC/AHA guidelines for exercise testing: A report of the American College of Cardiology/American Heart Association Task Force on Practice Guidelines. *J Am Coll Cardiol* 30:260–311, 1997.

103. McInnis KJ, Hayakawa S, Balady GJ: Cardivascular screening and emergency procedures at health clubs and fitness centers. *Am J Cardiol* 80:380–383, 1997.

104. Braith RW, Welsh MA, Mills RM, et al: Resistance exercise prevents glucocorticoid-induced myopathy in heart transplant recipients. *Med Sci Sports Exerc* 30:483–489, 1998.

105. Kenney L (ed.): *ACSM's Guidelines for Exercise Testing and Presciption* (5th ed), Media, PA: Williams & Wilkins, 1995.

106. Balady GJ, Weiner DA, McCabe CH, et al: Value of arm testing in detecting coronary artery disease. *Am J Cardiol* 55:37–39, 1985.

107. Kelemen MH, Stewart KG, Gillilan RE, et al: Circuit weight training in cardiac patients. *J Am Coll Cardiol* 7:38–42, 1986.

108. Wenger NK, Froelicher ES, Smith LK, et al: Cardiac Rehabilitation. Clinical Practice Guideline No.17. Rockville, MD: U.S. Department of Health and Human Services, Public Health Service, Agencies for Health Care Policy and Research, and the National Heart, Lung, and Blood Institute. AHCPR Publication No. 96–0672. October 1995.

109. Hagberg JM, Montain SJ, Martin WH: Effect of exercise training in 60–69-year-old persons with essential hypertension. *Am J Cardiol* 64: 348–353, 1989.

110. Stefanick M, Mackey S, Sheehan M, et al: Effects of diet and exercise in men and postmenopausal women with low levels of HDL cholesterol and high levels of LDL cholesterol. *N Engl J Med* 339:12–20, 1998.

111. Blair SN, Kampert JB, Kohl HW, et al: Influences of cardiorespiratory fitness and other precursors on cardiovascular disease and all-cause mortality in men and women. *JAMA* 276:205–210, 1996.

112. Stratton JR, Chandler WL, Schwartz RS, et al: Effects of physical conditioning on fibrinolytic variables in young and old healthy adults. *Circulation* 83:1692–1697, 1991.

113. Coats AJS: Exercise rehabilitation in chronic heart failure. *J Am Coll Cardiol* 22(Suppl A):172A–177A, 1993.

114. Charo S, Gokce N, Vita J: Endothelial dysfunction and coronary risk reduction. *J Cardiopul Rehabil* 18:60–67, 1998.

115. Haskell W, Alderman E, Fair J, et al: Effects of intensive multiple risk factor reduction on coronary atherosclerosis and clinical cardiac events in men and women with coronary artery disease: The Stanford Coronary Risk Intervention Project (SCRIP). *Circulation* 89:975–990, 1994.

116. Belardinelli R, Georgiu D, Purcaro A. Low dose dobutamine echocardiography predicts improvement in functional capacity after exercise training in patients with ischemic cardiomyopathy: Prognostic implication. *J Am Coll Cardiol* 31:1027–1034, 1998.

Chapter 8

MARFAN SYNDROME AND OTHER DISORDERS OF VASCULAR FRAGILITY: IMPLICATIONS FOR EXERCISE

Reed E. Pyeritz, M.D., Ph.D.

CLINICAL PRESENTATIONS OF VASCULAR FRAGILITY

Circulation of blood occurs through vessels of varying caliber and function. The wall of the vessel can be as highly complex as that of an elastic artery, or as simple as that of a capillary that consists of a single endothelial cell and a basement membrane. Blood vessels are subject to an array of pathologic processes, such as atherosclerosis, thrombosis, and calcification, that depend on the intrinsic properties of the vascular wall. This chapter deals with the common causes of dilatation, dissection and rupture of blood vessels of any caliber. The focus is on the young patient who might be at risk from vigorous exertion, so the degenerative conditions that are increasingly common in later life will be mentioned only in passing. The first section reviews the clinical presentations and consequences of these types of vascular problems. The second section considers specific disorders, their diagnoses, and their management in active people.

ARTERIAL ANEURYSM

The caliber of any given portion of any given artery normally varies as a function of age and body size. Standards, however, exist for major arteries, especially the aorta.[1,2] It should be noted that several terms cause confusion and unfortunately are often interchanged. *Aneurysm* can be a subjective term. What degree of dilatation constitutes an aneurysm varies among studies and clinical usage; for the aorta, a criterion of 1.5 times the expected normal diameter for the vessel at the specific location has been suggested.[3] However, an aneurysm is anatomically limited to a short region of a vessel, although an individual might have multiple aneurysms of the same vessel. *Ectasia* refers to an extensive dilatation, which may be confined to a single vessel, or be more generalized, even systemic. The symmetry of dilatation is also used to classify aneurysms: a *fusiform* aneurysm is symmetric and extends over at least 5 to 8 cm; a *saccular* aneurysm represents a defect of one portion of the arterial wall and is exemplified by the "berry" aneurysm commonly seen in the cerebral circulation. A *pseudoaneurysm* is not a true aneurysm, but a collection of blood (clotted, free-flowing, or both) that is extravascular; a common cause is a traumatic or pathologic rupture contained by organized thrombus and structures surrounding the artery. Occasionally the initial rupture is iatrogenic, such as by arterial cannulation.

The caliber of an artery can be abnormally large due to trauma, inflammation, infection, focal or generalized developmental defects, or generalized defects of one or another component of the vascular wall. The diameter of the ascending aorta increases modestly, but significantly, as a function of age. The causes of aneurysms vary with the type of artery and the location. The most common causes of aortic aneurysms, classified by location, are listed in Table 8.1. Since many of the causes involve systemic pathology, the discovery of one aneurysm should prompt a search for others.

Gradual dilatation of an artery is usually pain-

TABLE 8.1.   CAUSES OF AORTIC ANEURYSMS

Site	Cause
Root	Medial degeneration ("cystic medial necrosis") Marfan syndrome and other defects of fibrillin-1, bicuspid aortic valve, aortic coarctation, or both
	Aortic dissection
	Arteritis (e.g., polyarteritis, Beçhet, relapsing polychondritis, ankylosing spondylitis, psoriatic arthritis, Reiter syndrome)
Ascending	Medial degeneration (extension from root or primarily superior to the sinotubular junction)
	Syphilis (rare in developed countries)
	Aortic dissection
Arch	Extension from the ascending aorta
	Atherosclerosis
	Aortic dissection
	Trauma (especially distal arch)
Descending thoracic	Atherosclerosis
	Trauma (especially proximal)
	Dissection
Abdominal	Medial degeneration (inflammatory, often familial)
	? Atherosclerosis

less, although if the cause is a generalized condition, such as polyarteritis nodosum or adult polycystic kidney disease, the patient may be symptomatic in other ways. However, the chronic and progressive dilatation of the aortic root that occurs in Marfan syndrome, and of the abdominal aorta in the common forms of aneurysmal disease, are in and of themselves without symptoms even to large diameter (6–8 cm). The appearance of pain usually means rapid expansion or localized tearing, perhaps heralding rupture. Physicians ignore this clue at their patient's—and their own—peril.

Clinical sequelae of an aneurysm relate to its location and to the vascular forces acting on it. Complications include: dissection, rupture, or both (covered in the next section); local pressure on surrounding structures; and, in the case of the aortic root, aortic regurgitation. Even large aneurysms of the aorta rarely cause problems related only to their size. An exception is stretching of the recurrent laryngeal and vagus nerves that course around the aortic arch. Aneurysm is always in the differential of otherwise unexplained hoarseness because aortic arch aneurysms can affect the recurrent laryngeal nerve.

As a general rule of thumb, aneurysms of any part of the aorta that reach 55 mm in diameter should be repaired.[4–6]

ARTERIAL DISSECTION OR RUPTURE

A dissection is the entry of the circulation into the wall of a vessel. This usually occurs when the media is defective and an intimal tear occurs. Occasionally, rupture of the vasovasorum produces an intramural hematoma, which may stabilize or progress to a frank dissection. A dissection is fully contained within the vessel, and it may progress for any length antegrade or retrograde and even reenter the true lumen of the vessel. Complications of dissection include blockage of branch vessels (leading to myocardial infarction, stroke, limb ischemia, paraplegia, etc.), rupture, and aortic regurgitation (in ascending aortic dissection).[7] The causes of aortic dissection are listed in Table 8.2. The relation of LaPlace pertains, especially, to capacitance vessels such as the aorta. The tension on the vascular wall is directly related to the radius and the blood pressure and indirectly related to the thickness of the wall. In Marfan syndrome, as the radius increases the wall thins, and the tension on the wall increases markedly. This accounts for the well-documented increasing risk of dissection as the caliber of the aortic root increases, even if there is considerable individual variation in risk at equal aortic diameters. In syphilitic aortitis, in contrast, the wall becomes thickened and even calcified, and despite substantial dilatation, dissection is uncommon.

Because of location, the common and internal carotid arteries are susceptible to blunt and torsional trauma during athletic activities. Dissection can result in an acute cerebral ischemic event.[8] Intrinsic abnormalities of the aortic wall clearly predispose to such events.

Rupture is a tear through all layers of the vessel wall, and in the case of the aorta is often preceded by dissection. The causes of arterial rupture are shown in Table 8.3. The complications of rupture depend on the size of the vessel and the location of the tear. Dissection of the ascending aorta may extend retrograde and rupture into the pericardial sac, producing tamponade. Rupture of any other portion of the aorta stands a high risk of massive hemorrhage and hypovolemic shock. Occasionally aortic rupture occurs into the pulmonary artery, esophagus, or intestine. Focal rupture due to trauma, even of the aorta, may produce a pseudoaneurysm that remains contained, at least for a time. Rupture of a peripheral artery often produces a focal hematoma that may tamponade the vascular tear. One risk is that the hematoma will itself cause problems, such as compartment syndrome leading to myonecrosis or venous obstruction leading to edema.

VENOUS VARICOSITIES

Dilatation of veins is poorly understood as to cause and pathogenesis. Genetic factors clearly play a role, as varicosities of the superficial veins of the lower extremities occur with increased fre-

TABLE 8.2. CAUSES OF ARTERIAL DISSECTION

Medial degeneration often with preceding aneurysm
    Marfan syndrome
    Ehlers-Danlos syndrome (classic type)
    Familial aortic dissection
    Bicuspid aortic valve, aortic coarctation, or both
Pregnancy
Trauma (especially intraluminal hematoma)
Hypertension
Iatrogenic (intravascular procedures)

TABLE 8.3. CAUSES OF ARTERIAL RUPTURE

Intrinsic wall defects
    Ehlers-Danlos syndrome (vascular type)
    Berry aneurysms
Aortic dissection
Trauma (wall disruption)
Iatrogenic (e.g., cannulation)

quency in Marfan syndrome and in some families without an evident connective tissue disorder.[9] The process is clearly a vicious cycle; as a vein dilates, a valve becomes incompetent, which leads to pooling of blood and further intravascular pressure on the dependent (inferior) portion of the vein. Developmental defects of veins occur in several conditions, including Klippel-Trenaunay-Weber syndrome and the Noonan syndrome. Peripheral edema, especially of the legs, has early onset and persistence, despite aggressive treatment with compression stockings.

The complications of chronic venous varicosities include those of venous stasis: edema; skin changes of atrophy, loss of hair, and hyperpigmentation; and poor wound healing.

ARTERIOVENOUS MALFORMATIONS

All normal connections between the arterial and venous sides of the circulation occur through capillaries. Capillaries not only mediate the transfer of oxygen and nutrients to tissues in end organs and in uptake of carbon dioxide, but provide for the gradual diminution of arterial pressure to that of the venous system. Anytime the connection occurs at the level of arterioles and venules or resistance arteries and veins, then all functions of capillaries are lost. Arteriovenous malformations (AVMs) are most commonly developmental or traumatic. When developmental, multiple AVMs are likely. Table 8.4 lists the most frequent conditions associated with AVMs. Traumatic AVMs may occur from blunt trauma (usually of an extremity) or penetrating wounds. Iatrogenic AVMs may be unintentional (surgical misadventures) or intentional, such as shunts and fistulas for access for hemodialysis.

Complications of AVMs include high-output cardiac failure (usually associated with either multiple AVMs or a communication between a single large artery and vein); consequences of emboli (stroke, end-organ ischemia, abscess); systemic hypoxemia (pulmonary AVMs); and rupture usually of the vessel at the arterial side of the malformation.

CAPILLARY FRAGILITY

Generalized capillary fragility is usually associated with systemic disorders of connective tissue, such as Ehlers-Danlos syndrome, especially the vascular form. The most common cause of acquired capillary fragility is excess adrenocortical hormones, either through overproduction (e.g., Cushing syndrome) or exogenous sources.

The major complication is excessive bruising, with subsequent hyperpigmentation and skin atrophy.

DISORDERS THAT PREDISPOSE TO VASCULAR FRAGILITY

MARFAN SYNDROME

FEATURES, DIAGNOSTIC CRITERIA, AND NATURAL HISTORY

The Marfan syndrome is due to defects in the *FBN1* gene that encodes the microfibrillar protein, fibrillin-1.[10–13] Manifestations occur in many systems, especially the eye, the skeleton, the dura, the lung, and the cardiovascular system. The diagnosis is based largely on clinical criteria[14] (Table 8.4). No laboratory is currently offering analysis of the *FBN1* gene on a clinical basis.[15] The Marfan syndrome is more prevalent than was generally recognized; at least 1 per 5000 is affected, and all ethnic groups are equally affected.

GENETIC ASPECTS

No family that meets the clinical diagnostic criteria has failed to map to the *FBN1* locus, although the possibility continues to exist. The Marfan syndrome is inherited as an autosomal dominant trait, meaning that males and females are equally frequently affected, and an affected person has a 50–50 chance at each conception of passing the condition to an offspring.[11] However, about one-quarter or more of people with Marfan syndrome have neither parent affected; these so-called sporadic cases arise from a *de novo* mutation in the egg or sperm that result in that conception. The average age of fathers is advanced in sporadic cases,

TABLE 8.4. DIAGNOSTIC CRITERIA FOR THE MARFAN SYNDROME

Skeletal System

Major criteria (Presence of at least four of the following manifestations.)
  Pectus carinatum
  Pectus excavatum requiring or in need of surgery
  Reduced upper to lower segment ratio or arm span to height ratio greater than 1.05
  Positive wrist and thumb signs
  Scoliosis of ≥ 20 or spondylolithesis
  Reduced extension of the elbows (< 170)
  Medial displacement of the medial malleolus causing pes planus
  Protrusio acetabulae of any degree (ascertained on x-ray, CT, or MRI)
Minor criteria
  Pectus excavatum of moderate severity
  Joint hypermobility
  Highly arched palate with dental crowding
  Facial appearance (dolicocephaly, malar hypoplasia, enophthalmos, retrognathia, down-slanting palpebral
    fissures)
*For the skeletal system to be involved, at least two of the components comprising the major criterion or one
component comprising the major criterion plus two of the minor criteria must be present.*

Ocular System

Major criterion
  Ectopia lentis
Minor criteria
  Abnormally flat cornea (as measured by keratometry)
  Increased axial length of globe (as measured by ultrasound)
  Hypoplastic iris or hypoplastic ciliary muscle causing a decreased miosis
For the ocular system to be involved, at least two of the minor criteria must be present.

Cardiovascular System

Major criteria
  Dilatation of the ascending aorta with or without aortic regurgitation and involving at least the sinuses
    of Valsalva *or*
  Dissection of the ascending aorta
Minor criteria
  Mitral valve prolapse with or without mitral valve regurgitation;
  Dilatation of main pulmonary artery, in absence of valvular or peripheral pulmonic stenosis or any other
    obvious cause, below the age of 40 years;
  Calcification of the mitral annulus below the age of 40 years; *or*
  Dilatation or dissection of the descending thoracic or abdominal aorta below the age of 50 years
*For the cardiovascular system to be involved a major criterion or only one of the minor criteria must be
  present.*

Pulmonary System

Major criteria
  None
Minor criteria
  Spontaneous pneumothorax *or*
  Apical blebs (ascertained by chest radiography)
For the pulmonary system to be involved one of the minor criteria must be present.

TABLE 8.4. CONTINUED

Skin and Integument

Major criterion
  Lumbosacral dural ectasia by CT or MRI
Minor criteria
  Striae atrophicae (stretch marks) not associated with marked weight changes, pregnancy or repetitive stress
    or
  Recurrent or incisional herniae
  For the skin and integument to be involved the major criterion or one of the minor criteria must be present.

Family History

Major criteria
  Having a parent, child, or sibling who meets these diagnostic criteria independently;
  Presence of a mutation in *FBN1* known to cause the Marfan syndrome; *or*
  Presence of a haplotype around *FBN1,* inherited by descent, known to be associated with unequivocally
    diagnosed Marfan syndrome in the family
Minor criteria
  None
  For the family history to be contributory, one of the major criteria must be present.

Requirements of the Diagnosis of the Marfan Syndrome

For the index case
  Major criteria in at least 2 different organ systems and involvement of a third organ system
For a family member
  Presence of a major criterion in the family history and one major criterion in an organ system and involve-
  ment of a second organ system

Adapted with permission from DePaepe A, Dietz HC, Devereux RB, et al: Revised diagnostic criteria for the Marfan syndrome. *Am J Med Genet* 62:417, 1996.

a feature observed in many autosomal dominant conditions. Thus, the possibility of germinal mosaicism exists and has been documented in at least one case. This means that the unaffected parents of a sporadic case have only a small risk (~1/1000) chance of having a second affected child.

PATHOLOGY AND PATHOPHYSIOLOGY

The major risks to an athlete with Marfan syndrome concern the cardiovascular system.[16–18] This is due to the two primary defects, aortic root dilatation and mitral valve prolapse. Because the aortic root is usually dilated, even at an early age,[19,20] the risk of ascending aortic dissection is increased (Fig. 8.1). The degree of dilatation, and its progression during childhood and adolescence, can be assessed based on the body surface area.[2,21] The risk of dissection is roughly proportional to diameter, although the family history of early dissection is an important predictor.[22,23]

MANAGEMENT AND SPECIAL CONSIDERATIONS FOR THE ATHLETE

The major risks associated with physical exertion are an electrical event and aortic dissection. Dysrhythmia is almost always associated with mitral valve prolapse and often with a history of palpitations. A careful history and physical examination can usually detect those patients who need closer scrutiny, such as ambulatory electrocardiogram (ECG) monitoring or exercise testing.[24]

The aortic root dilates gradually, probably due to the repetitious stress of left ventricular ejection on the intrinsically weak arterial wall (Fig. 8.2). Thus, management should address three issues:

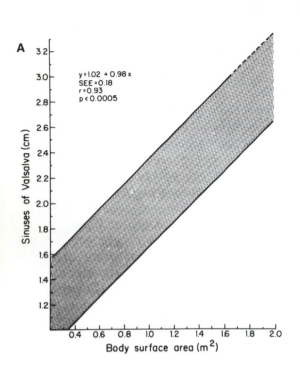

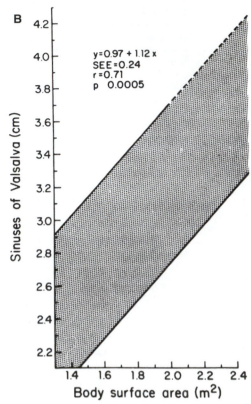

FIGURE 8.1. This shows 95% normal confidence intervals for aortic root diameter at the sinuses of Valsalva in relation to body surface area. A. Infants and children. B. Adults less than 40 years old. Adapted with permission from Roman MJ, Devereux RB, Karamer-Fox R, et al: Two-dimensional echocardiographic aortic root dimensions in normal children and adults. Am J Cardiol 64:507, 1989.

detecting aortic dilatation;[25,26] reducing the chance of a traumatic event that would suddenly damage the weakened aortic wall; and reducing the repetitive stresses acting to dilate the root. The cornerstones to each are avoiding contact sports that risk deceleration injury to the aorta; avoiding isometric exertion that greatly increases the blood pressure-heart rate product; and using β-adrenergic blockade to reduce inotropy and chronotropy.[27–29] Atenolol is a reasonable choice to begin; dosage must be individualized with a goal of keeping the resting pulse at 60 beats per minute or less, the submaximal exercise pulse less than 110 in an adult (e.g., after running up and down two flights of stairs), and the resting blood pressure in the

normal range. Pharmacological therapy and exercise restriction should be instituted as soon as the diagnosis is established. The larger the aortic root, the greater the exercise restriction. For those with minimal or mild aortic root dilatation, exertion at an aerobic pace is probably not harmful and may be beneficial in terms of self-esteem and general physical conditioning.

The life-expectancy of people with Marfan syndrome has been increased markedly through three advances: early diagnosis, exercise restriction and β-adrenergic blockade, and prophylactic aortic root surgery.[30] When adults with Marfan syndrome who have aortic root dilatation of moderate degree (50–55 mm) undergo prophylactic

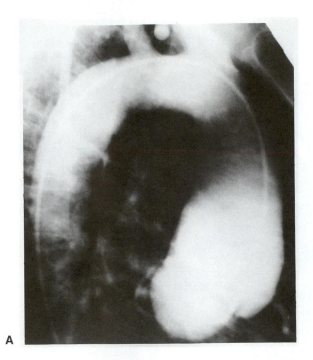

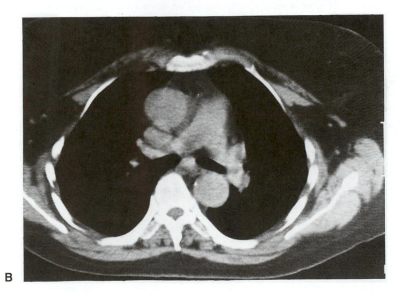

FIGURE 8.2. Imaging studies of the ascending aorta in a woman with Marfan syndrome. A. An aortogram at age 50 showing typical aortic root aneurysm in the Marfan syndrome. B. A CT scan also at age 50 showing dilatation limited to the ascending aorta.

(continues)

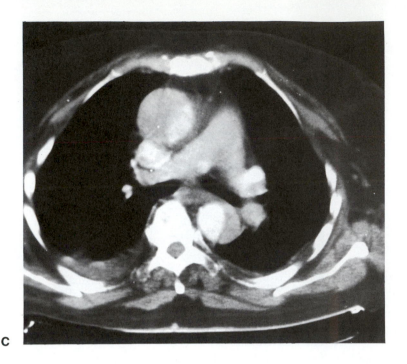

C

FIGURE 8.2. C. A CT scan at age 53 at the time of an acute type I dissection; note the double lumen in both the ascending and descending limbs of the thoracic aorta.

repair, the surgical risks are minimal (< 2% mortality[5]) and long-term survival into the seventh decade is becoming common.[30] For the past 25 years, the standard approach to prophylactic aortic root repair has been with a composite graft, which requires life-long anticoagulation with warfarin. This alone precludes activities that carry a risk of head injury or other trauma. An approach to root repair, the valve-sparing procedure, has now been used with good short- and intermediate-term results in people with Marfan syndrome who have no more than mild aortic regurgitation at the time of surgery.[5,31,32] Because the native valve is preserved, anticoagulation is not necessary. This proves particularly beneficial to young women who want to undertake pregnancy. However, given the uncertain natural history of the Marfan aorta above the graft,[5,33] avoidance of vigorous exertion is still advised. Most type I dissections that arise in the arch and extend distally have only the aortic root repaired,

leaving the rest of the dissected aorta to be treated medically even in Marfan syndrome. This is then followed by magnetic resonance imaging (MRI). Only when the diameter of any portion of the remaining aorta dilates markedly is repair performed. The value for surgical repair has been 55 mm. People with chronic type I dissections should avoid all but minimal exertion and lifting of more than about 20 lb.

FAMILIAL AORTIC ANEURYSM, DISSECTION, OR BOTH

Some families have an autosomal dominant tendency to develop aneurysms of the aortic root. The aneurysms are histologically and pathologically indistinguishable from those of the Marfan syndrome. Indeed, in some cases, mutations in *FBN1* have been found to cause the condition.[34] However, such families do not have Marfan syndrome,[14] although there may be mild skeletal changes (e.g., pectus excavatum, scoliosis, straight back), striae atrophicae, and mitral valve prolapse.[35] Such patients should be examined carefully for signs of a bicuspid aortic valve or an aortic coarctation, which would place them in the diagnostic category discussed in the next section. "Isolated" aortic root aneurysms should be managed as discussed earlier for Marfan syndrome, with the same indications for β-adrenergic blockade, routine echocardiography, limitation of exertion, and prophylactic surgery.

In a minority of families, the ascending aorta tends to dissect in the absence of much dilatation. Occasionally individuals with this susceptibility will have subtle skeletal changes, but it is unclear how reliable such features are for diagnosing the susceptibility to dissection. Mild aortic root dilatation is as sound a diagnostic criterion as currently available. Molecular markers or causes have not been found. Until they are, this will remain a difficult and frustrating clinical problem.

In the preparticipation evaluation of any athlete, family history is a key element.[18,36] This theme is repeated in several chapters in this book, such as for hypertrophic cardiomyopathy, long QT syndrome, and early coronary artery disease. Athletes should be questioned specifically about aneurysms and dissections, in addition to sudden death in general, in relatives 50 years or younger. Those with a positive history in a near relative (parent, sibling, cousin, or aunt/uncle) should undergo a more detailed physical examination and, potentially, electrocardiography and echocardiography.

AORTIC COARCTATION, BICUSPID AORTIC VALVE, AND ASCENDING AORTIC ANEURYSM

Morgagni first described the pathologic anatomy of aortic coarctation more than 2 centuries ago. The lesion is either a focal or more elongated narrowing of the proximal descending aorta. Signs and symptoms relate to both the site of the coarctation and its severity. Narrowings that produce little in the way of a pressure gradient are usually asymptomatic and clinically unrecognized. For

those that are symptomatic, the specific site of the narrowing is important. A *preductal coarctation* occurs in the distal aortic arch just proximal to the ductus arteriosus; circulation to the viscera and lower extremities is dependent on a patent ductus and right side of the heart flow. A *postductal coarctation* is more common, and distal circulation is dependent on the left side of the heart. In the developed world, severe coarctation is generally recognized early in life on account of the characteristic systolic murmur, pulse deficit, diminished blood pressure in the legs, or arterial hypertension. Repair is straightforward and in the infant or child currently can usually be performed via intravascular dilatation.

No one with an unrepaired coarctation should exercise vigorously. From the perspective of vascular fragility, however, two considerations are important in any person with a documented coarctation, repaired or not. First, the association with bicuspid aortic valve and ascending aortic aneurysm is well established.[37–39] Any person with a bicuspid aortic valve, regardless of function, should be followed regularly with echocardiography to detect the development of an ascending aortic dilatation. Any individual with a congenital bicuspid aortic valve is at increased risk of dissection of the ascending aorta. Some clinicians advocate prophylactic treatment with β-adrenergic blockade.[40]

This triad of bicuspid aortic valve, aortic coarctation, and ascending aortic aneurysm falls into the "left-sided flow defect" category of congenital heart disease[41] (Fig. 8.3). This is the category of congenital heart defects that has the highest risk of recurrence in offspring, verging on 25%.[42,43] No study has examined the prevalence in relatives of subtle coarctation; MRI would be the most sensitive method, although transthoracic or transesophageal echocardiography would be useful. Thus, the risk of recurrence may be higher than what has been reported. Studies are ongoing to try to identify a molecular or genetic defect in families with left-sided flow defects. Any patient with coarctation, including a repaired one, needs to have regular assessment of the aortic root with

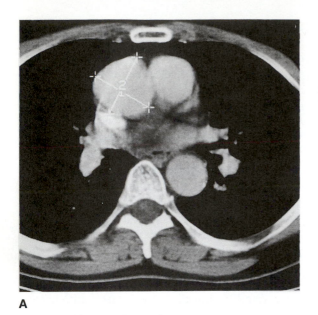

A

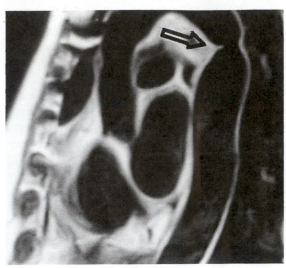

B

FIGURE 8.3. Imaging studies of a woman with coarctation, bicuspid aortic valve, and ascending aortic aneurysm. A. At age 54, a CT showing ascending aortic dilatation of 45 mm. (marked by the perpendicular lines). B. At age 57, an MRI showing a composite graft in the ascending aorta and a periductal aortic coarctation (indicated by the arrow).

echocardiography. If dilatation appears, the condition should be managed in the same way that Marfan syndrome is managed (*vide supra*).

The second risk of vascular fragility occurs in the postductal area, where dilatation of the aorta can occur. Echocardiography or MRI can be used to follow the anatomy at this site.

Finally, the patient who has had a dilatation procedure to relieve the gradient associated with the coarctation needs to have regular follow-up of the site, by computed tomography (CT), MRI, or transthoracic echocardiography from the suprasternal notch, into adulthood to ensure that focal stenosis or dilatation is not occurring.

EHLERS-DANLOS SYNDROMES

A new classification scheme for the Ehlers-Danlos syndromes has been advanced (Table 8.5).[44] The unifying theme is involvement of joints and skin; the individual types are distinguished by the severity of joint and skin mani-

festations and by the involvement of other tissues.[45,46] Joints tend to be hypermobile, both passively and actively. While dislocations are somewhat more common than in the general population, the risks of tendon and ligament rupture are clearly increased. Skin fragility leads to frequent lacerations and an inability to hold standard sutures. Healing is delayed, wounds gape, and scars are atrophic. Bruising is increased in all of the types, some more than others. No accurate prevalence estimates exist; fortunately, the vascular type occurs in less than 1 per 20,000.

In the classic type (formerly called Ehlers-Danlos syndrome I and II), there is an underrecognized tendency to develop dilatation of the ascending aorta;[47,47a] however, this is not as frequent or severe as in Marfan syndrome in most cases. Many people with classic Ehlers-Danlos syndrome do have mitral valve prolapse, occasionally associated with important mitral regurgitation, dysrhythmia, or both. Thus, any person with the classic form of Ehler-Danlos syndrome

TABLE 8.5.   CLASSIFICATION OF THE EHLERS-DANLOS SYNDROMES

Type	Former name	Clinical Features	Inheritance	OMIM #(s)[†]	Molecular Defect
Classical	EDS I & II	Joint hypermobility; skin hyperextensibility; atrophic scars; smooth, velvety skin; subcutaneous spheroids	AD	130000 130010	Structure of type V collagen ? *COL5A1, COL5A2*
Hypermobility	EDS III	Joint hypermobility; some skin hyperextensibility; ± smooth & velvety	AD	130020	?
Vascular	EDS IV	Thin skin; easy bruising; pinched nose; acrogeria; rupture of large & medium caliber arteries, uterus, & large bowel	AD	130050 (225350) (225360)	Deficient type III collagen
Kyphoscoliotic	EDS VI	Joint hypermobility, congenital, progressive scoliosis; scleral fragility with globe rupture; tissue fragility, aortic dilatation, MVP	AR	225400	
Arthrochalasia	EDS VII A & B	Joint hypermobility, severe, with subluxations; congenital hip dislocation; skin hyperextensibility; tissue fragility	AD	130060	No cleavage of *N*-terminus of type I procollagen 2 mutations in *COL1A1* or *COL1A2*
Dermatosparaxis	EDS VIIC	Severe skin fragility; decreased skin elasticity; easy bruising; hernias; premature rupture of fetal membranes	AR	225410	No cleavage of *N*-terminus of type I procollagen 2 deficiency of peptidase
Unclassified types	EDS V	Classical features	XL	305200	?
	EDS VIII	Classic features and periodontal disease	AD	130080	?
	EDS X	Mild classical features, MVP	?	225310	?
	EDS XI	Joint instability	AD	147900	?
	EDS IX	Classic features; occipital horns	XL	309400	Allelic to Menkes syndrome

EDS, Ehlers-Danlos syndrome; AD, autosomal dominant; AR, autosomal recessive; XL, X-linked, MVP, mitral valve prolapse.

Clinical features listed in order of diagnostic importance.

OMIM entries refer to Online Mendelian Inheritance in Man (http://www.ncbi.nlm.nih.gov/OMIM).

Adapted with permission from Pyeritz RE: Ehlers-Danlos syndrome, in Goldman L, Bennett JC (eds): *Cecil Textbook of Medicine*, 21st ed. Philadelphia, WB Saunders, 2000, p. 1119.

deserves a screening echocardiogram; this certainly should be performed before any participation in competitive athletics.

Vascular and viscus fragility is the main concern in the vascular form of Ehlers-Danlos syndrome (Fig. 8. 4). This condition is due to a functional or relative deficiency of type III collagen and is inherited most often as an autosomal dominant trait. Rupture of the bowel, uterus, and bladder can occur either spontaneously or with minimal blunt trauma.[46] Most affected individuals also have skin fragility, easy bruising, and poor wound healing. The most feared complication, however, is arterial rupture.[47] The vessels at most risk include the descending aorta and all of its major branches. Occasionally some dilatation precedes a rupture, but in most cases the artery simply tears, without dissection. For this reason, people with the vascular form of Ehler-Danlos syndrome should avoid all strenuous exertion (including pregnancy, during which the risk of arterial or uterine rupture is quite high[48]) and activities that carry a risk of deceleration injury.

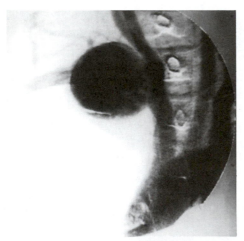

FIGURE 8.4. *A false aneurysm of the bifurcation of the innominate artery in a 16-year-old boy with the vascular form of Ehlers-Danlos syndrome*. *Adapted with permission from Pyeritz RE, Stolle CA, Parfrey NA, et al: Ehlers-Danlos Syndrome IV due to a novel defect in type III procollagen.* AM J Med Genet *19:607, 1984.*

PSEUDOXANTHOMA ELASTICUM

In pseudoxanthoma elasticum, another rare heritable disorder of connective tissue, the histopathologic hallmark is calcification and fragmentation of elastic fibers.[49,50] The result is widespread clinical features, especially in elastic arteries. The molecular cause of this condition is unknown, but the gene has been mapped to 16p13.1 for both the autosomal recessive (most common) and autosomal dominant forms.[51] Two major clinical sequelae stem from the arteriopathy. The first is occlusive arterial disease, which presents as stroke and myocardial infarction, often at an early age. The vascular narrowing results from an arteriolosclerosis, with intimal-medial thickening due to the calcified elastic laminae. The second is fragility of arterioles, particularly in the gastrointestinal tract. Once a vessel ruptures, the calcified media prevents vasoconstriction, so the bleeding tends to be profound. Additionally, the retina is more susceptible to degeneration and detachment. For all of these reasons, people with pseudoxanthoma elasticum should avoid contact sports and exertion at maximal capacity. A regular assessment of their coronary circulation is in order once adulthood is reached on account of the markedly increased risk of lumenal narrowing.

POLYCYSTIC KIDNEY DISEASE

Adult polycsytic kidney disease is one of the most common causes of end-stage renal disease and hemodialysis in the developed world. The condition is autosomal dominant and genetically heterogeneous, with at least 3 different genes, when mutated, causing the disease.[52,53] The most common cause is mutation of the *PKD1* locus on chromosome 16p13.3–p13.12, with mutation of the *PKD2* locus at 4q21–q23 accounting for about 10% of families. In adult polycystic kidney disease due to mutations in *PKD2,* the course of renal disease and hypertension is generally milder. People with this disease often develop mild dilatation of the aortic root, which rarely results in clinical problems and mitral valve prolapse.[54] The risk for abdominal aortic aneurysm may also be increased.[55] A much more important vascular feature is the occurrence of cerebral aneurysms of the "berry" type. Approximately 5% of people with adult polycystic kidney disease have clinically relevant but often asymptomatic berry aneurysms,[56] and a higher proportion have them at autopsy. It remains uncertain to what extent people with this disease should be screened for cerebral aneurysms, and by what method; one group recommends high-resolution CT.[56] The potential for such aneurysms is a strong motivation for controlling blood pressure, especially as renal function deteriorates. A strong argument could be made that any person with adult polycystic kidney disease should avoid activities that markedly increase the heart rate-blood pressure product.

Molecular testing is available to detect who in a family has inherited mutations of *PKD1* or *PKD2*. Alternatively, renal ultrasound can be used, but because the kidney cysts are age-dependent, it will not be clear in some cases until middle-age or later whether or not a person has inherited the mutant allele.

FAMILIAL INTRACRANIAL (BERRY) ANEURYSM

The frequency with which cerebral aneurysms are hereditary is unclear, but in some families, a clear autosomal dominant predisposition occurs. Several population surveys suggest a familial prevalence of 10 to 20%.[57,58] As a result, a routine question on the preparticipation medical screen for athletes should seek to identify relatives who have had stroke or cerebral hemorrhage under the age of 50 years. A positive response should prompt more scrutiny of the family history. However, the extent to which screening modalities such as CT or MRI can detect those at risk, especially adolescents or young adults, is unclear. Furthermore, whether asymptomatic, small aneurysms, once detected, require surgery is unclear.[59] Individuals with berry aneurysms should avoid vigorous exercise.

FAMILIAL ABDOMINAL AORTIC ANEURYSM

Aneurysms of the abdominal aorta are a disease of aging, with the prevalence among 50-year-olds quite low but among 70-year-olds about 5 to 10%. Males are much more frequently affected. Because of this age distribution, statistically aneurysms of the abdominal aorta pose little risk for the young competitive athlete. However, because the general population rarely distinguishes among "aneurysms," a positive response to a family history screening question about aneurysms will often reveal relatives with aneurysms of the abdominal aorta. While the information may have little relevance at that time to the athlete, it is worth noting that this disease clearly has a strong familial predisposition.[60] Although no data exist to support the following recommendations, individuals with aneurysms of the abdominal aorta of a caliber > 40 mm should avoid vigorous exercise and contact sports. Mounting evidence suggests that the underlying cause is inflammation, which induces apoptosis of vascular smooth muscle cells.[61] No causative gene has been identified.

HEREDITARY HEMORRHAGIC TELANGIECTASIA AND OTHER CAUSES OF ARTERIOVENOUS MALFORMATIONS

Hereditary hemorrhagic telangiectasia (Osler-Weber-Rendu syndrome) is more common than generally recognized, with at least 1 per 20,000 Caucasians in the United States affected. Angiodysplasia, including AVMs of various sizes, from telangiectases to large and complex communications in the lungs, arterial aneurysms, and phlebectasia, is the hallmark finding and result in the pleiotropic manifestations.[62] The classic telangiectases of the lips, oral mucosa, and fingertips should prompt the correct diagnosis. Epistaxis results from small AVMs in the nose and can lead to chronic anemia. The AVMs that lead to chronic gastrointestinal blood loss and anemia tend to be a bit larger. Cyanosis, polycythemia, clubbing, and dyspnea can result from pulmonary AVMs, although the first manifestation can be a cerebral event, either a stroke or an abscess, from the right-to-left shunting in the lungs. In one large series studied with MRI, 23% of people with hereditary hemorrhagic telangiectasia had cerebrovascular malformations,[63] although most central nervous system morbidity results from emboli.[64]

The main risk to people with this disease who exert themselves is likely an embolic event if pulmonary AVMs are present. Any person in whom hereditary hemorrhagic telangiectasia is diagnosed should have careful auscultation of the lungs, a chest radiograph, a measured hemoglobin level, and an arterial blood gas determination on room air.

The cause of most cases of this disease is a mutation in the gene that encodes endoglin on chromosome 9q34.1.[65] At least one other gene must be involved because hereditary hemorrhagic telangiectasia in some families does not map to the 9q locus; these families seem at much less risk for pulmonary AVMs.[66] Presymptomatic individuals can be detected in families either through linkage analysis or mutation detection.

Congenital AVMs occur outside of hereditary hemorrhagic telangiectasia, can affect any organ of the body, and can be simple or complex. Invariably the arterial wall is thinned and potentially prone to rupture. Depending on the size of the shunt, which depends on the caliber of a single AVM or the number of multiple AVMs, high-output cardiac failure can develop. A large AVM can affect development of a body part and result, for example, in limb hypertrophy. When AVMs are limited to the brain, the presentation is usually hemorrhage; subarachnoid bleeds have a better prognosis than do the intraparenchymal type.[67] For AVMs that were deemed unresectable, the risk of hemorrhage was 2 to 4% per year.[68] Anyone with a cerebral AVM should not engage in vigorous activity.

Cerebral cavernous malformations can occur as an autosomal dominant condition, which seems particularly prevalent (although not common) among Mexican Hispanics.[69] The most effective screening tool is MRI. Any person detected with such a defect should have imaging of the brain and liver (in which angiomas occur) and detailed retinoscopic evaluation. Because cavernous angioma tend to leak, causing neurologic problems, affected individuals should not engage in vigorous activities.

The gene for one form of cerebral cavernous malformations has been mapped to 7q11.2–q21, and additional loci at 7p15–p13 and 3q25.2–q27 have been reported.[70] Once an individual is detected, close relatives should be screened by MRI.

KLIPPEL-TRENAUNAY-WEBER SYNDROME

The clinical features of Klippel-Trenaunay-Weber (KTW) syndrome are cutaneous hemangiomata, hypertrophy of the underlying soft tissues and bone, and atresia or malformation of veins, which results in lymphedema. Varicose veins are common, and stripping should be avoided if the deep veins are atretic.[71] Hemangiomata can occur in organs and lead to acute or chronic hemorrhage.

The KTW syndrome has no known genetic basis, and most cases are sporadic occurrences in families. The suggestion has been made that KTW arises due to a somatic mutation (postzygotic) in a gene that controls angiogenesis.[72]

PERSONAL PERSPECTIVE

At least one-third of the people in whom I diagnose Marfan syndrome are serious athletes and are disappointed when I advise them to restrict their activity. I learned early in my career, first, to give options and, second, to be specific. I diagnosed Marfan syndrome in a 14-year-old boy with his parents present. He was a superb basketball player just entering high school; his entire perspective on life, and his personal identity, was linked to basketball. When I told him I would not clear him to play, he was crestfallen. I told him he could still be active and encouraged him to learn to play golf and to stay in shape through aerobic activity such as swimming. This did little to buoy his spirits in my office, and I wondered how he would cope. A year later when I saw him again, he was so thankful that I had given him an alternative to basketball. He had won the 100 m butterfly at the state swimming meet. Since then, I have learned to be specific about limits.

Occasionally, I learn from a parent or a spouse that my advice is unheeded. On follow-up evaluations, I might relate the story of Flo Hyman, the American volleyball player who won a silver medal playing for the United States in the 1984 Olympics. She died at age 31 in 1986 while playing a volleyball game in a professional league in Japan. Her parents insisted on an autopsy when her body was returned home; a dissection of her ascending aorta was found.

Her story is instructive for several reasons. First, it illustrates that vigorous athletics can be hazardous, and there is no way of predicting when tragedy might strike. Second, Flo Hyman had been evaluated specifically for her exceptional stature while an adolescent, and the diagnosis of Marfan syndrome had not been made. Nor had it been made on the 6'5" athlete throughout multiple medical evaluations associated with her national and Olympic team participation. The third point was brought home when, some months after Flo's death, I appeared on "Good Morning America" with her sister. I then learned about her mother who had died young of "rheumatic heart disease," of her maternal grandmother with a leaky mitral valve, and her athletic brother. I learned this from an exceptionally talented, tall, and lanky young woman who did not suspect that the condition that killed her sister might be present in her or her relatives. Her brother was convinced to undergo echocardiography and was found to have a large aortic root aneurysm; prophylactic surgery was successful. Flo Hyman's death may well have saved her brother's life.

REFERENCES

1. Kalath S, Tsipouras P, Silver FH: Non-invasive assessment of aortic mechanical properties. *Ann Biomed Eng* 14:513, 1986.

2. Roman MJ, Devereux RB, Kramer-Fox R, et al: Two-dimensional echocardiographic aortic root dimensions in normal children and adults. *Am J Cardiol* 64:507, 1989.

3. Johnston KW, Rutherford RB, Tilson MD, et al: Suggested standards for reporting on arterial aneurysms. *J Vasc Surg* 13:444, 1991.

4. Coady MA, Rizzo JA, Hammond GL, et al: What is the appropriate size criterion for resection of thoracic aortic aneurysms? *J Thorac Cardiovasc Surg* 113:476, 1997.

5. Gott VL, Greene PS, Alejo DE, et al: Surgery for ascending aortic disease in Marfan patients: A multi-center study. *N Engl J Med* 340:1307, 1999.

6. Weintraub AM, Gomes MN: Clinical Manifestations of abdominal aortic aneurysm and thoracoabdominal aneurysm, in Lindsay J Jr, Hurst JW (eds): *The Aorta*. New York, Grune & Stratton, 1979; p. 131.

7. Spittell PC: Diseases of the aorta, in Topol EJ (ed.): *Comprehensive Cardiovascular Medicine.* Philadelphia, Lippincott-Raven, 1998; p. 3031.

8. Mokri B: Spontaneous dissections of internal carotid arteries. *Neurologist* 3:104, 1997.

9. Matousek V, Prerovsky I: A contribution to the problem of the inheritance of primary varicose veins. *Hum Hered* 24:225, 1974.

10. Dietz HC, Pyeritz RE: Mutations in the human gene for fibrillin-1 (*FBN1*) in the Marfan syndrome and related disorders. *Hum Molec Genet* 4:1799, 1995.

11. Pyeritz RE: The Marfan syndrome and other disorders of the microfibril, in Rimoin DL, Connor JM, Pyeritz RE (eds.): *Principles and Practice of Medical Genetics,* 3rd ed. New York, Churchill Livingstone, 1997; p. 1027.

12. Pyeritz RE: Marfan syndrome, in Goldman L, Bennett JC (eds.): *Cecil Textbook of Medicine.* 21st ed. Philadelphia, WB Saunders, 2000, p. 1118.

13. Pyeritz RE, Dietz HC: The Marfan syndrome and other fibrillinopathies, in Royce PM, Steinmann B (eds.): *Connective Tissue and Its Heritable Disorders: Molecular, Genetic and Medical Aspects,* 2nd ed. New York, Wiley-Liss, 2001, in preparation.

14. DePaepe A, Deitz HC, Devereux RB, et al: Revised diagnostic criteria for the Marfan syndrome. *Am J Med Genet* 62:417, 1996.

15. Maron BJ, Moller JH, Seidman CE, et al: Impact of laboratory molecular diagnosis on contemporary diagnostic criteria for genetically transmitted cardiovascular diseases: Hypertrophic cardiomyopathy, long QT syndrome and Marfan syndrome. *Circulation* 98:1460, 1998.

16. Maron BJ, Shirani J, Poliac LC, et al: Sudden death in young competitive athletes: Clinical, demographic and pathological profiles. *JAMA* 276:199, 1996.

17. Braverman A: Exercise and the Marfan syndrome. *Med Sci Sports Exer* 30:S387, 1998.

18. Pyeritz RE: Enlargement and dissection of the aorta, in *Exercise Management for Persons with Chronic Diseases and Disabilities.* Champaign, IL: Am Coll Sports Med, 1997; p. 69.

19. Sisk HE, Zahka KG, Pyeritz RE: The Marfan syndrome in early childhood: Analysis of 15 patients diagnosed less than 4 years of age. *Am J Cardiol* 52:353, 1983.

20. Morse RP, Rockenmacher S, Pyeritz RE, et al: Diagnosis and management of Marfan syndrome in infants. *Pediatrics* 86:888, 1990.

21. Glesby MJ, Pyeritz RE: Association of mitral valve prolapse and systemic abnormalities of connective tissue: A phenotypic continuum. *JAMA* 262:523, 1989.

22. Silverman DI, Gray J, Roman MJ, et al: A family history of severe cardiovascular disease in the Marfan syndrome is associated with increased aortic diameter and decreased survival. *J Am Coll Cardiol* 26:1062, 1995.

23. Pyeritz RE: Predictors of dissection of the ascending aorta in Marfan syndrome. *Circulation* 84: II–351, 1991.

24. Maron BJ, Mitchell JH: Revised eligibility recommendations for competitive athletes with cardiovascular abnormalities. *J Am Coll Cardiol* 24:848, 1994.

25. Lewis JF, Maron BJ, Diggs JA, et al: Participation echocardiographic screening for cardiovascular disease in a large, predominantly black population of collegiate athletes. *Am J Cardiol* 64:1029, 1989.

26. Murry PM, Cantwell JD, Heath DL, et al: The role of limited echocardiography in screening athletes. *Am J Cardiol* 7:220, 1995.

27. Shores J, Berger KR, Murphy EA, Pyeritz RE: Chronic β-adrenergic blockade protects the aorta in the Marfan syndrome: A prospective, randomized trial of propranolol. *N Engl J Med* 330:1335, 1994.

28. Salim MA, Alpert BS, Ward JC, et al: Effect of beta-adrenergic blockade on aortic root rate of dilation in the Marfan syndrome. *Am J Cardiol* 74:629, 1994.

29. Desposito F, Cho S, Frias JL, et al: Health supervision for children with Marfan syndrome. *Pediatrics* 98:978, 1996.

30. Silverman DI, Burton KJ, Gray J, et al: Life expectancy in the Marfan syndrome. *Am J Cardiol* 75:157, 1995.

31. David TE: Aortic valve repair in patients with Marfan syndrome and ascending aorta aneurysms due to degenerative disease. *J Card Surg* 9(suppl):182, 1994.

32. Yacoub MH, Gehler P, Chandrasekaran V, et al: Late results of a valve-preserving operation in patients with aneurysms of the ascending aorta and root. *J Thor Cardiovasc Surg* 115:1080, 1998.

33. Clouse WD, Hallett JW Jr, Schaff HV, et al: Improved prognosis of thoracic aortic aneurysms: A population-based study. *JAMA* 280:1926, 1998.

34. Milewicz DM, Michael KC, Fisher N, et al: Fibrillin-1 mutations in patients with thoracic aortic aneurysms. *Circulation* 94:708, 1996.

35. Biddinger A, Rocklin M, Coselli JS, et al: Familial thoracic aortic aneurysms: A case-control study. *J Vasc Surg* 25:506, 1997.

36. Pelliccia A, Maron BJ: Preparticipation cardiovascular evaluation of the competitive athlete: Perspectives from the 30-year Italian experience. *Am J Cardiol* 75:827, 1995.

37. McKusick VA: Association of aortic valvular disease and cystic medial necrosis. *Lancet* I:1026, 1972.

38. Reifenstein GH, Levine SA, Gross RE: Coarctation of the aorta: A review of 104 autopsied cases of the "adult type," 2 years of age or older. *Am Heart J* 33:146, 1947.

39. Hahn RT, Roman MJ, Mogtader AH, et al: Association of aortic dilation with regurgitant, stenotic and functionally normal bicuspid aortic valves. *J Am Coll Cardiol* 19:283, 1992.

40. Burks JM, Illes RW, Keating EC, et al: Ascending aortic aneurysm and dissection in young adults with bicuspid aortic valve: Implications for echocardiographic surveillance. *Clin Cardiol* 21: 439, 1998.

41. Clark EB: Mechanisms in the pathogenesis of congenital cardiac malformations, in Pierpont MEM, Moller JH (eds.): *Genetics of Cardiovascular Disease.* Boston: Martinus Nijhoff, 1987, p. 3.

42. Glick BN, Roberts WC: Congenitally bicuspid aortic valve in multiple family members. *Am J Cardiol* 73:400, 1994.

43. Brenner JI, Berg KA, Schneider DS, et al: Congenital cardiovascular malformations in first degree relatives of infants with hypoplastic left heart syndrome. *Am J Dis Child* 143:1492, 1989.

44. Beighton P, De Paepe A, Steinmann B, et al:

Ehlers-Danlos syndromes: Revised nosology, Villefranche, 1997. *Am J Med Genet* 77:31, 1998.

45. Pyeritz RE: Ehlers-Danlos syndrome, in Goldman L, Bennett JC (eds.): *Cecil Textbook of Medicine.* 21st ed. Philadelphia, WB Saunders, 2000, p. 1119.

46. Byers PH: The Ehlers-Danlos syndromes, in Rimoin DL, Connor JM, Pyeritz RE (eds): *Principles and Practice of Medical Genetics,* 3rd ed. New York, Churchill Livingstone, 1997, p. 1067.

47. Pyeritz RE, Stolle CA, Parfrey NA, et al: Ehlers-Danlos syndrome IV due to a novel defect in type III procollagen. *Am J Med Genet* 19:607, 1984.

47a. Tiller GE, Cassidy SB, Wensel C, et al: Aortic root dilatation in Ehlers-Danlos syndrome types I, II and III. A report of five cases. *Clinical Genet* 53:460, 1998.

48. Rudd NL, Nimrod C, Holbrook KA, et al: Pregnancy complications in type IV Ehlers-Danlos syndrome. *Lancet* I:50, 1983.

49. Pope FM: Pseudoxanthoma elasticum, in Rimoin DL, Connor JM, Pyeritz RE (eds.): *Principles and Practice of Medical Genetics,* 3rd ed. New York, Churchill Livingstone, 1997, p. 1083.

50. Pyeritz RE: Pseudoxanthoma elasticum, in Goldman L, Bennett JC (eds): *Cecil Textbook of Medicine.* 21st ed. Philadelphia, WB Saunders, 2000, p. 1122.

51. Sturk B, Neldner KH, Rao VS, et al: Mapping of both autosomal recessive and dominant variants of pseudoxanthoma elasticum to chromosome 16p13.1. *Hum Molec Genet* 6:1823, 1997.

52. Germino GG, Barton NJ, Lamb J, et al: Identification of a locus which shows no genetic recombination with the autosomal dominant polycystic kidney disease gene on chromosome 16. *Am J Hum Genet* 46:925, 1990.

53. Daoust MC, Reynolds DM, Bichet DG, et al: Evidence for a third genetic locus for autosomal dominant polycystic kidney disease. *Genomics* 25:733, 1995.

54. Hossack KF, Leddy CL, Johnson AM, et al: Echocardiographic findings in autosomal dominant polycystic kidney disease. *N Engl J Med* 319:907, 1988.

55. Chapman JR, Hilson AJW: Polycystic kidneys and abdominal aortic aneurysms. *Lancet* I:646, 1980.

56. Chapman AB, Rubinstein D, Hughes R, et al: Intracranial aneurysms in autosomal dominant

polycystic kidney disease. *N Engl J Med* 327:916, 1992.

57. Ronkainen A, Hernesniemi J, Ryynanen M: Familial subarachnoid hemorrhage in east Finland, 1977–1990. *Neurosurg* 33:787, 1993.

58. Schievink WI, Schaid DJ, Rogers HM, et al: On the inheritance of intracranial aneurysms. *Stroke* 25:2028, 1994.

59. Caplan LR: Should intracranial aneurysms be treated before they rupture? *N Engl J Med* 339:1774, 1998.

60. Verloes A, Sakalihasan N, Koulischer L, et al: Aneurysms of the abdominal aorta: Familial and genetic aspects in three hundred thirteen pedigrees. *J Vasc Surg* 21:646, 1995.

61. Henderson LE, Geng Y-J, Sukhova GK, et al: Death of smooth muscle cells and expression of mediators of apoptosis by T lymphocytes in human abdominal aortic aneurysms. *Circulation* 97:96, 1999.

62. Guttmacher AE, Marchuk DA, White RI Jr: Hereditary hemorrhagic telangiectasia. *N Engl J Med* 333:918, 1995.

63. Fulbright RK, Chaloupka JC, Putman CM, et al: MR of hereditary hemorrhagic telangiectasia: Prevalence and spectrum of cerebrovascular malformations. *Am J Neuroradiol* 19:477, 1998.

64. White RI Jr, Lynch-Nyhan A, Terry P, et al: Pulmonary arteriovenous malformations: Techniques and long-term outcome of embolotherapy. *Radiology* 169:663, 1988.

65. McAllister KA, Grogg KM, Johnson DW, et al: Endoglin, a TGF-beta binding protein of endothelial cells, is the gene for hereditary haemorrhagic telangiectasia, type I. *Nature Genet* 8:345, 1994.

66. McAllister KA, Lennon F, Bowles-Biesecker B, et al: Genetic heterogeneity in hereditary haemorrhagic telangiectasia: Possible correlation with clinical phenotype. *J Med Genet* 31:927, 1994.

67. The Arteriovenous Malformation Study Group. Arteriovenous malformations of the brain in adults. *N Engl J Med* 340:1812, 1999.

68. Ondra SL, Troupp H, George ED, et al: The natural history of symptomatic arteriovenous malformations of the brain: A 24-year follow-up assessment. *J Neurosurg* 73:387, 1990.

69. Rigamonti D, Hadley MN, Drayer BP, et al: Cerebral cavernous angiomas of the brain: Observations in a four generation family. *N Engl J Med* 319:343, 1988.

70. Craig HD, Gunel M, Cepeda O, et al: Multilocus linkage identifies two new loci for a Mendelian form of stroke, cerebral cavernous malformation, at 7p15–13 and 3q25.2–27. *Hum Molec Genet* 7:1851, 1998.

71. Lindenauer SM: The Klippel-Trenaunay-Weber syndrome: Varicosity, hypertrophy and hemangioma with no arteriovenous fistula. *Ann Surg* 162:303, 1965.

72. Berry SA, Peterson C, Mize W, et al: Klippel-Trenaunay syndrome. *Am J Med Genet* 79:319, 1998.

Chapter 9

SUDDEN CARDIAC DEATH DUE TO HYPERTROPHIC CARDIOMYOPATHY IN YOUNG ATHLETES

Barry J. Maron, M.D.

Over the past several years, interest has heightened considerably in the medical community and with the lay public regarding the causes of sudden and unexpected deaths in young, trained athletes.[1,2] As a consequence, the underlying cardiovascular diseases responsible for these uncommon but devastating sudden events in trained athletes and others participating in sporting activities have been the subject of several reports and a large measure of clarification has resulted.[3–10] Recognition that athletic field deaths may be due to a variety of detectable (but usually unsuspected) cardiovascular lesions has also stimulated intense interest in preparticipation screening,[11] as well as issues related to the criteria for eligibility and disqualification from competitive sports.[12]

SUDDEN DEATH IN ATHLETES

PREVALENCE, IMPACT, AND SOCIETAL ISSUES

The frequency of sudden unexpected death during competitive sports in young athletes due to cardiovascular disease appears to be low, in the range of 1:200,000 per academic year for high school competitors;[13] lower estimates of the risk for sudden death have been calculated in apparently healthy male athletes, joggers, and marathon racers (i.e., 1:15,000 to 1:50,000).[14–16]

Such estimates could suggest to some that the intense and persistent public interest in these tragic events is perhaps disproportionate to their overall significance in the population. However, the emotional and social impact of athletic field catastrophes remains high. To most of the lay public and physician community (and the news media), the competitive athlete symbolizes the healthiest segment of our society and the unexpected collapse of such young people is a powerful event that inevitably strikes to the core of our sensibilities.[1] For these reasons, and despite its low event rate, sudden death in young athletes will probably continue to represent an important medical issue. Indeed, it is an important responsibility of the medical community to create a fully informed public and also, where prudent and practical, pursue early detection of the causes of catastrophic events in young athletes, as well as preventive measures. In contrast, because such events are uncommon relative to the vast numbers of athletes participating safely in sports, it is an important concern that information about athletic field deaths should not raise undue anxiety among youthful athletes and their families and, as a consequence, inhibit sports participation.

CAUSES

Several autopsy-based studies have documented the diseases responsible for sudden death in young competitive athletes or in youthful asymptomatic individuals with active life-styles.[3–10,17,18] These structural abnormalities are independent of the normal physiological adaptations in cardiac dimensions evident in many trained athletes, which usually consist of increased left ventricular end-diastolic cavity dimension or occasionally wall thickness.[19–24]

It is also important to be cautious in assigning strict prevalence figures for the occurrence of various cardiovascular diseases in studies of sudden death in athletes; patient selection biases and other issues unavoidably influence the acquisition of such data in the absence of an established systematic national registry. Indeed, the available published studies differ with regard to the methods used to document cardiovascular diagnosis and are derived from a variety of data bases.

Even with these limitations, it has been possible to demonstrate convincingly that the vast majority of sudden deaths in young athletes (< age 35) are due to a variety of primarily congenital cardiovascular diseases (over 20 in number; Fig. 9.1).[3,7] Indeed, virtually any disease capable of causing sudden death in young people may potentially do so in young competitive athletes.[3,7] Also, the lesions responsible for sudden death do not occur with the same frequency, with many responsible for only ≤ 5% of all deaths.[3] It should be emphasized that while these diseases may be relatively common in young athletes dying suddenly, each is rather uncommon within the general population.

HYPERTROPHIC CARDIOMYOPATHY

The single most common cardiovascular abnormality among the causes of sudden death in young athletes is hypertrophic cardiomyopathy (HCM),[3,7,9,10] usually in the nonobstructive form and with a prevalence in the range of 35% among these deaths (Fig. 9.2).[3] HCM is a primary and familial cardiac malformation with heterogeneous expression and diverse clinical course for which disease-causing mutations in 9 genes encoding proteins of the sarcomere have been reported.[25–32] HCM is a relatively uncommon cardiac malformation recognizable clinically in about 0.2% (1 in 500) of the general population.[33]

Sudden death in HCM has shown a predilection for young and asymptomatic individuals, occurring frequently during moderate or severe exertion similar to its demographic profile in athletic populations.[25,34] This clinical profile is

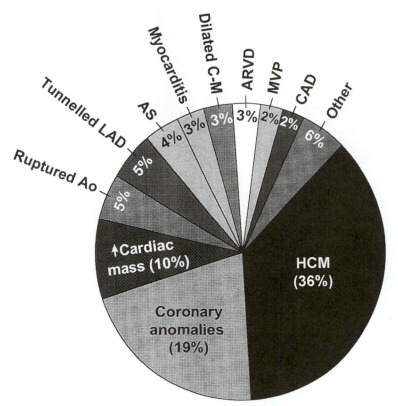

FIGURE 9.1. Causes of sudden cardiac death in young competitive athletes (median age, 17) based on systematic tracking of 158 athletes in the United States, primarily 1985 to 1995. In an additional 2% of the athletes, no evidence of cardiovascular disease that was sufficient to explain death was found at necropsy. ↑ *cardiac mass = hearts with increased weight and some morphologic features consistent with (but not diagnostic of) HCM. LAD, left anterior descending coronary artery; AS, aortic stenosis; C-M, cardiomyopathy; ARVD, arrhythmogenic right ventricular dysplasia; MVP, mitral valve prolapse; CAD, coronary artery disease.* Adapted with permission from the American Medical Association from Maron BJ, Shirani J, Poliac LC, et al: Sudden death in young competitive athletes: Clinical, demographic and pathological profiles. JAMA 276:199–204, 1998.

consistent with both the observation that HCM is a frequent cause of sudden death in athletes and the generally accepted and prudent recommendations of Bethesda Conference #26 to disqualify young competitive athletes with HCM from intense competitive sports.[12] Indeed, for a disease such as HCM in which there is a propensity for potentially lethal arrhythmias in some individuals, the stress of intense athletic training and

competition undoubtedly increases risk to some degree.

Despite intense investigation, however, reliable identification of the individual HCM patient (or athlete) at high risk remains a major challenge. This is due, in part, to the fact that most data on risk stratification have been assembled at referral institutions and are based on selected patient populations already judged to be at increased risk.[35]

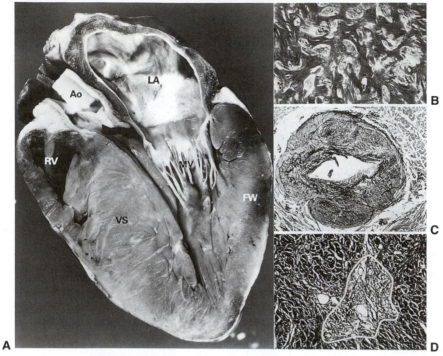

FIGURE 9.2. Morphologic components of the disease process in HCM, the most common cause of sudden death in young competitive athletes. A. Gross heart specimen sectioned in a cross-sectional plane similar to that of the echocardiographic (parasternal) long axis; left ventricular wall thickening shows an asymmetric pattern and is confined primarily to the ventricular septum (VS), which bulges prominently into the left ventricular outflow tract. Left ventricular cavity appears reduced in size. FW, left ventricular free wall. B, C, and D. Histologic features characteristic of left ventricular myocardium in HCM. B. Markedly disordered architecture with adjacent hypertrophied cardiac muscle cells arranged at perpendicular and oblique angles. C. An intramural coronary artery with thickened wall, due primarily to medial hypertrophy and apparently narrowed lumen. D. Replacement fibrosis in an area of ventricular myocardium adjacent to an abnormal intramural coronary artery. Ao, aorta; LA, left atrium; RV, right ventricle. Adapted with permission from Maron BJ: Hypertrophic cardiomyopathy. Lancet 350:127–133, 1997.

Nevertheless, disease variables that presently appear to identify young HCM patients at greatly increased risk include prior aborted cardiac arrest or sustained ventricular tachycardia, family history of sudden or other premature HCM-related death or identification of a high-risk genotype, multiple-repetitive or prolonged nonsustained ventricular tachycardia on ambulatory (Holter) electrocardiogram (ECG) recordings, recurrent or exertional syncope and massive left ventricular hypertrophy (≥ 30-mm wall thickness).[28,29] Magnitude of the left ventricular outflow tract pressure gradient has not been independently associated with an increased risk for sudden death since such events occur in both patients with and in patients without subaortic obstruction. Patients with HCM judged to be at high risk should be considered for primary prevention of sudden death with prophylactic implantation of the cardioverter-defibrillator.[36]

Of note are the investigations from the Veneto region in northeastern Italy, which report arrhythmogenic right ventricular dysplasia (ARVD), rather than HCM, to be the most common cause of sudden death in athletes.[5,6,37] ARVD is characterized morphologically by myocyte death in the right ventricular wall with replacement fibrous and/or adipose tissue formation as evidence of repair, often associated with myocarditis and apoptosis. This right ventricular disease process may be diffuse or, alternatively, segmental involving only limited portions of the wall. While ARVD is also a component of the experience with athletic field deaths in the United States, its frequency is clearly in the range of only < 5%.[3] Furthermore, the reason for the relatively *low* frequency with which HCM is apparently responsible for sudden death in Italian athletes is an interesting but also largely unresolved issue. Certainly, HCM appears to occur with reasonable frequency in Italy.[38,39] It is possible that the long-standing and systematic Italian national program for the cardiovascular assessment of competitive athletes[40] has had the effect of identifying and disqualifying disproportionate numbers of trained athletes with HCM, due to the fact that this cardiac malformation is

much more easily identifiable clinically than is a disease such as ARVD.[41,42]

MORPHOLOGY AND DIAGNOSIS

Left ventricular hypertrophy has traditionally been regarded as the gross anatomic marker and likely the determinant of many of the clinical features and course in most patients with HCM (Fig. 9.2)[25–27,29] Since the left ventricular cavity is usually small or normal in size, increased left ventricular mass is due almost entirely to an increase in wall thickness. Consequently, the clinical diagnosis of HCM has been based on the definition (by two-dimensional echocardiography) of the most characteristic morphologic feature of the disease—that is, left ventricular wall thickening associated with a nondilated cavity, and in the absence of another cardiac or systemic disease, capable of producing the magnitude of hypertrophy present (e.g., systemic hypertension or aortic stenosis)[25–27] (Fig. 9.3). Because the nonobstructive form of HCM is predominant,[27–29] the well-described clinical features of dynamic obstruction to left ventricular outflow, such as a loud systolic ejection mur-

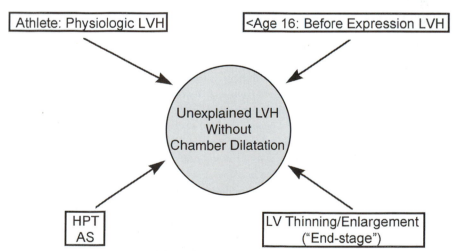

FIGURE 9.3. Basic morphologic definition of HCM showing those clinical conditions or circumstances which constitute exceptions that may obscure this diagnosis. AS, aortic stenosis; HPT, systemic hypertension; LV, left ventricular; LVH, left ventricular hypertrophy.

mur, systolic anterior motion of the mitral valve, or partial premature closure of the aortic valve, are not required for diagnosis.

Based on both echocardiographic and necropsy analyses in large numbers of patients, it is apparent that the HCM disease spectrum is characterized by vast structural diversity with regard to the patterns and extent of left ventricular hypertrophy[27,43] (Figs. 9.4 and 9.5). While the anterior ventricular septum is usually the predominant region of hypertrophy, virtually all possible patterns of left ventricular hypertrophy occur in HCM, and no single phenotypic expression can be considered "classic" or typical of this disease. Of note, although many patients show diffusely distributed hypertrophy, about 30% demonstrate localized wall thickening confined to only one segment of left ventricle.

Absolute thickness of the left ventricular wall varies greatly, although the average reported value is usually 21 to 22 mm.[27] Wall thickness is profoundly increased in many patients, including some showing the most severe hypertrophy observed in any cardiac disease (with 60 mm being the most extreme wall-thickness dimension reported to date).[44] In contrast, the HCM phenotype is not always expressed as a greatly thickened left ventricle, and some patients show only a mild increase of ≤ 15 mm, including a few genetically affected individuals with normal thicknesses (≤ 12 mm).[32,45] Patterns of wall thickening in HCM are often strikingly heterogeneous, involving noncontiguous segments of the left ventricle (i.e., with areas of normal thickness evident in between). Transitions between thickened areas and regions of normal thickness are often sharp and abrupt, not infrequently creating right-angled contours of the wall. The variability in morphologic expression of HCM is underlined by the fact that even first-degree relatives with the disease usually show considerable dissimilarities in the pattern of left ventricular wall thickening.[46]

FIGURE 9.4. *Variability of patterns of left ventricular hypertrophy in patients with HCM, shown in a composite of diastolic stop-frame images in parasternal short-axis plane. A, B, and D. Wall thickening is diffuse, involving substantial portions of ventricular septum and free wall. A. At papillary muscle level, all segments of the left ventricular wall are hypertrophied including posterior free wall (PW), but the pattern of thickening is asymmetric with the anterior portion of ventricular septum (VS) predominant and massive (i.e., 50 mm). B. The hypertrophy is diffuse, involving 3 segments of the left ventricle but with the posterior free wall spared and thin (< 10 mm; arrowheads) and with particularly abrupt changes in wall thickness evident (arrows). C. Marked hypertrophy in a pattern distinctly different from A, B, and D in which the thickening of posterior wall (PW) is predominant, and the ventricular septum is of near-normal thickness. D. Diffuse distribution of hypertrophy involving 3 segments of left ventricle similar to B, but without sharp transitions in the contour of the wall. E. Hypertrophy predominantly involving lateral free wall and only a small portion of contiguous anterior septum (arrows). F. Hypertrophy predominantly of posterior ventricular septum (PVS), and to lesser extent the contiguous portion of anterior septum (AVS). G. Thickening involving anterior and posterior septum to a similar degree, but with sparing of the free wall. Calibration dots are 1 cm apart. ALFW, anterolateral free wall; AML, anterior mitral leaflet; LFW, lateral free wall; PML, posterior mitral leaflet.* Adapted with permission of the American College of Cardiology from Klues HG, Schiffers A, Maron BJ: Phenotypic spectrum and patterns of left ventricular hypertrophy in hypertrophic cardiomyopathy: Morphologic observations and significance as assessed by two-dimensional echocardiography in 600 patients. J Am Coll Cardiol 26:1699–1708, 1995.

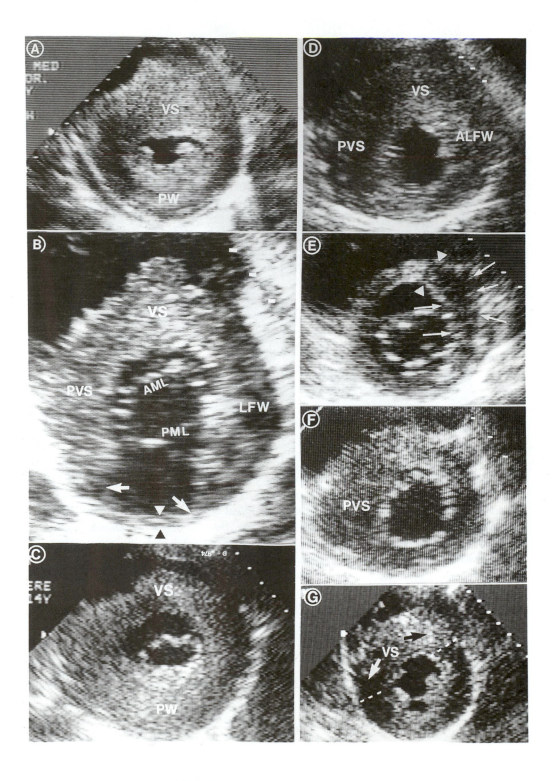

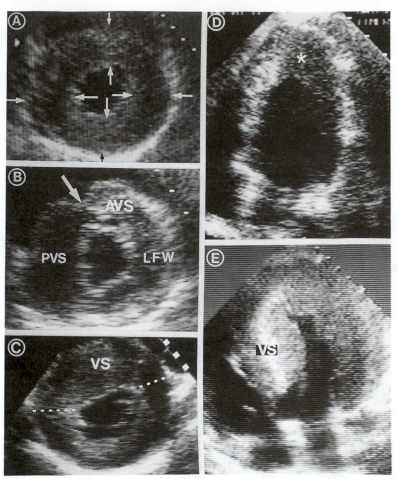

FIGURE 9.5. Heterogeneity in patterns of left ventricular hypertrophy in 5 patients with HCM, including examples of the uncommon concentric and apical forms. A, B, and C, Diastolic stop-frame images obtained in the parasternal short-axis plane. D and E, Apical four-chamber views. A. Relatively mild hypertrophy in a concentric (symmetric) pattern with each segment of septum and free wall having similar or identical thickness (paired arrows). B. "Butterfly" pattern with prominent indentation (arrow) and localized area of thinning interpositioned at the 11 o'clock position between adjacent thicker areas of ventricular septum. C. Hypertrophy of entire ventricular septum (VS) and sparing of free wall. D. Myocardial hypertrophy confined to left ventricular apex (asterisk). E. Image from another patient with hypertrophy involving the apex, as well as the basal ventricular septum and free wall. Calibration marks are 1 cm apart. AVS, anterior ventricular septum; LA, left atrium; LFW, lateral free wall; LV, left ventricle; PVS, posterior ventricular septum. *Adapted with permission of the American College of Cardiology from Klues HG, Schiffers A, Maron BJ: Phenotypic spectrum and patterns of left ventricular hypertrophy in hypertrophic cardiomyopathy: Morphologic observations and significance as assessed by two-dimensional echocardiography in 600 patients. J Am Coll Cardiol 26:1699-1708, 1995.*

DETECTION DURING PREPARTICIPATION SCREENING

While HCM may be suspected during preparticipation sports evaluations by the prior occurrence of exertional syncope, family history of the disease or premature cardiac death, or by a loud heart murmur, such clinical features are relatively uncommon among all individuals affected by this disease. Of note, most HCM patients have the nonobstructive form of this disease characteristi-cally expressed by no murmur or only a soft heart murmur.[29] Consequently, standard screening procedures with only history and physical examination cannot be expected to reliably and consistently identify this disease.[11] One retrospective study showed that potentially lethal cardiovascular abnormalities, including HCM, were suspected by the standard preparticipation history and physical examination in only 3% of 115 high school and collegiate athletes who ultimately died suddenly of such diseases[3] (Fig. 9.6).

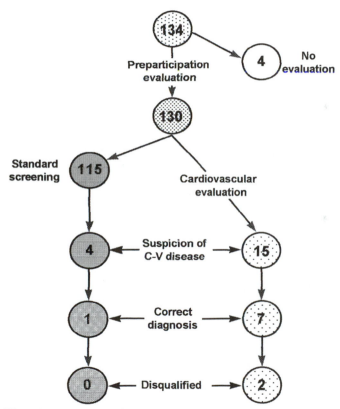

FIGURE 9.6. Flow-diagram showing impact of preparticipation medical history and physical examinations on the detection of structural cardiovascular (C-V) disease (and causes of sudden death), including HCM, as well as subsequent disqualification from competitive athletics. Cardiovascular evaluation indicates diagnostic testing (independent of standard school or institutional preparticipation screening), performed in 15 athletes because of symptoms, family history, cardiac murmur, or other physical findings suggestive of heart disease. Adapted with permission from the American Medical Association from Maron BJ, Shirani J, Poliac LC, et al: Sudden death in young competitive athletes: Clinical, demographic and pathological profiles. JAMA 276:199–204, 1998.

Even when noninvasive testing (i.e., echocardiography) is employed in screening athletes for HCM, false-negatives may occur when encountering individuals with this disease at a point of incomplete phenotypic expression, usually during adolescence.[47,48] Indeed, in young individuals with HCM (approximately less than age 13–15) left ventricular hypertrophy is often absent or mild, and therefore the echocardiographic findings (and phenotypic expression) may not be diagnostic at the time of preparticipation screening.

DIFFERENTIAL DIAGNOSIS OF HYPERTROPHIC CARDIOMYOPATHY AND ATHLETE'S HEART

Hypertrophy in some young athletes involving the anterior ventricular septum (wall thicknesses of 13–15 mm) is consistent with a relatively mild morphologic expression of HCM, and may be difficult to distinguish from the physiological form of left ventricular hypertrophy, which is an adaptation to athletic training (i.e., athlete's heart)[49] (Fig. 9.7). This distinction between athlete's heart[17–22,49] and cardiac disease[29,49] has particularly important implications, because identification of cardiovascular disease in an athlete may be the basis for disqualification from competition in an effort to minimize risk.[12] By the same token, the improper diagnosis of cardiac disease in an athlete may lead to unnecessary withdrawal from athletics, thereby depriving that individual of the varied benefits of sports.

For asymptomatic individuals within this morphologic "gray zone," the differential diagnosis between athlete's heart and HCM can be approached by clinical assessment and noninvasive testing[49] (Fig. 9.4). While this distinction cannot be resolved with certainty in some athletes, careful analysis of several echocardiographic and clinical features permits this diagnostic differentiation in most instances (Fig. 9.7).

WALL THICKNESS

In highly trained athletes, although the region of predominant left ventricular wall thickening al-

ways involves the anterior septum, the thicknesses of other segments of the wall are similar.[20] Absolute increases in left ventricular wall thickness within the "gray zone" due to athletic training have been identified most commonly in sports such as rowing and cycling, but not as a consequence of isometric training.[50] In HCM, while the anterior portion of septum is also usually the region of maximal wall thickening, areas other than the anterior septum (e.g., posterior septum and anterolateral free wall or apex) may show the most marked thickening.[27,43]

CAVITY DIMENSION

An enlarged left ventricular end-diastolic cavity dimension (> 55 mm) is present in more than one-third of highly trained elite male athletes.[22] Conversely, the diastolic cavity dimension is small (< 45 mm) in most patients with HCM and is > 55 mm only in those who evolve to the end-stage phase of the disease with progressive heart failure and systolic dysfunction.[51] Therefore, in some instances, it is possible to distinguish the athlete's heart from HCM solely on the basis of left ventricular diastolic cavity dimension.[49] For example, a cavity > 55 mm in an athlete with borderline wall thickness would constitute strong evidence against the presence of HCM; conversely a cavity dimension < 45 mm would be inconsistent with the athlete's heart in a highly trained individual. However, in those athletes in whom left ventricular cavity size falls between these extremes this variable alone cannot resolve the differential diagnosis with HCM.

DOPPLER TRANSMITRAL WAVEFORM

Abnormalities of left ventricular diastolic filling have been identified noninvasively with pulsed Doppler echocardiography.[52] Most patients with HCM, including those with relatively mild hypertrophy that could be confused with athlete's heart, show abnormal Doppler diastolic indexes of left ventricular filling and relaxation independently of whether symptoms or outflow obstruction are

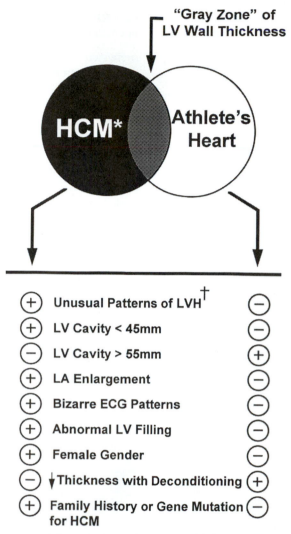

FIGURE 9.7. *Chart summarizing criteria used to distinguish hypertrophic cardiomyopathy (HCM) from athlete's heart when the left ventricular (LV) wall thickness is within the shaded gray zone of overlap (13–15 mm), consistent with both diagnoses. * Assumed to be the nonobstructive form of HCM, since the presence of substantial mitral valve systolic anterior motion would confirm, per se, the diagnosis of HCM in an athlete. † May involve a variety of abnormalities, including heterogeneous distribution of left ventricular hypertrophy (LVH) in which asymmetry is prominent, and adjacent regions may be of greatly different thicknesses, with sharp transitions evident between segments; also, patterns in which the anterior ventricular septum is spared from the hypertrophic process and the region of predominant thickening may be in the posterior portion of septum or anterolateral or posterior free wall. ↓ indicates decreased; LA, left atrial; ECG, electrocardiogram.* Adapted with permission of the American Heart Association from *Maron BJ, Pellicia A, Spirito P: Cardiac disease in young trained athletes: Insights into methods for distinguishing athlete's heart from structural heart disease with particular emphasis on hypertrophic cardiomyopathy.* Circulation *91:1596–1601, 1995.*

present.[52,53] In comparison, trained athletes have invariably demonstrated normal left ventricular filling patterns.[54–58] Consequently, in an athlete suspected of having HCM, a distinctly abnormal Doppler transmitral flow-velocity pattern strongly supports this diagnosis, while a normal Doppler study is compatible with either HCM or athlete's heart.[53]

GENDER

Sex differences with regard to cardiac dimensions and left ventricular mass have been identified in trained athletes.[19,59,60] For example, female athletes rarely show left ventricular wall thicknesses ≥ 12 mm (Fig. 9.8).[21] Therefore, female athletes with wall thicknesses within the gray zone between athlete's heart and HCM are most likely to have HCM.[21]

REGRESSION OF LEFT VENTRICULAR HYPERTROPHY WITH DECONDITIONING

Increased left ventricular cavity size or wall thickness can be shown to be a physiological consequence of athletic training by serial echocardiographic examinations, demonstrating a decrease in cardiac dimensions and mass after a short period of athletic deconditioning.[61–63] For example, elite athletes with left ventricular hypertrophy may show reduction in wall thickness (of about 2–5 mm) with 3 months of deconditioning[63] (Fig. 9.9). However, identification of such changes in wall thickness requires compliance from highly motivated competitive athletes to interrupt training, and also serial echocardiographic studies of optimal technical quality. An unequivocal decrease in left ventricular wall thickness with deconditioning is inconsistent with the diagnosis of pathologic hypertrophy and HCM.

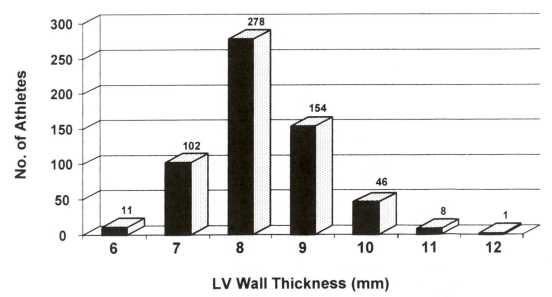

FIGURE 9.8. Distribution of maximal left ventricular (LV) wall thickness from 600 highly trained competitive women athletes participating in a variety of sporting disciplines. Of note, wall thickness did not exceed 12 mm and, therefore, did not fall into the equivocal gray-zone of overlap between the physiologic athlete's heart and pathologic hypertrophic cardiomyopathy. Adapted with permission of the American Medical Association from Pelliccia A, Maron BJ, Culasso F, et al: Athlete's heart in women: Echocardiographic characterization of highly trained elite female athletes. JAMA 276:211–215, 1996.

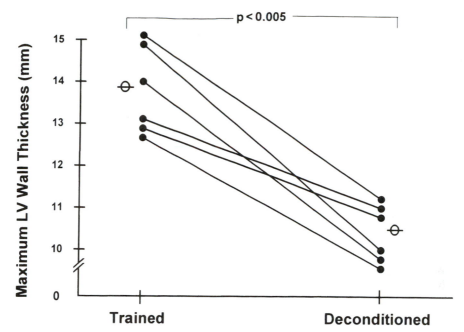

FIGURE 9.9. Changes in maximal left ventricular wall thickness associated with deconditioning in Olympic level rowers. Cardiac dimensions were obtained with two-dimensional echocardiography at peak training and subsequently after 6 to 34 weeks of deconditioning following the 1988 Olympic Games, with measurements made in a blinded fashion. Adapted with permission from Maron BJ, Pellicia A, Spartaro A, et al: Reduction in left ventricular wall thickness after deconditioning in highly trained Olympic athletes. Br Heart J 69:125–128, 1993.

ELECTROCARDIOGRAM

Because of the wide variety of ECG alterations present both in athletes without cardiovascular disease[64] and patients with HCM,[62] the 12-lead ECG is not particularly useful in distinguishing between these two entities. Furthermore, unusual and bizarre ECG patterns with, for example, strikingly increased voltages, prominent Q waves, or deep negative T waves are consistent with both HCM[65] and "athlete's heart."[64]

FAMILIAL TRANSMISSION AND GENETICS

The most definitive evidence for the presence of HCM in an athlete with increased wall thickness comes from the demonstration of the disease in a relative.[30–32,45,66–68] Therefore, in those athletes in

whom the distinction between HCM and athlete's heart cannot be achieved definitively by other methods, one potential approach for resolving this diagnostic uncertainty is by the echocardiographic screening of family members.[67] Absence of HCM in a family, however, does not exclude the diagnosis of HCM since the disease may be "sporadic" (i.e., absent in relatives other than the index case), presumably as a result of a *de novo* mutation.

Advances in the understanding of the genetic alterations responsible for HCM raise the possibility of DNA diagnosis in athletes suspected of having this disease. At present, mutations responsible for HCM have been identified in nine genes; each of which encode proteins of the sarcomere: β-myosin heavy chain, cardiac troponin T, troponin-I, myosin-binding protein C, α-tropomyosin, essential and regulatory myosin light chains, titin and actin, and well over 100 individual mutations (mostly of the missense variety).[30–32,45,66–71] This substantial genetic heterogeneity and the expensive, time intensive methodologies required, has made it difficult at present to use the techniques of molecular biology for the purpose of routinely resolving the differential diagnosis between athlete's heart and HCM in the clinical arena.

In addition, not infrequently encountered at autopsy, are hearts with increased mass (and wall thickness) and nondilated left ventricular cavity suggestive of HCM, but in which the objective morphologic findings are not sufficiently striking to permit a definitive diagnosis of this disease.[3] It is an uncertain but intriguing issue whether some of these cases (often referred to as idiopathic left ventricular hypertrophy, at autopsy)[8,10] represent a mild morphologic expression of HCM, or possibly unusual instances of athlete's heart with particularly marked physiological left ventricular hypertrophy associated with deleterious consequences.

Of note, in other selected athletes, marked left ventricular end-diastolic cavity enlargement (≥ 60 mm and up to 70 mm) may raise a consideration for the idiopathic dilated form of cardiomyopathy.[22] This differential diagnosis can usually be resolved by the absence of global or segmental left ventricular dysfunction (and cardiac symptoms) in the trained athlete.

DEMOGRAPHICS OF SUDDEN DEATH IN YOUNG ATHLETES

Based primarily on data assembled from broad-based United States populations, a profile of young competitive athletes who die suddenly has emerged.[3,4,7–10,72] Such athletes participated in a large number and variety of sports with the most frequent being basketball and football (about 70%), probably reflecting the high participation level in these popular team sports, and also their intensity. The vast majority of athletic field deaths occur in males (about 90%); the relative infrequency in females probably reflects a lower participation level, and sometimes less intense levels of training. Most athletes are of high school age at the time of death (about 60%); however, other sudden deaths occur in young athletes who have achieved collegiate or even professional levels of competition.

The vast majority of athletes who incur sudden death (with HCM or other diseases) have been free of symptoms during their lives and were not suspected to harbor cardiovascular disease. Sudden collapse usually occurs associated with exercise, predominantly in the late afternoon and early evening hours corresponding to peak periods of competition and training, particularly in organized team sports such as football and basketball (Fig. 9.10).[3] These findings for athletes with HCM contrast strikingly with prior findings

FIGURE 9.10. Hourly distribution of sudden cardiac deaths. Top Panel. Histogram showing time of death for 127 competitive athletes with either HCM (bold portion of bars) or a variety of other predominantly congenital cardiovascular malformations (lighter portions of bars). Death occurred predominantly in the late afternoon and early evening (2 pm to 9 pm), corresponding largely to the time of training and competition. Adapted with permission from the American Medical Association from Maron BJ, Shirani J, Poliac LC, et al: Sudden death in young competitive athletes: Clinical, demographic and pathological profiles. JAMA 276:199–204, 1998. *Bottom Panel. In contrast, shown for 94 patients recognized as having HCM (who were not athletes), demonstrating a prominent early peak between 7:00 am and 1:00 pm and a secondary peak in the early evening (most evident between 8:00 pm and 10:00 pm).* Adapted with permission of the American College of Cardiology from Maron BJ, Kogan J, Proschan MA, et al: Circadian variability in the occurrence of sudden cardiac death in patients with hypertrophic cardiomyopathy. J Am Coll Cardiol 23:1405–1409, 1994.

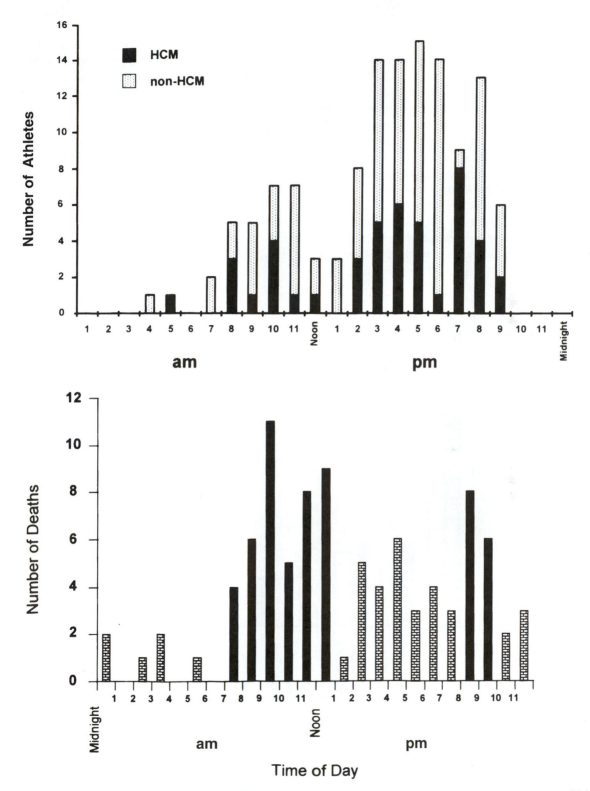

in patients with this disease (who were *not* competitive athletes) for whom a bimodal pattern of circadian variability over the 24-h day was evident, including a prominent early to mid-morning peak, similar to that described in patients with coronary artery disease (i.e., with sudden death, acute myocardial infarction, or angina) (Fig. 9.4).[73] Such observations substantiate that, in the presence of certain underlying structural cardiovascular diseases (including HCM and other cardiomyopathies), physical activity represents a trigger and an important precipitating factor for sudden collapse on the athletic field. In HCM, intense athletic participation may trigger potentially lethal tachyarrhythmias (usually primary ventricular tachycardia/fibrillation), given the underlying electrophysiologically unstable myocardial substrate comprised of disorganized cardiac muscle cells and replacement fibrosis (which is probably the consequence of ischemia).

Although the majority of reported sudden deaths in competitive athletes have been in white males, a substantial proportion (> 40%) are African-American athletes.[3,72,74] There is also evidence that HCM represents a common cause of sudden death in young African-American males (Fig. 9.11).[74] This substantial occurrence of HCM-related sudden death in young black male

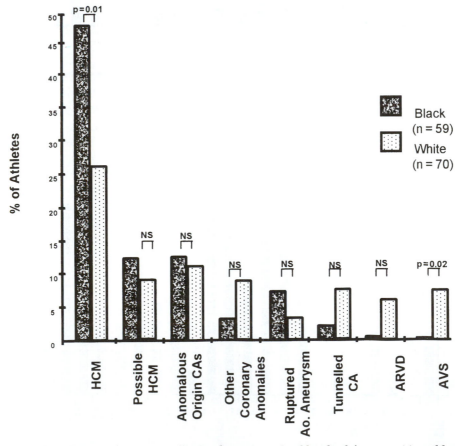

FIGURE 9.11. Impact of race on cardiovascular causes of sudden death in competitive athletes. Ao, aorta; AV, aortic valve stenosis; CA, coronary anomalies; HCM, hypertrophic cardiomyopathy; ARVD, arrhythmogenic right ventricular dysplasia.

athletes contrasts sharply with the very infrequent identification of black patients with HCM in hospital-based populations.[74] These data emphasize the disproportionate access to subspecialty health care between the African-American and white communities in the United States that makes it less likely for young black males to receive a relatively sophisticated cardiovascular diagnosis, such as HCM, compared with their white counterparts. Consequently, young African-American athletes with HCM are also less likely to be disqualified from competition, in accordance with the recommendations of the 26th Bethesda Conference[12] to reduce their risk for sudden death.

ELIGIBILITY CONSIDERATIONS FOR ATHLETES WITH HYPERTROPHIC CARDIOMYOPATHY

When a cardiovascular abnormality such as HCM is identified in a competitive athlete, the following considerations arise: (a) the magnitude of risk for sudden cardiac death associated with continued participation in competitive sports; and (b) the criteria to be implemented for determining whether individual athletes should be withdrawn from sports competition. In this regard, the 26th Bethesda Conference sponsored by the American College of Cardiology[12] offers prospective and consensus recommendations for athletic eligibility or disqualification, taking into account the severity of the cardiovascular abnormality as well as the nature of sports training and competition. The Bethesda Conference recommendations are predicated on the likelihood that intense athletic training will increase the risk for sudden cardiac death (or disease progression) in trained athletes with HCM, although at present it is not possible to quantify that risk in precise terms.

It is presumed that the temporary or permanent withdrawal of selected athletes from participation in certain sports is both prudent and beneficial by virtue of diminishing the perceived risk.

It is well recognized that all patients (or athletes) with HCM do not incur the same risk for sudden cardiac death.[28,29,34,72] However, the differentiation of subgroups of young athletes and patients with differing risks has proved challenging and remains largely unresolved. Although electrophysiological testing with programmed electrical stimulation has provided some measure of predictability with regard to outcome in high-risk patients with coronary artery disease, inferences from those data to patients with HCM are fraught with great uncertainty,[28,29] particularly with regard to the highly selected subset of trained athletes with this disease. Indeed, in a disease such as HCM in which there is a propensity for potentially lethal arrhythmias in some individuals, the stress of athletic training and competition as well as associated alterations in blood volume, hydration, and electrolytes that may occur make very tenuous any extrapolation of risk assessment from nonathletes with HCM directly to highly trained competitive athletes with this condition. These considerations are particularly relevant to a heterogeneous disease such as HCM, in which risk stratification remains imprecise.[28,29] That it is difficult at present to assess risk in individual athletes (or patients) with HCM is reflected in the Bethesda Conference recommendations for athletic eligibility that are necessarily conservative and homogeneous for most athletes with HCM:[75] "Athletes with the unequivocal diagnosis of HCM should not participate in most competitive sports, with the possible exception of those of low intensity. This recommendation includes those athletes with or without symptoms and with or without left ventricular outflow obstruction." [75]

The 26th Bethesda Conference report provides clear benchmarks for the expected standards of care that may be used in resolving medicolegal disputes in individual cases.[12] Indeed, the Bethesda Conference has been cited by a U.S. Court of Appeals (in Knapp v. Northwestern University) as a consensus reference document that the team physician should rely on in formulating disqualification decisions for competitive athletes with cardiovascular disease.[2]

DNA-based diagnosis has led to the identification of increasing numbers of children and adults with a preclinical diagnosis of HCM.[32,45,48,66,71] These individuals with a disease-causing genetic mutation, are nevertheless *without* clinical or phenotypic manifestations of HCM such as left ventricular wall thickening on echocardiogram or cardiac symptoms (a variety of alterations may, however, be evident on the 12-lead ECG).[48,71,76] Based on the available data, it is likely that most such genotype positive-phenotype negative children will develop left ventricular hypertrophy when achieving full body growth and maturation.[47,72]

Genetically affected adults without phenotypic expression of left ventricular hypertrophy appear to be relatively uncommon and largely confined to myosin-binding protein C[66,71,77] and cardiac troponin T mutations.[68] The clinical implications of a primary molecular diagnosis of HCM, and the appropriate management of such individuals, are largely unresolved issues. However, at present, there is no evidence to justify precluding most such genetically affected individuals without the HCM phenotype (i.e., without left ventricular hypertrophy on echocardiogram) from competitive athletics or most other life activities. However, a possible exception would be in those individuals with a family history of frequent HCM-related death or the documentation of a particularly malignant genotype where possible restriction from competitive sports may be justified.

REFERENCES

1. Maron BJ: Sudden death in young athletes: Lessons from the Hank Gathers affair. *N Engl J Med* 329:55–57, 1993.
2. Maron BJ, Mitten MJ, Quandt EK, et al: Competitive athletes with cardiovascular disease—The case of Nicholas Knapp. *N Engl J Med* 339:1632–1635, 1998.
3. Maron BJ, Shirani J, Poliac LC, et al: Sudden death in young competitive athletes: Clinical, demographic and pathological profiles. *JAMA* 276:199–204, 1996.
4. Burke AP, Farb A, Virmani R, et al: Sports-related and non-sports-related sudden cardiac death in young athletes. *Am Heart J* 121:568–575, 1991.
5. Corrado D, Thiene G, Nava A, et al: Sudden death in young competitive athletes: Clinicopathologic correlations in 22 cases. *Am J Med* 39:588–596, 1990.
6. Corrado D, Basso C, Schiavon M, et al: Screening for hypertrophic cardiomyopathy in young athletes. *N Engl J Med* 339:364–369, 1998.
7. Van Camp SP, Bloor CM, Mueller FO, et al: Nontraumatic sports death in high school and college athletes. *Med Sci Sports Exer* 27:641–647, 1995.
8. Maron BJ, Roberts WC, McAllister HA, et al: Sudden death in young athletes. *Circulation* 62:218–229, 1980.
9. Liberthson RR: Sudden death from cardiac causes in children and young adults. *N Engl J Med* 334:1039–1044, 1996.
10. Maron BJ, Epstein SE, Roberts WC: Causes of sudden death in the competitive athlete. *J Am Coll Cardiol* 7:204–214, 1986.
11. Maron BJ, Thompson PD, Puffer JC, et al: Cardiovascular preparticipation screening of competitive athletes. *Circulation* 94:850–856, 1996.
12. Maron BJ, Mitchell JH: 26th Bethesda Conference. Recommendations for determining eligibility for competition in athletes with cardiovascular abnormalities. *J Am Coll Cardiol* 24:845–899, 1994.
13. Maron BJ, Gohman T, Aeppli D: Prevalence of sudden cardiac death during competitive sports activities in Minnesota high school athletes. *J Am Coll Cardiol* 32:1881–1884, 1998.
14. Maron BJ, Poliac LC, Roberts WO: Risk for sudden cardiac death associated with marathon running. *J Am Coll Cardiol* 28:428–431, 1996.
15. Thompson PD, Funk EJ, Carleton RA, et al: Incidence of death during jogging in Rhode Island from 1975 through 1980. *JAMA* 247:2535–2538, 1982.
16. Siscovick DS, Weiss NS, Fletcher R, et al: The incidence of primary cardiac arrest during vigorous exercise. *N Engl J Med* 3111:874–877, 1984.
17. Shen W-K, Edwards WD, Hammill SC, et al: Sudden unexpected nontraumatic death in 54 young adults: A 30-year population-based study. *Am J Cardiol* 76:148–152, 1995.
18. Driscoll DJ, Edwards WD: Sudden unexpected

death in children and adolescents. *J Am Coll Cardiol* 5(Suppl B):118B–121B, 1985.

19. Maron BJ: Structural features of the athlete heart as defined by echocardiography. *J Am Coll Cardiol* 7:190–203, 1986.

20. Pelliccia A, Maron BJ, Spataro A, et al: The upper limit of physiologic cardiac hypertrophy in highly trained elite athletes. *N Engl J Med* 324:295–301, 1991.

21. Pelliccia A, Maron BJ, Culasso F, et al: Athlete's heart in women: Echocardiographic characterization of highly trained elite female athletes. *JAMA* 276:211–215, 1996.

22. Pelliccia A, Culasso F, Di Paolo F, et al: Physiologic left ventricular cavity dilatation in elite athletes. *Ann Intern Med* 130:23–31, 1999.

23. Shapiro LM, Smith RG: Effect of training on left ventricular structure and function: An echocardiographic study. *Br Heart J* 50:534–539, 1983.

24. Huston TP, Puffer JC, Rodney WM: The athletic heart syndrome. *N Engl J Med* 313:24–32, 1985.

25. Maron BJ, Bonow RO, Cannon RO, et al: Hypertrophic cardiomyopathy: Interrelation of clinical manifestations, pathophysiology, and therapy. *N Engl J Med* 316:780–789, 844–852, 1987.

26. Wigle ED, Sasson Z, Henderson MA, et al: Hypertrophic cardiomyopathy. The importance of the site and extent of hypertrophy. A review. *Prog Cardiovasc Dis* 28:1–83, 1985.

27. Klues HG, Schiffers A, Maron BJ: Phenotypic spectrum and patterns of left ventricular hypertrophy in hypertrophic cardiomyopathy: Morphologic observations and significance as assessed by two-dimensional echocardiography in 600 patients. *J Am Coll Cardiol* 26:1699–1708, 1995.

28. Spirito P, Seidman CE, McKenna SJ, et al: The management of hypertrophic cardiomyopathy. *N Engl J Med* 36:775–785, 1997.

29. Maron BJ: Hypertrophic cardiomyopathy. *Lancet* 350:127–133, 1997.

30. Marian AJ, Roberts R: Recent advances in the molecular genetics of hypertrophic cardiomyopathy. *Circulation* 92:1336–1347, 1995.

31. Schwartz K, Carrier L, Guicheney P, et al: Molecular basis of familial cardiomyopathies. *Circulation* 91:532–540, 1995.

32. Maron BJ, Moller JH, Seidman CE, et al: Impact of laboratory molecular diagnosis on contemporary diagnostic criteria for genetically transmitted cardiovascular diseases: Hypertrophic cardiomy-opathy, long-QT syndrome, and Marfan syndrome. *Circulation* 98:1460–1471, 1998.

33. Maron BJ, Gardin JM, Flack JM, et al: Assessment of the prevalence of hypertrophic cardiomyopathy in a general population of young adults: Echocardiographic analysis of 4111 subjects in the CARDIA study. *Circulation* 92:785–789, 1995.

34. Maron BJ, Roberts WC, Epstein SE: Sudden death in hypertrophic cardiomyopathy: A profile of 78 patients. *Circulation* 65:1388–1394, 1982.

35. Maron BJ, Spirito P: Impact of patient selection biases on the perception of hypertrophic cardiomyopathy and its natural history. *Am J Cardiol* 72:970–972, 1993.

36. Maron BJ, Shen W-K, Link MS, et al: Efficacy of implantable cardioverter-defibrillators for the prevention of sudden death in patients with hypertrophic cardiomyopathy. *N Engl J Med,* 342: 365–373, 2000.

37. Thiene G, Nava A, Corrado D, et al: Right ventricular cardiomyopathy and sudden death in young people. *N Engl J Med* 318:129–133, 1988.

38. Cecchi F, Olivotto I, Montereggi A, et al: Hypertrophic cardiomyopathy in Tuscany: Clinical course and outcome in an unselected regional population. *J Am Coll Cardiol* 26:1529–1536, 1995.

39. Spirito P, Rapezzi C, Bellone P, et al: Infective endocarditis in hypertrophic cardiomyopathy. Prevalence incidence, and indications for antibiotic prophylaxis. *Circulation* 99:2132–2137, 1999.

40. Pelliccia A, Maron BJ: Preparticipation cardiovascular evaluation of the competitive athlete: Perspectives from the 30 year Italian experience. *Am J Cardiol* 75:827–828, 1995.

41. Casolo GC, Rega L, Renzi PD: The diagnostic role of magnetic resonance imaging (MRI) in sports cardiology: MRI in right ventricular dysplasia. *Int J Sports Cardiol* 4:59–73, 1995.

42. McKenna WJ, Thiene G, Nava A, et al: Diagnosis of arrhythmogenic right ventricular dysplasia/cardiomyopathy. *Br Heart J* 71:215–218, 1994.

43. Maron BJ, Gottdiener JS, Epstein SE: Patterns and significance of the distribution of left ventricular hypertrophy in hypertrophic cardiomyopathy: A wide-angle, two-dimensional echocardiographic study of 125 patients. *Am J Cardiol* 48:418–428, 1981.

44. Maron BJ, Gross BW, Stark SI: Extreme left ventricular hypertrophy. *Circulation* 92:2748, 1995.

45. Charron P, Dubourg O, Desnos M, et al:

Diagnostic value of electrocardiography and echocardiography for familial hypertrophic cardiomyopathy in a genotyped adult population. *Circulation* 96:214–219, 1997.

46. Ciró E, Nichols PF, Maron BJ: Heterogeneous morphologic expression of genetically transmitted hypertrophic cardiomyopathy: Two-dimensional echocardiographic analysis. *Circulation* 67:1227–1233, 1983.

47. Maron BJ, Spirito P, Wesley YE, et al: Development and progression of left ventricular hypertrophy in children with hypertrophic cardiomyopathy. *N Engl J Med* 315:610–614, 1986.

48. Rosenzweig A, Watkins H, Hwang D-S, et al: Preclinical diagnosis of familial hypertrophic cardiomyopathy by genetic analysis of blood lymphocytes. *N Engl J Med* 325:1753–1760, 1991.

49. Maron BJ, Pelliccia A, Spirito P: Cardiac disease in young trained athletes: Insights into methods for distinguishing athlete's heart from structural heart disease with particular emphasis on hypertrophic cardiomyopathy. *Circulation* 91:1596–1601, 1995.

50. Spirito P, Pelliccia A, Proschan MA, et al: Morphology of the "athlete's heart" assessed by echocardiography in 947 elite athletes representing 27 sports. *Am J Cardiol* 74:802–806, 1994.

51. Maron BJ, Spirito P: Implications of left ventricular remodeling in hypertrophic cardiomyopathy. *Am J Cardiol* 81:1339–1344, 1998.

52. Maron BJ, Spirito P, Green KJ, et al: Noninvasive assessment of left ventricular diastolic function by pulsed Doppler echocardiography in patients with hypertrophic cardiomyopathy. *J Am Coll Cardiol* 10:733–742, 1987.

53. Lewis JF, Spirito P, Pelliccia A, et al: Usefulness of Doppler echocardiographic assessment of diastolic filling in distinguishing "athlete's heart" from hypertrophic cardiomyopathy. *Br Heart J* 68:296–300, 1992.

54. Colan SD, Sanders SP, MacPherson D, et al: Left ventricular diastolic function in elite athletes with physiologic cardiac hypertrophy. *J Am Coll Cardiol* 6:545–549, 1985.

55. Pearson AC, Schiff M, Mrosek D, et al: Left ventricular diastolic function in weight lifters. *Am J Cardiol* 58:1254–1259, 1986.

56. Fagard R, Van den Brocke C, Bielen E, et al: Assessment of stiffness of the hypertrophied left ventricle of bicyclists using left ventricular inflow Doppler velocimetry. *J Am Coll Cardiol* 9:1250–1254, 1987.

57. Finkelhor RS, Hanak IJ, Bahler RC: Left ventricular filling in endurance-trained subjects. *J Am Coll Cardiol* 8:289–293, 1986.

58. Nixon JV, Wright AR, Porter TR, et al: Effects of exercise on left ventricular diastolic performance in trained athletes. *Am J Cardiol* 68:945–949, 1991.

59. Milliken MC, Stray-Gundersen J, Pesock RM, et al: Left ventricular mass as determined by magnetic resonance imaging in male endurance athletes. *Am J Cardiol* 62:301–305, 1988.

60. Riley-Hagen M, Peshock RM, Stray-Gundersen J, et al: Left ventricular dimensions and mass using magnetic resonance imaging in female endurance athletes. *Am J Cardiol* 69:1067–1074, 1992.

61. Ehsani AA, Hagberg JM, Hickson RC: Rapid changes in left ventricular dimensions and mass in response to physical conditioning and deconditioning. *Am J Cardiol* 42:52–56, 1978.

62. Fagard R, Aubert A, Lysens R, et al: Noninvasive assessment of seasonal variations in cardiac structure and function in cyclists. *Circulation* 67:896–901, 1983.

63. Maron BJ, Pelliccia A, Spataro A, et al: Reduction in left ventricular wall thickness after deconditioning in highly trained Olympic athletes. *Br Heart J* 69:125–128, 1993.

64. Pelliccia A, Maron BJ, Culasso F, et al: Athlete's heart syndrome revisited: Prevalence and clinical significance of abnormal electrocardiographic patterns in trained athletes. *Circulation*, in press.

65. Maron BJ, Wolfson JK, Ciró E, et al: Relation of electrocardiographic abnormalities and patterns of left ventricular hypertrophy identified by two-dimensional echocardiography in patients with hypertrophic cardiomyopathy. *Am J Cardiol* 51:189–194, 1983.

66. Niimura H, Bachinski LL, Sangwatanaroj S, et al: Mutations in the gene for human cardiac myosin-binding protein C and late-onset familial hypertrophic cardiomyopathy. *N Engl J Med* 338:1248–1257, 1998.

67. Maron BJ, Nichols PF, Pickle LW, et al: Patterns of inheritance in hypertrophic cardiomyopathy: Assessment by M-mode and two-dimensional echocardiography. *Am J Cardiol* 53:1087–1094, 1984.

68. Watkins H, McKenna WJ, Thierfelder L, et al:

Mutations in the genes for cardiac troponin T and α-tropomyosin in hypertrophic cardiomyopathy. *N Engl J Med* 332:1058–1064, 1995.

69. Morgensen J, Klausen IC, Pedersen AK, et al: α-cardiac actin is a novel disease gene in familial hypertrophic cardiomyopathy. *J Clin Invest* 103:R39–R43, 1999.

70. Flavigny J, Richard P, Isnard R, et al: Identification of two novel mutations in the ventricular regulatory myosin light chain gene (MYL2) associated with familial and classical forms of hypertrophic cardiomyopathy. *J Mol Med* 76:208–214, 1998.

71. Maron BJ, Niimura H, Casey SA, et al: Hypertrophic cardiomyopathy in adult patients without left ventricular hypertrophy: Genotype-phenotype correlations for cardiac myosin binding protein-C mutations (abstract). *Circulation* 98 (Suppl I):I–596–I-597, 1998.

72. Maron BJ: Cardiovascular risks to young persons on the athletic field. *Ann Intern Med* 129:379–386, 1998.

73. Maron BJ, Kogan J, Proschan MA, et al: Circadian variability in the occurrence of sudden cardiac death in patients with hypertrophic cardiomyopathy. *J Am Coll Cardiol* 23:1405–1409, 1994.

74. Maron BJ, Poliac LC, Mathenge R: Hypertrophic cardiomyopathy as an important cause of sudden cardiac death on the athletic field in African-American athletes (abstract). *J Am Coll Cardiol* 29(Suppl A):462A, 1997.

75. Maron BJ, Isner JM, McKenna WJ: Hypertrophic cardiomyopathy, myocarditis and other myoperi-cardial diseases, and mitral valve prolapse, Task Force 3. *J Am Coll Cardiol* 14:880–885, 1994.

76. Panza JA, Maron BJ: Relation of electrocardiographic abnormalities to evolving left ventricular hypertrophy in hypertrophic cardiomyopathy. *Am J Cardiol* 63:1358–1365, 1989.

77. Charron P, Dubourg O, Desnos M, et al: Clinical features and prognostic implications of familial hypertrophic cardiomyopathy related to the cardiac myosin-binding protein C gene. *Circulation* 97:2230–2236, 1998.

CASE REPORT

Age 14 (height 5'7"), male competitive basketball player. Because of exercise-induced dyspnea, an echocardiogram was performed. It was judged to be most consistent with athlete's heart. Maximal left ventricular wall thickness was within normal limits (i.e., 11 mm), although mild systolic anterior motion of the mitral valve and associated mild mitral regurgitation were present. Left ventricular end-diastolic dimension was 46 mm. It was concluded that the athlete had exercise-induced asthma.

Age 17 (height 6'5"). During a high school basketball game the athlete stumbled off the court and collapsed. He was found to be pulseless and apneic. Cardiopulmonary resuscitation was initiated immediately by the boy's father (a cardiovascular surgeon) for about 5 min; ventricular fibrillation was documented and external defibrillation performed (3 times), ultimately restoring sinus rhythm. An echocardiogram performed the next day demonstrated a markedly increased left ventricular wall thickness (over the previous 27-month period): anterior ventricular septum of 25 mm; posterior septum of 21 mm; and posterobasal left ventricular free wall of 23 mm. Moderate mitral valve systolic anterior motion was present without mitral-septal contact or evidence of outflow obstruction under basal conditions; 12-lead electrocardiogram showed a bizarre pattern with evidence of left ventricular hypertrophy, including markedly increased voltages (e.g., $R_{v6} = 41$ mm) and giant T-wave inversion (up to 18 mm in depth). The patient recovered completely without neurologic impairment. An implantable cardioverter-defibrillator was placed for secondary prevention of sudden death. This case makes four important points regarding hypertrophic cardiomyopathy (HCM) and athletic participation:

- Sudden death not infrequently occurs in athletes with HCM during intense physical exertion (particularly, burst exertion), particularly in sports such as competitive basketball.

- Successful resuscitation from ventricular fibrillation (and survival) is possible, given that appropriate measures are undertaken promptly and by adequately trained bystanders.

- Genetically affected children with HCM usually show little or no left ventricular wall thickening in childhood and early adolescence (age ≤ 14 years). However, abrupt and marked increases in wall thickness may occur before age 18 coinciding with growth and maturation. This scenario may create diagnostic uncertainty when echocardiography is performed in the pre-hypertrophic phase, and represents a potential limitation for the identification of HCM in the context of preparticipation screening, even when expensive echocardiographic testing is incorporated.

- Systolic anterior motion of the mitral valve, albeit mild and unassociated with outflow obstruction, may be a clinical clue suggestive of HCM in the pre-hypertrophic phase during childhood.

Chapter 10

ELECTROCARDIOGRAPHIC VARIANTS AND CARDIAC RHYTHM AND CONDUCTION DISTURBANCES IN THE ATHLETE

N. A. Mark Estes III, M.D.   *Mark S. Link, M.D.*   *Munther Homoud, M.D.*
Paul J. Wang, M.D.

Changes in the surface electrocardiogram (ECG) are common in the athlete based on the physiological changes that occur in myocardial conduction, repolarization, and impulse formation in response to athletic conditioning and changes in autonomic tone. Because these changes can appear pathologic and be interpreted as representing underlying cardiac disease, interpretation of normal from abnormal findings on the athlete's ECG can represent a challenge to the physician[1–39] (Table 10.1). The athlete may be subject to diagnostic evaluations including a stress test, ambulatory monitoring, or invasive tests such as electrophysiological evaluation or cardiac catheterization based on such ECG abnormalities as ventricular hypertrophy, repolarization abnormalities, or bradycardias, which are physiological rather than pathologic. In some instances unnecessary restriction from exercise or unwarranted therapy may be recommended in the athlete.[40] In contrast, the ECG may manifest changes that indicate the potential for a life-threatening arrhythmia.

TABLE 10.1.   COMMON ELECTROCARDIO-GRAPHIC FINDINGS IN ATHLETES

Sinus bradycardia
Sinus arrhythmia
First-degree AV block
Second-degree Wenckebach AV block
Incomplete right bundle branch block
Notched P waves
Right ventricular hypertrophy by voltage criteria
Left ventricular hypertrophy by voltage criteria
Repolarization abnormalities including ST-segment elevation
    and depression
Corrected QT interval at the upper limit of normal
Tall, peaked, and inverted T wave

Based on these considerations it is particularly important for the physician to appreciate the ECG changes that can accompany athletic conditioning and those that serve as a marker of underlying structural heart disease or vulnerability to cardiac arrhythmias. A substantial body of data regarding ECG changes and arrhythmias is available and serves as a basis for interpretation of the athlete's ECG and evaluation and management of brady-arrhythmias and tachyarrhythmias in the athlete.[1–39] This chapter will review the available literature on ECGs and arrhythmias in the athlete to provide the clinician with an objective basis for decisions regarding evaluation and management. In this regard it is important to remember that an interpretation of an ECG or arrhythmia should always be evaluated in light of the patient's medical and family history, symptoms, physical examination, and, when appropriate, studies evaluating the presence of underlying structural heart disease.

SINUS BRADYCARDIA AND SINUS ARRHYTHMIA

There is a broad spectrum of normal brady-arrhythmias in the conditioned athlete due to heightened vagal tone and reduction in sympathetic tone that accompanies physical conditioning.[1–19] Among the most common findings in the

athlete's ECG is sinus bradycardia, which is defined as a heart rate less than 60 beats per minute (Fig. 10.1). Generally, in the absence of symptoms due to sinus bradycardia, evaluation and therapy are not warranted. Up to 91% of athletes will have sinus bradycardia at rest depending on the athletic activity sampled.[1–12] For endurance sports such as long-distance running, bicycling, and swimming, the resting heart rates become lower with the level of conditioning.[20] One study of 650 athletes documented average heart rates at rest of 56 beats per minute in runners, 57 beats per minute in cyclists, 62 beats per minute in swimmers, and 51 beats per minute in wrestlers.[21] Elite long-distance runners have a mean resting heart rate of 47 beats per minute[7] with asymptomatic resting rates as low as 25 beats per minute in a long-distance runner.[9] Sinus pauses greater than 2 s without symptoms are common in athletes.[1] It has been observed that at a given level of exercise athletes also have lower heart rates than nonathletes and that the heart rates return to resting levels more rapidly in trained individuals than they do in untrained people.[30]

With physical conditioning increased, vagal tone and decreased sympathetic tone contribute to the bradycardia. Interestingly, in athletes whose hearts have been pharmacologically denervated using atropine and beta blockers, the intrinsic heart rate is lower than that in sedentary controls. This suggests that physical conditioning has a primary influence on the sinus node.[39] Significantly longer sinus pauses have been documented in long-distance runners as compared to untrained controls.[17] In runners, pauses up to 2.55 s while awake and 2.8 s while asleep have been documented.[17] In the absence of symptoms related to the sinus bradycardia, deconditioning, further evaluation, and/or therapy is not warranted.[40,41] In those athletes with or without structural heart disease and a resting rate < 30 beats per minute, consideration should be given to assessing the adequacy of sinus node function with an exercise stress test or an ambulatory monitor during exercise. In the absence of symptoms from sinus bradycardia, there is no need to restrict the indi-

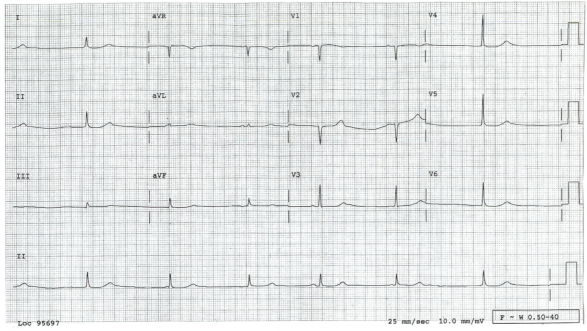

FIGURE 10.1. An asymptomatic 38-year-old female long-distance runner with marked sinus bradycardia and periods of junctional rhythm (note lead II rhythm strip). With exercise, her heart rate accelerated appropriately for age. Based on the absence of symptoms and appropriate increase in heart rate with exercise, no restriction on athletics or therapy was instituted.

vidual from athletic activity unless this restriction is based on underlying structural heart disease.[40,41]

Sinus arrhythmia, defined as respiratory variation in heart rate with an increase in heart rate with inspiration, is common in the athlete. It normally disappears with exercise.[9,21,31–35] Generally the younger the individual the more prominent the sinus arrhythmia. Interestingly, one study found no significant difference in the frequency of sinus arrhythmia in long-distance runners (100%) as compared to nonathletes (86%).[36a]

CONDUCTION ABNORMALITIES

Delay in conduction through the atrioventricular (AV) node with first-degree AV block defined as a PR interval ≥ .20 on the ECG is reported in 10 to

33% of athletes.[2,14,15] Similar to sinus bradycardia this is generally attributed to enhanced vagal tone. First-degree AV and Wenckebach-type block in the athlete typically normalizes with exercise or atropine as vagal tone is withdrawn.[3,7,12,15,18] In a review of 122,043 ECGs of healthy males in the military service, 6.5/1000 had first-degree AV block.[17]

Observations from ambulatory monitoring have documented that up to 40% of athletes with first-degree AV block will also demonstrate Möbitz type I or Wenckebach-type block with progressive PR prolongation before a nonconducted P wave followed by a shortening of the PR interval.[1,12] In a nonathlete population, the frequency of Möbitz type I block was noted to be 0.003%.[17] This type of AV block conduction has been noted to disappear with exercise and with deconditioning. In a group of 122 highly conditioned middle-aged cross-country skiers,[9,36b] the conclusion was reached that first-degree and Wenckebach-type block were changes seen as part of the spectrum of the "athletic heart syndrome" and were due to the training effect rather than to underlying coronary heart disease. Thus, various forms of vagally mediated heart block are more commonly seen in athletes than are in nonconditioned individuals and tend to disappear with exercise and deconditioning. Evaluation and therapy is generally warranted when there is underlying structural heart disease and the patient has clinically important symptoms.

The frequency in athletes with Möbitz type II block and advanced AV block with more than one consecutive nonconducted P wave is unknown but is rare compared to that of first-degree or Wenckebach-type block. Generally Möbitz type II block should be considered to be a potential marker of underlying heart disease and an indication for further evaluation of the athlete. Advanced AV block with more than one consecutive nonconducted P wave may occur at the level of the AV node due to the conditioning effect of vagal tone. It is frequently accompanied by prolongation of conduction through the AV node manifesting with first-degree AV block or Wenckebach-type block in association with the advanced AV block. Advanced AV block occurring in the setting of structural heart disease in the athlete or in the presence of significant conduction system disease below the level of the AV node may be a marker of high risk for progression to high degree AV block and often warrants permanent pacemaker implantation.

Complete heart block is extremely rare in the athlete. In a review of 15,000 ECGs of athletes,[1,9] only one single case of congenital complete heart block was noted. In another series, complete heart block was noted in 0.02% of the screened athletic population.[16] Not uncommonly with congenital complete heart block the junctional rhythm will accelerate to rates that allow the athlete to participate in athletics without symptoms. Congenital complete heart block is most commonly asymptomatic; it may be associated with certain types of

structural heart disease including L-transposition of the great vessels, which may be asymptomatic, and with maternal systemic lupus erythematosus. However, in one series up to 50% of cases had some identifiable structural heart disease.[1] In individuals with symptoms such as presyncope or syncope, participation in athletics should be restricted unless there is a period of 3 to 6 months of definitive therapy for the bradycardia.[40,41] In those instances where a permanent pacemaker is indicated, restriction from contact sports is recommended.[40,41]

In the absence of symptoms, worsening of the AV block with exercise, or underlying structural heart disease, there is no need to restrict athletic activity of those individuals with first-degree AV block or Wenckebach block. However, for individuals with Möbitz II or complete heart block permanent pacing is generally indicated regardless of underlying structural heart disease or symptoms. Athletes treated with a permanent pacemaker are restricted to those athletic activities in which there is no danger of bodily collision.[40,41]

INTRAVENTRICULAR CONDUCTION DELAYS

Incomplete right bundle branch block is the most common form of prolongation of intraventricular conduction and has been noted in up to 51% of athletes in some series.[2,12,15,20] Of 107 Olympic athletes, fully 51% had incomplete right bundle branch block.[2] In another analysis of 10 reports in 527 athletes, 16% had evidence of an incomplete right bundle branch block.[30] The physiological basis for incomplete right bundle branch block in the athlete remains unknown. It has been noted that this finding of incomplete right bundle branch block may represent right ventricular overload rather than true delayed conduction through the right bundle.[9] Prolongation of QRS conduction greater than 0.12 s due to a complete right bundle branch block or left bundle branch block is extremely rare.[1,16] This finding would prompt evaluation for underlying structural heart disease.

QRS AXIS

Generally the QRS frontal axis is between 0° and 90°.[12,20] In a study of 582 athletes, 78% had a frontal plane axis in this range.[38] In a report of 289 professional football players, the mean QRS axis was 56° with 5% manifesting right axis deviation of > 90°.[20,34] Left axis deviation with an axis < 0° is uncommon and, when present, should be considered as a possible marker of underlying structural heart disease particularly when accompanied by a bundle branch block.

P WAVE

Multiple studies have noted that the P-wave amplitude is greater in athletes than in an age-matched population of nonathletes.[2,3,7] The basis for this finding is unknown but may be due to atrial hypertrophy. In one series,[7] 25% of elite runners had P-wave voltage between 2.5 and 3 mm. In addition, it has been noted that there is a high frequency of "notched" P waves in athletes, with 18 of 25 runners[15] having this finding in one report. This contrasts with a lower frequency noted in a series of Finnish athletes in whom only 41 of 651 were noted to have notching of the P waves.[21]

VENTRICULAR HYPERTROPHY

It is common to find electrocardiographic criteria for either left or right ventricular hypertrophy in athletes.[12,20] The standard Sokolow-Lyon voltage criteria for right ventricular hypertrophy with R in V_1 + S in V_6 > 10.5 mm[22] were met in 9 of 46 Olympic athletes.[23] In a series of 3000 Israeli athletes, 20% met criteria for right ventricular hypertrophy[1] with a similar frequency noted of 18% in another series of 165 athletes.[24] Presumptively,

the basis for this relatively high frequency is physiological hypertrophy of the right ventricle, but there is little or no data correlating ECG evidence of right ventricular hypertrophy with echocardiographic or other assessment of right ventricular chamber enlargement or hypertrophy. A summary of 4 large series reporting on voltage criteria for right ventricular hypertrophy noted that criteria were met in 18 to 69% of athletes with a higher frequency noted in those with dynamic rather than static training.[14]

By contrast, ECG evidence of left ventricular hypertrophy has been studied extensively in athletes and correlated with echocardiographic measurements of left ventricular wall thickness.[12] Left ventricular hypertrophy is noted in up to 76% of athletes by standard ECG criteria.[2,3,5,6,7,13,15,25] In a series of world-class marathon runners, 76% were noted to have voltage criteria for left ventricular hypertrophy.[39] A summary of multiple studies involving 952 athletes found a 32% frequency of left ventricular hypertrophy.[38] In a series of professional football players, 35% were noted to have voltage criteria for left ventricular hypertrophy.[34] Sequential increases in voltage criteria have been noted with progressive training and regression of voltage with cessation of the training.[20] When endurance athletes are compared to sprinters, there is a significantly higher incidence of left ventricular hypertrophy in the endurance athletes with 44% of the former versus 32% of the latter having left ventricular hypertrophy.[6] In this study, both groups had similar dimensions of left ventricular cavity dilatation; however, the endurance group had greater wall thickness.[6] There has been no meaningful research on the extent to which chest wall musculature influences the frequency with which criteria for ventricular hypertrophy are met, but there is a general impression that the thinner chest wall in endurance athletes is associated with ECG evidence of left ventricular hypertrophy. Nonetheless, it is apparent that in the athlete, criteria for left ventricular hypertrophy are commonly met and can be considered physiological and within the spectrum of normal for this population.

REPOLARIZATION CHANGES IN THE ATHLETE

The patterns of repolarization seen in the athlete are commonly changed when compared to that of nonathletes. J-point elevation, ST-segment elevation, and T-wave changes are reported with high frequency[1,12,18,42] (Fig. 10.2). The patterns of ST-segment changes in the athlete include a high frequency of J-point elevation particularly in the inferior and precordial leads. In one series of 289 professional football players, 95% had J-point elevation of the ECG.[5] This typically ranged from 1 to 3 mm, but in isolated individuals as much as 5 mm of J-point elevation was noted. Repolarization changes have been noted in elite distant runners with 14 of 20 (70%) having J-point elevation.[7] Of 25 endurance athletes, 20 (80%) had J-point elevation compared to 37% of control subjects.[15] These and other series reporting a high frequency of J-point elevation in athletes[7,15,26] contrasts with a frequency of only 2.4% for J-point elevation in 49,000 healthy pilots who were not physically conditioned.[26] It has been reported that these J-point elevations normalize with exercise. It may be difficult to distinguish these changes on the ECG from those seen in acute pericarditis as the J-point elevation is commonly accompanied by ST-segment elevation. However, the clinical setting as well as the localization of the J-point changes to the inferior and anterior leads, in contrast to the global nature of the changes in pericarditis, can help distinguish the two.

ST-segment depression is unusual in the athlete. In the available literature, only one series noted this finding in athletes with 3% of bicyclists having 0.1 mm J-point and ST-segment de-

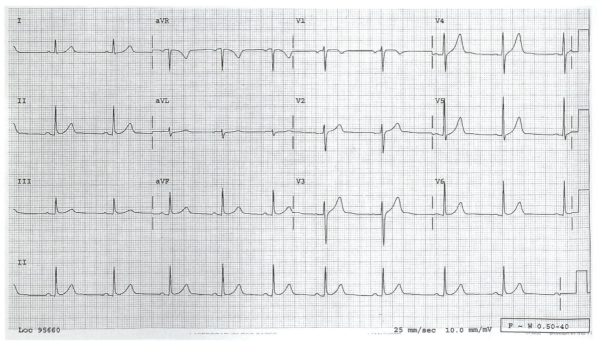

FIGURE 10.2. The electrocardiogram is shown from a 41-year-old asymptomatic athletic male referred for cardiac evaluation due to J-point and ST-segment evaluation in the inferior leads. This pattern is consistent with an early repolarization pattern. Evaluation with a stress test showed no evidence of ischemia and normalization of the repolarization changes.

pression.[14] By contrast T-wave changes with inversions in the precordial leads or limb leads are noted in up to 30% of endurance athletes.[1,2,4,7,15,27,29] The T waves may also be peaked and tall,[20] biphasic, or isoelectric. It has been reported that these T-wave changes normalize with exercise or with isoproterenol infusion.[18] Distinguishing these T-wave changes from metabolic or ischemic causes is based on the clinical setting.

SUPRAVENTRICULAR ARRHYTHMIAS

Premature atrial contractions have been noted in a high percentage of long-distance runners.[36,41] These are generally asymptomatic, but may be symptomatic or detected by the physician. A history, physical examination, and 12-lead ECG are recommended.[40–42] Without symptoms and in the absence of structural heart disease, additional evaluation and therapy is not recommended. When more severe symptoms are present, such as frequent or severe palpitations or light-headedness, beta-blocker therapy could be used as a first-line therapy. Because atrial premature contractions are frequently episodic in nature, it would be reasonable to treat them for a period of a few weeks with a long-acting beta blocker such as atenolol 25 to 50 mg daily. If the patient remains highly symptomatic, up-titration of beta blockers or changing to a long-acting calcium channel blocker such as verapamil-controlled-released preparation 120 to 240 mg daily would be reasonable. Without any significant cardiac disease, athletes with premature atrial contractions are not restricted from any athletic competition.[40–42]

Sustained supraventricular tachycardia (SVT) in the athlete is generally due to AV nodal reentry (AV nodal reentry tachycardia or AVRNT).[41] This generally manifests with a narrow complex tachycardia without visible P waves during the SVT. It typically starts abruptly and terminates abruptly. Triggers in the individual may include physical or emotional stress, caffeine, or alcohol. Valsalva

maneuvers or intravenous adenosine or verapamil are commonly used to terminate the acute episode. The dose of adenosine (Adenocard IV) is 6 mg intravenously given as a rapid bolus over 1 to 2 s. The dose should be given directly into a vein or in an intravenous line as close to the body as possible and followed by a fluid bolus. If the arrhythmia is not terminated within 1 to 2 min, a 12-mg bolus can be given and repeated a second time if needed. Doses higher than 12 mg are not recommended. Verapamil may be given intravenously in a dose of 5 to 10 mg over 1–2 min. Blood pressure and electrocardiographic rhythm should be continuously monitored. A second bolus dose may be given 30 min later. Alternatively, intravenous diltiazem may be administered as a bolus dose of 0.25 mg per kilogram of body weight over 1 to 2 min. If no response is seen in 15 min, a second bolus is given at 0.35 mg per kilogram of body weight over 1 to 2 min. A backup defibrillator should always be available. Both verapamil and diltiazem are vasodilators and may decrease the blood pressure.

When SVT occurs in the athletes during exercise, they may experience symptoms ranging from mild palpitations to syncope depending on a number of factors including the rate of the tachycardia and the blood pressure. The evaluation should include a history, physical examination, and invasive electrophysiological evaluation to define the tachycardia mechanism. Occasionally, stress testing will provoke the arrhythmia or an episode can be documented with ambulatory or loop monitoring. With success rates of over 95% with radiofrequency ablation and complication rates < 1%, a curative approach with radiofrequency ablation is the preferred initial approach.[41–43] For individuals who elect pharmacologic therapy of this arrhythmia, drug therapy should be proven effective for a period of 6 months before resuming competitive low-intensity athletics.[40–43] Pharmacologic therapy for patients with recurrent SVT secondary to AVNRT include beta blockers, calcium channel blockers, digoxin, and rarely, a class IA (quinidine, procainamide, disopyramide) or IC (flecainide, propafenone) antiarrhythmic agents. Verapamil can be given in divided dosages 3 or 4 times a day (total 240 to 480 mg daily) or the long-acting form can be given once or twice daily. The total daily dose of diltiazem is 240 to 360 mg given as divided doses of the short-acting form 3 or 4 times a day or of the long-acting form once daily. Digoxin is administered once daily in a dose of 0.25 mg daily. Serum levels help determine the need for higher doses in case the arrhythmia recurs. Rarely would one have to resort to therapy with class IA antiarrhythmic agents such as quinidine or procainamide or with class IC antiarrhythmic agents such as flecaninde or propafenone, especially considering the potential for developing proarrhythmia with these agents. If IA agents are started, this should be done in the hospital with continuous electrocardiographic monitoring. A stress test on individuals taking pharmacologic therapy to assess for arrhythmia or proarrhythmia recurrence is reasonable, although no prospective data are available regarding the predictive value of this approach. For athletes undergoing successful catheter ablation, resumption of all competitive athletics is permitted after 3 months.[40–43] For individuals with more severe symptoms related to the arrhythmia or for athletes involved in high-intensity competitive athletics, the radiofrequency catheter ablation technique would be preferred.

WOLFF-PARKINSON-WHITE SYNDROME

Wolff-Parkinson-White (WPW) syndrome is found in approximately 3 out of 1000 individuals. This condition manifests on the surface ECG with a short PR interval ($\leq .12$ s) and a δ wave represented as a slurred upstroke on the QRS complex from early activation of the ventricular myocardium (Fig. 10.3). The evaluation of the athlete with asymptomatic WPW remains controversial, although many experts recommend observation without restriction of athletic participation in asymptomatic subjects since the risk of sudden death is very low.[40–43] The risk of sudden cardiac

death in WPW syndrome is estimated at 1 in 1000 patients per year.[40–42] The mechanism is considered to be atrial fibrillation with rapid conduction down the accessory pathway resulting in ventricular fibrillation. Symptomatic patients with WPW syndrome should have an electrophysiological study done to establish potential for the bypass tract to conduct rapidly to the ventricle. Attempts at determining noninvasive indexes of the accessory bypass tract's potential for rapid antegrade conduction have not been conclusive. A history of syncope, the presence of multiple bypass tract, and an interval of 250 ms or less (equivalent to a heart rate of ≤ 240 beats per minute) between two maximally preexcited QRS complexes during atrial fibrillation are considered markers for increased risk of sudden death. Intermittent preexcitation, defined as the abrupt loss of preexcitation and the lengthening of the PR interval during a continuous electrocardiographic recording with minimal variation in the underlying sinus rate, is considered a sign that the accessory bypass tract has a prolonged effective refractory period.[40–42] Other electrocardiographic features described include "pre-excitation alternans" and "concertina" pre-excitation.[40–42] Some cardiologists and electrophysiologists recommend electrophysiological evaluation to define the properties and location of the bypass tract. If the bypass tract allows conduction to the ventricle at a rate greater than 240 beats per minute, radiofrequency ablation to eliminate the risk of future life-threatening arrhythmias would be a reasonable approach.[40–43]

Symptomatic arrhythmias due to WPW syndrome in the athlete may be due to AV-reciprocating tachycardia, atrial fibrillation, or, rarely, ventricular fibrillation. Typically the SVT seen with WPW syndrome is a narrow complex rhythm with P waves visible with a short RP interval during the tachycardia. Less commonly, the tachycardia proceeds antegrade through the bypass tract and retrograde via the AV node, resulting in a wide, complex preexcited tachycardia that can mimic ventricular tachycardia. A history, physical examination, ECG, 24-h ambulatory monitor, ex-

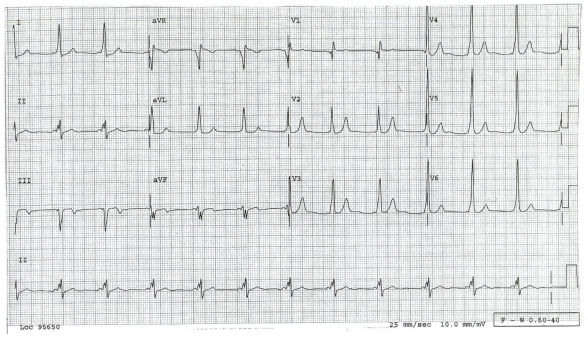

FIGURE 10.3. *This electrocardiogram is shown from a 25-year-old male who had recurrent episodes of palpitations and presyncope while playing basketball. The ECG shows a short PR interval and δ wave consistent with Wolff-Parkinson-White syndrome. At electrophysiological evaluation, atrioventricular reciprocating tachycardia was documented. The posterior septal bypass tract has been successfully ablated.*

ercise testing, and echocardiogram to exclude any underlying structural heart disease would be a reasonable initial approach.[40–43]

Manifest preexcitation may not be present on the surface ECG with a short PR interval and δ wave, but a retrograde bypass tract may still be identified at the time of electrophysiological evaluation. This "concealed" bypass tract allows retrograde conduction from the ventricle to the atrium during the tachycardia and serves as the substrate for the reentrant circuit. With success rates > 95% and complication rates < 1%, radiofrequency ablation is considered the preferred approach. Resumption of all athletic activities at 3 months is recommended after successful ablation. However, when drug therapy is used, a period of 6 months without recurrence is recommended before resumption of athletics.[40–43]

The commonest arrhythmia associated with WPW syndrome is orthodromic AV reentrant tachycardia (AVRT). This presents as a narrow complex tachycardia. It can be distinguished from AV nodal reentrant tachycardia associated with dual AV pathways by the presence of retrograde P waves inscribed in the ST segment or T waves of the tachycardia. Acute treatment of acute orthodromic AVRT is the same as for AV nodal tachycardia with intravenous adenosine 6 to 12 mg, intravenous beta blocker (metoprolol, 5 mg intravenously, total of 3 doses given 5 min apart) or calcium channel blockers (intravenous verapamil, 5 to 10 mg). These agents work by blocking the AV node, an essential component of the arrhythmia pathway. If these agents fail or the patient is hemodynamically compromised, synchronized direct current cardioversion should be employed.

First-line agents used in preventing recurrent SVT and WPW syndrome are the class IC agents, flecainide or propafenone. These agents work by prolonging the accessory bypass tract's refractory period. They also reduce the incidence of atrial and ventricular premature beats, known triggers of SVT. The starting dose of flecainide is 50 mg twice daily. Due to flecainide's long half-life, the dose can be increased in 50-mg increments no sooner than every 4 days. The maximum daily dose for SVT is 150 mg twice daily. Although propafenone has not been approved for the use in SVT, its beta-blocking effect may provide additional advantage in limiting recurrences. The starting dose is 150 mg 3 times a day. Dosage can be increased to a maximum of 300 mg 3 times daily. Changes in dosage should not be made until 3 to 4 days have elapsed since the last dose was increased. In patients with underlying structural heart disease, both agents have the potential to exacerbate preexisting arrhythmias. Great care should be exercised in excluding underlying cardiac disease, ischemic or otherwise, before these agents are initiated, preferably in a monitored, hospital setting. Although beta blockers can be used in patients with WPW syndrome, digoxin and calcium channel blockers are best avoided as chronic therapy. The potential for these agents to enhance conduction down an accessory bypass tract during atrial fibrillation while slowing conduction through the AV node limits their use to patients who have had electrophysiological studies documenting the safety of their use.

ATRIAL FIBRILLATION AND ATRIAL FLUTTER

Atrial fibrillation or atrial flutter in the athlete may be more common when compared with an age-matched population of nonathletes.[44] Atrial fibrillation can be either acute or chronic. By definition, atrial fibrillation lasting more than 2 weeks is chronic. A particular form of atrial fibrillation has been described in young patients with no underlying structural heart disease and paroxysmal atrial fibrillation. This arrhythmia's proclivity to start during sleep and after meals has led to the suggestion that it may be parasympathetically mediated. Digoxin, a drug commonly prescribed to patients with atrial fibrillation, would not be expected to have a favorable impact on this form of atrial fibrillation. Self-limited atrial fibrillation in young individuals often occurs after the heavy consumption of alcoholic beverages.

The incidence of atrial fibrillation increases with age and with underlying heart disease. Patients with atrial fibrillation younger than 65 years of age with no underlying cardiovascular disease or hyperthyroidism are labeled as having "lone atrial fibrillation." This group is characterized by a relatively low risk of thromboembolism. They constitute a distinct minority of patients with atrial fibrillation, however, young athletes with atrial fibrillation are likely to be in this group. The management of young patients with recently diagnosed atrial fibrillation should routinely include an ECG and an echocardiogram. An echocardiogram should be performed to exclude underlying cardiovascular disease.

Most cases of acute atrial fibrillation convert spontaneously within 24 h of their onset. However, cardioversion should not be delayed beyond the first 48 h of the arrhythmia's onset because of the increased risk of developing left atrial thrombus. If the duration of the atrial fibrillation exceeds 48 h or the patient cannot define the time of its onset, conversion to sinus rhythm should be deferred until 3 weeks of therapeutic anticoagulation has been achieved. Patients who have been in atrial fibrillation in excess of 48 h should also receive anticoagulation for at least 4 weeks after sinus rhythm has been restored.

Cardioversion is best accomplished with synchronized direct current shock after adequate sedation and analgesia have been provided. Care must be taken to exclude electrolyte disturbances and toxic levels of digoxin and other antiarrhythmic agents. Alternatively, the potassium channel blocker ibutilide (Corvert) may be used. It is given in a dose of 1 mg over 10 min. If this fails, a second 1-mg dose can be given 10 min after completion of the first dose. This drug has the potential to precipitate life-threatening ventricular arrhythmias in 2% of patients, usually within the first 4 h after administration. A corrected QT interval of less than 440 ms and serum potassium level of greater than 4.0 meq/L should be confirmed before ibutilide is started. Its administration should be followed by careful observation to defibrillate the patient in the event sustained ventricular arrhythmias occur. Other antiarrhythmics used to cardiovert patients with atrial fibrillation include procainamide, flecainide, propafenone, amiodarone, and sotalol.

Athletes may be predisposed to atrial fibrillation due to the high vagal tone resulting from training. A history, physical examination, ECG, echocardiogram, thyroid function tests, and test for illicit drug use should be completed. The maximal exertion rate of the atrial fibrillation or flutter should be assessed with an exercise tolerance test. An ambulatory monitor to assess maximal and minimal rates and the presence of any ventricular arrhythmias should also be performed. Options for therapy include rhythm control by reestablishing and maintaining normal sinus rhythm or rate control during atrial fibrillation. Rhythm control has the advantage of avoiding anticoagulation, but the potential disadvantage of risks and cost of the antiarrhythmic drug therapy.[45,46] If athletes have structural heart disease or other risk factors for embolic events, chronic anticoagulation with warfarin may be needed, which would then necessitate restriction from participation in any sport with a risk of bodily collision. Rate control of the ventricular response can also be difficult in athletes. In some competitive athletics, beta blockers are prohibited. Athletic participation is allowed despite persistent atrial fibrillation for athletes with or without structural heart disease who maintain a ventricular response during physical activity comparable to sinus rate with or without therapy. This recommendation must be within the guidelines recommended for their anticoagulation status and the limitations of their structural heart disease.[40,41] Catheter-based approach with radiofrequency ablation for atrial flutter and atrial tachycardia offers the potential for cure, but success rates are not as high as for AV nodal reentry or WPW arrhythmias.[43] When successful, athletic participation is allowed after 3 months without arrhythmia recurrence.[40,41]

VENTRICULAR ARRHYTHMIAS

Premature ventricular contractions in the athlete are common. Fortunately, they rarely cause symptoms that necessitate therapy. Without congenital or acquired structural heart disease, there is no increased risk of life-threatening cardiac arrhythmias. In athletes with premature ventricular contractions, a history, physical examination, ECG and echocardiogram should be performed. With congenital heart disease such as long QT syndrome hypertrophic cardiomyopathy, arrhythmogenic right ventricular dysplasia, anomalous origin of the coronary arteries, or acquired heart disease such as coronary artery disease or a dilated cardiomyopathy, further evaluation is needed.[46-57] Without structural heart disease, therapy with beta blockers may decrease symptoms with or without a reduction in the frequency of premature ventricular contraction. Drug therapy with other antiarrhythmic agents is not recommended unless the symptoms are severe and persist despite beta-blocker therapy. When the premature ventricular contractions do not cause symptoms with exertion or worsen with exercise, there are no athletic restrictions in the absence of structural heart disease.[40,41] Nonsustained ventricular tachycardia without structural heart disease indicates no additional risk of sudden cardiac death.[41,56-58] Nonsustained ventricular tachycardia is defined as ventricular tachycardia less than 30 s in duration. Management of these athletes is similar to those with premature ventricular contractions. However, those athletes with nonsustained polymorphic ventricular tachycardia may be at high risk for life-threatening ventricular arrhythmias, and therapy with beta blockers should be considered.[58]

Sustained ventricular tachycardia or prior episodes of ventricular fibrillation require a comprehensive evaluation of the athlete's cardiac status with history, physical exam, ECG, echocardiogram, and selective use of the stress test, cardiac magnetic resonance imaging, cardiac catheterization, and electrophysiological evaluation.[40,41,46,47] Sustained ventricular tachycardia in the absence of any identifiable structural heart disease can originate from the right ventricular outflow tract or other regions of the right or left ventricle (idiopathic ventricular tachycardia). Programmed ventricular stimulation supplemented by isoproterenol infusion can usually induce the arrhythmia to allow mapping and cure with radiofrequency ablation. When cured, these athletes can return to athletic competition in 3 months.[40,41]

Sustained ventricular tachycardia or ventricular fibrillation usually occurs in the presence of structural heart disease. In the athlete younger than 35 years, hypertrophic cardiomyopathy, right ventricular dysplasia, anomalous origin of the coronary arteries, or other congenital abnormalities[46–57] are the underlying heart diseases that most commonly predispose to sudden cardiac death. Since a risk of arrhythmia recurrence exists, antiarrhythmic therapy or an implantable cardioverter defibrillator (ICD) should be used. In athletes older than 35 years coronary artery disease is the most common cause of sudden cardiac death. The ICD confers superior protection for sudden death prevention in this patient population. Competitive athletics in patients with ICDs are generally prohibited by current guidelines. When an anomalous coronary artery is identified, competitive athletics can be resumed 6 months after bypass surgery.[40]

In many of the cardiovascular conditions known to predispose to sudden death, exercise may trigger the arrhythmia.[41,56,57] In both right ventricular outflow tract ventricular tachycardia and the sustained monomorphic ventricular tachycardia associated with right ventricular dysplasia, the arrhythmias are commonly exercise induced.[41] Similarly in patients with congenital abnormalities of the coronary arteries, exercise triggers sudden death.[56] In idiopathic ventricular fibrillation, approximately 15% of individuals have their cardiac arrest while exercising.[46,58,59] In the most common form of underlying structural heart disease associated with sudden cardiac death in the young—hypertrophic cardiomyopathy—the arrhythmias are exertionally induced in most of the individuals. There is evidence that restriction of athletic activity in this athletic population is a successful strategy for prevention of sudden death.[60] With the long QT syndrome, sudden death is generally exertional or immediately post-exertional.[61] In this condition beta blockers have been shown to decrease the frequency of syncope and sudden death. However the ICD provides better protection against sudden cardiac death, particularly with syncope or ventricular arrhythmia recurrence while patients are on beta-blocker therapy. Restriction from athletic activities is recommended even when effective therapy is identified.[40]

PARTICIPATION OF ATHLETES WITH LIFE-THREATENING VENTRICULAR ARRHYTHMIAS AND AN IMPLANTABLE CARDIOVERTER DEFIBRILLATOR

Although the ICD has proved to be an extremely effective device for the prevention of sudden cardiac death, its ability to terminate lethal arrhythmias under conditions of the vigorous physical activity associated with competitive athletics is unknown.[40] The ICD should not be placed to allow continued participation in athletic activity for individuals at risk for life-threatening ventricular arrhythmias. Generally, it is accepted that for individuals with an ICD all moderate and high-intensity sports are contraindicated.[40,41] In addition, it is recommended that low-intensity competitive sports, which do not constitute a significant risk to the ICD, be restricted for at least 6 months after the last ventricular arrhythmia, requiring intervention including pacing, cardioversion, or defibrillation.

ELECTROCARDIOGRAPHIC PATTERNS OF CARDIAC CONDITIONS ASSOCIATED WITH CARDIAC ARRHYTHMIAS IN THE ATHLETE

A number of underlying cardiac conditions may be detected based on characteristic electrocardiographic findings in the athlete (Table 10.2) These underlying cardiac conditions may predispose the athlete or nonathlete to life-threatening cardiac arrhythmias. Arrhythmogenic right ventricular dysplasia[62,63] is an uncommon form of congenital heart disease, which predisposes to sustained ventricular tachycardia and cardiac arrest in athletes (Fig. 10.4). It is pathologically characterized by adipose infiltration of the right ventricular myocardium and has characteristic electrocardiographic findings. In most patients, there is T-wave

TABLE 10.2.   ELECTROCARDIOGRAPHIC PATTERNS OF STRUCTURAL HEART DISEASE OR HIGH RISK FOR SUDDEN DEATH IN THE ATHLETE

Arrhythmogenic right ventricular dysplasia
Hypertrophic cardiomyopathy
Myocardial infarction
Brugada syndrome
Long QT syndrome

inversion in the precordial leads V_1 to V_3 commonly accompanied by an incomplete right-bundle-branch-block pattern. Less common, but more specific, are the small discrete late depolarization waves seen after the QRS complexes known as the ε waves. These are generally felt to be due to late depolarization of the right ventricle.[62,63]

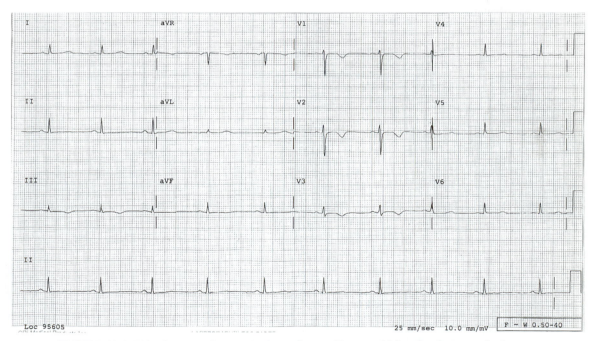

FIGURE 10.4. This electrocardiogram is shown from a 19-year-old female after resuscitation from a cardiac arrest while playing soccer. Note the T-wave inversions in leads V_1 to V_3 commonly found with arrhythmogenic right ventricular dysplasia. This diagnosis was subsequently confirmed with a right ventriculogram, and an implantable cardioverter defibrillator was placed. She has been restricted from athletic competition and has required antiarrhythmic therapy with amiodarone to suppress spontaneous ventricular arrhythmias resulting in ICD shocks.

Hypertrophic cardiomyopathy occurs with a frequency of 1 out of 500 in the population and as such represents the most common underlying structural heart disease predisposing to sudden death. There may be a family history of the condition or of sudden death. In many patients the physical examination is normal. Most athletes with the condition have an intraventricular conduction delay and voltage criteria for left ventricular hypertrophy with ST-segment depression and T-wave inversions (Fig. 10.5). Approximately 20% of patients with hypertrophic cardiomyopathy will show Q waves that can cause a "pseudoinfarct" pattern in the inferior or anterior precordial leads.[64] Unfortunately, the 12-lead ECG is normal in up to 20% of individuals with hypertrophic cardiomyopathy and the overlap with the spectrum of normal voltage criteria for

hypertrophy in the athlete is considerable. Accordingly, when the condition is suspected based on physical findings, family history, symptoms such as syncope, or electrocardiographic findings and echocardiogram, further evaluation is warranted. When the condition is definitively diagnosed, restrictions from athletics are recommended.[20]

In the athletic population over age 35 years, the most common cause of sudden death is underlying coronary artery disease.[46–57] In this patient population or in younger patients at risk for premature coronary artery disease, abnormalities on the surface ECG may serve as a marker of risk. Certainly in the presence of pathologic Q waves indicating a prior myocardial infarction, further evaluation stress testing and, if appropriate, coronary angiography should be considered. In some

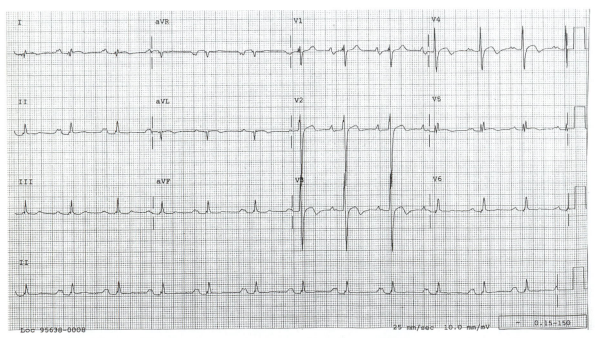

FIGURE 10.5. This electrocardiogram is shown from a 32-year-old male who suffered out-of-hospital cardiac arrest while playing basketball. Note the first-degree AV block, voltage criteria for left ventricular hypertrophy, and marked ST- and T-wave changes. Cardiac catheterization and echocardiography confirmed obstructive hypertrophic cardiomyopathy. Therapy with beta blockers and an implantable cardioverter defibrillator was started with restriction from athletic activities.

instances, pathologic Q waves may not be present, but only ST- or T-wave changes raising the possibility of underlying coronary artery disease may be present. In individuals with symptoms, risk factors or ECG changes sufficiently suggestive of coronary artery disease, appropriate restriction from athletics should be instituted until further evaluation is undertaken and, if appropriate, therapy is instituted.

In some athletes QT abnormalities may be detected with a prolonged QT interval, prominent U wave, or qualitative repolarization abnormalities suggesting one of the forms of congenital long QT syndrome[61] (Fig. 10.6). In such patients, exercise may be associated with a high risk of torsades de pointes, a rapid polymorphic ventricular tachycardia that can degenerate into ventricular fibrillation. The long QT syndrome is a heteroge-

neous genetic disorder affecting ionic channels of myocardial cells. It is characterized by prolongation of the corrected QT interval (QTc > 460 ms), recurrent syncope, sudden cardiac death, and a family history. In patients with borderline prolonged QTc intervals (QTc of 440–480 ms), ancillary ECG changes such as sinus bradycardia and T-wave alternans may help establish the diagnosis. Most patients are diagnosed during routine electrocardiographic evaluation or during screening of family members of a diagnosed individual. The heterogeneous nature of this hereditary defect is reflected in differing JT-segment morphology on electrocardiography and in the clinical precipitants of acute events.

Sudden cardiac death, one of the hallmarks of this disorder, may be one of this disorder's first presentations. Twenty percent of patients die

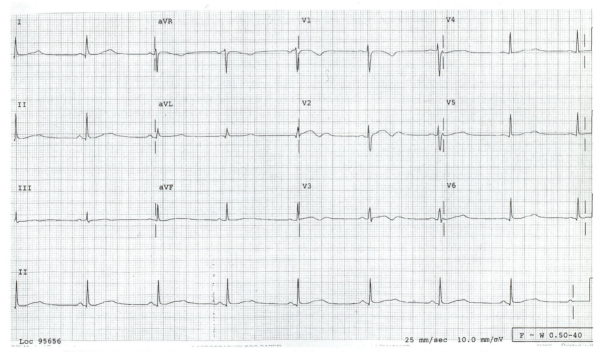

FIGURE 10.6. The 12-lead electrocardiogram is shown from a 17-year-old female with recurrent syncope with physical or emotional stress. The patient had two sisters with recurrent syncope with similar ECGs. The ECG shows sinus bradycardia (48 beats per minute) with a measured QT interval of 535 ms and a QTc of 478 with prominent U waves diagnostic of the long QT syndrome. Therapy with a permanent pacemaker and beta blockers has eliminated syncope.

within a year of the first syncopal spell; 50% within 10 years. Polymorphic ventricular tachycardia from abnormality in ventricular repolarization is the arrhythmia responsible for sudden death and recurrent syncope. This arrhythmia is often, but not invariably, precipitated by physical or emotional stress. The genetic basis of the long QT syndrome is now clearly established with mutations in 4 genes accounting for the majority of identified defects. Beta blockers are the mainstay of therapy, reducing the income of syncope by 75%. The 3-year mortality is reduced from 26 to 6% with beta blockers. Beta blockers should be administered to the point where the patient's heart rate does not exceed 130 beats per minute on exercise stress testing. Pacemakers are used when beta-blocker therapy results in symptomatic bradycardia. Patients considered at high risk for sudden cardiac death and markedly prolonged QTc (QTc > 520 ms) should be considered for ICDs. In most forms of the long QT syndrome, the QTc lengthens with exercise. Because effective therapy with beta blockers, pacemakers, and/or implantable cardioverter defibrillators along with restriction from athletic activities are available, establishing the diagnosis and instituting therapy are critically important.

A syndrome has been identified as the Brugada syndrome in which young healthy individuals develop idiopathic ventricular fibrillation, sometimes in association with exercise.[65] These individuals have a characteristic ST-segment elevation in lead V_1, which has been associated with a SCN5A sodium channel defect (Fig. 10.7A–7D). A challenge with a sodium channel blocking agent can make these repolarization changes more marked. These individuals typically have ventricular fibrillation induced at electrophysiological studies and should be treated with an ICD and restricted from athletic activity.

CONCLUSIONS

The athlete commonly shows a wide spectrum of heart rates, conduction intervals, and repolarization abnormalities on the surface ECG, related to the changes in autonomic tone and chamber hypertrophy that accompany athletic conditioning. These abnormalities include sinus bradycardia, sinus arrhythmia, first- and second-degree AV block, J-point and ST-segment elevation, T-wave peaking and inversion, incomplete right bundle branch block, and voltage criteria for right ventricular hypertrophy or left ventricular hypertrophy. Because of the overlap of normal physiological ECG changes with electrocardiographic abnormalities associated with forms of structural heart disease, it may be impossible to distinguish normal from abnormal ECGs without further evaluation of the individual athlete, including a personal and family medical history, a physical examination, and selective use of other tests including the echocardiogram. Atrial and ventricular arrhythmias may develop in the athlete and should be managed pharmacologically or non-

FIGURE 10.7. A. The 12-lead electrocardiogram is shown from a 51-year-old male with cardiac arrest while sleeping. He was found to have no structural heart disease but inducible ventricular fibrillation at electrophysiological evaluation. Notice the markedly abnormal ST segment in the precordial leads V_1 to V_3 with evidence of right bundle branch block with ST-segment elevation in V_1 to V_3. B. The same patient shown in A was challenged with oral flecainide, resulting in more marked repolarization changes in the inferior and anterior leads. Based on the prior cardiac arrest, inducible ventricular fibrillation at electrophysiological evaluation, and repolarization abnormalities, a diagnosis of Brugada syndrome was made and the patient was treated with an implantable cardioverter defibrillator.

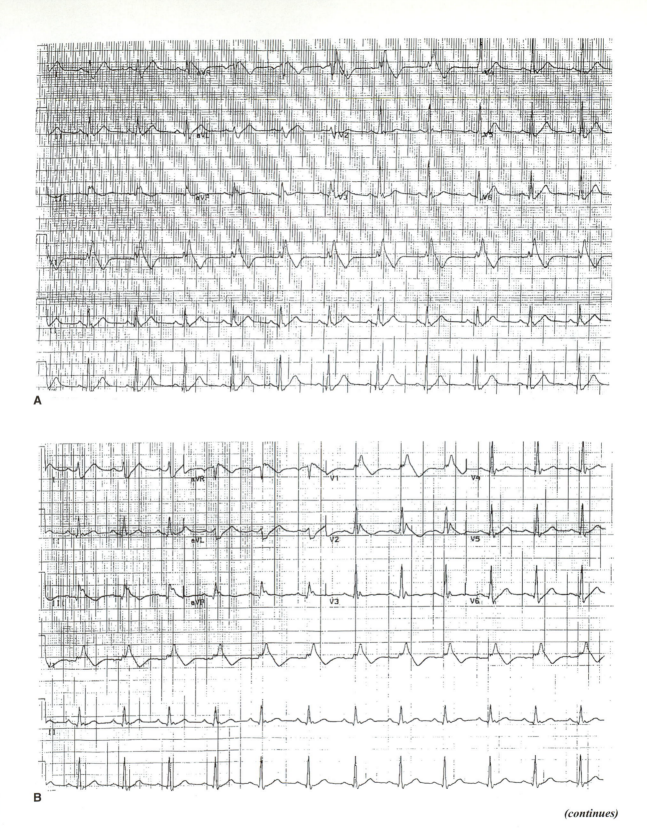

A

B

(continues)

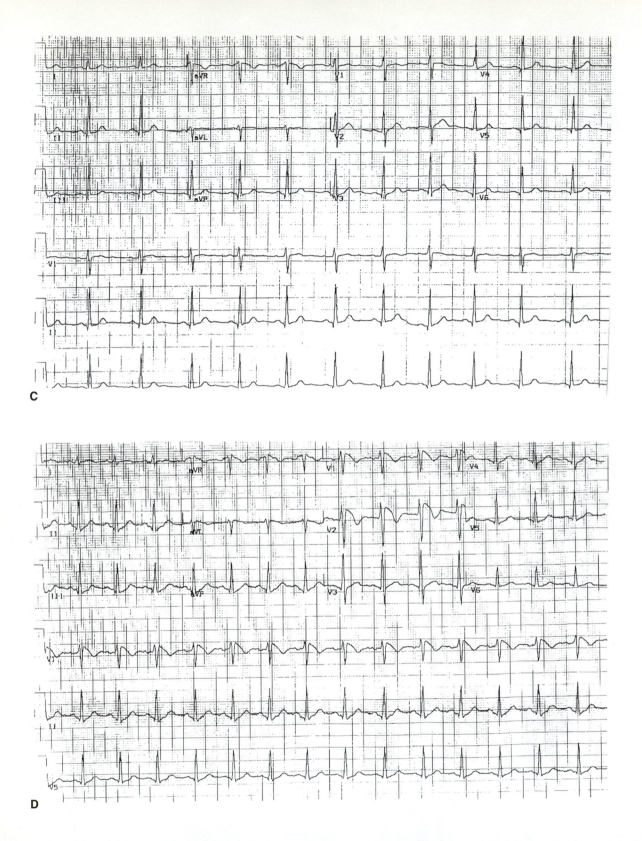

C

D

pharmacologically based on the specific arrhythmia, the patient's symptoms, the nature of the underlying structural heart disease, and the risks and benefits of the therapy. Guidelines for restricting athletes from exercise are available based on the best available information about the arrhythmias. It is particularly important for the physician to recognize the specific abnormalities on the ECG associated with a risk of serious or life-threatening arrhythmias.

SUMMARY

The physician evaluating the ECG and cardiac rhythm of the athlete should be aware of the wide range of normal. Resting bradycardia, prolongation of the PR interval, and occasionally high degrees of AV block are seen as related to the heightened vagal tone that accompanies athletic conditioning. Electrocardiographic criteria for left ventricular hypertrophy and repolarization changes including J-point and ST-segment elevation and T-wave inversion are also common. Electrocardiographic patterns of the long QT syndrome, arrhythmogenic right ventricular dysplasia, WPW syndrome, the Brugada syndrome, and hypertrophic cardiomyopathy should alert the clinician to the need for further evaluation, therapy, and restriction from athletics. When supraventricular arrhythmias are symptomatic or when WPW syndrome is identified, evaluation for cure with radiofrequency ablation may be appropriate. When clinically significant ventricular arrhythmias are present, evaluation of the underlying structural heart disease is generally needed before definitive therapy for the arrhythmia. In the set-

ting of sustained ventricular tachycardia or prior episodes of ventricular fibrillation, therapy with an ICD generally should be accompanied by restrictions from vigorous exertion. Further research is needed to effectively distinguish normal ECG changes from those changes that indicate underlying cardiac disease in the athlete. Improved methods of identifying athletes at risk of serious or life-threatening arrhythmias are also needed.

PERSONAL PERSPECTIVE

The evaluation and management of the athlete with a documented arrhythmia, symptoms of an arrhythmia, or an "abnormal" ECG remain a considerable challenge for the physician. It is important, as noted in this chapter, for every physician to appreciate the wide spectrum of ECG changes that can accompany athletic conditioning. It is essential also to recognize those changes on the ECG that can serve as markers of underlying heart disease or vulnerability to supraventricular or ventricular arrhythmias. Among these are the changes on the ECG of WPW syndrome, long QT syndrome, hypertrophic cardiomyopathy, arrhythmogenic right ventricular dysplasia, Brugada syndrome, and the many abnormalities that accompany a variety of forms of other congenital or acquired structural heart diseases. Any ECG, symptom, or arrhythmia should always be evaluated in the context of the athlete's family history, personal history, physical examination, and evidence of underlying structural heart disease. Selective use of additional testing, including an echocardiogram, stress test, ambulatory monitoring, cardiac catheterization, or electrophysiological evaluation, may be needed in a minority of athletes. Symptoms such as palpitations, light-headedness, dizziness, chest tightness, or shortness of breath are common in the athlete. There

---

FIGURE 10.7. C. The 21-year-old asymptomatic son of the patient represented in A and B had a screening ECG that showed subtle but nondiagnostic repolarization abnormalities in leads V$_1$ to V$_2$. D. When the 21-year-old son was challenged with oral flecainide, the repolarization changes became more marked, which is consistent with Brugada syndrome. It has been recommended that the patient receive a prophylactic ICD based on a high risk of sudden cardiac death.

remain no firm guidelines for interpretation, evaluation, and management of these common complaints. The athlete may be subject to diagnostic evaluations such as stress testing, tilt table testing, ambulatory monitoring, or even invasive testing to evaluate such complaints with a minimal preevaluation probability of any diagnostic abnormalities being identified. The risk of unnecessarily evaluating such common symptoms or imposing unwarranted restrictions is real. At the same time, not recognizing electrocardiographic findings or subtle abnormalities on physical examination could result in failure to more completely evaluate and diagnose a condition that predisposed to a life-threatening arrhythmia. In this respect, further research is needed on the optimal assessment techniques for the athlete presenting with symptoms, electrocardiographic abnormalities, or findings on physical examination to develop evaluation and management guidelines for the physician. When clear abnormalities are noted, such as frank syncope, abrupt onset of palpitations with presyncope, ventricular preexcitation on the ECG, or a harsh systolic murmur, the process of evaluation is more straightforward. However, in the more common "gray zone" cases with nondiagnostic symptoms, "borderline" ECG, or physical findings, more research is needed regarding appropriate evaluation. Despite the substantial body of observational data regarding the spectrum of ECG changes and arrhythmias in the athlete reviewed in this chapter, interpretation of the ECG, evaluation of symptoms, and management of arrhythmias remain largely generally dependent on the experience and judgment of the individual physician and much remains unknown.

Over the last several years there has been a growing collaboration amongst the pediatrician, family practitioner, internist, team physician, sports medicine physician, cardiologist, and athletic trainer in evaluating the individual athlete and advancing the state of our knowledge regarding ECG changes and arrhythmias in the athlete. Physicians with knowledge and experience in evaluating, treating, and dealing with the unique psychosocial and legal issues involved in evaluating athletes can play an invaluable role in these vexing cases. As more information becomes available on the ECG changes and arrhythmias in the athlete from applied research on epidemiology, pathophysiology, screening guidelines, recommendations for athletic participation, and the ethical, social, psychological, and legal issues, guidelines for optimal management will continue to evolve.

REFERENCES

1. Hanne-Paparo N, Drory Y, Schoenfeld YS, et al: Common ECG changes in athletes. *Cardiology* 61:267–278, 1976.
2. Venerando A, Rulli V: Frequency morphology and meaning of the electrocardiographic anomalies found in Olympic marathon runners and walkers. *J Sports Med Phys Fitness* 4:135–141, 1964.
3. Van Ganse W, Versee L, Eylenbosch W, et al: The electrocardiogram of athletes: Comparison with untrained subjects. *Br Heart J* 32:160–164, 1970.
4. Northcote R, Canning GP, Ballantyne D: Electrocardiographic findings in male veteran endurance athletes. *Br Heart J* 61:155–160, 1989.
5. Balady GJ, Cadigan JB, Ryan TJ: Electrocardiogram of the athlete: An analysis of 289 professional football players. *Am J Cardiol* 53:1339–1343, 1984.
6. Ikaheimo M, Palatsi I, Takkunen J: Noninvasive evaluation of the athletic heart: Sprinters versus endurance runners. *Am J Cardiol* 44:24–30, 1979.
7. Gibbons L, Cooper K, Martin R, et al: Medical examination and electrocardiographic analysis of elite distance runners. *Ann N Y Acad Sci* 301:283–296, 1977.
8. Bjornstad H, Storstein L, Dyre Meen H, et al: Electrocardiographic and echocardiographic findings in top athletes, athletic students and sedentary controls. *Cardiology* 82:66–74, 1993.
9. Chapman J: Profound sinus bradycardia in the athletic heart syndrome. *J Sports Med Phys Fitness* 22:45–48, 1982.
10. Hanne-Paparo N, Kellerman J: Long-term Holter ECG monitoring of athletes. *Med Sci Sports Exerc* 13:294–298, 1981.
11. Smith M, Hudson D, Graitzer H, et al: Exercise training bradycardia: The role of autonomic balance. *Med Sci Sports Exerc* 21:40–44, 1989.
12. Foote CB, Michaud G: The athletes electrocardiogram: Distinguishing normal from abnormal, in Estes NAM III, Salem D, Wang PJ (eds.): *Sudden Cardiac Death in the Athlete.* New York, Futura, 1998, pp. 101–1115.
13. Parker B, Londeree B, Cupp G, et al: The noninvasive cardiac evaluation of long-distance runners. *Chest* 73:376–381, 1978.
14. Huston T, Puffer J, Rodney WM: The athletic heart syndrome. *N Engl J Med* 313:24–32, 1985.
15. Nakamoto K: Electrocardiograms of 25 marathon

runners before and after 100 meter dash. *Jpn Circ J* 33:105–126, 1969.

16. Zehender M, Meinertz T, Keul J, et al: ECG variants and cardiac arrhythmias in athletes: Clinical relevance and prognostic importance. *Am Heart J* 119:1378–1391,1990.

17. Hiss R, Lamb L: Electrocardiographic findings in 122,043 individuals. *Circulation* 25:947–961, 1962.

18. Zippilli P, Fenici R, Sassasra M, et al: Wenckebach second degree AV block in top-ranking athletes: An old problem revisited. *Am Heart J* 100:281–294, 1980.

19. Storstein L, Bjornstad H, Hals O, et al: Electrocardiographic findings according to sex in athletes and controls. *Cardiology* 79:227–236, 1991.

20. Knowlan DM: The electrocardiogram in the athlete, in Waller B, Harvey WP (eds.) *Cardiovascular Evaluation of Athletes.* Newton, NJ, Laennec, 1993, pp. 43–59.

21. Klemola E: Electrocardiographic observations on 650 Finnish athletes. *Ann Med Finn* 40:121–132, 1951.

22. Sokolow M, Lyon T: The ventricular complex in right ventricular hypertrophy as obtained by unipolar precordial and limb leads. *Am Heart J* 38:273, 1949.

23. Arstila M, Koivikko A: Electrocardiographic and vectorcardiographic signs of left and right ventricular hypertrophy in endurance athletes. *J Sport Med Phys Fitness* 4:166–175, 1964.

24. Beckner G, Winsor T: Cardiovascular adaptations to prolonged physical effort. *Circulation* 9:835–846, 1954.

25. Douglas PS, O'Toole ML, Hiller DB, et al: Electrocardiographic diagnosis of exercise-induced left ventricular hypertrophy. *Am Heart J* 116:784–790, 1988.

26. Parisi A, Beckmann C, Lancaaster M: The spectrum of ST segment elevation in the electrocardiograms of healthy adult men. *J Electrocardiol* 4:137–144, 1971.

27. Oakley DG, Oakley CM: Significant of abnormal electrocardiograms in highly trained athletes. *Am J Cardiol* 50:985–989, 1982.

28. Hanne-Paparo N, Wendkos MH, Brunner D: T wave abnormalities in the electrocardiogram of top-ranking athletes without demonstrable organic heart disease. *Am Heart J* 81:743–747, 1971.

29. Zeppilli P, Pirrami MM, Sassara M, et al: T wave abnormalities in top ranking athletes: Effects of isoproterenol, atropine, and physical exercise. *Am Heart J* 100:213–222, 1980.

30. Lichtman J, O'Rourke RA, Klein A, et al: Electrocardiogram of the athlete. *Arch Intern Med* 123:763–770, 1973.

31. Beswick FW, Jordan RC: Cardiological observations at the sixth British Empire and Commonwealth Games. *Br Heart J* 23:113–129, 1961.

32. Hantzschel K, Dohrn K: The electrocardiogram before and after a marathon race. *J Sports Med Phys Fitness* 6:29–32, 1966.

33. Hunt BPE: Electrocardiographic study of 20 champion swimmers before and after 100 yard sprint swimming competition. *Can Med Assoc J* 88:1251–1253, 1963.

34. Viitasalo MT, Kala R, Eissalo A: Ambulatory electrocardiographic recordings in endurance athletes. *Br Heart J* 47:213–220, 1982.

35. Sargin O, et al: Wenckebach phenomenon with nodal and ventricular escape in marathon runners. *Chest* 57:102–105, 1970.

36a. Talan DA, Bauernfeind RA, Ashley WW, et al: Twenty-four hour continuous ECG recordings in long distance runners. *Chest* 92:19–24, 1982.

36b. Lie H, Erikssen J: Five year follow of ECG aberrations, latent coronary disease and cardiopulmonary fitness in various age groups of Norwegian cross-country skiers. *Acta Med Scand* 216:377–383, 1984.

37. Hanne-Paparo N, Drory Y, Kellerman JJ: Complete heart block and physical performance. *Int J Sports Med* 3:9–13, 1983.

38. Ferst JA, Chaitman BR: The electrocardiogram and the athlete. *Sport Medicine* 1:390–403, 1984.

39. Smith WG, Cullen KJ, Thorburn IO: Electrocardiograms of marathon runners in 1962 Commonwealth Games. *Br Heart J* 26:469–476, 1964.

40. 26th Bethesda Conference: Recommendations for Determining Eligibility for Competition in Athletes with Cardiovascular Abnormalities. *J Am Coll Cardiol* 24:854–899, 1994.

41. Link MS, Wang PJ, Estes NAM III: Cardiac arrhythmias and electrophysiologic observations in the athlete, in Williams RA (ed.): *The Athlete and Heart Disease.* Philadelphia, Lippincott, Williams & Wilkins, 1998, pp. 197–216.

42. Krahn AW, Klein GW, Yee R: The approach to the athlete with Wolff-Parkinson-White Syndrome:

Risks of sudden cardiac death, in Estes NAM, Salem D, Wang PJ (eds.): *Sudden Cardiac Death in the Athlete.* New York, Futura, 1998, pp. 232–252.

43. Manolis AS, Wang PJ, Estes NAM III: Radiofrequency ablation for cardiac tachyarrhythmias. *Ann Int Med* 121:452–461, 1994.

44. Furlanello F, Bertoldi A, Dallago M, et al: Atrial fibrillation in elite athletes. *J Cardiovasc Electrophysiol* 9:S63–S68, 1998.

45. Katcher MS, Foote CB, Homoud M, et al: Strategies for managing atrial fibrillation. *Cleve Clin J Med* 63:282–294, 1996.

46. Maron BJ, Shirani J, Poliac LC, et al: Sudden death in young competitive athletes: Clinical, demographic, and pathologic profiles. *JAMA* 276:199–204, 1996.

47. Corrado D, Thiene G, Nava A, et al: Sudden death in young competitive athletes: Clinicopathologic correlations in 22 cases. *Am J Cardiol* 89:588–596, 1990.

48. Liberthson RR: Sudden death from cardiac causes in children and young adults. *N Engl J Med* 334:1039–1044, 1996.

49. Maron BJ, Epstein SE, Roberts WC: Causes of sudden death in competitive athletes. *J Am Coll Cardiol* 7:204–214, 1986.

50. Maron BJ: Triggers for sudden cardiac death in the athlete. *Card Clin* 14:195–210, 1996.

51. Maron BJ, Fananapazir L: Sudden cardiac death in hypertrophic cardiomyopathy. *Circulation* 85 (Suppl I):I-57–63, 1992.

52. Maron BJ, Poliac LC, Kaplan JA, et al: Blunt impact to the chest leading to sudden death from cardiac arrest during sports activities. *N Engl J Med* 333:337–342, 1995.

53. Link MS, Wang PJ, Pandian NG, et al: An experimental model of sudden death due to low energy chest wall impact (commotio cordis). *N Engl J Med* 338(25):1805–1811, 1998.

54. Maron BJ, Thompson PD, Puffer JC, et al: Cardiovascular preparticipation screening of competitive athletes: A statement for health care professionals from the Sudden Death Committee (clinical cardiology) and Congenital Defects Committee (cardiovascular disorders in the young) American Heart Association. *Circulation* 94:85–86, 1996.

55. Maron BJ, Bodison S, Wesley YE, et al: Results of screening a large group of intercollegiate competitive athletes for cardiovascular disease. *J Am Coll Card* 10:1214–1222, 1987.

56. Katcher M, Salem DN, Wang PJ, et al: Mechanisms of sudden death in the athlete, in Estes NAM, Salem DN, Wang PJ (eds.): *Sudden Cardiac Death in the Athlete.* Armonk, NY: Futura Publishing Co., Inc, 1998, pp. 3–24.

57. Thompson PD, Funk EJ, Carleton RA, et al: Incidence of death during jogging in Rhode Island from 1975 through 1980. *JAMA* 247:2635–2638, 1982.

58. Kinder C, Tamburro P, Kopp D, et al: The clinical significance of nonsustained ventricular tachycardia: Current perspectives. *PACE* 17:637–664, 1994.

59. Eisenberg SJ, Scheinman MM, Dullet NK, et al: Sudden cardiac death and polymorphous ventricular tachycardia in patients with normal QT intervals and normal systolic cardiac function. *Am J Cardiol* 75:687–692, 1995.

60. Corrado D, Basso C, Schiavon M, et al: Screening for hypertrophic cardiomyopathy in young athletes. *N Engl J Med* 339:364–369, 1998.

61. Vincent GM, Jaisawal D, Timothy KW: Effects of exercise in heart rate, QT, QTc, QT/QS2 in the Romano-Ward inherited long QT syndrome. *Am J Cardiol* 68:498–503, 1991.

62. Marcus FI, Gontaine G: Arrhythmogenic right ventricular dysplasia, in Podrid PJ, Kowey PR (eds.): *Cardiac Arrhythmia: Mechanisms, Diagnosis, and Management.* vol. 1. Boston, Philadelphia: Williams & Wilkins: 1995, pp. 1121–1130.

63. Link MS, Wang PJ, Haugh CJ, et al: Arrhythmogenic right ventricular dysplasia: Clinical results with implantable cardioverter defibrillators. *J Inter Cardiovasc Elect* 1:41–48, 1997.

64. Savage D, Seides S, Clark C, et al: Electrocardiographic findings in patients with obstructive and nonobstructive hypertrophic cardiomyopathy. *Circulation* 58:402–408, 1978.

65. Brugada P, Brugada J: Right bundle branch block persistent ST segment elevation and sudden death: A distinct clinical and electrocardiographic syndrome. A multicenter report. *J Am Coll Cardiol* 20:1391–1396, 1992.

PART III

SPECIAL CLINICAL ISSUES IN ATHLETES

Chapter 11

SCREENING ATHLETES FOR CARDIOVASCULAR DISEASE

Antonio Pelliccia, M.D.   *Barry J. Maron, M.D.*

Sudden and unexpected deaths of competitive athletes are tragic and emotional events, which unavoidably raise great concern in the lay public, as well as in the medical community. Such events often assume a high public profile because of the intuitive perception that trained athletes represent the healthiest segment of society, with the deaths of well-known and elite athletes often exaggerating this visibility.[1] Although these athletic field catastrophes strike the core of our sensibilities and often galvanize to action, they also raise a number of practical and ethical issues, including the feasibility, appropriateness, and efficacy of preparticipation cardiovascular screening.

DEFINITIONS

For the purpose of this discussion, we define *sudden cardiac death* as the unexpected death of cardiovascular etiology, in which there is a loss of consciousness within 1 h from the onset of symptoms. Although the majority of the reported sud-

235

den cardiac deaths in athletes have occurred during or immediately after exercise, death can also occur at rest or while sleeping.[2–4]

An *athlete* is defined as an individual who participates in an organized team or individual sport requiring systematic training and regular competition against others, while placing a high premium on athletic excellence and achievement.[5] The elite and professional athletes represent a select subgroup of this population, distinguished not only for the intensity of conditioning required and the highest level of achievement, but also for the substantial economic rewards related to sports participation.

INCIDENCE OF SUDDEN DEATH IN ATHLETES

Sudden death in athletes is a rare event. Although the number of athletic field deaths is not known with certainty either in the United States and in Italy, the estimated risk in young (high school and college) athletes is about 1:200,000 and higher in males than in females.[6,7] Older athletes are apparently at higher risk than young athletes, and reasonably in the range of 1:15,000 to 1:50,000.[8,9] Considering such a relatively low incidence, the heightened awareness and intense interest in sudden death in athletes, often fueled by the news media, are perhaps disproportionate to its actual numerical impact as a public health problem.

CAUSES OF SUDDEN DEATH IN ATHLETES

A variety of cardiovascular abnormalities have been found to be responsible for sudden cardiac death in competitive athletes.[2–4,6–23] The exact prevalence of the various cardiovascular diseases differ in the available studies, due to differences in patient selection and methods used to document cardiovascular diagnosis. Even with these

limitations, it has been convincingly demonstrated that the lesions responsible for athletic field deaths differ with regard to age.[2–4]

In *young athletes* (i.e., $\leq$ 35 years), a broad spectrum of congenital or acquired cardiac lesions have been described as causes of sudden death (Fig. 11.1). Hypertrophic cardiomyopathy (HCM) is the predominant abnormality that accounts for more than one-third of all cases;[4,8,20,23] this proportion would increase further if athletes who died with unexplained left ventricular hypertrophy, but without unequivocal evidence of HCM, were also considered.[4,8] The second most frequent cause of death is the congenital coronary anomalies, particularly anomalous origin of the left main coronary artery from the right (anterior) sinus of Valsalva.[4,11] Taken together, HCM and the coronary anomalies represent about two-thirds of all causes of sudden cardiac death in athletes. Several other diseases occur less frequently, including myocarditis, ruptured aortic aneurysm (usually in the context of Marfan syndrome), idiopathic dilated cardiomyopathy, aortic valve stenosis, mitral valve prolapse, and arrhythmogenic right ventricular cardiomyopathy (ARVC).[4,18–20,23] The rare occurrence of ARVC in pathologic series published in the United States contrasts sharply with the experience of Italian investigators, who have come to regard ARVC as the most common cause of sudden death in Italian competitive athletes (approximately 25%) based on the experience in the Veneto region.[24] In conclusion, it can be reliably estimated that all the congenital cardiac lesions responsible for sudden death *in young athletes* (the target of cardiovascular screening) account for a prevalence of about 0.2% in the general athletic population.[25]

In *adult and senior athletes* the most common cause of sudden death is ischemic heart disease.[9,12–15,17] Available studies describe significant atherosclerotic coronary artery narrowing (> 75% cross-sectional luminal area) of 2 or 3 major epicardial coronary arteries in the majority of these deaths; only a minority of athletes show lesions confined to one major epicardial artery (usually,

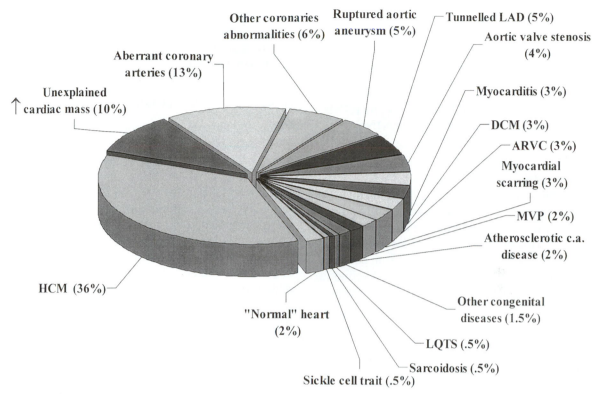

**FIGURE 11.1 Causes of sudden death in young competitive athletes, based on systematic track-
ing of 134 athletes in the United States HCM, hypertrophic cardiomyopathy; LAD, left anterior
descending; DCM, dilated cardiomyopathy; ARVC, arrhythmogenic right ventricular cardiomyopathy; MVP, mitral valve prolapse; LQTS, long QT syndrome.** *Adapted with permission from
Maron BJ, Shirani J, Poliac L, et al: Sudden death in young competitive athletes: Clinical, demographic and pathologic profiles.* JAMA *276:199–204, 1996.*

the left anterior descending).[12–15,17,26] Less commonly, idiopathic dilated cardiomyopathy, HCM,
or valvular heart disease are responsible for death
in the older age group.[12–15]

The occurrence of sudden cardiac death in
young athletes is greater in the sports with the
highest participation levels (i.e., basketball and
football in the United States and soccer in
Italy).[4,7,18,19] Older athletes usually die during jogging and running, but not infrequently during
squash, tennis, or soccer.[9,12–15,17]

The time of sudden death in young athletes is
clustered between 3:00 pm and 9:00 pm, corresponding to the period usually spent in training
and competition. This pattern differs, for example, from sedentary subjects dying of HCM, in
which the peak occurs in the morning (between
7:00 am and 1:00 pm).[4,27] Deaths are most common from August through January, corresponding
to the competitive seasons for basketball and
football in the United States. Indeed, the vast majority of athletes (up to 90%) collapse during or
immediately after a training session or in an official athletic contest; only a minority die while

sedentary (including sleeping) or during mild physical activity unrelated to sports.[4,23,27] These relationships underline the role of intense physical exertion as a trigger for sudden death.

GOAL, FEASIBILITY, AND LIMITATIONS OF CARDIOVASCULAR SCREENING

GOAL

The objective of preparticipation cardiovascular screening is the early identification of pathologic cardiac lesions with the potential risk for sudden death (or disease progression) in competitive athletes. The identification of such at-risk individuals should result in disqualification from competitive sports, in an effort to reduce the likelihood, and possibly prevent, the occurrence of athletic field deaths.[28]

RATIONALE OF THE SCREENING

The appropriateness and feasibility of preparticipation screening, however, are not unanimously accepted, and a number of issues are still debated. Major considerations against screening include: (a) the low prevalence of the cardiovascular diseases that represent the target of investigation (approximately, 0.2%);[25] (b) the identification of most of these diseases requiring clinical suspicion and diagnostic testing (i.e., imaging techniques), not universally available and often prohibitively expensive; and (c) the substantial number of competitive athletes (about 25 million individuals in the United States and 6 million in Italy) that should be screened.[25]

In comparison, in favor of screening are the following points: (a) most athletes at risk are completely asymptomatic, and sudden death is their initial clinical event; therefore, only preparticipation screening may allow identification of such at-risk individuals; (b) since most sudden deaths are precipitated by exertion, it is likely that disqualification from training and competition may diminish mortality (or disease progression). Also, certain diseases, such as aortic aneurysm in the context of Marfan syndrome, or congenital wrong aortic sinus origin of coronary arteries, may be amenable to surgical treatment if detected in a timely fashion.

SCREENING STRATEGIES

There is uncertainty regarding the most appropriate strategy for screening. Controversial issues related to diagnostic accuracy, cost-efficacy, legal implications, and feasibility of diagnostic tests impact on this decision (Fig. 11.2). Although history and physical examination are relatively easy to be implemented in screening large athlete populations, the potential for identifying cardiovascular diseases with such preparticipation screening is probably limited. The addition of noninvasive diagnostic testing, such as 12-lead electrocardiogram (ECG) and echocardiography, would enhance the diagnostic efficacy of screening, but require huge financial efforts to be implemented in large athletic populations. Indeed, inclusion of diagnostic tests makes the screening procedure more complex, creates the likelihood of false-positive and false-negative results, and raises medicolegal issues, related to possibly unwarranted exclusion of the athlete from professional sport activity.

LEGAL AND ADMINISTRATIVE BACKGROUND

The circumstances surrounding the implementation of preparticipation athletic screening are remarkably different in Italy and the United States.

ITALY

At present, Italy is one of the few countries where a state law specifically addresses this issue. In 1971, the Italian government conceived and passed legislation intended to provide medical surveillance to citizens engaged in official athletic events. This legislation, known as Tutela Sanitaria delle Attività Sportive (Medical Protection of

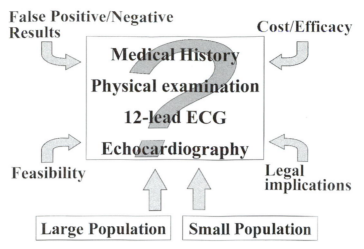

FIGURE 11.2 Flow chart showing the different factors that may affect the strategy of preparticipation cardiovascular screening. ECG, electrocardiogram.

Athletic Activities), legislates preventive medical evaluations for the purpose of identifying potentially deleterious disease and, specifically, dictates "every citizen engaged in official competitive sport activities must successfully pass periodic preventive examinations intended to evaluate his/her eligibility for sports participation."[29] The primary objective of the Italian law is to offer benevolent protection to the athlete population, which is considered to be consistently exposed to enhanced risk by virtue of the regular commitment to intensive exercise training and competition. In this context, the large proportion (about 10%) of the Italian population involved in competitive athletics is regarded as a valued segment of society and worthy of specific legislative protection. This law is an example of the preventive medical approach of the Italian national health system that is committed to safeguard all members of society.

Indeed, in 1982 the Italian Ministry of Health provided detailed guidelines for implementation of the preparticipation screening of competitive athletes. Specifically, it stipulated that medical evaluation should include history, physical examination, 12-lead resting ECG, and, for most of the athletic disciplines, a submaximal exercise test (step-test).[30] Implementation of the 12-lead ECG in the screening design is made possible in Italy because of the limited cost (the global cost of the screening including 12-lead ECG is about US$50).

UNITED STATES

In contrast, no federal law governing preparticipation screening exists in the United States and, therefore, there is no mandatory legal obligation for competitive athletes to undergo preparticipation medical evaluations and receive clearance for sports participation. Only customary practice and local directives have been implemented in most states, usually requiring an examination prior to participation in high school athletics.[31]

Another question concerns who should be responsible for the decision-making process in determining the eligibility of an athlete with cardiovascular disease.

In Italy, the medical clearance of athletes is an exclusive function of a specialist in sports medicine, which is an accredited multidisciplinary academic specialty, with a postgraduate 4-year residency program, implemented in several Italian medical schools. Sports medicine programs place a particular emphasis on the cardiovascular system and screening procedures, according to the dictates of the Italian law. Under Italian legislation, the specialist in sport medicine is the responsible party who must determine, with a reasonable degree of medical certainty, which medical risk an athlete is safe to assume. The legislation denies this right to the athlete, the family, the school, or athletic associations, when medical issues and decisions are involved. The specialist in sport medicine is responsible for the accuracy of medical assessment and is the final judge of the athlete's clearance for sport activity, by issuing the *certification of eligibility,* which represents for the Italian law "the necessary condition for the athlete's participation in official competitive athletic activities."[30] Consequently, the specialist is also considered responsible in the case of misdiagnosis or negligence that ultimately results in the athlete's death; in this instance, the physician is likely to be prosecuted on criminal and civil charges. In fact, some judicial proceedings have been held in Italy in the last decade, resulting from incidents in which elite and professional athletes with cardiovascular disease died suddenly. In a few instances, physicians who have engaged in negligent professional conduct have been subjected to compensatory financial damages.

In the United States, no systematic academic programs in sports medicine exist, and there are no criteria providing assurance that the examining physician has an adequate level of expertise in screening athletes for cardiovascular diseases. Indeed, although most states formally require that physicians should be responsible for the preparticipation examination, about 50% allow alternative clinicians, such as nurse practitioners, physician assistants, and even chiropractors to provide clearance for sports competition.[31] Therefore, the legal responsibility of the examining physician is less defined in the United States and the ultimate decision regarding the medical clearance of an athlete with a cardiovascular abnormality often represents the product of different opinions (and interests) among the team physician, the consulting cardiologists, the athlete, and the school or athletic association.[1,32] These conflicting perspectives have represented the legal framework of several judicial cases involving athletes with cardiovascular abnormalities and only recently the decision in the case of *Knapp v. Northwestern University*[32] indicated that the medical determination of eligibility to participate in competitive college sports *should be* the domain of team physicians and schools, not of the courts, as long as the decision-making process is carried out reasonably and is based on reliable scientific evidence.

IMPLEMENTATION AND EFFICACY OF CARDIOVASCULAR SCREENING

HISTORY AND PHYSICAL EXAMINATION

In 1996, the American Heart Association (AHA) provided a consensus panel statement for health professionals with guidelines for preparticipation cardiovascular screening of competitive athletes.[28] The AHA recommendations specifically state

> A complete and careful personal and family history and physical examination designed to identify (or raise the suspicion of) those cardiovascular lesions known to cause sudden death or disease progression in young athletes is the best available and most practical approach to screening populations of competitive sports participants, regardless of age. Such cardiovascular screening is an obtainable objective and should be mandatory for all athletes.[28]

The AHA statement also provides specific recommendations for the history and physical examination, based on the perception that the efficacy of screening ultimately depends on the accuracy of this process.

Implementation of these recommendations in the United States is, however, far from complete. Of the 51 state jurisdictions, only 43 provide approved history and physical examination questionnaires to be used by the examiner. Composition of these questionnaires varies greatly with respect to content, length, and comprehensiveness, and only 17 (40%) of the 43 state forms contain a number of items regarded as sufficient to identify (or raise suspicion of) cardiovascular disease, according to the recommendations of the AHA.[31]

Assessment of the efficacy of the history and physical examination in the preparticipation screening of athletes is difficult, because no prospective data on a national basis are available to provide the results of screening. In the retrospective analysis of Maron et al,[4] conducted in 134 young athletes who died suddenly of cardiovascular disease (see Fig. 9.6), the majority of these athletes (86%) had undergone a preparticipation medical evaluation as part of high school or college athletic programs, comprised of medical history and physical examination. In only 4 athletes (3%) did the examination arouse suspicion of cardiac disease and in just 1 (with Marfan syndrome) was the correct diagnosis ultimately made. It is of particular note that only 1 of the 48 athletes with HCM in that series had a correct diagnosis made during life.[4] Therefore, the preparticipation screening process based solely on history and physical examination appears to lack sufficient power to consistently recognize clinically important cardiovascular diseases. This opinion is also supported by the AHA panel, that confirmed that "history and physical examination alone (without noninvasive testing) is not sufficient to guarantee detection of many critical cardiovascular abnormalities in large population of young trained athletes" and that "detection of hypertrophic cardiomyopathy by standard screening is unreliable."[28]

THE 12-LEAD ELECTROCARDIOGRAM

Addition of the 12-lead ECG will likely increase the diagnostic efficacy of screening. The ECG has the potential to identify HCM (since over 90% of patients with this disease who die suddenly have an abnormal ECG pattern), with the most common changes including marked increase in R- or S-wave voltages, deep Q waves, ST-T changes,

markedly inverted T waves, left axis deviation, and atrial enlargement.[33] Also, subjects dying with arrhythmogenic right ventricular cardiomyopathy (ARVC) often show inverted T waves in the anterior precordial leads, ε wave, and increased QT-interval dispersion.[34] The 12-lead ECG has, moreover, the potential to identify most individuals with Wolff-Parkinson-White (WPW) and long QT syndromes.

Important limitations to the efficacy of the 12-lead ECG in screening athletes arise, however, from the variety of abnormalities present in highly trained subjects which are regarded as an expression of the athlete's heart.[35] Several of the ECG characteristics of athlete's heart may mimic cardiac pathologic conditions, including increased R- and/or S-wave voltages, deep Q waves, and markedly inverted T waves.[36-40] To clarify the clinical significance of abnormal 12-lead ECGs in athletes, Pelliccia et al evaluated the ECG patterns in a large cohort of 1005 highly trained athletes and compared these tracings directly with cardiac morphology and function, as assessed by echocardiography.[41] It was found that 40% of the athletes had abnormal ECG patterns, in particular 145 (14% of the study population) had particularly abnormal or bizarre ECGs, but only 10% of these athletes had evidence of structural cardiovascular abnormalities. Therefore, in highly trained athletes, abnormal ECG patterns are quite common findings, but convey only a low probability for cardiac disease.

The efficacy of routine 12-lead ECG in the setting of preparticipation screening has been evaluated by a few studies in the United States.[42-45] The number of subjects identified with cardiovascular abnormalities varied according to the size of the study population and the length of investigation, but did not exceed 10% of the examined athletes.[45] Most were only minor abnormalities that did not require disqualification from training and competition, and none had an unequivocal diagnosis of HCM, ARVC, or congenital coronary anomalies.[42-45]

However, the Italian experience suggests that the 12-lead ECG (in addition to medical history and physical examination) increases the diagnostic efficacy of the preparticipation screening and, specifically, may allow the identification of many athletes with HCM. Corrado et al[24] reported results of preparticipation screening for athletes living in the Veneto region of northeastern Italy. From a large population of 33,735 young athletes that entered the screening program in the period 1979 to 1996, about 2% were disqualified for cardiovascular abnormalities (Fig. 11.4). Of particular relevance, 22 subjects with HCM were identified as a result of the screening and most (73%) because of an abnormal 12-lead ECG. According to the Italian guidelines[46] (closely resembling those of the 26th Bethesda Conference Recommendations[5]), all these athletes with HCM were disqualified from training and competition and survived over the 8-year follow-up period.

In the same time period, 269 sudden cardiac deaths occurred in young subjects (< 35 years), including 49 in competitive athletes (Fig. 11.5). The most common causes in athletes were arrhythmogenic right ventricular cardiomyopathy (22%), premature atherosclerotic coronary artery disease (18%), and anomalous origin of a coronary artery from the wrong aortic sinus (12%); less frequently, HCM (2%) was found. Of note, HCM was a less frequent cause of death in athletes than it was in nonathletes (2 vs. 7%).[24]

ECHOCARDIOGRAPHY

Use of an echocardiogram would significantly enhance the diagnostic efficacy of screening by allowing identification of the majority of the causes of sudden cardiac deaths in young competitive athletes. Specifically, HCM can be easily identified in most affected athletes, with the only possible exception being those young family members (usually < 14 years of age) who have not yet manifested full phenotypic expression of their disease.[21,47] Wrong aortic sinus origin of a coronary artery can potentially be identified by a careful imaging study of the proximal aortic root and visualization of the coronary artery ostium with transthoracic echocardiography.[48] Echocardiography may raise the suspicion of ARVC,[49,50] although other investigations (e.g., magnetic resonance imaging) are usually necessary

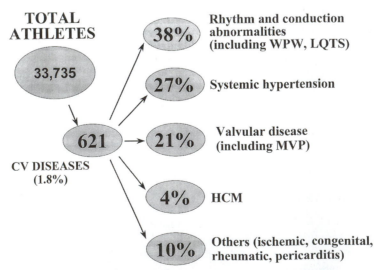

FIGURE 11.4 Results of preparticipation medical evaluation and cardiovascular conditions causing disqualification from competitive sports in athletes of the Veneto region of Italy. Adapted with permission from Corrado D, Basso C, Schiavon M, et al: Screening for hypertrophic cardiomyopathy in young athletes. N Engl J Med 339:364–369, 1998.

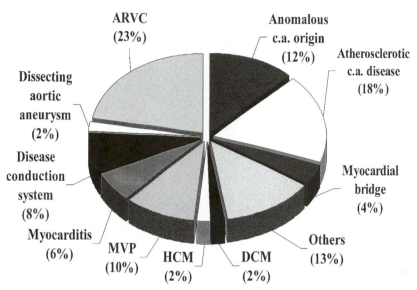

FIGURE 11.5 Causes of sudden death in young competitive athletes (< 35 years) in the Veneto region of Italy, 1979 to 1996. See Figure 11.1 for abbreviations. Adapted with permission from Corrado D, Basso C, Schiavon M, et al: Screening for hypertrophic cardiomyopathy in young athletes. N Engl J Med 339:364–369, 1998.

to confirm the diagnosis. Indeed, echocardiography would be expected to identify most of the athletes with aortic root dilatation (associated with cystic medial necrosis and Marfan syndrome), aortic valvular stenosis, mitral valve prolapse, and myocarditis with left ventricular dysfunction.

Few studies have evaluated the efficacy of echocardiography in the screening for cardiovascular disease in athletes.[42,44,45,51–53] Maron et al[42] examined 501 athletes with history, physical examination, and 12-lead ECG; of the 90 athletes with a suspicion of a cardiovascular abnormality who underwent echocardiography, 15% showed mitral valve prolapse, 1% had systemic hypertension, and 3% showed unexplained left ventricular hypertrophy. In a larger cohort of 5615 high school athletes examined by Fuller et al,[45] 10% had an echocardiographic study because of the abnormal findings found either with history, physical examination, or 12-lead ECG. Of these echocardiograms, < 1% showed minor abnormalities, such as bicuspid aortic valve and minimal left ventricular hypertrophy; only 1 athlete

showed an important abnormality, severe aortic regurgitation, and was disqualified from training and competition.

Lewis et al[44] evaluated 265 predominantly African-American college athletes by echocardiography and found 11% with increased left ventricular wall thickness (but no other evidence of HCM). In addition, another 13% had mitral valve prolapse, systemic hypertension, or a small atrial septal defect. Feinstein et al[51] assessed the feasibility and efficacy of a limited echocardiographic study confined to the parasternal long axis view; of the 1570 junior and senior high school athletes examined in a 3-year program, none showed HCM or any other cardiac disease that would preclude them from sports participation. Murry et al[52] used a similar limited echocardiographic study in 125 freshman athletes and found 10% with either mitral valve prolapse or bicuspid aortic valve, but none with evidence of HCM or Marfan syndrome. In a large cohort of 2997 high school athletes routinely examined by echocardiography, Weidenbener et al[53] described 2% of athletes with morphologic cardiac abnormalities (mostly mitral valve prolapse and bicuspid aortic valve), but none with Marfan syndrome or HCM.

Indeed, implementation of echocardiography in a large population screening is hampered by the cost of this test, which averages $600 and ranges up to $1000 in the United States In the experience of Weidenbener et al[53] and Murry et al,[52] the costs were remarkably low (less than $20 per study) due to the limited imaging protocol and the volunteered time and equipment; however, these examples represent a noteworthy exception in the usual United States scenario and are unlikely to be implemented on a scale necessary for consistently screening large athlete populations.

A different perspective has been derived from the experience of the Institute of Sports Science in Rome,[54] where Italian elite athletes undergo periodic physiological and medical evaluations. A comprehensive and multidisciplinary medical program specifically designed for these athletes has been implemented since 1963, and the cardiovascular evaluation is a part of this program routinely including medical history, physical examination, 12-lead and exercise ECG, and (since 1985) two-dimensional and Doppler echocardiography. The implementation of this program, which has been made possible by the financial support of the Italian Olympic Committee, administered up to 1000 athletes per year, with the global cost for a cardiovascular evaluation about $700 per athlete.

Although this evaluation does not represent true preparticipation screening, because the majority of the elite/professional Italian athletes have already been examined (at younger ages) in peripheral sports medicine centers, this program represents a unique cardiovascular program involving routine echocardiography in a large athlete population[54] and permits definition of the athlete's heart syndrome.[55,56]

During the 7-year period (1990 to 1996), about 4000 athletes were evaluated at the Institute of Sports Science and 30 subjects (0.8%) were identified with a structural cardiovascular abnormality at risk for sudden cardiac death and, consequently, were disqualified from participation in training and competition. The most frequent cardiac lesions detected were aortic aneurysm and Marfan syndrome ($n = 7$), HCM ($n = 6$), and myocarditis ($n = 6$). Less frequently, dilated cardiomyopathy, coronary artery disease, and ARVC were identified. Specifically, echocardiographic abnormalities were found in 97% of these subjects, while ECG abnormalities in only 67%.

In the same time period, only 2 of the 4000 examined athletes died suddenly. Deaths occurred during physical exertion, and both individuals had been considered normal at the cardiovascular evaluation: one was a hockey player who had a blunt chest blow resulting in a commotio cordis event,[57] and the other was a basketball player with a thrombotic stroke (on the basis of a congenital cerebrovascular abnormality). No deaths occurred among the 30 athletes with cardiovascular abnormalities, who had been disqualified from competition.

EXERCISE ELECTROCARDIOGRAPHY

The principal utility of exercise ECGs in athlete screening is the identification of occult atherosclerotic coronary artery disease.

In *young* asymptomatic athletes, the likelihood of significant coronary artery disease is extremely low (with the possible exception for individuals with a strong family history of premature coronary artery disease or known familial dyslipidemias), limiting the utility of exercise testing. Congenital coronary anomalies may be identified as well, but the predictive accuracy of exercise ECGs is very low.[58]

In asymptomatic *adult* athletes ($\geq$ 35 years), exercise ECGs have a low predictive accuracy, especially in those subjects with a low pretest probability of coronary disease. A number of studies have demonstrated that identification by exercise ECG of subjects at risk in a large population of asymptomatic individuals conveys only marginal benefit, due to the greater incidence of future cardiac events (including sudden death) among subjects screened with negative exercise ECGs.[9,59,60] For example, Siscovick et al[60] evaluated over 3600 individuals with an abnormal lipid profile; in the follow-up, 62 subjects had an exercise-related myocardial infarction or sudden cardiac death, but less than 20% of these individuals had a prior positive exercise test. Therefore, even in a high-risk population, exercise testing would fail to identify the majority of individuals who will have exercise-related cardiac events.[61]

Despite these limitations, exercise ECG is recommended by the American College of Sports Medicine[62] in high-risk individuals prior to engaging in vigorous exercise training and competition. Individuals at high risk are considered men over age 40 and women over age 50, in the presence of risk factors, either multiple or single (but markedly abnormal), or with known coronary artery disease. The American Heart Association, however, considers exercise testing prior to exercise programs an unresolved issue.[63]

PERSONAL PERSPECTIVE

Screening athletes for cardiovascular disease is a benevolent and ambitious project, which presents implicit difficulties and limitations related to costs and feasibility. An effort to screen several million athletes requires enormous financial support and raises innumerable challenges in terms of organization, implementation, and efficacy.

However, the long-standing Italian experience with medical screening implemented in a large population of competitive athletes is worthy of note for its objectives and results. The Italian experience suggests: (a) that a nationwide screening program is feasible, and (b) that inclusion of the 12-lead ECG conveys the potential to identify some of the most common causes of sudden cardiac death in young athletes, especially HCM.

Whether other societies will find the Italian approach to preventive medicine for competitive athletes an attractive strategy is uncertain. The Italian experience represents a challenging effort aimed to protect and improve the quality of the life for competitive athletes, which has been made possible by unique legislative initiatives, specifically designed for athletes.

Finally, because of the great variety of cardiac lesions potentially responsible for sudden death, it should be emphasized that medical clearance may not preclude the possibility of all potentially lethal cardiovascular diseases in individual athletes and, therefore, we should not encourage a false sense of security on the part of the examining physician and the general public with regard to the efficacy of the athletic screening.

REFERENCES

1. Maron BJ: Sudden death in young athletes. Lessons from the Hank Gathers affair. *N Engl J Med* 329:55–57, 1993.
2. Maron BJ, Roberts WC, McAllister HA, et al: Sudden death in young athletes. *Circulation* 62:218–229, 1980.
3. Maron BJ, Epstein SE, Roberts WC: Causes of sudden death in competitive athletes. *J Am Coll Cardiol* 7:204–214, 1986.
4. Maron BJ, Shirani J, Poliac LC, et al: Sudden death in young competitive athletes: Clinical, demographic and pathological profiles. *JAMA* 276:199–204, 1996.
5. Maron BJ, Mitchell JH: 26th Bethesda Conference: Recommendations for determining eligibility for competition in athletes with cardiovascular abnormalities. *J Am Coll Cardiol* 24:845–899, 1994.
6. Maron BJ, Gohman TE, Aeppli D: Prevalence of sudden cardiac death during competitive sports activities in Minnesota high school athletes. *J Am Coll Cardiol* 32:1881–1884, 1998.
7. Van Camp SP, Bloor CM, Mueller FO, et al: Nontraumatic sports death in high school and college athletes. *Med Sci Sports Exerc* 27:641–647, 1995.
8. Burke AP, Farb V, Virmani R, et al: Sports-related and non-sports-related sudden cardiac death in young adults. *Am Heart J* 121:568–575, 1991.

9. Thompson PD: The cardiovascular complications of vigorous physical activity. *Arch Intern Med* 156:2297–2302, 1996.

10. James TN, Froggatt P, Marshall TK: Sudden death in young athletes. *Ann Intern Med* 67:1013–1021, 1967.

11. Cheitlin MD, De Castro CM, McAllister HA: Sudden death as a complication of anomalous left coronary origin from the anterior sinus of Valsalva: A not-so-minor congenital anomaly. *Circulation* 50:780–787, 1974.

12. Thompson PD, Stern MP, Williams P, et al: Death during jogging or running: A study of 18 cases. *JAMA* 242:1265–1267, 1979.

13. Waller BF, Roberts WC: Sudden death while running in conditioned runners aged 40 years or over. *Am J Cardiol* 45:1292–1300, 1980.

14. Virmani R, Robinowitz M, McAllister HA Jr: Nontraumatic death in joggers: A series of 30 patients at autopsy. *Am J Med* 72:874–882, 1982.

15. Thompson PD, Funk EJ, Carleton RA, et al: Incidence of death during jogging in Rhode Island from 1975 through 1980. *JAMA* 247:2535–2538, 1982.

16. Tsung SH, Huang TY, Chang HH: Sudden death in young athletes. *Arch Pathol Lab Med* 106:168–170, 1982.

17. Northcote RJ, Flannigan C, Ballantyne D: Sudden death and vigorous exercise: A study of 60 deaths associated with squash. *Br Heart J* 55:198–203, 1986.

18. Thiene G, Nava A, Corrado D, et al: Right ventricular cardiomyopathy and sudden death in young people. *N Engl J Med* 318:129–133, 1988.

19. Corrado D, Thiene G, Nava A, et al: Sudden death in young competitive athletes: Clinicopathologic correlations in 22 cases. *Am J Med* 89:588–596, 1990.

20. McCaffrey FM, Braden DS, Strong WB: Sudden cardiac death in young athletes: A review. *Am Dis Child* 145:177–183, 1991.

21. Maron BJ: Hypertrophic cardiomyopathy. *Lancet* 350:127–133, 1997.

22. Maron BJ, Poliac LC, Roberts WO: Risk for sudden cardiac death associated with marathon running. *J Am Coll Cardiol* 28:428–431, 1996.

23. Maron BJ: Triggers for sudden cardiac death in the athlete. *Card Clin* 2:195–210, 1996

24. Corrado D, Basso C, Schiavon M, et al: Screening for hypertrophic cardiomyopathy in young athletes. *N Engl J Med* 339:364–369, 1998.

25. Katcher MS, Maron BJ, Homoud MK: Risk profiling and screening strategies, in Estes III M, Salem DN, Wang PJ (eds.): *Sudden Cardiac Death in the Athlete.* Armonk, New York: Futura Publishing Co., 1998, pp. 57–85.

26. Ciampricotti R, Deckers JW, Taverne R, et al: Characteristics of conditioned and sedentary men with acute coronary syndromes. *Am J Cardiol* 73:219–222, 1994.

27. Maron BJ, Kogan J, Proschan MA, et al: Circadian variability in the occurrence of sudden cardiac death in patients with hypertrophic cardiomyopathy. *J Am Coll Cardiol* 23:1405–1409, 1994.

28. Maron BJ, Thompson PD, Puffer JC, et al: Cardiovascular preparticipation screening of competitive athletes. A statement for health professionals for the Sudden Death Committee (Clinical Cardiology) and Congenital Cardiac Defects Committee (Cardiovascular Disease in the Young) American Heart Association. *Circulation* 94:850–856, 1996.

29. Tutela Sanitaria delle Attività Sportive. Gazzetta Ufficiale della Repubblica Italiana. December 23, 1971: 8162–8164.

30. Norme per la tutela sanitaria della attività sportiva agonistica. Gazzetta Ufficiale della Repubblica Italiana. March 5, 1982: 1715–1719.

31. Glover DW, Maron BJ: Profile of preparticipation cardiovascular screening for high school athletes. *JAMA* 279:1817–1819, 1998.

32. Maron BJ, Mitten MJ, Quandt EF, et al: Competitive athletes with cardiovascular disease. The case of Nicholas Knapp. *N Engl J Med* 339:1632–1635, 1998.

33. Maron BJ, Wolfson JK, Cirò E, et al: Relation of electrocardiographic abnormalities and patterns of left ventricular hypertrophy identified by 2-dimensional echocardiography in patients with hypertrophic cardiomyopathy. *Am J Cardiol* 51:189–194, 1983.

34. McKenna WJ, Thiene G, Nava A, et al: Diagnosis of arrhythmogenic right ventricular dysplasia/cardiomyopathy. *Br Heart J* 71:215–218, 1994.

35. Huston P, Puffer JC, MacMillan RW: The athletic heart syndrome. *N Engl J Med* 315:24–32, 1985.

36. Venerando A, Rulli V: Frequency, morphology and meaning of the electrocardiographic anomalies

found in Olympic marathon runners. *J Sports Med* 3:135–141, 1964.

37. Hanne-Paparo N, Wendkos MH, Brunner DT: T wave abnormalities in the electrocardiograms of top-ranking athletes without demonstrable organic heart disease. *Am Heart J* 81:743–747, 1971.

38. Lichtman J, O'Rourke RA, Klein A, et al: Electrocardiogram of the athlete: Alterations simulating those of organic heart disease. *Arch Intern Med* 132:763–770, 1973.

39. Oakley DG, Oakley CM: Significance of abnormal electrocardiograms in highly trained athletes. *Am J Cardiol* 50:985–989, 1982.

40. Zehender M, Meinertz T, Keul J, et al: ECG variants and cardiac arrhythmias in athletes: Clinical relevance and prognostic importance. *Am Heart J* 119:1378–1391, 1990.

41. Pelliccia A, Maron BJ, Culasso F, et al: Clinical significance of abnormal electrocardiographic patterns in trained athletes. *Circulation,* 2000 (in press).

42. Maron BJ, Bodison SA, Wesley YE, et al: Results of screening a large group of intercollegiate athletes for cardiovascular disease. *J Am Coll Cardiol* 10:1214–1221, 1987.

43. LaCorte MA, Boxer RA, Gottesfeld IB, et al: EKG screening program for school athletes. *Clin Cardiol* 12:42–44, 1989.

44. Lewis JF, Maron BJ, Diggs JA, et al: Preparticipation echocardiographic screening for cardiovascular disease in a large, predominantly black population of collegiate athletes. *Am J Cardiol* 64:1029–1033, 1989.

45. Fuller CM, McNulty CM, Spring DA, et al: Prospective screening of 5,615 high school athletes for risk of sudden cardiac death. *Med Sci Sports Exerc* 29:1131–1138, 1997.

46. Comitato Organizzativo per l'Idoneità allo Sport (COCIS). Protocolli cardiologici per il giudizio di idoneità allo sport agonistico. *G Ital Cardiol* 19:250–272, 1989.

47. Maron BJ, Spirito P, Wesley Y, et al: Development and progression of left ventricular hypertrophy in children with hypertrophic cardiomyopathy. *N Engl J Med* 315:610–614, 1986.

48. Pelliccia A, Spataro A, Maron BJ: Prospective echocardiographic screening for coronary artery anomalies in 1,360 elite competitive athletes. *Am J Cardiol* 72:978–979, 1993.

49. Kisslo J: Two-dimensional echocardiography in arrhythmogenic right ventricular dysplasia. *Eur Heart J* 10(Suppl D):22–26, 1989.

50. Scognamiglio R, Fasoli G, Nava A, et al: Relevance of subtle echocardiographic findings in the early diagnosis of the concealed form of right ventricular dysplasia. *Eur Heart J* 10 (Suppl D): 27–28, 1989.

51. Feinstein RA, Colvin E, Kim OM: Echocardiographic screening as a part of a preparticipation examination. *Clin J Sports Med* 3:149–152, 1993.

52. Murry PM, Cantwell JD, Heath DL, et al: The role of limited echocardiography in screening athletes. *Am J Cardiol* 76:849–850, 1995.

53. Weidenbener EJ, Krauss MD, Waller BF, et al: Incorporation of screening echocardiography in the preparticipation exam. *Clin J Sports Med* 5: 86–89, 1995.

54. Pelliccia A, Maron BJ: Preparticipation cardiovascular evaluation of the competitive athlete: Perspective from the 30-year Italian experience. *Am J Cardiol* 75:827–829, 1995.

55. Pelliccia A, Maron BJ, Spataro A, et al: The upper limit of physiologic cardiac hypertrophy in highly trained elite athletes. *N Engl J Med* 324:295–301, 1991.

56. Pelliccia A, Culasso F, Di Paolo FM, et al: Physiologic left ventricular cavity dilatation in elite athletes. *Ann Intern Med* 130:23–31, 1999.

57. Maron BJ, Poliac LC, Kaplan JA, et al: Blunt impact to the chest leading to sudden death from cardiac arrest during sports activities. *N Engl J Med* 333:337–342, 1995.

58. Basso C, Maron BJ, Corrado D, et al: Clinical profile of congenital coronary artery anomalies with origin from the wrong aortic sinus leading to sudden death in competitive athletes. *J Am Coll Cardiol,* 2000 (in press).

59. McHenry PL, O'Donnel J, Morris SN, et al: The abnormal exercise electrocardiogram in apparently healthy men: A predictor of angina pectoris as an initial coronary event during long-term follow-up. *Circulation* 70:547–551, 1984.

60. Siscovick DS, Ekelund LG, Johnson JL, et al: Sensitivity of exercise electrocardiography for acute events during moderate and strenuous physical activity. The Lipid Research Clinics Coronary Primary Prevention Trial. *Arch Intern Med* 151: 325–330, 1991.

61. Thompson PD: Sudden death in the athlete: Atherosclerotic coronary artery disease, in Estes III M, Salem DN, Wang PJ (eds.): *Sudden Cardiac Death in the Athlete.* Armonk, New York: Futura Publishing Co., 1998, pp. 393–402.

62. Mahler DA, Froelicher VF, Miller NH, et al: Health screening in risk stratification, in Kenney WL, Humphrey RH, Bryant CX (eds.): American College of Sports Medicine Guidelines for Exercise Testing and Prescription. 5th edition. Baltimore: Williams & Wilkins, 1995, pp. 25.

63. Schlant RC, Blomqvist CG, Brandemburg RO, et al: Guidelines for exercise testing: A report of the Joint American College of Cardiology/American Heart Association Task Force on Assessment of Cardiovascular Procedures (subcommittee on exercise testing). *Circulation* 74:653A–667A, 1986.

Chapter 12

SUDDEN DEATH AND OTHER CARDIOVASCULAR MANIFESTATIONS OF CHEST WALL TRAUMA IN SPORTS

Mark S. Link, M.D.   *Barry J. Maron, M.D.*   *Paul J. Wang, M.D.*
N. A. Mark Estes III, M.D.

Sudden death of an athlete is a rare event. Over the last few years it has become apparent that a significant proportion of deaths on the athletic field are due to chest wall impact in which death is sudden, resuscitation is difficult, and cardiologic pathologic abnormalities are absent (commotio cordis). Chest blows causing sudden death have been predominantly observed in baseball, with an impact velocity relatively normal for the age group involved. Higher levels of energy that impact the chest (than that of baseball impact), such as horse kicks and football injuries, have been reported to cause myocardial infarctions and aneurysm formation. Increasing the energy of impact, as is seen in motor vehicular accidents, can cause myocardial contusions and rupture as well as multiple ventricular arrhythmias. Thus, the degree of cardiac pathologic damage appears to be related to the energy of the impact. However, and somewhat surprisingly, impacts that do not cause cardiac pathologic abnormalities can cause sudden death. In this chapter we will focus primarily on lower energy impacts as these are the most commonly observed during sporting activities.

COMMOTIO CORDIS

DEFINITION

Commotio cordis, or *cardiac concussion,* is a term initially used to describe the cardiac manifestations of chest impact in an animal model producing no or minimal cardiac damage.[1] These cardiac manifestations included ST-segment elevation and arrhythmias, including ventricular tachycardia, ventricular fibrillation, heart block, asystole, and sinus bradycardia.[2–10] Despite descriptions of various arrhythmias in an animal model, the first well-documented case of death due to low-energy blunt chest impact was in 1978, and involved a 7-year-old boy struck in the chest by a baseball during a T-ball game.[11] In the 1980s and 1990s, case reports documented several other occurrences of sudden death due to chest impact, not only in baseball,[12,13] but also in hockey,[14] lacrosse,[15] and softball,[16,17] as well as from fist blows to the chest.[13]

In 1984 the United States Consumer Product Safety Commission reported 23 deaths due to baseball chest impact and found that there were more deaths in baseball from chest impact than there were from head impact.[18] In 1995, Maron et al provided the first comprehensive analysis of the commotio cordis phenomenon.[19] Since that time, reports from the Commotio Cordis Registry[20] and the development of an experimental model of sudden death with low-energy chest wall impact[21] have contributed to a fuller understanding of the mechanisms and prevention of sudden death with chest wall impact.

HUMAN OBSERVATIONS

Commotio cordis shows a predilection for the youthful athlete. In the Commotio Cordis Registry, the mean age is 12 years, with 70% less than age 16.[20] The oldest individual reported to date is a 43-year-old cricket player.[22] It is thought that the increased risk in young athletes is due to a more pliable chest wall that facilitates the transmission of energy to the myocardium upon impact. As the athlete ages, the thoracic cage stiffens and the chest wall absorbs more of the impact energy. However, there may be other variables that explain this predilection for young people such as the experimental finding that lower energies of impact, such as that encountered with youthful participants, may increase the risk of sudden death.[23] The overwhelming majority of the victims are male, with only one female appearing in the Commotio Cordis Registry.[20] The reason for this gender predominance is not clear. It is unlikely that the ratio of male-to-female baseball, softball, hockey, and other sports participants is as high as that in the registry; therefore, the male gender predominance is not entirely explained by the higher frequency of male sports participants. It likely may be a fundamental and relevant biological difference between the sexes, possibly including that of differences in repolarization, hormonal influences, or chest wall anatomy, which is, as of yet, unknown.

The most common sports in which commotio cordis has been reported are baseball, softball, and ice hockey (Fig. 12.1).[20] In addition, cases of commotio cordis have been reported occasionally in many other sports including football, lacrosse, kickboxing, and karate, as well as non–sports-related contact with a fist. In some of these other cases, a body part, usually a hand, foot, or elbow, creates the impact.[20] In all of these sports, it appears to be essential that the chest is impacted by a relatively hard object. Commotio cordis has never been reported with chest impact by a pneumatic ball (including soccer, football, tennis, and racquetball). In sports such as soccer or football, where commotio cordis deaths have occurred, the impact object has been a knee, fist, or helmet.

The energy or force of chest blows in victims of commotio cordis is difficult to quantify. However, it is fair to estimate that in all cases, the energy level of impact (velocity of the impact object) is not of unusual force for the sport in-

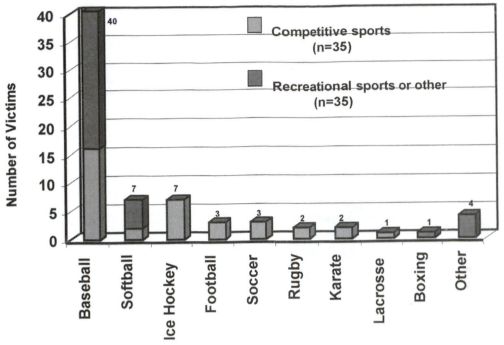

FIGURE 12.1. Bar graph documenting the frequency of sports (and ratio of competitive to recreational play) during which commotio cordis has been documented. More than one-half of the deaths have been due to baseball impacts. Adapted with permission from Maron BJ, Link MS, Wang PJ, et al: Clinical profile of commotio cordis: An under-appreciated cause of sudden death in the youth during sports and other activities. J Cardiovasc Electrophysiol *10:114–120, 1999.*

volved. For example, most of the victims died while playing with their peers, not while playing with much older individuals. None of the reported cases had chest wall or cardiac damage sufficient to explain their death, in contrast to the cases of death reported in motor vehicular accidents in which myocardial contusion or more severe cardiac and thoracic damage occurs.[24]

In commotio cordis victims, the chest blows strike the left chest (Fig. 12.2). Most of these blows reportedly occur directly over the cardiac silhouette; however, the exact location of the chest wall strike cannot always be determined with precision.[19] To our knowledge, there has never been a case of commotio cordis with a chest blow to the right chest or back.

Instantaneous collapse occurs in approxi-

mately one-half of the victims. In the others, collapse follows a brief period of consciousness often marked by extreme light-headedness.[19] When a rhythm is documented, it is most commonly ventricular fibrillation,[11,12,14,25–27] but one case of complete heart block[14] and idioventricular rhythm (after 10 min)[16] has also been reported. After resuscitation, the 12-lead ECG may show marked ST-segment elevation, especially in the anterior leads (Fig. 12.3).[26] However, the electrocardiographic manifestations of commotio cordis can resolve over time, without the development of Q waves, and myocardial enzymes are not elevated.[26]

Survival in commotio cordis appears to approach 10%.[20,25] As with other causes of ventricular fibrillation, the most important determinant of

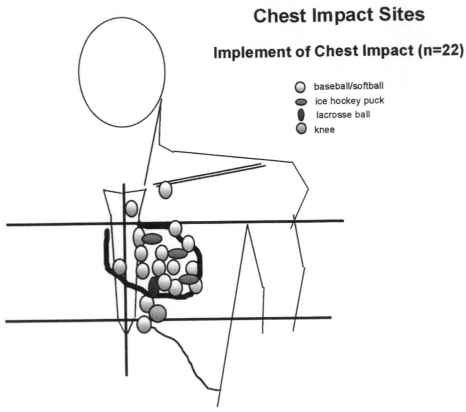

FIGURE 12.2. Location of chest wall impact that caused commotio cordis in Maron's original series of 25 individuals. The location of impact was ascertained by chest wall bruises. Note that the impacts were centered over the cardiac silhouette. Reproduced with permission from Maron BJ, Poliac LC, Kaplan JA, et al: Blunt impact to the chest leading to sudden death from cardiac arrest during sports activities. N Engl J Med *33:337–342, 1995.*

survival is early resuscitation. Of the 70 cases reported from the Commotio Cordis Registry, 11 survived to the hospital.[20] However, 4 of these patients ultimately expired due to severe end-organ damage. Of the 7 who survived to hospital discharge, 5 have had a complete neurologic recovery. In these 7 individuals, basic life support had been initiated within 1 min in 5 of the 6 and the other had spontaneous resolution of his event (and presumably his arrhythmia). Thus far, no person is known to have experienced commotio cordis more than once.

EXPERIMENTAL MODELS OF CHEST WALL TRAUMA

As the entity of sudden death with low energy chest wall impact was not generally appreciated until 20 years ago, early experimental efforts focused on more severe chest wall trauma, which was typically seen with victims of motor vehicular accidents, falls from heights, and bomb blasts. These models were therefore limited in their applicability to commotio cordis by the severity of the cardiac damage resulting from the substantial

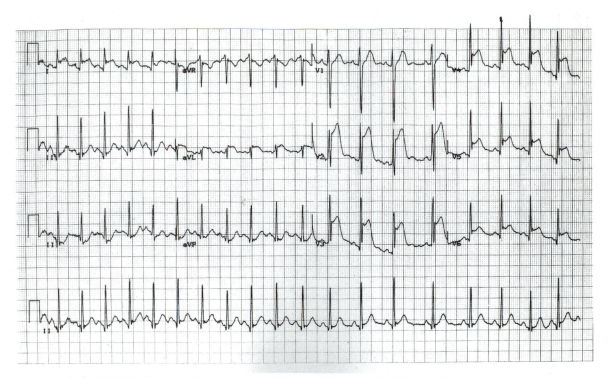

FIGURE 12.3. Electrocardiogram from a 14-year-old boy obtained 35 min after resuscitation from ventricular fibrillation caused by a knee blow to the chest in a game of football. Note the marked ST-segment elevation in the anterior leads. This patient underwent immediate cardiac catheterization, which documented normal coronary arteries. Myocardial infarction was ruled out, and the ST-segment elevation normalized over several days without the development of Q waves. Reproduced with permission from Link MS, Ginsburg SH, Wang PJ, et al: Commotio cordis: Cardiovascular manifestations of a rare survivor. Chest 114:326–328, 1998.

impact energies. Nevertheless, in these models, sudden death was occasionally described (both bradyarrhythmic and tachyarrhythmic) and ascribed to heightened vagal stimulation,[7] coronary spasm,[28] and myocardial contusion.[2]

In the first experiments using graded force, ventricular arrhythmias frequently resulted from marked impact energies.[6,8,10] However, most animals that died were found to have severe cardiac abnormalities that could account for their death and thus these experiments evaluated cardiac contusion, not true commotio cordis. Only one experiment gated the chest impact to the cardiac cycle and, although ventricular fibrillation was more

commonly seen with T-wave impacts, the energies of impact (on average, equivalent to a 123 mi/h baseball) caused relatively severe chest wall trauma.[10] In the early 1990s, a swine model of chest wall impact was developed utilizing a 95 mi/h baseball.[9] In this experiment bradyarrhythmias and tachyarrhythmias were seen, but no correlation to the cardiac cycle was noted, and animals suffered relatively severe thoracic and cardiac abnormalities.

It was concluded that these models were not necessarily reflective of the mechanisms of commotio cordis because they utilized high-energy projectiles with resultant chest wall and cardiac abnormalities.[21] Therefore, to study the patho-physiology of commotio cordis, a model was developed in which low-energy chest wall blows were gated to the cardiac cycle. In this model a 30 mi/h wooden sphere (subsequently baseballs) was utilized to deliver chest blows to 8- to 12-kg swine directly over the cardiac silhouette.[21] Swine were anesthetized with ketamine and isoflurane and suspended in a sling in order to approximate physiological cardiac anatomy and function (Fig. 12.4). The impact was directed to the papillary muscle of the left ventricle using transthoracic echocardiographic guidance and gated to the cardiac cycle using an electrophysiological stimula-tor. In addition to quantifying the electrophysio-logical effects of low energy (30 mi/h) chest wall trauma, wall motion abnormalities were evaluated with transthoracic echocardiography and myocar-dial blood flow with ^{99m}Tc- Sestamibi imaging and coronary angiography. It was found that the electrophysiological consequences of chest wall impact are largely dependent on the portion of the cardiac cycle during which impact occurs (Table 12.1). In this initial study, impacts occurring dur-ing repolarization on a particularly vulnerable portion of the T wave (15 to 30 ms prior to the peak) reproducibly and immediately caused ven-tricular fibrillation (Fig. 12.5). Subsequent exper-

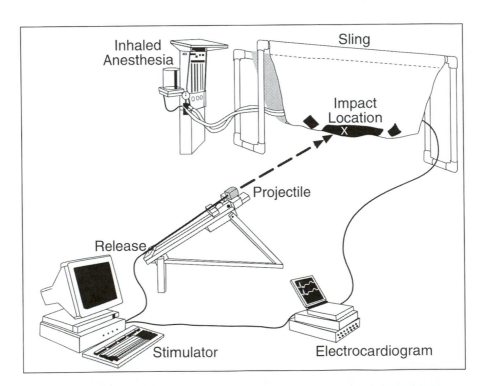

FIGURE 12.4. Experimental room setup showing the pronated swine in a sling attached to a standard 6-lead electrocardiogram. The impact is directed by transthoracic echocardiography to the area of the chest wall directly over the papillary muscles. The baseball is affixed to an alu-minum shaft propelled by a spring. With a known flight time of 130 ms and the release able to be adjusted according to the cardiac cycle, impact could be given anytime in the cardiac cycle.
Reproduced with permission from Link MS, Wang PJ, VanderBrink BA, et al: Selective activation of the K+ATP channel is a mechanism by which sudden death is produced by low-energy chest wall impact (commotio cordis). Circulation 100:413–418, 1999.

TABLE 12.1.   ELECTROPHYSIOLOGICAL CONSEQUENCES OF CHEST WALL IMPACT[a]

	Ventricular Fibrillation	Polymorphic Ventricular Tachycardia	Transient Heart Block	Left Bundle Branch Block	ST-Segment Elevation
T wave strikes from 15 to 30 ms prior to T peak (n = 10)	9	0	0	0	1
T wave strikes at other portions of T wave (n = 7)	0	2	0	1	2
QRS strikes (n = 10)	0	0	4	10	10
ST segment strikes (n = 4)	0	0	0	1	3

[a] Incidences shown in the first 28 animals studied with 30 mi/h impacts.

Adapted with permission from Link MS, Wang PJ, Pandian NG, et al: An experimental model of sudden death due to low energy chest wall impact (commotio cordis). *N Engl J Med* 338:1805–1811, 1998.

iments have shown that the vulnerable window extends to 10 ms prior to the T peak (Table 12.2). Blows during other portions of the cardiac cycle did not produce ventricular fibrillation, but caused ST elevations and transient complete heart block (Fig. 12.6). Transient wall motion abnormalities were observed in the apex of the heart, an area distant from the area of impact. In addition, mild apical perfusion defects in one-fourth of the animals were noted on Sestamibi imaging,

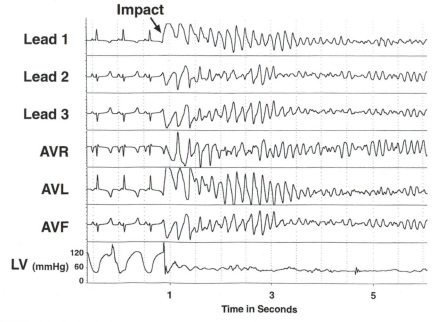

FIGURE 12.5. Six-lead electrocardiogram of a 9-kg swine undergoing chest wall impact with a 30 mi/h object the shape and weight of a standard baseball. With impact within the vulnerable zone of repolarization (10 to 30 ms prior to the T peak), ventricular fibrillation is immediately produced. *Reproduced with permission from Link MS, Wang PJ, Pandian NG, et al: An experimental model of sudden death due to low energy chest wall impact (commotio cordis). N Engl J Med 338:1805–1811, 1998.*

TABLE 12.2.   INCIDENCE OF VENTRICULAR FIBRILLATION WITH IMPACTS DURING DIFFERENT SEGMENTS OF THE CARDIAC CYCLE[a]

	QRS	ST	−40 to −31 ms to T peak	−30 to −21 ms to T peak	−20 to −10 ms to T peak	−9 to −1 ms to T peak	T downslope
Total impacts	59	89	46	287	196	17	34
VF induced	0	0	2	77	65	2	0
% VF	0%	0%	4%	27%	33%	11%	0%

[a] Ventricular fibrillation (VF) was only produced with impact on the upslope of the T wave, a vulnerable area of repolarization.

but no epicardial coronary artery abnormalities were found with coronary angiography performed within 1 min of the blow.[21]

In further experiments, other variables relevant to the risk of ventricular fibrillation were explored. First, the incidence of ventricular fibrillation was directly correlated with the hardness of the impact object (Fig. 12.7), with firmer objects more likely to cause ventricular fibrillation.[21] In experiments evaluating the energy of impact, it

was found that an energy level exists (20 mi/h) that is insufficient to cause ventricular fibrillation (commotio lower limit of vulnerability).[23] As the impact velocity was increased, the risk of ventricular fibrillation increased, up to 100% at 40 mi/h. At velocities over 40 mi/h, however, the incidence of ventricular fibrillation decreased to 80% at 50 mi/h and 20% at 60 mi/h (commotio upper limit of vulnerability). It has been shown that the induction of ventricular fibrillation with electrical

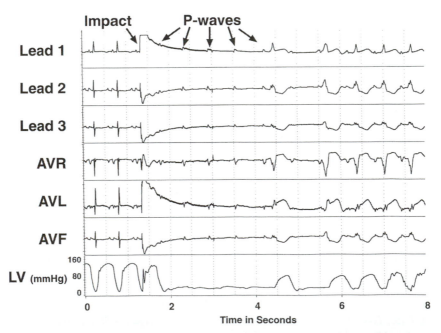

FIGURE 12.6. Six-lead electrocardiogram of a 8-kg swine undergoing chest wall impact with a 30 mi/h object the shape and weight of a standard baseball. Transient heart block is produced by impact during the QRS segment. Reproduced with permission from Link MS, Wang PJ, Pandian NG, et al: An experimental model of sudden death due to low energy chest wall impact (commotio cordis). N Engl J Med 338:1805–1811, 1998.

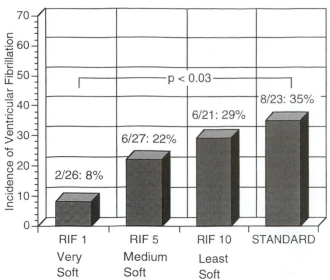

FIGURE 12.7. Incidence of ventricular fibrillation with chest wall impacts at 30 mi/h with a regulation baseball compared to softer-than-standard (safety) baseballs of 3 different grades of hardness. Reproduced with permission from Link MS, Wang PJ, Pandian NG, et al: An experimental model of sudden death due to low energy chest wall impact (commotio cordis). N Engl J Med 338:1805–1811, 1998.

shocks also exhibits a bell-shaped curve, with energies too low and energies too high to cause ventricular fibrillation.[29-31] In these experiments with the electrical induction of ventricular fibrillation, the upper limit of vulnerability is related to the defibrillation threshold. Thus, it is proposed that the reason the upper limit of vulnerability and the defibrillation threshold are similar relate to the homogeneity of the myocardium after the electrical shock. If the shock energy causes the entire myocardium to be homogeneously depolarized, then ventricular fibrillation will be extinguished if it is present, and if sinus rhythm is present, ventricular fibrillation cannot be induced. With shocks below the upper limit of vulnerability the depolarization of the myocardium is inhomogeneous and, therefore, ventricular fibrillation can result. Whether the mechanisms for the decreased vulnerability at higher impact velocities in commotio cordis are similar to the mechanism with the electrical induction of ventricular fibrillation remains unresolved.

Finally, the area of impact in both the model and in the human condition was directly over the heart. In the model, transthoracic echocardiography was used to define the area of the chest wall in which the ventricle was in closest approximation to the chest wall, which proved to be the left ventricle anterior lateral papillary muscle.[21] Impacts at sites on the left and right chest wall that did not overlie the cardiac silhouette never caused ventricular fibrillation. In fact, there was even a difference in those sites directly over the cardiac silhouette, with impacts directly over the left ventricular papillary muscle causing a higher frequency of ventricular fibrillation (30%) as compared to those over the base of the left ventricle (13%) and those over the apex of the heart (4%).

MECHANISMS

With the findings in humans and the experimental data, it is apparent that ventricular fibrillation is the cause of death with low-energy chest wall trauma. Since the ventricular fibrillation is virtually instantaneous, it is unlikely due to ischemia, heart block, or myocardial hemorrhage but rather due to a primary electrical event. Therefore, the possibility that specific ion channels are activated by the mechanical impact was considered. A candidate channel is the K^+_{ATP} channel, given that it is thought responsible for the ST-segment elevation and contributes to the risk of ventricular fibrillation in myocardial ischemia. This channel is normally inactivated by physiological concentrations of adenosine triphosphate (ATP). When ATP decreases and the adenosine diphosphate (ADP) increases, as in myocardial ischemia, the channel is opened, and potassium exits the cell. The increased extracellular potassium leads to ST-segment elevation and increases the risk of ventricular fibrillation. Because of the similarities of the electrocardiographic changes and arrhythmias in commotio cordis and myocardial ischemia, it was hypothesized that the K^+_{ATP} channel may play a role in the genesis of the immediate electrical findings in the model of commotio cordis. Indeed, it was found that a specific blocker of the K^+_{ATP} channel (glibenclamide) reduced the magnitude of the ST-segment elevation and the incidence of ventricular fibrillation.[32] Of 18 impacts in control animals, there were 6 episodes (33%) of ventricular fibrillation, while in 27 impacts in animals pretreated with glibenclamide, there was only 1 episode (4%) of ventricular fibrillation ($p = 0.01$). Whether activation of other channels or the autonomic nervous system play a role in commotio cordis is not yet known.

TREATMENT

In the human victims of commotio cordis, successful resuscitation has occurred in approximately 10%. As in other mechanisms of sudden death, the major determinant of survival would appear to be earlier resuscitation efforts and, especially, early defibrillation. In the 7 known resuscitated victims of commotio cordis, cardiopulmonary resuscitation began within 1 min in 5 of the 6 (the other had a spontaneous resolution of

consciousness).[20] In the commotio cordis experimental model, early defibrillation was also found to be critical to the survival of the animal.[33] All animals defibrillated under 2 min survived, while only 3 of 7 animals defibrillated after 4 min survived. In this model, a frequent occurrence of heart block and ST-segment elevation after defibrillation was found, suggesting that these factors may also play a role in the poor resuscitation outcomes of commotio cordis victims. Therefore, an important implication of these data would be for coaches and other sporting personnel (including parents) to be trained in basic life support and to consider obtaining ready access to automatic external defibrillators.

PREVENTION

Since resuscitation is so seldom successful, the primary prevention of commotio cordis should be stressed. In Maron's series of 25 victims of commotio cordis, 7 were wearing a commercially available chest wall protector (4 were hockey players, 1 was a football player, 1 was a baseball catcher, and 1 a lacrosse goalie).[19] Two other commotio cordis deaths in hockey have been reported despite chest protection.[14] Yet, it appears that in some of these victims wearing chest protection, lifting of the arms prior to impact nevertheless exposed the area over the heart.[19] Animal models have been used to evaluate safety baseballs (softer than standard) and chest wall protection in two laboratories. In one laboratory utilizing a 95 mi/h baseball impact with 6 swine, there were minor reductions in fatalities when a softer-than-standard baseball was used in combination with commercially available chest wall protectors.[34] However, chest wall protectors in combination with standard baseballs had little effect on the incidence of fatalities. In experiments with a dummy model, increased values for force and momentum were observed with the combination of softer-than-standard baseballs thrown at 95 mi/h and chest protectors.[34] Thus, these investigators suggested that softer-than-standard baseballs may actually enhance the risk of sudden death with chest wall impact. However, the marked impact energies employed, the varied electrophysiological results produced, and the limited number of animals used in this experiment limit the applicability of the findings. In a 1998 publication by this same group evaluating the risk of cardiac injury from 40, 50, and 60 mi/h impacts, 8 safety baseballs were evaluated and compared to a regulation baseball.[35] In this study utilizing dummy models, 6 of the 8 safety balls tested had a significantly lower viscous criterion than the standard baseball at at least 1 of the velocities tested. One of the 8 balls had no differences from the standard baseball, and 1 of the 8 baseballs had no difference in viscous criterion at 2 of the velocities and had a significantly greater viscous criterion at 60 mi/h.

Experiments with a 30 and 40 mi/h baseball impacts in our swine model showed a statistically significant reduction in the risk of fatal ventricular arrhythmias with safety baseballs (Fig. 12.7). The softest ball (Reduced Injury Factor, RIF, 1, Worth Inc., Tullahoma, TN), marketed for use in T-ball for youths aged 5 to 7, has the hardness similar to that of a tennis ball. In Link et al's model,[21] this ball had an incidence of ventricular fibrillation of 8% at 30 mi/h and 8% at 40 mi/h. The medium soft balls (RIF 5), marketed for use in children 8 to 10 years, had a ventricular fibrillation incidence of 22% at 30 mi/h and 23% at 40 mi/h. Balls with a hardness slightly less than regulation baseball (RIF 10), had an incidence of 29% at 30 mi/h and 20% at 40 mi/h. Finally, regulation baseballs had an incidence of ventricular fibrillation of 35% at 30 mi/h and 69% at 40 mi/h. At all velocities the safety baseballs reduced the incidence of ventricular fibrillation when compared to that of regulation baseballs. The differences between Link et al's experiment and Janda et al's experiment is likely related to the hypothesis that as the velocity of the impact object increases, the softness of the object may not be able to protect against commotio cordis. Thus, at 95 mi/h, a safety baseball may not offer much protection. However, baseball velocities of 95 mi/h are extremely unlikely in youth baseball where the average velocity of a pitched ball is in

the range of 30 to 50 mi/h. Thus, at lower velocities such as those more applicable to youth baseball, it appears that safety balls will reduce the risk of cardiac injury and sudden death.

CONTUSIO CORDIS

Contusio cordis is to be differentiated from commotio cordis by the presence of myocardial contusion. While this myocardial contusion can only be demonstrated with certainty at autopsy (intramyocardial hemorrhage and necrosis, similar to that seen with myocardial infarction[36]), its presence can be inferred clinically by segmental wall motion defects on echocardiography or by the measurement of increased serial cardiac enzymes.[24] In practice, the types of chest wall injury that cause myocardial contusions are those incurred by motor vehicular accidents, falls from heights, or in bomb blast victims.[24,37–40] Individuals involved in sports are rarely subjected to chest wall impact of the energy levels seen in cardiac contusion. Exceptions would be the occasional horse kick to the chest,[41–43] and motor vehicular accidents in sports car drivers. Sometimes a clear demarcation between commotio cordis and contusio cordis cannot always be made since chest impact energies that lie between blows inflicted by a little league baseball and a motor vehicular accident could cause myocardial hemorrhage in some individuals and no myocardial hemorrhage in others.

In individuals dying from myocardial contusion, a wide variety of cardiac arrhythmias have been reported, including ventricular fibrillation, ventricular tachycardia, asystole, and pulseless electrical activity.[44] These arrhythmias are frequently seen in association with pericardial tamponade and myocardial or valvular rupture; thus, the arrhythmias are secondary to severe myocardial dysfunction, hypotension, hypoxia, and cardiac ischemia. Nearly all of the patients with myocardial contusion have associated thoracic abnormalities including rib fractures, pulmonary contusions, pneumothorax, and hemothorax.[24]

Animal models of contusio cordis have found that the pathologic damage and the arrhythmias observed generally correlate with the amount of energy to which the chest wall is subjected.[6,8,10,45] The arrhythmias seen in cardiac contusion can be immediate, as in commotio cordis, or can be delayed (up to 12 to 24 h). Delayed arrhythmias are likely secondary to the pathologically damaged myocardium, similar to that observed with acute myocardial infarction.[24,44]

Electrocardiograms in individuals with myocardial contusion show changes similar to those seen in myocardial ischemia, including T-wave peaking, ST-segment elevation, depression, and even prolonged QT intervals.[3,24,36,46,47] However, these electrocardiographic changes are neither sensitive nor specific for cardiac contusion.[40,48,49] Echocardiograms will often document segmental wall motion abnormalities and are useful in the documentation of pericardial tamponade, myocardial rupture, aortic dissection, and acute valvular disease.[24] Management of these patients includes careful hemodynamic monitoring, cardiac ECGs, echocardiograms, and often admission to the hospital.[24,39] Whether admission to the hospital is necessary is not based solely on electrocardiographic abnormalities, but also the extent of trauma and echocardiographic abnormalities.[24,40] Individuals with mild chest trauma (i.e., most sports-related trauma) and no ECG abnormalities can usually be safely discharged home after a brief observation in the emergency department.

MYOCARDIAL INFARCTION

Although myocardial infarction due to atherosclerotic coronary disease often occurs with exertion in sporting events, chest wall trauma causing acute myocardial infarction is unusual. In a review of 40 myocardial infarctions reportedly occurring secondary to chest wall trauma, 21 were due to motor vehicular accidents and 14 were due to chest wall impact during sporting activities, including chest blows with softballs, soccer balls, basketballs, and as a consequence of fistfights.[50]

In addition to the cases reported in this article, there are an additional 6 reports of myocardial infarction presumptively caused by chest impact in sports.[43,51–54] It is from these reports that the demographic information on myocardial infarction secondary to chest wall trauma is drawn. Of the 20 patients, there were 2 females. The mean age was 32 ± 11 years (range of 10 to 53). The most common sports involved included boxing/fistfights ($n = 6$), soccer ($n = 4$), and rugby, skiing, and horse kicks (2 each). In 7 of the patients, the chest pain and myocardial infarction was immediate; in others it appeared hours or days later (median time of 455 min). Whether preexisting atherosclerosis increases the risk of traumatic myocardial infarction is not clear, but it is likely that the hardened atheromatous plaque is susceptible to traumatic rupture from chest wall trauma.[55] Still, several of the individuals with acute myocardial infarction were young, and normal coronary arteries had been documented in several others. Thus, preexisting coronary artery disease is not a prerequisite for these events. In distinction from commotio cordis, chest wall trauma causing myocardial infarction occurs with an older age group, is more common with fistfights than it is with baseball, has a time from impact to presentation that is highly variable, and has energies of impact that appear to be greater.

The management of an individual with a traumatic myocardial infarction is similar to that of any patient with a myocardial infarction. Beta blockade, aspirin, nitrates, and admission to a monitored setting should be routine. However, given the difficulty with diagnosis and the concern about other thoracic injuries, thrombolytics should be avoided in most cases. Immediate cardiac catheterization with angioplasty or stent placement should be considered.[43]

SUMMARY

Although sudden deaths of athletes are rare, it has lately become apparent that a significant percentage of deaths on the athletic field are due to chest wall impact (commotio cordis). This phenomenon has been reported in over 70 individuals and may be significantly underreported. It is most frequently observed in the young athlete (age 4 to 18), but has also been reported in several individuals over the age of 20 years. The most common projectile is a baseball, but commotio cordis has also been described in hockey, lacrosse, softball, fistfights, and with any activity that can have chest impact with a hard object. Victims are most often found in ventricular fibrillation, and resuscitation is more difficult than expected given the young age and excellent health of the victims. Autopsies are notable for the lack of any significant cardiac or thoracic abnormalities.

In an experimental model of commotio cordis, ventricular fibrillation could be produced by a 30 mi/h baseball strike, but only if impact occurred during a 20 ms window on the upslope of the T wave. Other important variables in this model include the energy of impact, the hardness of the impact object, and the location of the impact.

Chest impact at high energy levels can occasionally cause myocardial contusions. These impacts are typically produced by motor vehicular accidents, but can also be seen in horse kicks. Myocardial infarctions, even in the presence of normal coronary arteries, can be produced by chest wall trauma. Evaluation of myocardial contusion includes echocardiography to document structural heart pathology, electrocardiograms (ECGs), and electrocardiographic monitoring. Traumatic myocardial infarctions are best treated with beta blockade, aspirin, and immediate coronary angiography, if available. Thrombolytics should be avoided.

REFERENCES

1. Schlomka G, Schmitz M: Experimentelle untersuchungen uber den einfluss stumpfer brustkorbtraumen auf das electrokardiogramm. *S Ges Exp Med* 85:171–190, 1932.
2. Bright EF, Beck CS: Nonpenetrating wounds of the heart. A clinical and experimental study. *Am Heart J* 10:293–321, 1935.
3. Kissane RW, Fidler RS, Koons RA: Electrocardiographic changes following external chest injury to dogs. *Ann Intern Med* 11:907–935, 1937.
4. Moritz AR, Atkins JP: Cardiac contusion: An experimental and pathologic study. *Arch Path* 25:445–462, 1938.
5. Louhimo I: Heart injury after blunt thoracic trauma. An experimental study on rabbits. *Act Chir Scand* 380:7–60, 1967.
6. Liedtke AJ, Gault JH, Demuth WE: Electrographic and hemodynamic changes following nonpenetrating chest trauma in the experimental animal. *Am J Physiol* 226:377–382, 1974.
7. Meola F: La commozione toracica. *Gior Internaz Sci Med* 1879.
8. Viano DC, Artinion CG: Myocardial conducting system dysfunctions from thoracic impact. *J Trauma* 18:452–459, 1978.
9. Viano DC, Andrzejak DV, Polley TZ, et al: Mechanism of fatal chest injury by baseball impact: Development of an experimental model. *Clin J Sport Med* 2:166–171, 1992.
10. Cooper GJ, Pearce BP, Stainer MC, et al: The biomechanical response of the thorax to nonpenetrating impact with particular reference to cardiac injuries. *J Trauma* 22:994–1008, 1982.
11. Dickman GL, Hassan A, Luckstead EF: Ventricular fibrillation following baseball injury. *Phys Sport Med* 6:85–86, 1978.
12. Abrunzo TJ: Commotio cordis, the single, most common cause of traumatic death in youth baseball. *Am J Dis Child* 145:1279–1282, 1991.
13. Frazer M, Mirchandani H: Commotio cordis, revisited. *Am J Forensic Med Path* 5:249–251, 1984.
14. Kaplan JA, Karofsky PS, Volturo GA: Commotio cordis in two amateur ice hockey players despite the use of commercial chest protectors: Case reports. *J Trauma* 34:151–153, 1993.
15. Edlich RF, Mayer NE, Fariss BL, et al: Commotio cordis in a lacrosse goalie. *J Emerg Med* 5:181–184, 1987.
16. Green ED, Simson LR, Kellerman HH, et al: Cardiac concussion following softball blow to the chest. *Ann Emerg Med* 9:155–157, 1980.
17. Froede RC, Lindsey D, Steinbronn K: Sudden unexpected death from cardiac concussion (commotio cordis) with unusual legal complications. *J Foren Sci* 24:752–756, 1979.
18. Rutherford GW, Kennedy J, McGhee L: Baseball and softball related injuries to children 5–14 years

of age. Washington DC: United States Consumer Product Safety Commission, 1984.

19. Maron BJ, Poliac LC, Kaplan JA, et al: Blunt impact to the chest leading to sudden death from cardiac arrest during sports activities. *N Engl J Med* 333:337–342, 1995.

20. Maron BJ, Link MS, Wang PJ, et al: Clinical profile of commotio cordis: An under-appreciated cause of sudden death in the young during sports and other activities. *J Cardiovasc Electrophysiol* 10:114–120, 1999.

21. Link MS, Wang PJ, Pandian NG, et al: An experimental model of sudden death due to low energy chest wall impact (commotio cordis). *N Engl J Med* 338:1805–1811, 1998.

22. Haq CL: Letter to the editor. *N Engl J Med* 339:1399, 1998.

23. Link MS, Wang PJ, Pandian NG, et al: Upper and lower energy limits of vulnerability to sudden death with chest wall impact (commotio cordis) (abstract). *Circulation* 98:I–51, 1998.

24. Tenzer ML: The spectrum of myocardial contusion: A review. *J Trauma* 25:620–627, 1985.

25. Maron BJ, Strasburger JF, Kugler JD, et al: Survival following blunt chest impact induced cardiac arrest during sports activities in young athletes. *Am J Cardiol* 79:840–841, 1997.

26. Link MS, Ginsburg SH, Wang PJ, et al: Commotio cordis: Cardiovascular manifestations of a rare survivor. *Chest* 114:326–328, 1998.

27. Van Amerongen R, Rosen M, Winnik G, et al: Ventricular fibrillation following blunt chest trauma from a baseball. *Pediatr Emerg Care* 13:107–110, 1997.

28. Schlomka G: Commotio cordis und ihre folgen. *Med Kinderheilk,* 47, 1934.

29. Chen P-S, Shibata N, Dixon EG, et al: Comparison of the defibrillation threshold and the upper limit of ventricular vulnerability. *Circulation* 73:1022–1028, 1986.

30. Fabritz CL, Kirchhof PF, Behrens S, et al: Myocardial vulnerability to T wave shocks: Relation to shock strength, shock coupling interval, and dispersion of ventricular repolarization. *J Cardiovasc Electrophysiol* 7:231–242, 1996.

31. Swerdlow CD, Peter CT, Kass RM, et al: Programming of implantable cardioverter-defibrillators on the basis of the upper limit of vulnerability. *Circulation* 95:1497–1504, 1997.

32. Link MS, Wang PJ, VanderBrink BA, et al:

Selective activation of the K+ATP channel is a mechanism by which sudden death is produced by low-energy chest-wall impact (commotio cordis). *Circulation* 100:413–418, 1999.

33. Link MS, Wang PJ, Pandian NG, et al: Resuscitation in a biological model of commotio cordis, sudden death from low energy chest wall impact (abstract). *J Am Coll Cardiol* 31:403A, 1998.

34. Janda DH, Viano DC, Andrzejak DV, et al: An analysis of preventive methods for baseball-induced chest impact injuries. *Clin J Sport Med* 2:172–179, 1992.

35. Janda DH, Bir CA, Viano DC, et al: Blunt chest impacts: Assessing the relative risk of fatal cardiac injury from various baseballs. *J Trauma* 44:298–303, 1998.

36. Kissane RW: Traumatic heart disease: Nonpenetrating injuries. *Circulation* 6:421–425, 1952.

37. Parmley LF, Manion WC, Mattingly TW: Nonpenetrating traumatic injury of the heart. *Circulation* 28:371–396, 1958.

38. Ritchie AJ, Gibbons JRP: Life threatening injuries to the chest caused by plastic bullets. *Br Med J* 301:1027, 1990.

39. Rothstein RJ: Myocardial contusion. *JAMA* 250:2189–2191, 1983.

40. Pretre R, Chilcott M: Blunt trauma to the heart and great vessels. *N Engl J Med* 336:626–632, 1997.

41. Pontillo D, Capezzuto A, Achilli A, et al: Bifascicular block complicating blunt cardiac injury: A case report and review of the literature. *Angiology* 45:883–890, 1994.

42. Fox KM, Rowland E, Krikler DM, et al: Electrophysiologic manifestations of non-penetrating cardiac trauma. *Br Heart J* 43:458–462, 1980.

43. Marcum JL, Booth DC, Sapin PM: Acute myocardial infarction caused by blunt chest trauma: Successful treatment by direct coronary angioplasty. *Am Heart J* 132:1275–1277, 1996.

44. Healey MA, Brown R, Fleiszer D: Blunt cardiac injury: Is this diagnosis necessary? *J Trauma* 30:137–146, 1990.

45. Anderson AE, Doty DB: Cardiac trauma: An experimental model of isolated myocardial contusion. *J Trauma* 15:237–244, 1975.

46. Cane RD, Schamroth L: Prolongation of Q-T interval with myocardial contusion. *Heart Lung* 7:652–656, 1978.

47. Potkin RT, Werner JA, Trobaugh GB, et al: Evaluation of noninvasive tests of cardiac damage in suspected myocardial contusion. *Circulation* 66:627–631, 1982.

48. Blair E, Topuzlu D, Davis JH: Delayed or missed diagnosis in blunt chest trauma. *J Trauma* 11: 129–145, 1971.

49. Schick ECJ: Nonpenetrating cardiac trauma. *Card Clin* 13:241–247, 1995.

50. Neiman J, Hui WKK: Posteromedial papillary muscle rupture as a result of right coronary artery occlusion after blunt chest injury. *Am Heart J* 123:1694–1699, 1992.

51. Borodkin HD, Massey FC: Myocardial trauma produced by nonpenetrating chest injury. *Am Heart J* 53:795–801, 1957.

52. Ledley GS, Yazdanfar S, Friedman O, et al: Acute thrombotic coronary occlusion secondary to chest trauma treated with intracoronary thrombolysis. *Am Heart J* 123:518–521, 1992.

53. Hedinger C: Contusio cordis mit spatrupter der linken herzkammer. *Cardiologia* 12:46–48, 1948.

54. Singh R, Nolan SP, Schrank JP: Traumatic left ventricular aneurysm: Two cases with normal coronary angiograms. *JAMA* 234:412–413, 1975.

55. Roberts WC, Maron BJ: Sudden death while playing professional football. *Am Heart J* 102: 1061–1063, 1981.

Chapter 13

EXERCISE IN CHILDREN AFTER SURGERY FOR CONGENITAL HEART DISEASE

Jeffrey Alan Conwell, M.D.   J. Timothy Bricker, M.D.

Congenital heart disease is the most common congenital defect, occurring in approximately 0.8% of all live births. The high incidence of congenital heart disease makes it likely that clinicians and exercise physiologists will evaluate, treat, and make exercise recommendations regarding congenital heart disease patients during their years of practice. Many patients will have undergone surgical repair or cardiac catheterization intervention for their structural defect. Health care providers need to know the more common cardiac defects, their treatment, and potential residual defects, as well as postoperative complications following repair or cardiac catheterization intervention to better advise and treat these patients. Most congenital heart disease patients will be followed by a pediatric or adult cardiologist, but some patients may not have had a recent evaluation.

Guidelines for sports participation have been published in the past for "competitive" athletes with congenital heart disease.[1–4] However, most patients with congenital heart disease will not be participating in competitive athletics and are more likely to have an active lifestyle and to participate in sports at a recreational level for enjoyment or health benefits. Few guidelines have been developed for participation in recreational, vocational, or rehabilitative exercise.[5,6] Guidelines for competitive athletics were developed because of well-publicized deaths among high school, college, and professional athletes and with the identification of congenital heart disease patients as a high-risk group.

Advances in pediatric cardiothoracic surgery over the last 20 to 30 years have allowed a change from predominantly palliative types of cardiac surgery to complete cardiac repair. Along with the increase in complete cardiac repairs, there have been improvements in the medical management of patients, with a resultant decrease in the morbidity and mortality associated with cardiac surgery. The survival of children with complex congenital heart disease is increasing, as is their life span. Therefore, the probability is progressively increasing that the general pediatrician and internal medicine physician will see patients with repaired cardiac disease during their careers.

As patients with congenital heart disease age and their life expectancy increases, the incidence of adult diseases will increase in this patient population. Diseases such as atherosclerotic coronary artery disease, hypertension, and diabetes are more likely to develop. Consequently, preventive cardiology becomes even more important because there may be underlying structural or functional abnormalities that can make the congenital heart disease patient more susceptible to these degenerative disease processes. Patients with repaired or palliated congenital heart disease require guidance to avoid smoking, to follow a heart-healthy diet, and, most of all, to participate in a regular exercise program. This guidance should be similar to that which is given to all individuals during health maintenance visits[7–11] (Table 13.1).

Regular exercise may provide other benefits to congenital heart disease patients. People involved in regular exercise have an improved sense of well-being, increased exercise tolerance, and possibly, even a decreased number of illnesses. These results are even more important in this patient group since they may have limited exercise toler-

TABLE 13.1.   AMERICAN HEART ASSOCIATION HEALTHY PHYSICAL ACTIVITY STANDARDS

1. Regular walking, bicycling, and backyard play; use of stairs, playgrounds, and gymnasiums; interaction with other children.
2. Less than 2 h per day watching television (includes video games and videotapes).
3. Weekly participation in age-appropriate organized sports, lessons, clubs, or sandlot games.
4. Daily school or day care physical education, including at least 20 min of coordinated large muscle exercise.
5. Regular participation in household chores.
6. Weekly family outings that involve walking, cycling, swimming, or other recreational activities.
7. Positive role modeling for a physical lifestyle by parents, other caretakers, physicians, and school personnel.

Adapted with permission from Subcommittee on Atherosclerosis and Hypertension in Childhood, Council on Cardiovascular Disease in the Young, American Heart Association. Integrated cardiovascular health promotion in childhood. *Circulation* 85:1638–1650, 1992.

ance and may not tolerate frequent illness. Also, the psychological benefits of exercise may assist in the long-term patient care.[8,11]

The diagnosis of congenital heart disease is made in the first few years of life (98% by 4 years of age), making the likelihood of a school-aged child with significant undiagnosed cardiac disease unlikely. However, because of the well-publicized sudden deaths of young athletes—some with congenital cardiac abnormalities—there is always a level of concern that a significant cardiac defect may be missed.

Children with congenital heart disease are, in general, at low risk for sudden death during exercise. There are a few exceptions to this generalization, including such defects as severe aortic valve stenosis, hypertrophic cardiomyopathy, coronary artery abnormalities, long QT-interval syndromes, Marfan syndrome, and myocarditis.[12–16] These cardiac defects are, fortunately, very uncommon, but identification of cases and prediction of risk may be difficult.

Guidelines for congenital heart disease patients in the past have been predominantly of a restrictive nature without guidance about the health benefits. This chapter will try to address some of these issues and suggest recommendations for recreational sport participation for various cardiac defects. These recommendations will take into consideration the current knowledge about exercise and congenital heart disease, but will also include practical recommendations based on clinical experience when more definitive data are not available.

This chapter will also discuss the more common congenital cardiac defects along with some less common types that have similar cardiac repairs; it, however, is limited to structural cardiac defects. Exercise both before and after surgical repair or nonoperative intervention will also be discussed.

EVALUATION

The impact of a patients' other medical conditions should be considered in any decision re-garding athletic participation. As with all patient evaluations, a complete history and physical examination should be included in the evaluation prior to participation in any athletics. Additional cardiac testing should be directed by specific historical and physical examination findings. Patients must be evaluated in their entirety and not just as the cardiac defect in isolation.[1,2,17]

Although there are many diagnostic tools available for evaluation prior to exercise participation, the most important remains the history and physical examination. Patients with postoperative congenital heart disease sometimes have residual defects that are hemodynamically significant, such as ventricular dysfunction, pulmonary hypertension, or cardiac arrhythmias. Some patients may be on medications, which can influence recommendations (such as anticoagulants) or have pacemakers or implanted defibrillators. The effects of the activity on the hemodynamic aspects of a cardiac repair need to be considered.

HISTORY

The cardiac history before sports participation should be thorough for all athletes. Many states have questionnaires that are required for sports physicals. These alone may not be adequate for evaluation of the cardiovascular system in children with congenital heart disease. A complete history should include questions about current physical status, past medical history, and family history (Table 13.2).

The past medical history of cardiac patients should include inquiry as to the type of cardiac defect, surgical repair, or intervention in the cardiac catheterization laboratory; complications and residual defects from the intervention or repair; and the use of medication. In addition, information regarding prior evaluations or restrictions should be elicited.

Current health status history should include questions about (a) presence of chest pain or chest discomfort with exercise; (b) history of syncope or near-syncope; (c) excessive, unexplained or unexpected shortness of breath or fatigue with

TABLE 13.2.   CARDIAC HISTORY
IN CONGENITAL HEART DISEASE

Patient history	Type of cardiac defect
	Repair or intervention
	Chest pain/discomfort with exercise
	Shortness of breath with exercise
	Excessive fatigue
	History of murmur
	Hypertension
	Elevated cholesterol
	Palpitations
	Syncope/near-syncope
Family history	Coronary artery disease in family members
	< 50 years of age
	Hypertension
	Long QT syndrome
	Sudden or early death
	Cardiomyopathy
	Marfan syndrome
	Arrhythmias
	Elevated cholesterol
Social	Tobacco use

exercise; (d) history of a cardiac murmur; (e) history of systemic hypertension or high blood pressure; and (f) presence of palpitations.[17]

Family history of all athletes should be carefully addressed. Questions about cardiac disease in family members less than 50 years old, hypertension, long QT syndrome, deafness, sudden or early deaths, cardiomyopathy, syncope, Marfan syndrome, arrhythmias, and hyperlipidemias should be included. Any of these could be a clue to risk of cardiac complication.

PHYSICAL EXAMINATION

A complete physical examination of the cardiovascular system should include inspection, precordial palpation, auscultation, and percussion. Vital signs should include both arm and leg blood pressure. If patients are cyanotic or have a history of a cyanotic cardiac defect, their oxygen saturation, while breathing room air, should be measured by pulse oximetry.

Inspection should assess color, the presence of clubbing in cyanotic patients, respiratory rate and

effort, and chest wall symmetry. All pulses should be palpated, and the pulses in the upper and lower extremities should be simultaneously palpated to determine if there is any radial-femoral pulse delay. Precordial palpation should assess the location and quality of the apical impulse and the point of maximal impulse, the presence of any heaves or taps which may signify right ventricular hypertrophy, and the presence of any thrills. Auscultation should include the rate and regularity of the rhythm, the normal heart sounds, any extra systolic or diastolic sounds, and the characterization of any murmurs (Table 13.3).

LABORATORY STUDIES

Individuals with known cardiac disease or who have heart disease suspected after history and physical examination may require additional testing prior to sports participation. Findings on the chest x-ray, electrocardiogram (ECG), echocardiogram, exercise test, or cardiac catheterization may be important in making sports-related decisions. These tests are discussed in the sections to follow on specific cardiac defects. Not all patients with suspected heart disease will need testing. In fact, most heart murmurs are found in individuals with a normal heart and do not require more than an examination by an experienced individual who can confidently identify a functional murmur. Testing should be done with specific questions in mind. The practitioner requesting the testing and making the sports participation decision has the responsibility to assure that the crucial questions were answered and that the quality of the examination was adequate. Occasionally, further testing is required to reassure patients or parents that there is no cardiac defect present.

SPECIFIC STUDIES

Chest Radiograph.   The standard chest x-ray is often very useful in evaluating patients following cardiac surgery since this procedure provides information on cardiac size, pulmonary vascularity, and other cardiac or pulmonary abnormalities

TABLE 13.3.   PHYSICAL EXAMINATION

Vital Signs	Inspection	Palpation	Auscultation
Heart rate	Color	Peripheral pulses	Rate and regularity
Respiratory rate	Clubbing	Apical impulse	Heart sounds
Blood pressure (4 extremity)	Respiratory rate and effort	Location and diffuseness	Intensity
Oxygen saturation if cyanotic	Diaphoresis	Point of maximal impulse	Quality
	Chest wall symmetry or deformities	Heave or tap	Gallops
		Thrills	Systolic and diastolic sounds
			Clicks
			Opening snap
			Murmur
			Intensity
			Timing
			Location
			Transmission
			Quality

warranting evaluation prior to determining recommendations regarding exercise.

Electrocardiogram and Holter Monitor.   A 12- or 15-lead ECG provides invaluable information on the predominant rhythm (sinus or other), conduction abnormalities, and chamber hypertrophy or enlargement. Holter monitoring is useful primarily to evaluate symptomatic athletes with possible arrhythmias during their usual daily activities. Patients with certain cardiac repairs may require Holter monitoring due to the increased incidence of arrhythmias associated with the repair, even though they may be asymptomatic.

Exercise Testing.   Exercise testing is useful in children to determine their exercise capacity, evaluation of exercise-related symptoms, and to reassure families and physicians about the safety of exercise in patients after cardiac interventions. The testing protocol should be adapted for children as the normal values for exercise parameters differ in children as compared to adults.[18–20]

Other Studies.   Various other studies, either invasive or noninvasive, may provide information that will assist in making recommendations regarding sports participation. Tests that can be used include nuclear medicine studies for ventric-ular function, cardiac catheterization for anatomic and hemodynamic information, and computed tomography (CT) or magnetic resonance imaging (MRI) to provide anatomic detail of some lesions.

SPORTS DEFINITIONS FOR EXERCISE RECOMMENDATIONS

Sports vary in the amount of workload and stress exerted on the cardiovascular system. During exercise, changes occur in blood flow, blood pressure, body temperature, and peripheral vascular resistance. (This is discussed in Chapter 1.) These changes may have a significant impact on patients with congenital heart disease in their risk for sudden death, life-threatening cardiovascular alterations, and possibly progression of the disease.

In order to make recommendations for sports participation, a discussion concerning the different types of exercise and the classification of sports is necessary. Sports can be classified according to the type and intensity of exercise performed.[1,20] Further division can be made based on the risk of bodily injury from collision or the risk of injury if syncope occurs while participating. These definitions apply to organized athletic participation, are quite restrictive, and, consequently, are less applicable to recreational sports, job-related activities, and rehabilitative exercise.

The classification of physical intensity used by the Bethesda Conferences was made for competitive athletic participation.[1,21] Exercise can also be divided into four broad groupings, including competitive sports (i.e., professional or school athletics), recreational sports, therapeutic exercise, and vocational activities. Competitive exercise is generally organized team or individual sports, which usually require a degree of training and practice. There is often a trainer or a coach overseeing and encouraging further effort by the athlete. Recreational exercise is sports participation for enjoyment or to maintain health. There is minimal regular training or practice involved, and the athlete can stop and rest when needed. However, the athletes themselves may push themselves in both competition and training even though the competition is intended to be minimized. Therapeutic exercise is for recovery from injuries or rehabilitative in nature. Lastly, exercise can be related to vocation.

Exercise can also be classified as either static or dynamic in nature. Dynamic exercise is defined as rhythmic movement, which produces changes in muscle length, joint movement, and develops a relatively small intramuscular force. Static exercise has minimal change in muscle length or joint movement but generates a large intramuscular force. No sport is purely dynamic or purely static in nature and most activities are a combination of dynamic and static components. An example of an activity that is predominantly dynamic with a low static component would be long-distance running. A predominantly static activity is weightlifting, which has a relatively low dynamic component.[1]

Dynamic exercise causes increases in oxygen consumption, cardiac output, heart rate, and stroke volume during the activity. The increase in these measurements during a predominantly dynamic exercise are usually much greater than the same measurements during a predominantly static exercise. Systolic blood pressure increases in both types of exercise, but the diastolic blood pressure decreases with dynamic exercise but may increase during static exercise. Peripheral vascular resistance decreases during dynamic exercise but remains the same throughout static exercise (see Table 13.1).

Table 13.4 shows the American Heart Association classification of sports into different categories by the 26th Bethesda Conference based on the amount of static and dynamic exercise required by the activity. The categories are based on the demands for participation in the actual sporting event and do not take into consideration other variables, such as training. Other variables that can impact the cardiovascular demand during sports participation include the emotional state of the athlete, position played, environmental factors (altitude, temperature, and pollution), and the demands of training for the particular sport. Emotional state may cause significant increases in sympathetic activity resulting in increased catecholamines. Training for a sport often exceeds the demands of the particular sports participation. Such factors must be considered in sports participation recommendations.

COMMON CONGENITAL CARDIAC DEFECTS

A complete discussion of congenital cardiac defects is beyond the scope of this chapter, but more common cardiac defects will be discussed in brief so that recommendations for sports participation can be placed in context.

ATRIAL SEPTAL DEFECTS

Atrial septal defect is a frequent cardiac defect, occurring as an isolated defect in about 5 to 10% of all congenital heart disease. Atrial septal defects are characterized by a direct communication between the right and left atria, allowing blood to shunt from one side to the other, depending on the pressures in each chamber. The size of the defect can vary along with the location in the atrial septum. Depending on location, defects are clas-

TABLE 13.4.   CLASSIFICATION OF SPORTS (BASED ON PEAK ISOTONIC AND ISOMETRIC COMPONENTS DURING COMPETITION)

	Low Isotonic	Moderate Isotonic	High Isotonic
Low isometric	Billiards	Baseball	Badminton
	Bowling	Softball	Cross-country skiing (classic technique)
	Cricket	Table tennis	Field hockey[a]
	Golf	Tennis (doubles)	Race walking
	Riflery	Volleyball	Racquetball
			Running (long distance)
			Soccer[a]
			Squash
			Tennis (singles)
Moderate isometeric	Archery	Fencing	Basketball[a]
	Auto racing[a,b]	Field events (jumping)	Ice hockey[a]
	Diving[a,b]	Figure skating[a]	Cross-country skiing (skating technique)
	Equestrian[a,b]	Football (American)[a]	Football (Australian rules)[a]
	Motorcycling[a,b]	Rodeoing[a,b]	Lacrosse[a]
		Rugby[a]	Running (middle distance)
		Running (sprint)	Swimming
		Surfing[a,b]	Team handball
		Synchronized swimming	
High isometric	Bobsledding[a,b]	Body building[a,b]	Boxing[a]
	Field events (throwing)	Downhill skiing[a,b]	Canoeing/kayaking
	Gymnastics[a,b]	Wrestling[a]	Cycling[a,b]
	Karate/judo[a]		Decathlon
	Sailing		Rowing
	Rock climbing[a,b]		Speed skating
	Waterskiing[a,b]		
	Weightlifting[a,b]		
	Windsurfing[a,b]		

[a] Danger of bodily collision.

[b] Increased risk if syncope occurs.

sified as primum, secundum, sinus venosus, or coronary sinus atrial septal defects.

Atrial septal defects can be divided into small, medium, and large based on size and the amount of shunting across the defect. Small defects do not cause right ventricular dilation, which is secondary to volume overload from left-to-right shunting across the atrial septal defect. Moderate or large atrial septal defects will cause right ventricular volume overload with right ventricular dilation. In the presence of large left-to-right shunts, changes can occur in the pulmonary vasculature leading to elevated pulmonary vascular resistance and pulmonary hypertension. The inci-

dence of elevated pulmonary vascular resistance increases with increasing age of the patient. Other complications associated with atrial septal defects are paradoxical embolism caused by a thrombus from the right side of the heart or venous system crossing the atrial septal defect and embolizing "paradoxically" to the arterial system.

Symptoms associated with atrial septal defect rarely appear in childhood. The majority of patients who develop symptoms related to the atrial septal defect do so in their 20s and 30s, or significantly later. Evander Holyfield, the heavyweight boxer, had a small atrial septal defect discovered incidentally during an evaluation for atrial flutter.

He had trained for many years without symptoms prior to his episode of flutter. Symptoms may include easy fatigue, increased number of respiratory illnesses, and symptoms of congestive heart failure including shortness of breath, paroxysmal nocturnal dyspnea, edema, and pulmonary hypertension. The increased blood flow to the right side of the heart may result in right atrial and right ventricular enlargement. Over time, the increased blood flow may cause changes in the pulmonary arteries leading to development of pulmonary vascular occlusive disease.

Physical examination may reveal a normal first heart sound, a murmur associated with increased blood flow across the pulmonary valve, wide and fixed splitting of the second heart sound, and a tricuspid area diastolic flow rumble. The ECG may show evidence of right ventricular enlargement or right atrial enlargement, but can be normal. A chest radiograph may show mild cardiomegaly from right atrial and right ventricular enlargement, increased pulmonary vascular markings, and a prominent main pulmonary artery if the shunt is large.

Arrhythmias can be associated with atrial septal defects in both the preoperative and postoperative state. The rhythm disturbances are usually of atrial origin and can occur because of dilation of the atria or from sinus node damage resulting from repair of the defect. Atrial arrhythmias are more common in patients whose defect was repaired later in life (> 25 years of age). Patients should be queried about possible tachycardias (palpitations) during their clinic visits and during the preparticipation examination.

Patients who are older than 25 years of age can show decreased working capacity because of pulmonary hypertension. If the pulmonary artery pressures are near normal, however, there should be near-normal working capacity. There is decreased cardiac capacity associated with resting systolic pulmonary artery pressures $\geq$ 50 mmHg or a mean pulmonary artery pressure of $\geq$ 30 mmHg. Cardiac work capacity is also decreased with a pulmonary artery resistance of $\geq$ 3 Wood units. Exercise capacity may also be limited with large left-to-right shunts despite normal pulmonary vascular resistance.[22–32] Patients may also have a decreased work capacity secondary to inactivity.

Postoperatively, adult patients show a minimal increase in work capacity after surgical closure compared to their preoperative work capacity. Children have normal work capacity following surgical repair. Late repairs have a higher incidence of residual hemodynamic abnormalities than do early repairs. There is a decreased heart rate response at various levels of exercise and an increased systolic blood pressure present at peak exercise in some adult patients.

Current recommendations for treatment of atrial septal defects are for closure sometime during childhood to prevent development of right ventricular failure from pulmonary hypertension later in life and to eliminate the risk of paradoxical embolism. Atrial septal defects can be closed by open heart surgery or by transcatheter procedures.

Following repair of a secundum atrial septal defect, 18% of adults will have atrial flutter and 39% may develop sinus node dysfunction. After sinus venosus atrial septal defect repair, 60 to 70% of patients will have atrial arrhythmias and approximately 50% will have sinus node dysfunction. Exercise-induced arrhythmias are rare, and most arrhythmias classically associated with atrial septal defects are well-tolerated and not life-threatening.

There is no evidence that sports participation causes more rapid progression of the disease process in patients with atrial septal defect. Patients with small atrial septal defects and without pulmonary hypertension can participate in all sports. If pulmonary hypertension or a right-to-left shunt at the atrial septal defect is present, patients should be restricted to low intensity sports only (Class IA). If there is markedly elevated right side of the heart pressures, patients should not participate in competitive sports.[1–3] (See pulmonary hypertension guidelines.)

Evaluation of athletes after closure of an atrial septal defect should include history, physical ex-

TABLE 13.5. GENERAL GUIDELINES FOR EXERCISE PARTICIPATION IN POSTOPERATIVE CONGENITAL HEART DISEASE

1. No sports participation for 6 months after surgery.
2. No sports with a risk of collision for patients on anticoagulants.
3. Patients with arrhythmias should be restricted by the underlying heart disease in addition to the arrhythmia restrictions.
4. Congenital heart disease patients are in general at low risk for sudden cardiac death with exercise.
5. No sports with risk of collision if pacemaker or implanted defibrillator.

amination, chest x-ray, and ECG. Care should be taken to ask about the possibility of arrhythmias (palpitations, heart racing, syncope, or presyncope). If cardiomegaly is present on chest x-ray, evaluation with an echocardiogram should be considered to evaluate for residual shunting and to estimate right ventricular pressure. In patients with a history of pulmonary hypertension, an echocardiogram should be performed to assess right ventricular and pulmonary artery pressures and cardiac catheterization should be considered to determine pulmonary vascular resistance.[1–3]

Following surgical or percutaneous closure of the atrial septal defect, patients should not participate in competitive sports for 6 months. If after 6 months there is no evidence of pulmonary hypertension, symptomatic arrhythmias, or myocardial

dysfunction, athletes may participate in all sports.[1] (See Tables 13.5 and 13.6.)

VENTRICULAR SEPTAL DEFECTS

Ventricular septal defect is the most common congenital heart defect, accounting for 15 to 20% of all congenital heart disease. A ventricular septal defect is a direct communication between the right and left ventricles of the heart. Blood usually shunts from the higher pressure left ventricle to the lower pressure right ventricle. Symptoms and findings on physical examination are related to the amount of blood shunting across the defect. A small ventricular septal defect may have a loud cardiac murmur on examination but rarely produces symptoms or cardiac chamber enlargement. Moderate or large ventricular septal defects allow a large volume of blood to flow from the left ventricle to the right ventricle, producing dilation of the left ventricle and left atrium from the increased pulmonary venous return.

Ventricular septal defects also vary in location and may require closure because of potential effects on the aortic valve, rather than because of the degree of shunting. Small ventricular septal defects diagnosed in infancy may close spontaneously or have no hemodynamic significance and therefore require no intervention. Those defects still present by the time a child reaches school age are unlikely to close spontaneously.

TABLE 13.6. ATRIAL SEPTAL DEFECT EXERCISE RECOMMENDATIONS

	Size	Signs/Symptoms	Sports
Preoperative	Small	Asymptomatic No pulmonary hypertension	All
	Moderate/Large	Symptomatic Right-to-left shunt Pulmonary hypertension	IA
		Markedly elevated pulmonary artery pressure	None
Postoperative	No significant residual defect	Asymptomatic No arrhythmias No pulmonary hypertension Normal ventricular function ≥ 6 Months after repair	All

Symptoms associated with ventricular septal defects are secondary to the increased amount of pulmonary blood flow and include tachypnea, poor weight gain, and congestive heart failure. In larger defects, the increased blood flow may lead to development of elevated pulmonary vascular resistance and a subsequent decrease in the amount of shunting. In school-aged children, there rarely are symptoms related to the ventricular septal defect. Symptomatic ventricular septal defects are commonly closed in infancy or early childhood.

Physical examination reveals a holosystolic murmur along the left sternal border. Larger ventricular septal defects may have an increased precordial impulse and a palpable thrill associated with the murmur. With increased ventricular septal defect size and flow, a diastolic flow rumble across the mitral valve may also be present.

Findings on ECG and chest radiograph are nonspecific. The ECG may show left ventricular hypertrophy or possibly biventricular hypertrophy in larger defects. The chest radiograph can show cardiomegaly with increased pulmonary vascular markings, and there may be a left ventricular contour to the heart.

Small ventricular septal defects have no hemodynamic significance and there is at least one National Football League linebacker who competes despite a small ventricular septal defect. Patients with small ventricular septal defects have no symptoms, are acyanotic, have no exercise intolerance, and grow normally. If patients have normal heart size and normal pulmonary artery pressure and no signs or symptoms of pulmonary edema, no further evaluation is needed and they may participate in all sports. Most patients with a ventricular septal defect will likely have had an evaluation performed by a pediatric cardiologist in the past and the size of the defect determined. If a pediatric cardiologist has not evaluated the athlete in the last 3 to 5 years, referral to such a specialist before sports participation is appropriate. Although the ventricular septal defect does not enlarge over time, subtle aortic insufficiency may develop if the defect is near the aortic valve.

Moderate or large defects require the same evaluation as small defects, but might need an echocardiogram to assess size of the defect and to estimate right ventricular pressure. If differentiation between a moderate or large defect cannot be made by noninvasive studies, cardiac catheterization may be necessary to evaluate the cardiac pressures and pulmonary vascular resistance. Patients with moderate-sized defects, without pulmonary hypertension, may participate in all sports; those with large defects may participate in low intensity competitive sports (Class IA). Moderate and large defects should be referred for surgical closure if the pulmonary vascular resistance is low. If elevated pulmonary pressures are present, patients should be restricted according to the guidelines for the pulmonary hypertension. [See section, "Elevated Pulmonary Resistance (Pulmonary Hypertension)".] In reality, most ventricular septal defects will have been treated surgically well before the age when children become active in sports.[1–3]

Postoperatively, these patients may have residual defects (up to 20% in old reports), arrhythmias, decreased ventricular function (rare), right bundle branch block, or residual pulmonary hypertension if pulmonary hypertension was present prior to repair. Many postoperative complications are hemodynamically or clinically insignificant and would not restrict participation. Right bundle branch block is rarely of any clinical significance unless there is progression to complete heart block with exercise. Surgical closure of a ventricular septal defect is now usually performed via an atrial approach across the tricuspid valve, with closure performed from the right ventricular side of the septum. In the past, closures were performed through a ventriculotomy through the right or left ventricle resulting in impaired ventricular function over time. Serious postoperative arrhythmias are rare following ventricular septal defect closure.[26,27,29,33,34]

Patients are considered to have a successful ventricular septal defect repair if there are no symptoms, no cardiomegaly on chest x-ray, no arrhythmias, and normal pulmonary artery pressures.

Small residual defects are usually of no concern other than that they require subacute bacterial endocarditis (SBE) prophylaxis in accordance with American Heart Association Guidelines.

Echocardiogram may be useful after surgery in selected circumstances to evaluate right-sided pressures, to assess residual defects, and to evaluate ventricular function. If the evaluation reveals cardiomegaly, myocardial dysfunction, or the presence of possible pulmonary artery hypertension, further quantitative assessment is necessary. An exercise treadmill test and a cardiac catheterization may be required to determine recommendations for sports participation (Table 13.7).

Some patients (3–14%) develop late postoperative abnormalities including mild mitral regurgitation, subaortic stenosis, and aortic regurgitation. Pulmonary hypertension rarely occurs if the defect is repaired by the teenage years. Left ventricular shortening fraction by echocardiogram is normal in 61% and is increased in 17% of patients. The left ventricular end-diastolic dimension is normal in 86% of patients, whereas 10% will have left ventricular enlargement. Those patients with decreased shortening fractions have abnormal septal wall motion. Arrhythmias following surgical closure of ventricular septal defects are rare. Electrocardiograms were normal in 51%: 93% had normal sinus rhythm, 5% had an atrial rhythm, 32% had right bundle branch block pattern, and 2% had surgical atrioventricular block requiring a pacemaker. Late mortality after repair was about 2%. Greater than 80% of patients will have a normal exercise tolerance following surgical closure of a ventricular septal defect.[33,34]

Athletes should not participate in athletics for 6 months after surgical repair. After 6 months, those patients with no or small residual ventricular septal defect, no symptoms, no evidence of pulmonary hypertension, no arrhythmia, and normal cardiac function may participate in all sports. If there is a moderate-sized residual defect, participation in low intensity sports may be allowed. If pulmonary hypertension is present, the patient should not participate in sports [see section, "Elevated Pulmonary Resistance (Pulmonary Hypertension)"]. It is rarely necessary to restrict patients with a repaired ventricular septal defect from any recreational or vocational activity unless pulmonary hypertension is present.

PATENT DUCTUS ARTERIOSUS

Patent ductus arteriosus accounts for 5 to 10% of all congenital heart disease in full-term infants and occurs as an isolated defect in 1 in 2500 to 5000 live births. The ductus arteriosus is a normal connection between the pulmonary artery and the aorta in the fetus that allows blood to bypass the lungs in the fetal circulation. The ductus arteriosus usually closes within several hours after birth

TABLE 13.7.   VENTRICULAR SEPTAL DEFECT EXERCISE RECOMMENDATIONS

	Size	Signs/Symptoms	Sports
Preoperative	Small	Asymptomatic	All
	Moderate/large	No pulmonary hypertension	All
		Pulmonary hypertension (mild)	IA
Postoperative	No residual defect or only small residual defect	Asymptomatic Normal ventricular function No pulmonary hypertension No arrhythmias ≥ 6 Months after repair	All
	Moderate/large		IA

when exposed to increased oxygen and expansion of the lungs. If a ductus arteriosus remains patent, there is usually left-to-right shunting of blood from the aorta to the pulmonary artery. This increased blood flow to the lungs can lead to left atrial and left ventricular dilation from the increased pulmonary venous return to the left side of the heart. With the increased blood flow to the pulmonary arteries, patients may develop pulmonary vascular disease. Also, in the presence of a patent ductus arteriosus there is an increased risk for infective endocarditis occurring at the ductus. Patients with patent ductus arteriosus undergo closure to eliminate the lifetime risk of infective endocarditis.

There is no typical history for a patent ductus arteriosus. Physical examination will usually show a widened pulse pressure and prominent carotid arterial pulsations. There is a continuous, machinery-like murmur heard best at the left upper sternal border. The ECG is usually normal, but may show left ventricular hypertrophy in the presence of a moderate-to-large shunt. The chest x-ray varies with the amount of left-to-right shunting. With increased shunting there is increased pulmonary vascular markings and possibly a double density from an enlarged left atrium.

Patent ductus arteriosus patients are rarely symptomatic when the ductus is small. A large shunt patent ductus arteriosus may cause signs and symptoms of congestive heart failure and lead to pulmonary vascular occlusive disease and pulmonary hypertension. A small patent ductus arteriosus will have a characteristic continuous murmur with normal heart size on chest radiograph and no chamber enlargement on echocardiogram.

Postoperative complications from patent ductus arteriosus repair are rare. A residual patent ductus arteriosus, which is usually clinically insignificant, damage to the recurrent laryngeal nerve or the phrenic nerve, and persistence of elevated pulmonary artery pressure can occur.

Patients with a small patent ductus arteriosus can participate in all sports. Patients with a moderate or large patent ductus arteriosus generally have ventricular enlargement and should have the patent ductus arteriosus closed. Patients with pulmonary hypertension should be restricted from sports participation. [See "Elevated Pulmonary Resistance (Pulmonary Hypertension)."]

Athletes with no evidence of pulmonary hypertension or cardiac enlargement following closure of the patent ductus arteriosus may participate in all sports. Patients should wait approximately 3 months after surgical correction or 1 month after interventional cardiac catheterization before competing. If residual pulmonary hypertension is present, patients should be restricted as discussed in "Elevated Pulmonary Resistance (Pulmonary Hypertension)" (Table 13.8). Similarly, patients with a closed patent ductus arteriosus and no pulmonary hypertension do not need to be restricted in their recreational or occupational activities unless pulmonary hypertension is present.

TABLE 13.8.   PATENT DUCTUS ARTERIOSUS EXERCISE RECOMMENDATIONS

	Size	Signs/Symptoms	Sports
Preoperative	Small	None	All
	Moderate/large	Ventricular enlargement Pulmonary hypertension (mild)	IA
Postoperative	No significant residual shunting	≥ 3 Months from surgery ≥ 1 Month from cardiac catheterization No pulmonary hypertension No chamber enlargement	All

COARCTATION OF THE AORTA

Coarctation of the aorta is a narrowing of the aorta at the level of the juxtaductal or juxtaligamental area, which is located between the distal transverse aortic arch and the proximal descending thoracic aorta. It occurs as an isolated defect in 8 to 10% of all congenital heart disease. Elevated blood pressure occurs in the arms with a lower blood pressure in the legs. In neonates, the transverse aortic arch may be hypoplastic and contribute to the obstruction. Patients with successful coarctation repair have participated in competitive sports including one nationally ranked gymnast, Chris Waller. Indeed, since coarctation patients often have a reduced development of the lower limbs, coarctation may actually confer a slight competitive advantage in sports such as gymnastics where a lengthened lower body segment is a disadvantage. Mr. Waller was the 1992 U.S. Men's National Champion on the pommel horse.

Normally, the blood pressure in the lower extremities is 10 to 20 mmHg higher than it is in the upper extremities due to amplification of the pulse wave as it travels toward the periphery. The arm-to-leg blood pressure gradient, a focused physical examination, exercise testing, and echocardiogram can assess severity of the coarctation. Coarctation patients may require restriction of their activity because of the elevation of blood pressure that occurs with exercise.

Patients with coarctation may present during infancy with left ventricular decompensation from pressure overload as the ductus arteriosus closes and the ventricle faces elevated peripheral resistance from the coarctation. Most cases present after infancy with a murmur or hypertension. Patients who present after infancy rarely have symptoms related to the coarctation, but may complain of nonspecific symptoms such as cold feet and leg cramps, nosebleeds, or headaches.

Physical examination reveals a discrepancy between the upper and lower extremity pulses and an arm-to-leg blood pressure difference. Patients may also be hypertensive. A murmur from collaterals may be present that is continuous in nature

and is maximal in the left infraclavicular area. The ECG is often normal, but may demonstrate left ventricular hypertrophy. The chest radiograph usually demonstrates a normal heart size with normal pulmonary vascular markings. A dilated ascending aorta visible to the right of the sternum may be present. Rib notching may be seen on chest x-ray in individuals greater than 5 years of age with uncorrected coarctation of the aorta, if there are large collateral vessels in the anterior chest wall. Prior to surgical repair, patients may have elevated blood pressures in the arms at rest. Exercise duration during exercise testing can be decreased and the systolic blood pressure response, at all stages of exercise, is usually significantly increased.

Postoperatively, patients often have residual systemic hypertension at rest and during exercise. Patients who are normotensive after repair are at increased risk to develop systemic hypertension later in life. This persistent hypertension has several potential causes including increased vascular resistance from changes in the vessels proximal to the coarctation site; transverse aortic arch gradients caused by residual obstruction or poor growth of this segment; increased arterial stiffness; or persistently increased left ventricular contractility after the repair. During exercise testing patients may develop an arm-to-leg blood pressure difference even if no gradient is present at rest. Indeed, approximately 8 to 20% of patients have a significant gradient evidenced only by exercise testing.[35–42]

Correction of the coarctation is performed either percutaneously in the cardiac catheterization laboratory or surgically. The usual surgical repair involves end-to-end anastomosis of the aorta after removal of the area of coarctation. Other types of repairs include a subclavian flap repair or patch angioplasty of the coarctation segment. In the presence of a hypoplastic transverse aortic arch, the descending aorta may be mobilized and anastomosed to the underside of the aortic arch relieving any transverse aortic arch narrowing. Repair is usually considered adequate if there is less than a 20 mmHg residual gradient between the upper and lower extremity blood pressures. Most patients will have repair performed during childhood with more patients having coarctation repair earlier in infancy or the first year of life. It is unknown how this earlier repair will affect the subsequent clinical course.

Problems following repair include residual stenosis, ventricular hypertrophy, systemic hypertension, and residual obstruction only evident with exercise. Neonates reportedly have a 15 to 20% rate of recoarctation and approximately 5% of older patients will develop a recoarctation after surgical repair.

Preoperative patients with mild coarctation may participate in all sports if they do not have collateral vessels or severe aortic root dilation, their exercise performance is normal, and they have less than a 20 mmHg difference between the upper and lower extremities and a peak systolic blood pressure of ≤ 230 mmHg during exercise. If the arm-to-leg gradient is > 20 mmHg or the peak blood pressure is > 230 mmHg during exercise, the athlete should engage only in low physical intensity (Class IA) sports until the coarctation is treated[1-3] (Table 13.9).

Evaluation after repair should include a history and physical examination, blood pressures in all 4 extremities, a chest radiograph, ECG, exercise study, and echocardiographic evaluation of left ventricular function. Patients with residual gradients of > 20 mmHg, decreased ventricular function, or exercise-induced hypertension should be restricted to low physical intensity (Class IA) sports. Athletes should be restricted from high intensity static exercises (Classes IIIA, IIIB, and IIIC) and sports with danger of collision during the first year after surgery. If after a year, athletes remain asymptomatic and without hypertension or an arm-to-leg pressure gradient > 20 mm Hg, they can participate in all sports except power lifting.[1-3] (Table 13.9)

Recommendations for participation in recreational activity are similar to those for competitive athletics. The evaluation should also include an exercise test to evaluate for hypertension with exercise. Vocations that have a high static component such as heavy lifting should be discouraged.

If significant aortic dilation, aortic wall thinning, or aneurysm formation is present, the athlete should be restricted to Class IA activities. Athletes

TABLE 13.9.   COARCTATION OF THE AORTA EXERCISE RECOMMENDATIONS

	Degree of Coarctation	Signs/Symptoms	Sports
Preoperative	Mild (≤ 20 mmHg)	Normal blood pressure Systolic blood pressure with exercise ≤ 230 mmHg No aneurysm No large collateral vessels	All
	Moderate (> 20 mmHg)	Hypertension Systolic blood pressure with exercise > 230 mmHg Aneurysm or aortic wall thinning	IA
Postoperative	≤ 20 mmHg residual gradient	≥ 6 Months after treatment Normal blood pressure at rest Systolic blood pressure with exercise ≤ 230 mmHg ≥ 12 Months after treatment Asymptomatic Normal blood pressure at rest and exercise	No high static sports (IIIB, IIIC) All except power lifting
	> 20 mmHg residual gradient	Aortic root dilation Aortic wall thinning Aneurysm	IA

with coarctation repair who were markedly hypertensive or had repair in adolescence or later should have cranial magnetic resonance angiography to rule out an aneurysm of the circle of Willis prior to isometric sports or training.

TETRALOGY OF FALLOT

Tetralogy of Fallot is defined by 4 abnormalities: a large nonrestrictive ventricular septal defect, aortic override of the ventricular septal defect, infundibular pulmonic stenosis, and right ventricular hypertrophy. Tetralogy of Fallot occurs in about 6% of all congenital heart disease and is the most common form of cyanotic cardiac disease. Symptoms in tetralogy of Fallot vary with the degree of pulmonary stenosis and range from severe hypoxemia to no symptoms. The degree of infundibular stenosis influences hypoxemia and symptoms because it largely determines the amount of shunting of "blue" blood from the right ventricle to the left ventricle across the ventricular septal defect. Patients may have episodic hypoxic or cyanotic spells, also called "Tet" spells, that occur prior to complete repair. Patients often learn to self-manage these hypoxemic episodes by squatting, which increases systemic vascular resistance, increases left side of the heart pressures, and reduces the right-to-left shunting across the ventricular septal defect.

Physical examination reveals a systolic crescendo-decrescendo murmur from the pulmonary stenosis. The second heart sound is usually single. The ECG characteristically shows right axis deviation and right ventricular hypertrophy. Radiography of the chest classically reveals a normal heart size but a boot-shaped heart or *coeur en sabot* shape to the cardiac silhouette. A right aortic arch is present in 25% of patients.

Some patients with tetralogy of Fallot require placement of an aorta-to-pulmonary artery shunt during infancy to provide adequate pulmonary blood flow. Complete repair of this defect is usually performed in the first year of life. Some older patients may have been palliated with a surgical shunt alone and are not completely repaired.

Palliated patients will typically remain cyanotic to some degree and may have developed pulmonary hypertension, depending on the type of shunt placed. Exercise recommendations for these patients are those for palliated cyanotic lesions. (See section on "Specific Surgical Reports—Unoperated or Palliated Cyanotic Heart Disease.")

Repair of tetralogy of Fallot includes closure of the ventricular septal defect and opening up of the right ventricular outflow tract. The latter often requires a transannular pulmonary incision and placement of a pericardial patch on the right ventricular outflow tract. In addition, there is commonly a need to augment the main and branch pulmonary arteries by placing patch material in these locations as well. The patch on the outflow tract crosses the pulmonary valve annulus and usually no valve is inserted at the time of repair, resulting in pulmonary insufficiency in patients undergoing complete repair. Postoperative complications include residual ventricular septal defect, residual right ventricular outflow tract obstruction, pulmonary artery stenosis, arrhythmias of either atrial or ventricular origin, conduction problems, most commonly right bundle branch block and rarely complete atrioventricular block, and ventricular dysfunction.

Tetralogy of Fallot patients show impaired exercise responses, especially if only surgical palliation was performed. Palliated patients hyperventilate at rest, and there is an increased ventilatory response with exercise. Following intracardiac repair, 80 to 85% of patients have a normal working capacity with exercise testing. Decreased exercise capacity is related to the degree of pulmonary insufficiency and the presence of abnormal right ventricular function. Patients with severe pulmonary insufficiency will often show an increase in exercise capacity following placement of a valve conduit in the right ventricular outflow tract. The heart rate response to exercise is decreased at maximal and submaximal levels of exercise and may be secondary to sinus node dysfunction. After complete repair, the cardiac output is normal at rest and may be normal in response to exercise.[29,35,43–50]

Patients with mild pulmonary insufficiency and mild residual right ventricular outflow tract obstruction have no functional limitations. Ventricular arrhythmias occur in up to 73% of patients after repair in some studies and are related to the outcome of surgery and the length of time since the repair. Supraventricular tachycardia occurs in up to 34% of patients.[51–53]

Evaluation of the athlete following repair of tetralogy of Fallot includes a history and physical examination, ECG, chest radiograph, and exercise testing. In contrast to most other postrepair congenital heart disease groups, a Holter monitor should be obtained because cardiac arrhythmias are frequent after tetralogy of Fallot repair. Most patients with minimal or no residual stenosis and only mild or moderate pulmonary insufficiency will be asymptomatic.

Further investigation may be necessary in those patients with cardiomegaly on chest x-ray, residual stenosis, residual ventricular septal defect, or with history of arrhythmia. This includes echocardiography or cardiac catheterization. Patients with normal or near-normal right side of the heart pressures, only mild right ventricular volume overload, no residual shunt, and no arrhythmia may participate in all competitive sports. Patients with marked pulmonary regurgitation, right ventricular pressure ≥ 50% systemic, or rhythm abnormalities should be restricted to low physical intensity (Class IA) activities only[1–3] (Table 13.10).

Patients with good surgical results can participate in recreational sports and vocations requiring intense exertion. Those with significant residual defects need to be limited. Residual pulmonary gradients in the mild range of < 40 mmHg and without symptoms may participate fully in all sports. Small residual ventricular septal defects do not necessitate restriction of activities. If ventricular function is mildly depressed, participation in static exercise activities should be restricted to low intensity static exercises only (Classes IA, IB, and IC).[1–3]

Continued follow-up by a cardiologist experienced in congenital heart disease is recommended for all patients after tetralogy of Fallot repair.

UNCOMMON CONGENITAL CARDIAC DEFECTS

ATRIOVENTRICULAR SEPTAL DEFECT

A complete atrioventricular (AV) septal defect (also known as an AV canal defect) is character-

TABLE 13.10.   TETRALOGY OF FALLOT EXERCISE RECOMMENDATIONS

	Signs/Symptoms	Sports
Preoperative or palliated	Oxygen saturation > 80% with exercise No arrhythmia No symptomatic ventricular dysfunction Near-normal working capacity on exercise testing	IA
Postoperative	Asymptomatic Only mild right ventricular volume overload Normal or near-normal right side of the heart pressure No significant shunt No arrhythmia on Holter or exercise testing	All
	Marked pulmonary regurgitation Right ventricular pressure ≥ 50% systemic Arrhythmias More than mild right ventricular volume overload	IA

ized by the presence of a primum atrial septal defect, an inlet ventricular septal defect, and a common (single) AV valve. This is a form of endocardial cushion defect, which is the embryologic term. There are also various intermediate forms of AV canal defects, which can involve only a cleft in one AV valve and/or the presence of a primum atrial septal defect. Atrioventricular septal defects are uncommon, accounting for approximately 2% of all congenital heart disease. Thirty percent of AV septal defect patients also have Down syndrome (Trisomy 21). In Down syndrome, endocardial cushion defects account for about 40% of the cardiac defects seen.

Patients with complete AV canal defects usually have signs and symptoms of congestive heart failure in early childhood. They have a history of retarded growth and repeated respiratory infections. Physical examination shows tachycardia and tachypnea. The precordium is hyperactive, and the heart sounds are accentuated. There may be a systolic murmur associated with AV valve regurgitation. Signs of congestive heart failure including hepatomegaly and a gallop rhythm are often present. The chest x-ray shows cardiomegaly with increased pulmonary vascular markings. The ECG usually demonstrates a superiorly oriented QRS frontal plane axis with a counterclockwise depolarization pattern, first-degree AV block, and right ventricular hypertrophy. Partial AV canal defects usually have clinical findings similar to other atrial septal defects but ECG findings will be similar to complete AV canal defects.

Patients with complete AV septal defects usually have surgical repair between 3 and 8 months of age. The operation involves closure of the primum atrial septal defect and inlet ventricular septal defect and reconstruction of the AV valves. Without surgery, these patients tend to develop early pulmonary vascular disease and pulmonary hypertension related to the increased blood flow. Unrepaired patients older than 2–3 years of age may have findings of pulmonary hypertension on physical examination.

Surgical repair of the defect requires closure of both the atrial septal defect and the ventricular

septal defect along with valvuloplasty of the AV valve in order to make 2 valves out of 1. The success of surgery depends on the degree of pulmonary artery hypertension present and the amount of left-sided AV valve (mitral valve) regurgitation. Postoperatively, approximately 10% of patients have AV valve regurgitation (mitral regurgitation). They can also have pulmonary artery hypertension, decreased ventricular function, and a residual ventricular septal defect. Atrial arrhythmias may develop postoperatively.

Recommendations for exercise are similar to those for patients after atrial septal defect and ventricular septal defect repair. Additionally, the amount of AV valve regurgitation is an important issue. Most patients should be restricted to Class IA activities if significant mitral regurgitation is present. Activities that increase the systemic arterial blood pressure and peripheral vascular resistance increase the left ventricular afterload and may increase the amount of mitral regurgitation. The increased afterload may also stress the AV valve repair. Repetitive increases in left ventricular afterload may over time cause progression of the AV valve regurgitation and produce deterioration in cardiac function[1–3] (Table 13.11).

If mitral regurgitation is not present, low and moderate static and low and moderate dynamic exercise (Classes IA, IB, IIA, and IIB) is permissible. If left ventricular enlargement or dysfunction is present, patients should be restricted from sports. Recreational sports may also require activity restriction based on the amount of mitral regurgitation and left ventricular dysfunction present.

Patients with complete AV canal defects require follow-up by a pediatric cardiologist or by an adult cardiologist with training or experience with congenital heart disease in adults.

TRANSPOSITION OF THE GREAT ARTERIES

Transposition of the great arteries occurs in about 5% of all patients with congenital heart disease. In this defect, the aorta (along with the coronary arteries), which should arise posteriorly, arises

TABLE 13.11.   ATRIOVENTRICULAR SEPTAL DEFECT EXERCISE RECOMMENDATIONS

Residual Defects	Signs/Symptoms	Sports
No significant atrial septal defect	≥ 6 Months after repair	IA
No significant ventricular septal defect	Asymptomatic	With selected patients IB, IIA, IIB
No mitral regurgitation	No arrhythmias	Avoid sports with risk of bodily collision
	No pulmonary hypertension	
	Normal ventricular function	
Mitral regurgitation		IA
Left ventricular dysfunction		None

anteriorly from the right ventricle, and the pulmonary artery which should arise anteriorly, arises posteriorly from the left ventricle, giving parallel circuits instead of circulation in series. A ventricular septal defect is present in 30 to 40% of patients and may be located anywhere in the ventricular septum. Patients with transposition of the great arteries are usually extremely cyanotic during infancy and have had surgery early in life with either baffling in the atria (Mustard or Senning procedure) or an arterial switch operation.

The arterial switch operation is most commonly used at present. Surgery involves transecting the great vessels (aorta and pulmonary artery) above the valve annulus and anastomosing them to the proximal end of the other great artery. The coronary arteries must also be transferred as a separate part of the procedure involving taking a button of tissue around the coronary ostia and then anastomosing the coronary to the aorta now repositioned over the left ventricle. There is a risk that the coronaries can be kinked or become stenotic after reimplantation. Coronary stenosis may occur as a long-term complication and appears to occur more frequently when the pattern of the coronary arteries is complicated or if there is an associated single coronary. Other postoperative complications include narrowing of the pulmonary artery at the anastomotic site in 5 to 10% of patients, complete heart block in 5 to 10%, and aortic regurgitation as a late development in up to 20% of patients.

Patients who have had an atrial baffle procedure continue to use the anatomic right ventricle as the systemic ventricle. The pulmonary venous drainage is baffled to the systemic right ventricle and the systemic venous drainage to the left ventricle. This allows "blue" blood to be pumped out the pulmonary artery by the left ventricle and the "red" blood out the aorta by the right ventricle. Complications associated with these procedures include baffle obstruction; dilation and poor function of the right ventricle; pulmonary stenosis or pulmonary hypertension; tricuspid insufficiency (which is the systemic AV valve); and significant atrial or ventricular arrhythmias. The functional reserve and durability of the right ventricle is intrinsically less than that of the left ventricle. Changes resulting from exercise in a systemic right ventricle, which must support peripheral blood flow and pressure, are unknown. Changes in the left ventricle with exercise training include increased mass of the ventricle and enlargement of the chamber for an increased stroke volume. It is not known if similar changes occur in the right ventricle functioning as the systemic ventricle in patients who have had atrial baffle repair. It is possible that enlargement of the systemic right ventricle by participating in exercise may provoke or worsen tricuspid valve regurgitation, leading to decreased ventricular function.

Patients with atrial baffle procedures often are asymptomatic when performing usual levels of activity. These individuals generally lead normal lives and participate in school or have jobs.

Nevertheless, more than one-half of these patients will have important abnormalities present with exercise testing. They demonstrate a decreased cardiac output and decreased exercise performance secondary to limited stroke volume and a blunted heart rate response. They also fatigue sooner than control subjects. Work performance is approximately 72% of normal and maximal heart rate is 86% of normal. Approximately 70% have a low resting heart rate. Sinus rhythm is present in 77% of patients with an atrial baffle at 5 years and 40% at 20 years after repair. The systemic ventricular function is abnormal in 60% of patients, and 84% will have an abnormal right (systemic) ventricular ejection fraction. Baffle obstruction occurs in 10 to 20% of patients, with pulmonary venous obstruction in approximately 5%.[54–62]

Athletic evaluation of the patient with transposition of the great arteries and an atrial baffle procedure (Mustard or Senning) should include a history and physical examination, chest radiograph, ECG, echocardiogram, Holter monitor, and exercise testing. Cardiac catheterization may be necessary if there is ventricular dysfunction,

evidence of baffle obstruction, or other hemodynamic problems that cannot be fully evaluated noninvasively.

Patients with normal heart size on chest x-ray, no history of atrial or ventricular arrhythmias, no history of syncope, and a normal exercise test may participate in low and moderate intensity (Classes IA and IIA) sports. Patients with atrial flutter should not participate in sports for at least 6 months after the last episode of flutter. Those with a sinus bradycardia may participate in low and moderate intensity (Classes IA or IIA) sports if there is an appropriate heart rate response to exercise. If a pacemaker is needed, the patients should not engage in sports where collision and trauma to the pacing system is a possibility (Table 13.12).

Patients who have undergone an arterial switch operation appear to have a lower incidence of ventricular dysfunction, symptomatic arrhythmias, and hemodynamic sequela than do those patients with defects repaired with either a Mustard or Senning (atrial baffle) procedure. Following an arterial switch, patients may develop stenosis at the anastomotic site of both the

TABLE 13.12.   TRANSPOSITION OF THE GREAT ARTERIES EXERCISE RECOMMENDATIONS

Operation	Signs/Symptoms	Sports
Atrial switch (Mustard or Senning)	≥ 6 Months after repair No significant cardiac enlargement No atrial flutter or ventricular arrhythmia No syncope Normal exercise test	IA, IIA
Arterial switch operation	≥ 6 Months after repair Normal heart size No residual defects Normal ventricular function Normal exercise test No arrhythmias Asymptomatic	All except high static sports (IIIA, IIIB, IIIC)
	≥ 6 Months after repair More than mild residual defects Ventricular dysfunction Normal exercise test Asymptomatic	IA, IB, IC, IIA

aorta and pulmonary arteries. There is concern over the long-term effects of sports, especially those with a high static component, and the effect that this will have on the neoaortic or systemic valve (previously the pulmonic valve). Sports with a high static component may place increased stress on the aortic valve, leading to, or causing more rapid progression of aortic regurgitation and ultimately requiring valve replacement. Long-term function of the pulmonary valve as the systemic valve is unknown.[63-65]

Patients should have a history, physical examination, chest radiograph, ECG, Holter monitor, echocardiogram, and exercise testing performed as part of the evaluation. Patients with a normal heart size, no residual defects, normal ventricular function, no arrhythmias, and normal exercise testing may participate in all sports except those with a high static component (Classes IIIA, IIIB, and IIIC). If there are only minor hemodynamic abnormalities or ventricular dysfunction, patients should be restricted to Class IA, IB, IC, and IIA sports (Table 13.12).

Occupations requiring heavy lifting or with a high static component should be discouraged. Recreational activities may not require as much restriction or as much evaluation, but patients should be cautioned against weightlifting and other exercises with high static load since such exertion could theoretically lead to early onset, or worsening of, aortic regurgitation.

SINGLE VENTRICLE (AND THE FONTAN OPERATION)

Patients with a single ventricle vary according to their underlying cardiac defect, including hypoplastic left side of the heart syndrome, tricuspid atresia, pulmonary atresia with intact ventricular septum, and indeterminate single ventricle. Older patients, in their late teens or older, may have had either a palliative shunt procedure to provide adequate pulmonary blood flow or more recently undergone the Fontan procedure, which creates a complete cavopulmonary anastomosis. Typical palliative shunt procedures include anas-

tomosis of the aorta to the pulmonary arteries (Waterston or Potts shunts), anastomosis of the subclavian or brachiocephalic artery to the pulmonary artery (Blalock-Taussig shunt), or anastomosis of the superior vena cava to the right pulmonary artery (Glenn shunt). Emphasis of surgery now is a staged approach to reaching a Fontan at completion. This typically takes 2 to 3 cardiac surgeries to achieve.

The Fontan procedure attempts to separate the blue blood from the red blood by a combination of prior surgeries. This is accomplished by attaching the superior vena cava to the right pulmonary artery and baffling the inferior vena cava to the pulmonary arteries. This procedure shunts venous blood directly to the pulmonary arteries thereby bypassing the heart. Oxygenated blood returns to the heart via pulmonary veins and is pumped by the single ventricle to the body. There is no right-sided pump following the Fontan operation. A fenestration may be made in the baffle, allowing blood to shunt from the venous circuit to the systemic circuit (right-to-left shunt).

The exercise tolerance of patients with single ventricles is decreased compared to patients with structurally normal hearts. Right-to-left intracardiac shunting and chronotropic insufficiency contributes to the decreased exercise tolerance. Exercise requiring high static loads may also be poorly tolerated because of the anatomy of the underlying ventricle, especially when the ventricle has right ventricular morphology or is of indeterminate morphology. Patients with a right ventricle Fontan appear to have a fixed stroke volume and only increase their cardiac output by increasing their heart rate. Following the Fontan procedure, there is an increased risk of atrial arrhythmias because of extensive atrial surgery involved in the repair. Other postoperative complications include poor ventricular function, baffle obstruction, and the development of pulmonary arteriovenous fistula, which cause increasing cyanosis. Modifications of surgical techniques are used to reduce the risk of atrial arrhythmias.[35,66-69]

Evaluation of the patient who has had the Fontan procedure should include a careful history, physical examination, ECG, chest x-ray, Holter monitor, and exercise stress testing. Since single-ventricle physiology may result from a variety of different anatomic defects, there are no invariable findings on physical exam or laboratory studies.

Patients with the single-ventricle or Fontan procedure generally should participate only in low intensity sports (Class IA). Consideration regarding participation in either moderate- or low-static-demand exercise can be considered if there is normal or near-normal ventricular function, normal oxygen saturation, and near-normal exercise tolerance on exercise testing. Any activity with a high static load should be avoided. Patients with arrhythmias should also have this considered in the decision regarding sports participation. Some studies suggest that a rehabilitation program helps improve the overall exercise function of these patients, but caution is necessary since changes, from exercise training, to the right ventricle functioning as the systemic ventricle may not be beneficial[1–3] (Table 13.13).

The right ventricle functioning as the systemic ventricle cannot adapt to exercise activity in the same manner as can the left ventricle. In fact, the increased ventricular size that occurs in the left ventricle with chronic exercise may also occur in the systemic, but anatomically right ventricle, and may decrease right ventricular function or exacerbate tricupsid (systemic AV valve) regurgitation, since the tricuspid valve was not designed to function in a high-pressure ventricle.

Patients with single-ventricle physiology are better suited for sedentary work and should be discouraged from pursuing careers that require high levels of activity. Each case must be considered on an individual basis when making the exercise plan.

CONGENITAL CORONARY ABNORMALITIES

Coronary artery abnormalities occur as either isolated defects or in combination with other forms of congenital heart disease. With increased activity, there may be compression of the coronary artery as it courses between the aorta and the pulmonary artery, causing partial occlusion and decreased blood flow to a portion of the heart. This could lead to acute ischemia, myocardial infarction, or death from ventricular arrhythmias. Alternatively, the acutely angled takeoff of the coronary artery from the aorta, in some coronary artery anomalies, may contribute to cardiac ischemia. This hypothesis maintains that the increase in stroke volume with exertion increases the diameter of the aortic root, compressing the origin of the coronary artery because of its acute, initial angulation. If coronary artery anomalies are identified, these patients should be referred for surgical intervention. Identification is difficult, however, and most cases are not recognized

TABLE 13.13.   SINGLE VENTRICLE AND FONTAN EXERCISE RECOMMENDATIONS

Condition	Signs/Symptoms	Sports
Palliation	≥ 6 Months after surgery Oxygen saturation > 80% No arrhythmias Near-normal work capacity with exercise testing	IA
Fontan	≥ 6 Months after surgery Asymptomatic No arrhythmias Normal or near-normal ventricular function Normal or near-normal oxygen saturation Normal or near-normal exercise tolerance on exercise testing	IA Selected patients IB, IC, IIA, IIB

before death. Unfortunately, the history, physical examination, ECG, and Holter monitor are usually normal.

Following repair of these defects, the coronary artery may have an increased likelihood of late stenosis. Evaluation of congenital coronary malformations postoperatively requires history, physical examination, ECG, echocardiography, Holter monitor, and exercise testing to evaluate for possible ischemia. If there is concern regarding possible coronary stenosis by either history or by testing, myocardial perfusion studies or coronary angiography is warranted. Patients may participate fully in all sports if no abnormalities are present (Table 13.14). If there has been a myocardial infarction, then participation should be restricted by those guidelines. (See Chapter 7.)

SPECIFIC SURGICAL REPAIRS

PALLIATIVE SURGERY

SHUNTS

Surgical shunts are used as palliative procedures in the treatment of congenital heart disease and may be used as staging for a more definitive repair in the future. Most patients are now taken to complete repair (a 2-ventricle repair) or scheduled for a Fontan operation (single ventricle repair).

The most common type of shunt used is a Blalock-Taussig shunt, either classic or modified. The classic form involves anastomosing the right subclavian artery to the right pulmonary artery to provide for pulmonary blood flow. In the modified form, a Gore-Tex tube is used in place of the subclavian artery to connect the subclavian artery or brachiocephalic trunk to the pulmonary artery.

Other shunts previously used were direct anastomosis of the ascending aorta to the right pulmonary artery (Waterston) or the descending aorta to the left pulmonary artery (Potts). Patients with these shunts continue (usually) to be cyanotic and may develop pulmonary vascular disease over time. Due to the chronic cyanosis, these patients frequently have polycythemia and may require therapeutic phlebotomies on a regular basis. Most patients will not have a normal exercise tolerance and will be voluntarily restricted in their activities.[70–72] Patients with a Glenn shunt will also exhibit marked decrease in exercise tolerance.

Following palliative procedures, patients may participate in Class IA sports if the arterial saturation is > 80%, symptomatic arrhythmias are not present, and the patient has near-normal physical work capacity on exercise testing[1] (Table 13.15).

Recreational and vocational activities are likely to be significantly limited in this patient group.

PULMONARY ARTERY BANDING

A pulmonary artery band is a narrowing placed above the pulmonary valve on the main pulmonary artery in an effort to restrict pulmonary blood flow. Pulmonary artery banding is

TABLE 13.14.   CONGENITAL CORONARY ARTERY ABNORMALITIES EXERCISE RECOMMENDATIONS

	Signs/Symptoms	Sports
Preoperative		None
Postoperative[a]	≥ 6 Months after repair No ischemia with maximal exercise testing No myocardial infarction	All
	Myocardial infarction	(See coronary artery disease recommendations.)

[a]Periodic evaluation is necessary postoperatively.

TABLE 13.15. UNOPERATED OR PALLIATED CYANOTIC HEART DISEASE

Condition	Signs/Symptoms	Sports
Unoperated	Oxygen saturation > 80% with exercise No symptomatic ventricular dysfunction Near-normal working capacity with exercise testing	IA
Palliated	Oxygen saturation > 80% with exercise No symptomatic arrhythmias No symptomatic ventricular dysfunction Near-normal working capacity on exercise testing	IA

still occasionally performed in infancy in lesions that are better addressed when the patient is larger. These patients are usually cyanotic at rest and do not have a normal exercise tolerance. They should be restricted to Class IA sports participation. Exercise recommendations are similar to those in patients with palliative shunts (Table 13.15).

UNOPERATED OR PALLIATED CYANOTIC HEART DISEASE

Patients with cyanotic heart disease that has either not been repaired or has only had palliation continue to be cyanotic. They have limited exercise tolerance and will have progressive hypoxemia with increasing effort. The majority of patients self-limit their activities.

Each patient in this category requires an individual assessment prior to any sports participation. Evaluation should include a complete history and physical examination, chest x-ray, ECG, and probably an echocardiogram. Exercise testing is also necessary. Further surgical treatment may help some in this category. Even Class IA sports should only be allowed if the arterial saturation remains > 80% with exercise, symptomatic arrhythmias are not present, and the patient has a near-normal physical work capacity on exercise testing (Table 13.15).

VALVAR DISEASE

Valvar disease is discussed in greater detail elsewhere (see Chapter 14). We will briefly review recommendations for congenital valvar problems and limit our discussion to the aortic and pulmonary valves since congenital mitral valve stenosis is an uncommon lesson.

PULMONARY VALVE STENOSIS

Pulmonary valve stenosis accounts for 8 to 12% of all congenital heart disease and is usually well tolerated. The stenosis may be at the valvar, subvalvar, or supravalvar level. Our discussion is limited to the valvar type of stenosis, which is the most common. Patients with moderate or severe disease have usually had either surgical or percutaneous cardiac catheterization intervention. Most patients are asymptomatic, but those with moderate or severe disease may have exertional dyspnea or easy fatigue. Stenosis is characterized by a systolic ejection murmur heard best at the left upper sternal border, an ejection click associated with the abnormal pulmonic valve, and possibly a right ventricular tap on physical examination. Laboratory studies show either a normal ECG or the presence of mild right ventricular hypertrophy. The chest x-ray shows normal heart size and possibly a prominent main pulmonary artery segment.

Pulmonic stenosis involves a fixed obstruction to right ventricular outflow. There is increased right ventricular systolic pressure and increased myocardial oxygen demand at rest. In mild pulmonic stenosis, exercise tolerance is normal, but exercise tolerance is usually decreased with moderate or severe disease. Patients may have a decreased cardiac output at rest that does not increase adequately with exercise. The gradient increases as a squared function of cardiac output during exercise (based on Gorlin formula for calculation of aortic valve area). Myocardial oxygen demand of the right ventricle is determined by the right ventricular systolic pressure, mass, and heart rate. During exercise, coronary blood flow may not meet the metabolic demands, resulting in right ventricular ischemia, dysfunction, and, ultimately, fibrosis.

Preoperatively, working capacity and endurance time are usually decreased, whereas the heart rate response to exercise is normal. The decreased exercise tolerance is probably due to reduced stroke volume and cardiac output. In severe stenosis, there is a low resting stroke volume index and no increase in stroke volume with exercise.

Postoperatively, patients have a decreased right ventricular systolic pressure with exercise. Children often have no abnormal findings during postoperative testing and have a near-normal exercise tolerance. Adults, however, show impaired exercise tolerance compared to that of children with a similar degree of stenosis, despite successful repair. Ventricular arrhythmias are common postoperatively; and 24% of patients have premature ventricular contractions during exercise, 3% have multiform premature ventricular contractions, 2% have couplets, and 0.5% have ventricular tachycardia.

Pulmonic stenosis is differentiated by the gradient across the valve. Mild pulmonary stenosis has a peak transvalvar gradient of < 40 mmHg, moderate stenosis 40 to 70 mmHg, and severe stenosis > 70 mmHg. Patients are usually referred for balloon valvuloplasty when the right ventricular pressure exceeds 50 mmHg. Patients who continue with high gradients across the valve are at increased risk for sudden death with exercise.[27,35,73,74]

Asymptomatic patients with gradients < 50 mmHg and normal right ventricular function may participate in all sports. If the gradient is > 40 mmHg, referral to a cardiologist is indicated. Annual reevaluation is needed for both patient groups.

If the gradient is > 50 mmHg, participation in low intensity sports is permissible. Patients with high gradients or high right ventricular pressures are at risk for arrhythmias, and the right ventricle may not be able to increase cardiac output during periods of exercise.

Following treatment, with either a surgical operation or percutaneous intervention, patients may participate in all sports 1 month after the percutaneous and 3 months after surgical intervention. If there is a persistent gradient > 50 mmHg, the same guidelines as before the intervention should be followed. If there is significant pulmonary insufficiency, the criteria for this abnormality should be considered as well (Table 13.16).

TABLE 13.16. PULMONARY STENOSIS EXERCISE RECOMMENDATIONS

	Degree	Signs/Symptoms	Sports
Preoperative	< 50 mmHg	Asymptomatic Normal right ventricular function	All
	> 50 mmHg	Asymptomatic	IA
Postoperative	≤ 50 mmHg	≥ 3 Months after surgery or ≥ 1 month after catherterization Normal ventricular function Asymptomatic	
	> 50 mmHg		Same as preoperative recommendations
		Pulmonary regurgitation Right ventricular enlargement	Individual assessment

AORTIC VALVE STENOSIS, CONGENITAL

Congenital aortic stenosis is often identified in early childhood and accounts for 3 to 6% of all congenital heart disease. Mild and moderate degrees of aortic stenosis are often asymptomatic, but may have some exercise intolerance or exertional chest pain. The physical examination findings reveal a systolic murmur heard best at the right upper sternal border, an ejection click possibly heard at the apex, and possibly a thrill palpable at the right upper sternal border. The ECG shows left ventricular hypertrophy, and the chest x-ray is usually normal.

The stenosis is classified as mild, moderate, or severe. Mild aortic stenosis has a peak gradient of ≤ 20 mmHg, moderate 21 to 49 mmHg, and severe ≥ 50 mmHg. Aortic stenosis may progress and requires regular follow-up and evaluation by a cardiologist. The classification for congenital aortic stenosis is different than that used for acquired aortic stenosis, which is based on the mean gradient across the aortic valve.

The increased stroke volume with exercise and the fixed aortic obstruction result in increased left ventricular pressure and an increased aortic valve gradient. Patients with aortic valve stenosis are at increased risk for sudden death with exercise.

Patients with severe disease or with symptoms related to the stenosis are also at increased risk for sudden death.[27,35,75–77]

Evaluation of the patient with aortic stenosis should include history, physical examination, ECG, echocardiogram, and exercise testing.

Patients with mild aortic stenosis may participate in all sports if the ECG is normal; there is normal exercise tolerance; and there is no history of exercise-related chest pain, syncope, or arrhythmia. Patients with moderate stenosis should be restricted to Class IA, IB, and IIA sports. They must also have only mild or no left ventricular hypertrophy; no evidence of left ventricular strain on ECG; normal exercise tolerance on exercise testing; and no symptoms. In cases of severe aortic stenosis, no sports are allowed and the patient should be referred for intervention.

Following repair, assessment for residual stenosis and the presence of aortic insufficiency should be made. Evaluation should include ECG, physical examination, and echocardiogram. Exercise testing may be considered if the degree of stenosis or the effect of regurgitation is not clearly determined by the preceding studies. Patients with residual stenosis should follow the same restrictions as prior to intervention. Patients with mild or moderate aortic regurgitation and normal or only mildly increased left ventricular size may participate in all sports. If left ventricular enlargement is present, participation in Class IA, IB, IC, IIA, IIB, and IIC sports may be considered on an individual basis (Table 13.17).

If there are arrhythmias associated with mild-to-moderate aortic insufficiency, only Class IA sports should be allowed. Patients with symptoms or with a dilated ascending aorta should not participate in any sports.

POSTOPERATIVE VALVE REPLACEMENT

AORTIC VALVE

Ross Procedure. The Ross procedure is performed in those patients with aortic stenosis or regurgitation who have a normal pulmonic valve. The pulmonary root and valve are harvested and transferred to the aortic position, and a homograft valve is placed in the pulmonary position. In addition, the coronary arteries are implanted into the pulmonary autograft. This procedure is more common in children than it is in adults and better results seem to be obtained in the pediatric population.

Advantages of this repair, compared to repair with prosthetic valves, include avoidance of anticoagulation, the valve growth with the patient, and there seems to be long-term durability of the pulmonic valve in the aortic position. Postoperative complications include aortic regurgitation (usually mild), stenosis of the homograft in the pulmonary position, and deterioration of the neoaortic valve. There is concern that high static sports may cause progression or induce regurgita-

TABLE 13.17. AORTIC STENOSIS EXERCISE RECOMMENDATIONS

	Degree	Signs/Symptoms	Sports
Preoperative[a]	Mild (≤ 20 mmHg peak)	Normal ECG Normal exercise test No exercise-related chest pain, syncope, or arrhythmia	All
	Moderate (21–49 mmHg)	Mild or no left ventricular hypertrophy by echocardiography No left ventricular hypertrophy or strain on ECG Normal exercise test Asymptomatic	IA, IB, IIA
	Severe (≥ 50 mmHg)		None
Postoperative	Residual stenosis	≥ 3 Months after surgery ≥ 1 Month after cardiac catheterization	Same as preoperative recommendations
		Mild or moderate aortic insufficiency Normal or only mildly increased left ventricular size Asymptomatic	All
		Mild or moderate aortic insufficiency Arrhythmias	IA
		Symptomatic and mild to moderate aortic insufficiency Severe aortic insufficiency Aortic insufficiency and marked dilation of ascending aorta	None

[a] Applies to patients with discrete subaortic stenosis and supravalvar stenosis.

tion in the pulmonic valve in the aortic position after surgery.[78]

Following surgery, the patients should be restricted from participation in sports for 6 months. Evaluation should include history, physical examination, ECG, chest x-ray, exercise testing, and an echocardiogram to evaluate the aortic valve and ventricular function. High static sports may be injurious to the aortic valve and may lead to or worsen aortic regurgitation. If there is no valvular dysfunction (stenosis or regurgitation) and normal or near-normal left ventricular function, participation may be considered for Class IA sports. Also, selected patients may participate in low and moderate static and low and moderate dynamic sports (Classes IA, IB, IIA, and IIB) (Table 13.18).

Similar recommendations should be followed for bioprosthetic (homograft) valves in the aortic position. Bioprosthetic valves are more likely to deteriorate over time and to calcify than are pulmonic valves in the aortic position following a Ross procedure.

TABLE 13.18. POSTOPERATIVE ROSS PROCEDURE EXERCISE RECOMMENDATIONS

Signs/Symptoms	Sports
≥ 6 Months postoperatively	IA
Normal valve function	Selected patients IB, IIA, IIB
Normal left ventricular function	(No high static sports)

PROSTHETIC OR BIOPROSTHETIC VALVE REPLACEMENT

Patients requiring valve replacement have an increased long-term mortality compared to that of the normal population of similar age. Even though most patients improve following surgery, there is still a residual valve gradient of varying severity. These patients also have abnormal hemodynamic response to exercise. Anticoagulants are necessary in patients with mechanical valves, but not necessarily with bioprosthetic valves.

Patients who have a prosthetic valve in either the aortic or mitral position and are taking anticoagulation therapy should avoid sports with the possibility of bodily injury.

Selected patients with a bioprosthetic valve in the aortic position may participate in selected Class IA, IB, IIA, and IIB sports if they are not taking anticoagulation therapy and have normal left ventricular function and no valvar stenosis or regurgitation (Table 13.19).

Patients with a prosthetic mitral valve who are not on anticoagulation with near-normal or normal valvular function and normal or near-normal left ventricular function may be considered for participation in low and moderate static and low and moderate dynamic competitive sports (Classes IA, IB, IIA, and IIB).

TABLE 13.19.   POSTOPERATIVE PROSTHETIC OR BIOPROSTHETIC VALVE

Valve	Signs/Symptoms	Sports
Aortic	> 6 Months after surgery Normal left ventricular function Normal valve function	IA Selected patients IB, IIA, IIB
	Anticoagulation	No sports with risk of collision
Mitral	≥ 6 Months after surgery Normal valve function Normal left ventricular function	IA, IB, IIA, IIB
	Anticoagulation	No sports with risk of collision

There is minimal information regarding exercise in postoperative valve replacement patients, particularly, the long-term health effects of exercise.

RASTELLI REPAIR

A Rastelli operation is a biventricular repair of defects requiring construction of a right ventricular outflow tract from the right ventricle to the pulmonary artery. Either a homograft or a man-made conduit is used for the construction of the outflow tract. This repair is commonly performed for patients with truncus arteriosus, pulmonary atresia with ventricular septal defect, transposition of the great arteries with severe pulmonary stenosis, or in some forms of double-outlet right ventricle. Since the conduit is attached to the right ventricle with a ventriculotomy, there may be an impact on right ventricular function. In addition, a Rastelli repair usually involves closure of a ventricular septal defect.

Long-term complications associated with this type of repair include conduit stenosis and branch pulmonary artery stenosis. There may also be the need to replace the conduit as the patient grows. Complete heart block is a rare complication. Aortic homografts used as conduits commonly calcify and may become stenotic. Synthetic conduits with a porcine valve have problems with valve deterioration and stenosis of the conduit. Patients may have elevated right ventricular pressures secondary to pulmonary artery or conduit stenosis. The risk of postoperative ventricular arrhythmias is unknown, but is likely similar to that seen in tetralogy of Fallot repaired with a right ventriculotomy.

Exercise is impaired in the presence of right ventricular hypertension. There is a decreased maximal oxygen consumption in about 50% of patients as compared to 70 to 75% of patients with tetralogy of Fallot.[79]

Evaluation of these patients requires the input of a pediatric cardiologist and should include a complete history, physical examination, ECG, chest x-ray, echocardiogram, Holter monitor, exercise testing, and possibly cardiac catheterization. Patients may need to be restricted to Class IA sports and follow restrictions that apply to patients following repair of the ventricular septal defect and pulmonary stenosis. Exercise recommendations should be made with consideration to prolonging the life of the conduit or homograft (Table 13.20).

VENTRICULAR DYSFUNCTION AFTER SURGERY

Ventricular dysfunction can be seen following any type of cardiac surgery, both simple and complex. Poor ventricular function of either the right or left ventricle affects exercise performance. Patients with ventricular dysfunction require regularly scheduled follow-up visits with a cardiologist to monitor cardiac function.

Evaluation includes history, physical examination, chest x-ray, ECG, echocardiogram, exercise testing, and possibly nuclear medicine study to evaluate ventricular function. Patients with normal or near-normal ventricular function may participate fully in sports. Patients with mildly depressed ventricular function should participate only in low intensity static exercise (Classes IA, IB, and IC). Athletes with moderately depressed function should only participate in low intensity sports (IA)[1] (Table 13.21).

ELEVATED PULMONARY RESISTANCE (PULMONARY HYPERTENSION)

Patients with pulmonary vascular disease resulting from underlying cardiac disease have an increased risk of sudden death with intense exercise. As the disease progresses, patients go from being relatively asymptomatic to progressively cyanotic. This contrasts with pulmonary hypertension not associated with intracardiac shunts, where cyanosis is a late symptom. The cyanosis in congenital heart disease patients worsens with physical activity, and the majority of patients self-limit their activities because of fatigue with exercise. Defects that may lead to pulmonary hypertension are those with unrestricted pulmonary blood flow such as large ventricular septal defects, double-outlet right ventricle, truncus arteriosus, and large atrial septal defects.

The history often reveals a decreased exercise tolerance. Care needs to be taken to ask about syncope or near-syncope in these patients, which may be seen with worsening disease. The physical examination may show cyanosis with or without clubbing, the presence of a right ventricular tap or lift, a single second heart sound with a loud P_2 component, and signs of right-sided heart failure. The resting ECG may show right axis deviation, right ventricular hypertrophy, and right atrial enlargement. The chest x-ray shows a normal or

TABLE 13.20.   POSTOPERATIVE RASTELLI REPAIR[a]

Signs/Symptoms	Sports
≥ 6 Months postoperatively	IA
Asymptomatic	
No pulmonary stenosis	
No residual ventricular septal defect	
Normal ventricular function	
No arrhythmias	

[a] Right ventricle to pulmonary artery conduit with ventricular septal defect closure.

TABLE 13.21.   VENTRICULAR DYSFUNCTION EXERCISE RECOMMENDATIONS[a]

Ventricular Function	Sports
Normal or near-normal	All
Mild depression	IA, IB, IC
Moderate depression	IA

[a] Restrictions of the underlying cardiac disease must also be considered. Periodic evaluation needed to follow for possible deterioration of function over time.

slightly enlarged cardiac silhouette with dilated proximal lung vessels and clear lung fields.

Patients with suspected elevated pulmonary artery pressures after surgery or cardiac intervention require follow-up by a pediatric cardiologist. Cardiac output may not increase with exercise testing. There may be no increase in systolic blood pressure or even a decrease in systolic blood pressure with exercise, because the right ventricle cannot provide adequate cardiac output. A decrease in blood pressure with exercise is a poor prognostic sign. Exercise testing should be used with caution in these patients since they are at risk for sudden death with exercise.[80–82]

Evaluation should include a history, physical examination, ECG, chest radiograph, echocardiogram for assessment of right ventricular pressures, and possibly a cardiac catheterization.

Patients with peak pulmonary artery pressure < 40 mmHg can participate in all sports. If peak pulmonary artery pressure is > 40 mmHg, individual assessment is necessary[1–3] (Table 13.22).

POSTOPERATIVE ARRHYTHMIAS

Postoperative management must include at least a brief discussion of arrhythmias. Many of the cardiac surgical repairs may cause rhythm disturbances or changes on ECG that need to be considered when making exercise recommendations. In general, athletes will be limited by the restrictions of the underlying cardiac disease and not by any arrhythmia that may be present. If the arrhythmia requires that the patient be on anticoagulation therapy, sports with a risk of bodily injury should be avoided.

The following discussion applies to patients

with congenital heart disease who have had intervention for the cardiac defect. Sinus node dysfunction including sinus pauses, sinoatrial exit block, and sick sinus syndrome may occur following atrial surgery. These patients' sports participation should not be limited if there is a normal response of the heart rate to exercise and no symptoms related to the arrhythmia. In comparison, if they experience symptomatic tachycardia or bradycardia syndrome or inappropriate sinus tachycardia, they should be medically treated for 3 to 6 months and allowed to participate in Class IA sports if they are then asymptomatic. Premature atrial contractions are common and require no specific restriction of activity. Most patients with isolated premature ventricular contractions may participate in all sports. Patients with congenital heart disease and atrial flutter may participate in low intensity sports (Class IA) only if it has been 6 months or more since the last episode of atrial flutter.

Atrial fibrillation may participate in sports and vigorous activity if the ventricular rate is comparable to an appropriate sinus tachycardia during the activity; they are not taking drugs; or they are rate controlled with digoxin, beta blockers, or calcium channel blockers. They should only participate in sports consistent with the underlying structural cardiac disease and, if anticoagulated, should avoid sports with risk of bodily injury.

Athletes are generally limited by the restrictions of their underlying cardiac disease and not by any arrhythmia that may be present. For a discussion of arrhythmias in patients without underlying structural cardiac disease, see Chapter 10, "Electrocardiographic Variants and Cardiac Rhythm and Conduction Disturbances in the Athlete." Recommendations for exercise in patients with postoperative congenital heart disease and arrhythmias are summarized in Table 13.23.

SUMMARY

Several studies have shown an improved exercise capacity in postoperative patients when these pa-

TABLE 13.22. PULMONARY HYPERTENSION EXERCISE RECOMMENDATIONS

Peak Pulmonary Artery Pressure	Sports
≤ 40 mmHg	All
> 40 mmHg	Individual assessment

TABLE 13.23.   SPORTS AND ARRHYTHMIAS IN POSTOPERATIVE CONGENITAL HEART DISEASE

Rhythm Disturbance	Criteria to Participate in Sports	Class of Sport
Sinus node dysfunction	No symptoms Normal heart rate increase with exercise	All
Junctional escape rhythm or junctional escape beats	Normal heart rate response to exercise	All
Tachycardia/bradycardia syndrome or inappropriate sinus tachycardia	Treatment for 3–6 months No symptoms	IA
Premature atrial contractions	No sustained tachycardia No worsening with exercise	All
Atrial flutter	Treatment for 6 months No episodes of atrial flutter Asymptomatic Absence of Wolff-Parkinson-White (WPW) syndrome	IA
Atrial fibrillation	No medications, or on digoxin, beta blocker, or calcium channel blocker Ventricular response to exercise is normal Absence of WPW	IA If on anticoagulation, no sports with risk of collision
Atrial and sinus node reentry tachycardia	No WPW	All
Premature junctional contractions	No sustained tachycardia	All
Premature ventricular contractions	Not a high-risk group With or without treatment	IA
Ventricular tachycardia	No episodes for 6 months Controlled on medication	IA
Ventricular fibrillation	Treatment ≥ 6 months No episodes	IA
First-degree atrioventricular (AV) block	No worsening with exercise	All
Second-degree AV block, type I	No worsening with exercise	All
Second-degree AV block, type II	Treat as complete AV block Needs pacemaker	No sports with risk of collision
Complete AV block	Pacemaker Appropriate heart rate response to exercise	No sports with risk of collision
Left bundle branch block	Electrophysiology study showing normal conduction through AV node	All
Right bundle branch block	No ventricular arrhythmias No AV block with exercise Asymptomatic	All
Supraventricular tachycardia	Treatment > 6 months No recurrence	IA
Congenital long QT interval syndrome		No sports

tients are enrolled in a monitored exercise program. Most studies have only followed the patients over a short time and the long-term effects of exercise are not known. It may be that having a rehabilitation program with scheduled follow-up over a longer time frame increases the likelihood that patients with congenital heart disease will maintain a more active lifestyle and potentially reap the health and psychological benefits of regular exercise.[83–88]

PERSONAL PERSPECTIVE

In our clinic, we provide guidance for expected exercise performance and tolerance very early in our evaluation and treatment of patients. We make specific recommendations regarding sports participation in any of the patients with congenital heart disease. Recommended sports or activities are discussed and patients are encouraged to develop other interests outside of athletics. The expectations and interests of the family and patient must be considered along with the expected clinical course of the disease. Patients with single-ventricle physiology are therefore not encouraged to participate in rigorous sports such as football, basketball, and track and field, since they will not have normal exercise tolerance. In contrast, patients with mild congenital heart disease or with good surgical repairs are reassured and encouraged to lead a fully normal life of physical activity.

REFERENCES

1. Maron BJ, Mitchell JH: 26th Bethesda Conference: Recommendations for determining eligibility for competition in athletes with cardiovascular abnormalities. *J Am Coll Cardiol* 24:846, 1994.

2. Kaplan S, Perloff JK: Exercise and athletics before and after cardiac surgery or interventional catheterization, in Perloff JK, Child JS (eds.): *Congenital Heart Disease in Adults*. Philadelphia: WB Saunders Company, 1991.

3. Liberthson RR: Arrhythmias in the athlete with congenital heart disease: Guidelines for participation. *Ann Rev Med* 50:441, 1999.

4. Koster NK: Physical activity and congenital heart disease. *Nurs Clin North Am* 29:345, 1994.

5. Gutgesell HP, Gessner IH, Vetter VL, et al: Recreational and occupational recommendations for young patients with heart disease: A statement for physicians by the committee on congenital cardiac defects of the council on cardiovascular disease in the young, American Heart Association. *Circulation* 74:1195A, 1986.

6. Freed MD: Recreational and sports recommendations for the child with heart disease. *Pediatr Clin North Am* 31:1307, 1984.

7. Fletcher GF, Balady G, Blair SN, et al: Statement on exercise: Benefits and recommendations for physical activity programs for all Americans. A statement for health professionals by the committee on exercise and cardiac rehabilitation of the council on clinical cardiology, American Heart Association. *Circulation* 84:857, 1996.

8. Franklin WH, Allen HD, Fontana ME: Sports, physical activity, and school problems, in Emmanouilides GG, Riemenschneider TA, Allen HD, et al (eds.): *Heart Disease in Infants, Children and Adolescents Including the Fetus and Young Adult*, 5th ed. Baltimore: Williams & Wilkins, 1995, pp. 673–683.

9. Fletcher GF, Balady G, Froelicher VF, et al: Exercise standards: A statement for health professionals from the American Heart Association, writing group. *Circulation* 91:580, 1995.

10. Fletcher GF: How to implement physical activity in primary and secondary prevention: A statement for healthcare professionals from the task force on risk reduction, American Heart Association. *Circulation* 96:355, 1997.

11. Strong WB, Raunikar RA: Physical activity, in Emmanouilides GG, Riemenschneider TA, Allen HD, et al (eds.): *Heart Disease in Infants, Children and Adolescents Including the Fetus and Young Adult*, 5th ed. Baltimore: Williams & Wilkins, 1995, pp. 643-649.

12. Berger S, Anwer D, Friedberg DZ: Sudden cardiac death in infants, children, and adolescents. *Pediatr Clin North Am* 46:221, 1999.

13. Virmani R, Burke AP, Farb A, et al: Causes of sudden death in young and middle-aged competitive athletes. *Card Clin* 15:439, 1997.

14. Kitchner D: Physical activities in patients with congenital heart disease. *Heart* 76:6, 1996.

15. Silka MJ, Hardy BG, Menashe VD, et al: A population-based prospective evaluation of risk of sudden cardiac death after operation for common con-

genital heart defects. *J Am Coll Cardiol* 32:245, 1998.

16. Liberthson RR: Sudden death from cardiac causes in children and young adults. *N Engl J Med* 334:1039, 1996.

17. Maron BJ, Thompson PD, Puffer JC, et al: Cardiovascular preparticipation screening of competitive athletes: A statement for health professionals from the Sudden Death Committee (clinical cardiology) and Congenital Cardiac Defects Committee (cardiovascular disease in the young). American Heart Association. *Circulation* 94:545, 1986.

18. Washington RL, Bricker JT, Alpert BS, et al: Guidelines for exercise testing in the pediatric age group: From the committee on atherosclerosis and hypertension in children, council on cardiovascular disease in the young, the American Heart Association. *Circulation* 90:2166, 1994.

19. Driscoll DJ: Exercise testing, in Emmanouilides GG, Riemenschneider TA, Allen HD, et al (eds.): *Heart Disease in Infants, Children and Adolescents Including the Fetus and Young Adult,* 5th ed. Baltimore: Williams & Wilkins, 1995, pp. 293-310.

20. Braden DS, Carroll JF: Normative cardiovascular responses to exercise in children. *Pediatr Cardiol* 20:4, 1999.

21. Mitchell JH, Blomquist CG, Haskell WL, et al: Classification of sports. *J Am Coll Cardiol* 6:1198, 1985.

22. Matthys D: Pre- and postoperative exercise testing of the child with atrial septal defect. *Pediatr Cardiol* 20:22, 1999.

23. Helber U, Baumann R, Seboldt H, et al: Atrial septal defect in adults: Cardiopulmonary exercise capacity before and 4 months and 10 years after defect closure. *J Am Coll Cardiol* 29:1345, 1997.

24. Meijboom F, Hess J, Szatmari A, et al: Long-term follow-up (9 to 20 years) after surgical closure of atrial septal defect at a young age. *Am J Cardiol* 72:1431, 1993.

25. Rosenthal M, Redington A, Bush A: Cardiopulmonary physiology after surgical closure of asymptomatic secundum atrial septal defects in childhood. Exercise performance is unaffected by age at repair. *Eur Heart J* 18:1816, 1997.

26. Frick MH, Punsar S, Somer T: The spectrum of cardiac capacity in patients with nonobstructive congenital heart disease. *Am J Cardiol* 17:20, 1966.

27. Cumming GR: Maximal exercise capacity of children with heart defects. *Am J Cardiol* 42:613, 1978.

28. Bink-Boelkens MTE, Meuzelaar KJ, Eygelaar A: Arrhythmias after repair of secundum atrial septal defect: The influence of surgical modification. *Am Heart J* 115:629, 1988.

29. Fratellone PM, Steinfeld L, Coplan NL: Exercise and congenital heart disease. *Am Heart J* 127:1676, 1994.

30. Perrault H, Drblik SP: Exercise after surgical repair of congenital cardiac lesions. *Sports Med* 7:18, 1989.

31. Gurses HN, Gurses A, Arikan H: Exercise testing in children with congenital heart disease before and after surgical treatment. *Pediatr Cardiol* 12:20, 1991.

32. Driscoll DJ, Wolfe RR, Gersony WM, et al: Cardiorespiratory responses to exercise of patients with aortic stenosis, pulmonary stenosis, and ventricular septal defect. *Circulation* 87(suppl I):I–102, 1993.

33. Meijboom F, Szatmari A, Utens E, et al: Long-term follow-up after surgical closure of ventricular septal defect in infancy and childhood. *J Am Coll Cardiol* 24:1358, 1994.

34. Moller JH, Patton C, Varco RL, et al: Late results (30 to 35 years) after operative closure of isolated ventricular septal defect from 1954 to 1960. *Am J Cardiol* 68:1491, 1991.

35. Reybrouck T, Rogers R, Weymans M, et al: Serial cardiorespiratory exercise testing in patients with congenital heart disease. *Eur J Pediatr* 154:801, 1995.

36. Ruttenberg HD: Pre- and postoperative exercise testing of the child with coarctation of the aorta. *Pediatr Cardiol* 20:33, 1999.

37. Pelech AN, Kartodihardjo W, Balfe JA, et al: Exercise in children before and after coarctectomy: Hemodynamic, echocardiographic, and biochemical assessment. *Am Heart J* 112:1263, 1986.

38. Connor TM: Evaluation of persistent coarctation of aorta after surgery with blood pressure measurement and exercise testing. *Am J Cardiol* 43:74, 1979.

39. Moskowitz WB, Schieken RM, Mosteller M, et al: Altered systolic and diastolic function in children after "successful" repair of coarctation of the aorta. *Am Heart J* 120:103, 1990.

40. Clarkson PM, Nicholson MR, Barratt-Boyes BG, et al: Results after repair of coarctation of the aorta beyond infancy: A 10 to 28 year follow-up with particular reference to late systemic hypertension. *Am J Cardiol* 51:1481, 1983.

41. Balderston SM, Daberkow E, Clarke DR, et al: Maximal voluntary exercise variables in children with postoperative coarctation of the aorta. *J Am Coll Cardiol* 19:154, 1992.

42. Pelech AN, Kartodihardjo W, Balfe JA, et al: Exercise in children before and after coarctectomy: Hemodynamic, echocardiographic, and biochemical assessment. *Am Heart J* 112:1263, 1986.

43. Carvalho JS, Shinebourne EA, Busst C, et al: Exercise capacity after complete repair of tetralogy of Fallot: Deleterious effects of residual pulmonary regurgitation. *Br Heart J* 67:470, 1992.

44. Walsh EP, Rockenmacher S, Keane JF, et al: Late results in patients with tetralogy of Fallot repaired during infancy. *Circulation* 77:1062, 1988.

45. Wessel HU, Paul MH: Exercise studies in tetralogy of Fallot: A review. *Pediatr Cardiol* 20:39, 1999.

46. Mulla N, Simpson P, Sullivan NM, et al: Determinants of aerobic capacity during exercise following complete repair of tetralogy of Fallot with a transannular patch. *Pediatr Cardiol* 18:350, 1997.

47. Perrault H, Drblik SP, Montigny M, et al: Comparison of cardiovascular adjustments to exercise in adolescents 8 to 15 years of age after correction of tetralogy of Fallot, ventricular septal defect or atrial septal defect. *Am J Cardiol* 64:213, 1989.

48. Rhodes J, Dave A, Pulling MC, et al: Effect of pulmonary artery stenoses on the cardiopulmonary response to exercise following repair of tetralogy of Fallot. *Am J Cardiol* 81:1217, 1998.

49. Meijboom F, Szatmari A, Deckers JW, et al: Cardiac status and health-related quality of life in the long term after surgical repair of tetralogy of Fallot in infancy and in childhood. *J Thorac Cardiovasc Surg* 110:883, 1995.

50. Tomassoni TL, Galioto FM Jr, Vaccaro P: Cardiopulmonary exercise testing in children following surgery for tetralogy of Fallot. *Am J Dis Child* 145:1290, 1991.

51. Garson A, Gillette PC, Gutgesell HP, et al: Stress induced ventricular arrhythmia after repair of tetralogy of Fallot. *Am J Cardiol* 46:1006, 1980.

52. Chandar JS, Wolff GS, Garson A, et al: Ventricular arrhythmias in postoperative tetralogy of Fallot. *Am J Cardiol* 65:655, 1990.

53. Roos-Hesselink J, Perlroth MG, McGhie J, et al: Atrial arrhythmias in adults after repair of tetralogy of Fallot. Correlations with clinical, exercise, and echocardiographic findings. *Circulation* 91: 2214, 1995.

54. Peterson RJ, Franch RH, Fajman WA, et al: Comparison of cardiac function in surgically corrected and congenitally corrected transposition of the great arteries. *J Thorac Cardiovasc Surg* 96:227, 1988.

55. Paul MH, Wessel HU: Exercise studies in patients with transposition of the great arteries after atrial repair operations (Mustard/Senning): A review. *Pediatr Cardiol* 20:49, 1999.

56. Page E, Perrault H, Flore P, et al: Cardiac output response to dynamic exercise after atrial switch repair for transposition of the great arteries. *Am J Cardiol* 77:892, 1996.

57. Helbing WA, Hansen B, Ottenkamp J, et al: Long-term results of atrial correction for transposition of the great arteries: Comparison of Mustard and Senning operations. *J Thorac Cardiovasc Surg* 108: 363, 1994.

58. Douard H, Labbe L, Barat JL, et al: Cardiorespiratory response to exercise after venous switch operation for transposition of the great arteries. *Chest* 111:23, 1997.

59. Weindling SN, Wernovsky G, Colan SD, et al: Myocardial perfusion, function and exercise tolerance after the arterial switch operation. *J Am Coll Cardiol* 23:424, 1994.

60. Sagin-Saylam G, Somerville J: Palliative Mustard operation for transposition of the great arteries: Late results after 15-20 years. *Heart* 75:72, 1996.

61. Gelatt M, Hamilton RM, McCrindle BW, et al: Arrhythmia and mortality after the Mustard procedure: A 30-year single-center experience. *J Am Coll Cardiol* 29:194, 1997.

62. Meijboom F, Szatmari A, Deckers JW, et al: Long-term follow-up (10 to 17 years) after Mustard repair for transposition of the great arteries. *J Thorac Cardiovasc Surg* 111:1158, 1996.

63. Bowyer JJ, Busst CM, Till JA, et al: Exercise ability after Mustard's operation. *Arch Dis Child* 65:865, 1990.

64. Massin M, Hovels-Gurich H, Dabritz S, et al:

Results of the Bruce treadmill test in children after arterial switch operation for simple transposition of the great arteries. *Am J Cardiol* 81:56, 1998.

65. Hovels-Gurich HH, Seghaye MC, Dabritz S, et al: Cardiological and general health status in pre-school- and school-age children after neonatal arterial switch operation. *Eur J Cardiothorac Surg* 12:593, 1997.

66. Driscoll DJ, Durongpisitkul K: Exercise testing after the Fontan operation. *Pediatr Cardiol* 20:57, 1999.

67. Gewillig MH, Lundstrom UR, Bull C, et al: Exercise responses in patients with congenital heart disease after Fontan repair: Patterns and determinants of performance. *J Am Coll Cardiol* 15:1424, 1990.

68. Gewillig M, Wyse RK, de Leval MR, et al: Early and late arrhythmias after the Fontan operation: Predisposing factors and clinical consequences. *Br Heart J* 67:72, 1992.

69. Driscoll DJ, Danielson GK, Puga FJ, et al: Exercise tolerance and cardiorespiratory response to exercise after the Fontan operation for tricuspid atresia or functional single ventricle. *J Am Coll Cardiol* 7:1087, 1986.

70. Giannico S, Santoro G, Marino B, et al: Bidirectional cavopulmonary anastomosis in congenital heart disease. Functional and clinical outcome. *Herz* 17:234, 1992.

71. Casey FA, Craig BG, Mulholland HC: Quality of life in surgically palliated complex congenital heart disease. *Arch Dis Child* 70:382, 1994.

72. Sietsema KE: Cyanotic congenital heart disease: Dynamics of oxygen uptake and ventilation during exercise. *J Am Coll Cardiol* 18:322, 1991.

73. Steinberger J, Moller JH: Exercise testing in children with pulmonary valvar stenosis. *Pediatr Cardiol* 20:27, 1999.

74. Krabill KA, Wang Y, Einzig S, et al: Rest and exercise hemodynamics in pulmonary stenosis: Comparison of children and adults. *Am J Card* 56:360, 1985.

75. Whitmer JT, James FW, Kaplan S: Exercise testing in children before and after surgical treatment of aortic stenosis. *Circulation* 63:254, 1981.

76. Atwood JE, Kawanishi S, Myers J, et al: Exercise testing in patients with aortic stenosis. *Chest* 93:1083, 1988.

77. James FW, Schwartz DC, Kaplan S, et al: Exercise electrocardiogram, blood pressure, and working capacity in young patients with valvular or discrete subvalvular aortic stenosis. *Am J Cardiol* 50:769, 1982.

78. Oury JH, Doty DB, Oswalt JD, et al: Cardiopulmonary response to maximal exercise in young athletes following the Ross procedure. *Ann Thoracic Surg* 66(6 Suppl):S153, 1998.

79. Barber G, Danielson GK, Puga FJ, et al: Pulmonary atresia with ventricular septal defect: Preoperative and postoperative responses to exercise. *J Am Coll Cardiol* 7:630, 1986.

80. Garofano RP, Barst RJ: Exercise testing in children with primary pulmonary hypertension. *Pediatr Cardiol* 20:61, 1999.

81. D'Alonzo GE, Barst RJ, Ayres SM, et al: Survival in patients with primary pulmonary hypertension: Results from a national prospective registry. *Ann Intern Med* 115:343, 1991.

82. Nixon PA, Joswiak ML, Fricker FJ: A six-minute walk test for assessing exercise tolerance in severely ill children. *J Pediatr* 129:362, 1996.

83. Goldberg B, Fripp RR, Lister G, et al: Effect of physical training on exercise performance of children following surgical repair of congenital heart disease. *Pediatrics* 68:691, 1981.

84. Ruttenberg HD, Adams TD, Orsmond GS, et al: Effects of exercise training on aerobic fitness in children after open heart surgery. *Pediatr Cardiol* 4:19, 1983.

85. Calzolari A, Pastore E: Exercise testing as a rehabilitative/training tool. *Pediatr Cardiol* 20:85, 1999.

86. Longmuir PE, Turner JAP, Rowe RD, et al: Postoperative exercise rehabilitation benefits children with congenital heart disease. *Clin Inv Med* 8:232, 1985.

87. Vaccaro P, Gallioto FM, Bradley LM: Development of a cardiac rehabilitation program for children. *Sports Med* 1:259, 1984.

88. Günther T, Mazzitelli D, Haehnel CJ, et al: Long-term results after complete repair of atrioventricular septal defects: Analysis of risk factors. *Ann Thorac Surg* 65:754, 1998.

Chapter 14

EVALUATING AND MANAGING ATHLETES WITH VALVULAR HEART DISEASE

Paul D. Thompson, M.D.

Aortic stenosis was implicated in 8% of the nontraumatic, exertion-related deaths reported by Jokl and Melzer in their review of medical reports published between 1921 and 1939.[1] Unfortunately, despite the widespread appreciation of the dangers of exertion with valvular aortic stenosis, this entity remains an important cause of exercise-related cardiac deaths and still accounts for 4% of sudden deaths among young athletes.[2,3] Furthermore, the evaluation of cardiac murmurs and valvular abnormalities remains a frequent reason for cardiology consultation. This chapter will address the evaluation and management of valvular heart disease in competitive and recreational athletes.

Evaluating valvular heart disease in athletes is not easy. The physiological cardiac adaptations to exercise training create innocent flow murmurs that are difficult to differentiate from those that are abnormal. Blood flow is laminar and without turbulence until a critical Reynolds number (Re) is exceeded. Re is determined by the following formula:

$$Re = \frac{\text{Average Velocity} \times \text{Tube Diameter} \times \text{Fluid Density}}{\text{Fluid Viscosity}^4}$$

Laminar flow is disrupted above an Re of 2000, creating turbulence and murmurs. Endurance exercise training reduces resting heart rate but enhances cardiac performance. Since oxygen demand determines cardiac output and since resting oxygen demand remains relatively constant before and after exercise training, resting cardiac output is also relatively constant. This means that the same cardiac output is delivered via a slower than normal heart rate and a larger stroke volume. Much of the larger stroke volume is delivered more vigorously in early systole by a more dynamic ventricle. This increases blood velocity. Neither the pulmonic nor aortic valve orifice increases with exercise training, and reductions in blood density with training are not sufficient to prevent the development of turbulence and cardiac "flow murmurs." Such flow murmurs in young athletes are due to flow across the pulmonic valve and often vary with respiration. Athletes aged $\geq$ 50 years may have mild sclerosis of the aortic valve leaflets. Flow murmurs in old endurance athletes are often due to aortic valve turbulence from the physiological changes of exercise training and the aortic valve sclerosis. These murmurs in senior athletes are less "innocent" because they may progress to important aortic stenosis, especially in athletes with other risk factors for atherosclerosis such as hypercholesterolemia.[5,6] Treatment of these risk factors may reduce the development of important aortic stenosis, but this has not been studied. Nevertheless, this author often recommends 3-hydroxy-3-methylglutaryl coenzyme A (HMG CoA) reductase inhibitors in patients with noncritical aortic stenosis of the adult in the hope of preventing such progression.

Further complicating the treatment of valvular disease in athletes is the lack of studies evaluating various management strategies in such patients. Indeed, there are few trials of valvular heart disease treatment approaches in nonathletic populations, and much of the available literature is based on single-center reports.[7] An additional problem is that athletes, because of their exercise activity, may present at earlier disease stages than other patients. This is a major issue because the appearance of symptoms is an important indicator that valvular repair or replacement may be necessary. Physicians do not want to intervene too soon in athletes with symptoms produced by extreme exertion because of the immediate risk of surgery, the finite life of many valvular prostheses, and the need for life-long anticoagulant therapy after some valve replacements.

The athlete's attitude can also complicate the decision. Some athletes deny symptoms and try to avoid surgery even with life-threatening conditions. Others prefer early intervention if waiting would mean restricted physical activity or reduced athletic performance. The latter patients need to understand the immediate risks of surgery versus its long-term benefits and also that few valvular repair procedures produce the performance characteristics of a normal native valve. In the final analysis there is no substitute for a sympathetic explanation and definitive recommendations as to how and why athletes should proceed for their best interest. Second opinions should be recommended if athletes seem reluctant to follow a recommended plan. Referrals and scheduling assistance should be provided to ensure athletes are evaluated by reputable physicians at recognized institutions.

CARDIAC EXAMINATION

A complete description of the cardiac examination of athletes is beyond the scope of this chapter. The following section emphasizes clinical principles useful in evaluating athletes for suspected valvular disease.

The examination of athletes with possible valvular disease is more complete than the often cursory examination routinely performed as part of the preparticipation physical. All cardiac evaluations should start with an accurate blood pressure measurement in both arms. The blood pressure should be measured by someone trained to avoid the digit selection and rounding to 10s that is common in most blood pressure "determinations." The average systolic pressure is several millimeters higher in the right arm probably because of the more direct course of the pulse wave to the inominate and right subclavian arteries. A systolic pressure > 15 mm higher in the right arm if associated with a systolic ejection murmur suggests supravalvular aortic stenosis,[8] which is an occasional cause of exercise-related sudden cardiac death.[3] A widened pulse pressure suggests a regurgitant murmur such as aortic insufficiency. The high-pitched diastolic murmur of aortic insufficiency can be difficult to hear without special attention, but a pulse pressure > 40 mmHg should prompt a careful search for this murmur with the patient leaning forward and holding his or her breath at end expiration. The aortic insufficiency murmur is often best heard over the sternum because bone transmits the high-frequency murmur more readily.

Elevated blood pressure in a young athlete requires simultaneous palpation of the radial and femoral pulses to exclude a radial-femoral pulse delay suggestive of aortic coarctation. It is often incorrectly assumed that the mere presence of a femoral pulse excludes coarctation, but some patients can reconstitute a palpable femoral pulse via collaterals. In these patients it is the delayed impulse between the radial or brachial and femoral pulse that suggests the diagnosis.[9]

Evaluating the carotid pulse is the most important palpation maneuver in athletes because aortic stenosis remains a frequent, easily identified cause of sudden cardiac death. A carotid pulse that is low volume, has a slow upstroke, or is difficult to locate should increase suspicion of important aortic stenosis.

Cardiac auscultation is an important part of evaluating valvular disease in athletes even in the present era of echocardiography. It is possible to both over- and underestimate the severity of valvular lesions with either echocardiography or the physical examination. The best decisions are made when the results of several examination techniques are compared for agreement or discrepancies. The physician should avoid relying exclusively on clinical, echocardiographic, or catheterization data alone. Consequently, the physical examination is a key component both in deciding who requires further study and in evaluating the additional data.

During cardiac auscultation, the examiner should ignore any obvious murmur and proceed with a sequential systematic examination of the heart sounds, possible gallops and clicks, diastolic murmurs, and finally systolic murmurs. If too much attention is given initially to any obvious finding, such as a systolic murmur, it is often difficult to appreciate more subtle findings that can contribute to the correct diagnosis. The auscultatory examination should start with an assessment of the intensity of S_1, which is produced by closure of the mitral and tricuspid valves. The intensity of S_1 is partly determined by the degree of leaflet separation at the onset of ventricular contraction. If the leaflets are widely separated to accommodate delayed ventricular filling such as with mitral stenosis, the valve leaflets travel farther at the onset of systole and S_1 is loud. In contrast, if the leaflets have been partially closed by the regurgitant jet of aortic insufficiency, S_1 is soft. Both aortic insufficiency and isolated mitral stenosis are notoriously difficult to hear and often require special maneuvers. The intensity of S_1 helps indicate when these additional maneuvers are required.

S_2 is produced by closure of the aortic followed by the pulmonic valves. During inspiration filling of the right ventricle is augmented. The larger volume of blood in the right ventricle shifts the intraventricular septum leftward, compromises left ventricle filling, and reduces the left ventricular stroke volume.[10] This hastens aortic closure so that the aortic valve closes earlier in the cardiac cycle during inspiration. On the right side, the larger right ventricular volume delays pulmonic valve closure. Both the earlier aortic closure and the delayed pulmonic closure increase the splitting of S_2 during inspiration. This is best appreciated in the seated position. In the supine position venous return from the legs can nearly maximize right ventricular filling so that any additional increase in the splitting of S_2 is difficult to detect. This is especially true in endurance athletes whose plasma volume can average 800 ml larger than in comparison subjects.[11] Part of this increased plasma volume shifts to the central circulation in the supine position. During the expiratory phase of the cardiac cycle, aortic and pulmonic closure occurs almost simultaneously and S_2 should be single or nearly so. If there is an intracardiac connection between the right and left sides of the heart such as an atrial septal defect, there is no or little differential in right and left cardiac filling during respiration. Right ventricular filling is also increased from left to right intracardiac shunting, which increases the right ventricular stroke volume. S_2, therefore, is often widely split, does not move during respiration, and fails to close during expiration. Atrial septal defects often are accompanied by a systolic murmur that has many of the characteristics of a pulmonic flow murmur. The behavior of S_2 is useful in separating these two conditions.

The examiner should then listen in diastole for an S_3 or S_4 gallop and in systole for any ejection clicks suggestive of pulmonic or aortic valvular stenosis or for any midsystolic clicks suggestive of mitral valve prolapse. Many athletes have S_3 and S_4 gallops, which are of no importance unless the gallops are loud or associated with other abnormalities. The examiner should then listen in diastole for the murmurs of aortic insufficiency and mitral stenosis and finally to any systolic murmurs. Systole should be examined last because these murmurs are usually the most obvious.

The initial auscultatory exam is performed with the athlete seated. As discussed previously, this reduces the chance of producing a flow murmur, facilitates hearing aortic insufficiency, and maximizes splitting of the second sound. In addition, the upright position reduces ventricular volume and increases the chance of detecting a murmur in obstructive hypertrophic cardiomyopathy. The sequence of auscultation is then repeated in the supine and left lateral positions. The later position facilitates detecting the murmurs of mitral stenosis and regurgitation. If there is any suspicion of either hypertrophic cardiomyopathy or mitral valve prolapse, the athletes should also be examined standing and squatting. Variations in ventricular volume alter the timing of midsystolic clicks in mitral valve prolapse and thereby facilitate its identification. Squatting increases ventricular afterload, which decrease the murmur of obstructive hypertrophic cardiomyopathy, whereas standing often increases the murmur if obstruction is present.

The electrocardiogram (ECG) in athletes is often not very useful in following athletes with valvular abnormalities because athletes may normally show evidence of right ventricular and left ventricular enlargement, T-wave abnormalities, and atrial abnormalities. Nevertheless, the ECG is a low-cost alternative in following asymptomatic or mildly symptomatic athletes between routine echocardiographic studies. Charting the ECG voltage in leads V_5 and V_6, as well as the T-wave configuration in athletes with aortic insufficiency or mitral regurgitation, helps identify changes in the cardiac status. Any changes in ECG voltage or T-wave orientation should prompt repeat echocardiographic examination to ensure that the lesion has not progressed unexpectedly.

Doppler echocardiography is the primary mechanism used to both evaluate valvular lesions at presentation and follow these conditions over time. Most cardiologists routinely refer athletes with possible valvular involvement for echocardiography unless the murmur is unquestionably a flow murmur on careful physical examination. Flow murmurs both in young and older athletes are generally grade 1 or 2 in intensity, systolic, associated with normal splitting of S_2, not associated with other abnormal sounds or diastolic murmurs, and not altered by the Valsalva maneuver.[7] The major limitation with Doppler echocardiography is that it is often too sensitive and detects trivial mitral regurgitation in 69% of athletes and trivial tricuspid regurgitation in 76%.[12] Physicians unaware of this fact and uncertain of the findings on physical examination may overestimate the importance of the echocardiographic results.

MANAGEMENT

The American College of Cardiology and the American Heart Association published "Guidelines for the Management of Patients with Valvular Heart Disease" in 1998.[7] This document provides an excellent summary[7] on how to manage this problem in the general patient. "Recommendations for Determining Eligibility for Competition in Athletes with Cardiovascular Abnormalities, the 26th Bethesda Conference" were published by the same two organizations in 1994 and included a section on athletes with acquired valvular heart disease.[13] The following section will summarize issues from these two documents and provide additional information relevant to physicians caring for athletes.

VALVULAR AORTIC STENOSIS

Valvular aortic stenosis remains a frequent cause of exertion-related sudden death in young athletes and an occasional cause of exercise-related deaths in adults. The normal aortic valve orifice is approximately 3 to 4 cm^2 and must be reduced by 75% of normal before causing significant hemodynamic obstruction.[7] Mild aortic stenosis is classified as an aortic valve area > 1.5, moderate as 1–1.5, and severe as < 1.0 cm^2. Severe aortic stenosis should produce a mean resting gradient of at least 50 mmHg if cardiac output is normal. These values are not normalized for body surface area. The hemodynamic significance of any specified aortic valve area depends on the cardiac output. Since muscle mass is a determinant of resting cardiac output, larger individuals may have more severe hemodynamic impairment despite a larger absolute aortic valve area. This may be an issue in athletes with an increased body size and muscle mass. Consequently, the calculated aortic valve area and classification of the severity of dis-

ease should be considered as only estimates and must be correlated with other findings.

Aortic stenosis is typified by a long asymptomatic period. Common symptoms of severe aortic stenosis when they do occur include angina, syncope or near-syncope, and heart failure. Sudden cardiac death may also be the first symptom, but this is rare. This presentation is more frequent in younger subjects with congenital aortic stenosis, but does occur in adults. The incidence of sudden death without prior symptoms is estimated to be < 1% of aortic stenosis patients per year.[7] The rate of narrowing of the aortic valve in individual patients is highly variable and unpredictable. Over 50% of patients with aortic stenosis show little or no progression over 3 to 9 years, but the average rate of aortic valve narrowing is 0.12 cm^2 per year.[7] Consequently, patients with aortic stenosis, once identified, require careful follow-up.

The initial evaluation of aortic stenosis patients requires a physical examination, ECG, and Doppler echocardiographic study. Estimation of the severity of aortic stenosis is based on an evaluation of the results from all 3 examination modalities, although the aortic valve area is based primarily on Doppler echocardiographic results. Cardiac catheterization is required to help clarify the severity of the aortic stenosis if the noninvasive testing and clinical evaluations are contradictory. Even cardiac catheterization can incorrectly assess the aortic valve area especially if the oxygen uptake value used to calculate the Fick cardiac output is estimated from body size and not directly measured by expired gas collection. In addition, the degree of stenosis can be overestimated by gradient calculations with concomitant aortic insufficiency since the regurgitant volume increases stroke volume beyond that measured by the Fick calculation as forward flow. Coronary angiography is required before valve surgery to detect any coronary artery disease.

Athletes with mild aortic stenosis can participate in all competitive sports if they are asymptomatic and have a normal exercise response.[13] Athletes with moderate aortic stenosis should be restricted to sports with low static and dynamic requirements (see Table 13.4 for examples of intensity classifications), although selected athletes can participate in moderate static and dynamic intensity sports provided they have a normal ST segment, cardiac rhythm, and blood pressure response to exercise testing and they are not symptomatic. Athletes with severe aortic stenosis should be restricted from competitive athletics even if they are asymptomatic. Exercise testing in these athletes is useful in documenting that they are truly without symptoms and in ensuring that they do not develop exercise-induced hypotension. Exercise-induced hypotension is a bad prognostic sign and should prompt consideration for aortic valve surgery even in the absence of symptoms.

Aortic valve replacement is advocated for patients with severe aortic stenosis once symptoms appear. This decision can be more difficult in athletes; they are at an undefined, but definite risk of sudden death during exercise, and they may present with symptoms earlier in their disease course because vigorous exercise provokes symptoms. There are no studies to address the issue as to whether valve replacement can be delayed if symptoms occur only with extreme exertion. Clinicians must balance the immediate and delayed risk of valve replacement against the risks of not proceeding. Despite such considerations, our bias is to proceed fairly promptly to surgery in athletes with severe aortic stenosis at the onset of symptoms. There is little additional benefit to waiting since surgery is inevitable in this situation. Also, there is the risk inherent in waiting and the possibility that left ventricular hypertrophy will develop or worsen. Left ventricular hypertrophy is in its own right a risk factor for sudden cardiac death in the general population and among athletes.[14]

The decision is considerably more complex in athletes who are asymptomatic and yet have severe aortic stenosis. It is generally thought that the immediate risk of surgery and the risks associated with a valvular prosthesis, such as anticoagulation, outweigh the benefits of proceeding.

Among the asymptomatic patient group, those with exercise-induced hypotension, systolic dysfunction, and marked left ventricular hypertrophy are probably at increased risk and should be considered for valve replacement. Some experts also consider exercise ST depression to represent an additional risk factor and suggest that sudden death is extremely rare in children with aortic stenosis who have no ST depression with exercise.[15] Asymptomatic athletes with severe aortic stenosis should undergo exercise testing to document their lack of symptoms and should be restricted from competing and training. This author's bias even in these asymptomatic athletes is to proceed to aortic valve replacement in the near future for the following reasons: surgery has relatively low risk in healthy subjects; prolonged pressure overload has deleterious effects on the left ventricle; and many active patients are reluctant to avoid vigorous exercise for a prolonged period of time.

CHRONIC AORTIC INSUFFICIENCY

Chronic aortic insufficiency can be well tolerated for decades, but many patients with moderate and severe regurgitation experience a gradual progression from normal to abnormal left ventricular function characterized by left ventricular enlargement, reduced contractility, and decreased ejection fraction. Most patients developing left ventricular dysfunction present with early symptoms of heart failure including exercise intolerance, dyspnea, and exercise-induced presyncope before left ventricular function is severe. Some patients, however, do not develop sentinel symptoms and present with marked left ventricular enlargement and a severely dysfunctional left ventricle.[7]

Early in the course of left ventricular dysfunction the left ventricle can recover after aortic valve replacement probably because the dysfunction was primarily due to volume overload. If the volume overload has been persistent and produced severe chamber enlargement with left ventricular dysfunction, the myocardial dysfunction is not wholly reversible despite correction of the valvular lesion. Consequently, the severity of left ventricular dilatation and dysfunction are the key determinants of postoperative ventricular function and survival.

Athletes with aortic insufficiency should be carefully questioned for exercise-induced signs of early heart failure. The physical examination should include a search for stigmata of Marfan syndrome since many Marfan patients have important aortic insufficiency. They should also have a baseline ECG, echocardiogram with careful measurement of left ventricular and left atrial diameters, and an exercise stress test. The baseline ECG is used to evaluate left ventricular voltage and T-wave changes over time. The exercise test is to document functional capacity and the absence of symptoms and exercise-induced arrhythmia. It is useful to chart the ECG voltage and T waves in leads II, aV_L, V_5, and V_6, as well as the echocardiographic left ventricular and left atrial dimensions. These can then be followed sequentially for evidence of early left ventricular dysfunction.

The general population of patients with moderate-to-severe aortic insufficiency, no symptoms, and normal left ventricular function has a reasonably good near-term prognosis. Among 7 studies including 490 patients who were followed for a mean of 6.4 years, sudden death occurred in only 6 and progression to symptoms or left ventricular dysfunction occurred at a rate of 4.3% per annum.[7] This is not a trivial rate of progression, however, since 21% of patients worsened over 5 years. It is not clear how exercise training would affect these results. Dynamic exercise acutely increases heart rate, which shortens diastole and the time available for aortic regurgitation. In contrast, exercise training in normal people induces bradycardia, which prolongs aortic insufficiency and theoretically hastens left ventricular dysfunction. This author is unaware of studies that have examined the effects of endurance training in aortic insufficiency patients so the ultimate effect of athletic training and competition on aortic insufficiency has not been determined. Patients with important aortic insufficiency are routinely advised to avoid static exertion because the increased afterload acutely increases aortic regurgitation, although whether static effort actually affects prognosis has not been examined.

Athletes with mild or moderate aortic insufficiency, minimal left ventricular enlargement, and normal left ventricular function can participate in all sports.[13] They should be cautioned to report any new symptoms. They should have a repeat echocardiogram 6 to 12 months after the initial visit to document disease stability and then every 2 to 3 years thereafter.[7]

Selected athletes with moderate aortic insufficiency and moderate left ventricular enlargement can participate in sports requiring moderate static and high dynamic effort.[13] These patients should also be cautioned to report new symptoms, have a repeat echocardiogram 6 months after the initial visit to document stability, and have repeat evaluations yearly thereafter.[7]

Asymptomatic athletes with severe aortic insufficiency should be restricted from competition and training and followed closely.[13] They should have a repeat echocardiogram 3 months after the initial visit and every 6 to 12 months subsequently. Asymptomatic athletes with moderate-to-severe aortic insufficiency and left ventricular dysfunction or marked dilatation due to the aortic insufficiency should undergo valve replacement.[7] *Left ventricular dysfunction* is defined as an ejection fraction (LVEF) of < 50%.[7] *Marked enlargement* is defined as a left ventricular end-diastolic volume > 75 mm or an end-systolic volume > 55.[7] Women with aortic insufficiency develop symptoms with less severe left ventricular dysfunction and enlargement than do men,[7] suggesting that smaller individuals may require valve replacement at smaller ventricular volumes. Aortic valve replacement should be strongly considered if there is progressive left ventricular dilation and dysfunction in asymptomatic patients even if the left ventricle does not achieve the preceding parameters. An LVEF of 50% already represents considerable left ventricular dysfunction in aortic insufficiency patients because the normal ventricular response to aortic insufficiency is to increase the LVEF above the normal 55 to 65%. Also, once the left ventricle is markedly dilated, there is the possibility that the left ventricle has been permanently altered and will not return to normal function.

Athletes with severe aortic insufficiency who are symptomatic should undergo aortic valve replacement. The timing of the aortic valve replacement can be varied depending on the effort level required to produce symptoms, as well as left ventricular function and dimensions.

It is generally recommended that patients with moderate-to-severe aortic insufficiency and systolic hypertension should be treated with afterload-reducing agents such as hydralazine, nifedipine, or angiotensin-converting enzyme (ACE) inhibitors to achieve a normal systolic pressure. There is no conclusive evidence that treating normotensive patients with aortic insufficiency is beneficial. Nevertheless, the present author routinely places patients with moderate-to-severe aortic insufficiency on ACE inhibitors in the hope of delaying the development of left ventricular dysfunction.

AORTIC VALVE REPLACEMENT IN ATHLETES

The management of athletes after valvular replacement was discussed in the 26th Bethesda Conference.[13] In general, athletes with normal left ventricular function after aortic valve replacement can participate in low-intensity sports, with selected athletes participating in moderate intensity static and dynamic sports. Athletes taking anticoagulants should not engage in sports with any risk of bodily contact. These recommendations[13] reflect concern about the aortic valve replacement techniques commonly available at that time. Until recently, nearly all aortic valve replacements were performed using a porcine heterograph, a cadaveric homograph, or a mechanical prosthesis. The mechanical prostheses required life-long anticoagulation and had an effective valve area of only 1.2 to 3.2 cm^2.[16] Both heterographs and homographs required anticoagulation for only 3

months unless there were other factors predisposing to systemic embolization. Unfortunately, the techniques to preserve these bioprostheses affected their durability, and 30% of heterographs and 10 to 20% of homographs had to be replaced in 10 to 20 years.[16] Bioprosthesis failure was most frequent in patients under age 40 years.[16]

In 1967, Ross described an autograft approach to aortic valve replacement in which the normal pulmonic valve was used to replace the diseased aortic valve. There was a fairly high early mortality rate to the operation of 7.4% over the first 24 years of its use.[17] Ross attributed this to the steep learning curve required for the operation.[17] In 1976, the procedure was altered to using the pulmonic valve with the pulmonic trunk in the replacement. This advancement eliminated many of the technical problems inherent in the earlier technique and helped reduce the current mortality rate to < 1%.[17] The Ross procedure has multiple advantages over other aortic valve replacement techniques. The tissue used is viable because it is not subjected to sterilization and preservation procedures required for heterographs and homographs. This viability means that the replacement should last indefinitely, and the new aortic root can actually enlarge with somatic growth of the child.[18] As with heterografts and homografts, long-term anticoagulation is not required and the hemodynamic performance of the autograft is equal or superior to all other replacements.[17] These advantages have lead many surgeons to conclude that the Ross procedure is the treatment of choice in otherwise healthy subjects with more than a 20-year life expectancy.[17] The procedure is especially attractive in athletes. Several high-profile athletes have competed successfully after a Ross replacement including Jesse Sapolo, the center of the San Francisco 49ers American football team.[19]

There are limitations to this operation. It is not indicated for Marfan syndrome patients or other patients with connective tissue disorders since the same process could affect the pulmonic valve in the aortic position. The operation is complicated and quite often long since it is really a "double valve procedure for a single valve disease"[17] and in addition requires reimplantation of the coronary arteries into the autograft. Finally, it has not been widely used and few surgeons have extensive experience with the technique. It is not clear that the excellent published mortality results will be replicated by less experienced surgeons. Nevertheless, if performed by an experienced operating team, the Ross procedure is probably the aortic valve replacement of choice for children, physiologically young adults, and athletes.

MITRAL STENOSIS

Mitral stenosis is almost always a consequence of rheumatic fever. Severe mitral stenosis is rarely seen in competitive athletes. The increase in heart rate with exercise decreases the ventricular diastolic filling time, increasing left atrial, pulmonary capillary wedge, and pulmonary artery pressures. This produces exercise dyspnea and, rarely, exercise-induced pulmonary edema.

Once mitral stenosis is suspected, the evaluation as to the severity is primarily based on symptoms and Doppler echocardiographic results. Doppler echocardiography can accurately estimate mitral valve area in isolated mitral stenosis and can also estimate pulmonary artery systolic pressure from the velocity of the tricuspid regurgitant jet. The same technique can be used with exercise to determine changes in pulmonary artery pressure with exertion. The echocardiographic study is also used to evaluate the approach to operative intervention. Catheter valvotomy using a venous approach across the atrial septum is often possible if the mitral leaflets are pliable and have minimal subvalvular commissural fusion.[7] A mitral valve that appears favorable to percutaneous valvotomy generally permits a more aggressive approach in patients with Doppler evidence of important mitral stenosis and mild symptoms.

The normal mitral valve area is 4 to 5 cm^2 (Table 14.1). A reduction to 2.5 cm^2 is required for symptoms.[7]

TABLE 14.1.   CLASSIFICATION OF MITRAL STENOSIS

Severity	Valve Area (cm^2)	Pulmonary Arterial Systolic Pressure (mmHg)
Mild	> 1.5	< 35
Moderate	1.1–1.4	< 50
Severe	< 1.1	> 50

Adapted with permission from Cheitlin MD, Douglas PS, Parmley WW: 26th Bethesda Conference: Recommendations for determining eligibility for competition in athletes with cardiovascular abnormalities. Task Force 2: Acquired valvular heart disease. *J Am Coll Cardiol* 24, 1994, pp. 874–880.

The Bethesda Conference recommends that athletes in normal sinus rhythm with mild mitral stenosis and no symptoms can participate in all sports.[13] Athletes with mild mitral stenosis and atrial fibrillation or with moderate mitral stenosis can participate in moderate static and dynamic sports as long as their exercise pulmonary systolic pressure remains below 50 mmHg. If the pulmonary pressure exceeds 50, these athletes should be restricted to moderate static and low dynamic sports. Patients with moderate or severe mitral stenosis plus symptoms on moderate exertion should be considered for percutaneous valvotomy if they have suitable anatomy or open valve repair or replacement if their anatomy appears unfavorable for a percutaneous approach.[7] Athletes with mild mitral stenosis and symptoms appearing with vigorous exertion could also be considered for percutaneous valve repair depending on the clinical circumstances. There is no evidence that this will improve their long-term prognosis. It is also possible that percutaneous valvotomy will produce significant mitral regurgitation and make a minimally symptomatic patient more symptomatic.

CHRONIC MITRAL REGURGITATION

In contrast to mitral stenosis, the common etiologies of chronic mitral regurgitation are multiple and include mitral valve prolapse, healed endocarditis, rheumatic heart disease, Marfan syndrome, and ischemic papillary muscle dysfunction. The left ventricle adapts to chronic mitral regurgitation by increasing its end-diastolic volume, but sustained volume overload in severe mitral regurgitation eventually leads to left ventricular systolic dysfunction. The left ventricle afterload in chronic mitral regurgitation is reduced because the left ventricle can "unload" into the relatively low-resistance left atrium. This reduced afterload can mask left ventricular dysfunction because the LVEF may be near normal. In chronic mitral regurgitation, however, the "normal" LVEF should be in excess of 60%. Mitral valve repair or replacement removes this low pressure escape for left ventricular ejection and may unmask a dysfunctional left ventricle.

Survival after mitral valve repair is reduced in patients whose preoperative LVEF is < 60%.[7]

The evaluation of patients with mitral regurgitation includes a history, physical examination, ECG, Doppler echocardiogram, and stress test. The history and exercise test should attempt to elicit symptoms of early heart failure since there is consensus that patients with symptoms should proceed to corrective surgery. Doppler echocardiography study is useful in defining left ventricular dimensions and performance, left atrial size, pulmonary systolic pressure, and the severity of the mitral regurgitation (Fig. 14.1). The Doppler echocardiographic study alone is not sufficient to determine the mitral regurgitation severity since the regurgitant jet can be missed and the interpre-

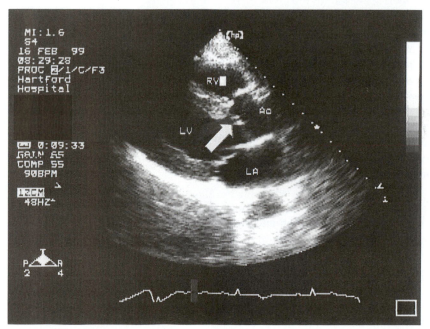

FIGURE 14.1. Long axis echocardiogram. The arrow points to eccentric aortic valve leaflets. The leaflet closure should be central, and the eccentricity is suggestive of a bicuspid aortic valve. The Doppler study revealed moderate aortic regurgitation. RV, right ventricle; Ao, aortic root; LV, left ventricular chamber; LA, left atrium. The patient was asymptomatic with left ventricular end-diastolic and systolic dimensions of 58 and 39 mm, respectively. He was treated with quinapril 10 mg daily and is followed with yearly echocardiograms.

tation is somewhat subjective. Consequently, the results of the echocardiography should be correlated with other findings. An exercise echocardiographic study may be especially useful in athletes with symptoms and mild-to-moderate mitral regurgitation at rest. The increased heart rate during exercise increases the frequency of regurgitation and decreases left ventricle diastolic filling time. Both factors may increase exercise pulmonary pressure and account for the symptoms.

Symptomatic athletes with moderate or severe mitral regurgitation should undergo corrective surgery. The timing of the operation can vary depending on the severity of the symptoms and cardiac dysfunction, but there is little benefit in waiting once symptoms have appeared and can be unequivocally attributed to the mitral regurgitation. Asymptomatic athletes with normal sinus rhythm and normal left ventricular function may participate in all sports.[13] They should have a repeat echocardiography in 6 months to document stability of the mitral regurgitation and then every 1 to 2 years thereafter. Asymptomatic athletes with normal left ventricular function and mild left ventricular enlargement can participate in moderate static and moderate dynamic activities. Selected athletes with these characteristics can participate in all sports. All patients with mild left ventricular enlargement should have echocardiography performed in 3 months to establish a stable clinical course and then yearly thereafter.

Mitral valve repair is the procedure of choice since it avoids long-term anticoagulation and preserves the mitral valve apparatus. Preserving the papillary muscles and chordal structures helps preserve left ventricular function.[7] The next best choice is valve replacement preserving the valve apparatus.

Athletes with left ventricular dysfunction or significant left ventricular enlargement should proceed to corrective surgery. The standard criteria for left ventricular function and surgical repair are an LVEF < 60% or a left ventricle end-systolic diameter > 45 mm.[7] Nevertheless, athletes with progressive increases in their left ventricular dimensions or decreases in LVEF should also be referred for surgery. Many centers recommend mitral repair for severe mitral regurgitation even in asymptomatic patients without left ventricular changes if there is a high chance the valve can be repaired.[20] Similarly, some centers strongly consider mitral valve surgery if atrial fibrillation has occurred even transiently.[7] The appearance of atrial fibrillation indicates left atrial dysfunction. Atrial fibrillation may also become permanent if the left atrium continues to face a volume and pressure overload. Chronic atrial fibrillation requires long-term anticoagulation, thereby eliminating one of the benefits of valvular repair.

The decision to intervene in severe mitral regurgitation with no or minimal symptoms depends greatly on the skill of the surgeon in valve repair. Valve repair has many benefits over replacement, but failure of the repair almost always leads to replacement. Consequently, the ability of available surgeons influences the decision when to proceed to surgery.

There is only theoretical support for the use of afterload reducing agents in normotensive patients with moderate-to-severe mitral regurgitation. Despite this, this author routinely recommends ACE inhibitors to such patients in the hope of preserving normal left ventricular function until corrective surgery.

EXERCISE AFTER MITRAL
VALVE SURGERY

Athletes with mitral valve replacements with normal ventricular function who are not taking anticoagulant medications can participate in moderate dynamic and static sports.[13] Athletes on anticoagulant medications should avoid sports with a high risk of bodily collision.[13] Athletes who have undergone mitral valve repair can participate in all competitive sports if they have no or minimal mitral regurgitation and normal left ventricular function. Since many of the young athletes who require mitral repair have mitral valve prolapse and since bodily collision can rupture elongated chordae tendinae, this author prohibits contact sports in mitral valve prolapse patients who have undergone valvular repair.

MITRAL VALVE PROLAPSE

Mitral valve prolapse (MVP) is the most common cause of significant mitral regurgitation in the United States and affects approximately 4 to 6% of the population.[7] Mitral valve prolapse has also been one of the most frequently overdiagnosed cardiac conditions, although this is changing with the use of stricter diagnostic echocardiographic criteria. The prognosis of MVP is generally benign. It is a rare cause of sudden cardiac death in the general population and responsible for only 1% of exercise-related cardiac deaths among high school and college athletes.[3] Atypical chest discomfort is a common complaint in individuals eventually diagnosed with mitral valve prolapse, but rarely has important sequelae. Palpitations from premature atrial or ventricular beats are also frequent in MVP patients. The important cardiac complications associated with MVP include cardiac arrhythmia, syncope, and sudden death; endocarditis; and significant mitral regurgitation usually produced by chordal rupture. Neurological events can also occur in MVP patients probably from cardiac emboli.[21,22] The serious cardiac complications are more frequent in patients with extensive valvular pathology including redundant and thickened valve leaflets, a systolic murmur, and left atrial enlargement.[23,24]

Mitral valve prolapse is usually detected during a routine physical examination or in patients undergoing echocardiography as part of an evaluation for chest pain or palpitations. The characteristic auscultatory findings include a midsystolic click and/or a late systolic murmur. Classically, the click and murmur are variable with position, respiration, and other maneuvers. This variability often leads to the diagnosis. Maneuvers that reduce ventricular volume such as standing move the click and the start of the murmur earlier in systole, whereas maneuvers that increase ventricular volume delay the onset of the click and murmur. Since MVP is common in Marfan syndrome, the physical examination of patients with MVP should include a search for stigmata of this condition. There is no requirement for echocardiographic confirmation of MVP if the findings are classic, the murmur does not indicate severe regurgitation, and the patient is asymptomatic. Some authorities recommend echocardiography in all subjects to detect valvular abnormalities associated with a more serious prognosis.[7] If echocardiography is performed at baseline, patients with moderate mitral regurgitation, left atrial enlargement, and thick or redundant leaflets should have the study repeated at 1 to 2 year intervals. Patients without evidence of serious valvular pathology should be restudied approximately every 5 years.

The management of athletes with MVP depends on the severity of the mitral regurgitation, the presence of symptoms, and the pathologic appearance of the valve. Athletes with moderate or severe mitral regurgitation should be evaluated and followed as discussed in the section, "Chronic Mitral Regurgitation." According to the Bethesda Conference,[25] the athlete with uncomplicated MVP can participate in all competitive sports. Athletes with MVP and arrhythmogenic syncope, a family history of sudden cardiac death associated with MVP, repetitive supraventricular or ventricular arrhythmia, or prior embolic events should be restricted to low-intensity dynamic and static sports.[25] Athletes with supraventricular arrhythmia can usually be well-managed with low-dose β-adrenergic blockade or with a strong chronotropic calcium channel blocker such as verapamil. Athletes with nonthreatening ventricular arrhythmia can similarly be managed with beta blockade. Such athletes should undergo exercise stress testing and should be cautioned to report any change in symptoms. The general recommendation is that patients with MVP and prior neurological events should be placed on aspirin therapy.[7] Although the risk of a stroke is extremely low, this author recommends that all patients with MVP use at least an 80-mg aspirin daily. The cost and risk of aspirin therapy is low, and the potential benefit is great.

TRICUSPID REGURGITATION AND TRICUSPID STENOSIS

Trivial tricuspid regurgitation may be detected by Doppler echocardiography in up to 76% of athletes and is not associated with any valvular pathology.[12] The most frequent cause of important tricuspid regurgitation among young adults in most medical centers is valvular damage secondary to acute endocarditis associated with intravenous drug use.[7] Congenital valvular abnormalities are the most frequent cause of tricuspid regurgitation in children and are often produced by Ebstein's anomaly of the tricuspid valve. Tricuspid regurgitation can also be caused by rheumatic heart disease and by right ventricular dilatation from volume or pressure overload. There is no evidence that isolated tricuspid regurgitation increases the risk of exercise and the effect of exercise training on the prognosis in tricuspid regurgitation has not been examined. Nevertheless, athletes with isolated tricuspid regurgitation and without markedly elevated right atrial pressures determined by neck vein examination can participate in all sports.

Tricuspid stenosis is generally produced by rheumatic fever and is almost always associated with mitral stenosis. Recommendations for sports participation in athletes with tricuspid regurgitation and mitral stenosis should be based on the severity of the mitral stenosis.

PULMONIC STENOSIS AND PULMONIC REGURGITATION

Valvular pulmonic stenosis and pulmonic regurgitation are almost always congenital in origin. Children and adolescents with pulmonic stenosis are often asymptomatic even with severe obstruction.[7] Adults and some children may have symptoms of exertional dyspnea, syncope, and presyncope although exercise-related sudden death is rare. Doppler echocardiography is used to determine the severity of pulmonic stenosis. A peak pulmonary valve gradient < 40 mmHg implies mild pulmonic stenosis. Peak values of 40 to 70 mmHg indicate moderate pulmonic stenosis and > 70 mmHg indicates severe pulmonic stenosis.[26]

Athletes with peak systolic gradient < 50 and normal right ventricular function can participate in all sports.[26] They should be reevaluated annually and undergo repeat echocardiographic studies every 2 to 3 years. Athletes with gradients > 50 should be referred for valvuloplasty.

Pulmonic regurgitation is usually due to congenital idiopathic dilation of the pulmonary artery.[7] Symptoms or exercise limitations are unusual from pulmonic regurgitation alone, although a rare patient may develop right ventricular enlargement and require pulmonic valve replacement. No exercise restrictions are placed on asymptomatic athletes with pulmonic regurgitation.

OTHER CONSIDERATIONS

ENDOCARDITIS PROPHYLAXIS

Subacute bacterial endocarditis is most frequent in valvular lesions where high velocity blood flow enters a lower pressure chamber. High velocity flow into a lower pressure chamber disrupts laminar blood flow and creates areas of platelet, fibrin, and bacterial deposition. This physiological profile applies to all of the valvular lesions discussed earlier with the exception of pure mitral stenosis. Antibiotic endocarditis prophylaxis should be prescribed for all athletes with valvular heart disease. The only exception is in athletes with tricuspid or pulmonic regurgitation when a murmur is not detected. Right-sided pressures are lower than left-sided pressures, which reduces the risk of bacterial deposition. Furthermore, tricuspid and pulmonary regurgitation detected only by Doppler is common. This author provides athletes with the wallet-sized instruction cards available in bulk at minimal cost from the Heart Association, 7272 Greenville Avenue, Dallas, TX 75231-4596.

The role of endocarditis prophylaxis in MVP has been controversial. Antibiotic prophylaxis is generally recommended only if a murmur is present.[7] In patients with only a midsystolic click, the general recommendation is to use endocarditis prophylaxis only in the presence of signs of severe valvular pathology as discussed earlier.[7] This author's approach is to place all patients with definite MVP on endocarditis prophylaxis before procedures associated with bacteremia. Mitral regurgitation is often intermittent in patients with MVP and can be missed on a single examination. Also as many as 33% of patients with MVP, but without mitral regurgitation at rest, can induce mitral regurgitation with exercise.[27] The cost and risk of endocarditis prophylaxis in MVP patients is small and the potential benefit, if endocarditis is prevented, great.

RHEUMATIC FEVER PROPHYLAXIS

Guidelines for the prevention of rheumatic fever have been published.[28] Rheumatic fever prophylaxis is extremely important in patients who have had rheumatic carditis. Recurrent episodes of rheumatic carditis exacerbate the valvular injury, increase the severity of the valvular lesion and may hasten the need for valvular surgery. Patients with prior rheumatic fever who develop streptococcal pharyngitis are at high risk for recurrent rheumatic fever, and the infection need not be symptomatic to restart the carditis. Also, rheumatic fever can occur after a streptococcal infection even when the infection is treated promptly and correctly. Individuals exposed to groups, such as athletes on athletic teams and their coaches, are more likely to acquire a streptococcal infection. For all of these reasons, any athlete or coach with documented rheumatic valvular disease should receive antibiotic prophylaxis until at least age 40 and probably for life if the athlete continues to be exposed to groups of athletes.

The best prophylactic treatment is 1.2 million U of benzathine penicillin G intramuscularly every 3 weeks.[28] Oral treatment with 250 mg of penicillin V twice a day is acceptable, but much less dependable as a prophylaxis because of reduced compliance. Patients allergic to penicillin can be treated with sulfadiazine 1 g daily or erythromycin 250 mg twice daily. Erythromycin

is usually a better choice in athletes because of the photosensitivity that can occur with sulfur containing compounds.

SUMMARY

Knowledge of the evaluation and management of active individuals with valvular heart disease is a critical component of sports cardiology. Valvular aortic stenosis continues to account for approximately 4% of exercise-related sudden deaths among young athletes. The presence of a cardiac murmur or the possibility of cardiac symptoms among young athletes is a frequent reason for cardiac referral. The most common cause of cardiac murmurs in athletes is a flow murmur across the pulmonic valve related to the cardiovascular adaptations that occur with exercise training. In adults, physiological flow murmurs are often related to aortic sclerosis, but this condition may not be as benign as flow murmurs in children because aortic sclerosis is accompanied by other risk factors for atherosclerosis such as hyperlipidemia.

Severe aortic stenosis may present with exercise-induced syncope, angina, heart failure, and, rarely, sudden death. Athletes with severe aortic stenosis should be restricted from competition and encouraged to undergo aortic valve replacement. Active subjects with moderate-to-severe aortic insufficiency require careful follow-up and periodic echocardiograms to detect early signs of heart failure or progressive left ventricular dilatation. Surgical repair should be performed with the onset of symptoms, marked cardiac enlargement, or progressive left ventricular dilatation. Athletes with moderate or severe mitral regurgitation should be followed in a fashion similar to that for aortic insufficiency and repair performed for symptoms or progressive left ventricular dilatation. Active individuals with mitral stenosis should undergo mitral valvuloplasty with the onset of symptoms. All athletes with valvular heart disease should receive antibiotic prophylaxis for endocarditis. Athletes whose valvular disease is secondary to rheumatic fever should receive streptococcal infection prophylaxis until age 40 or for as long as they are exposed to possible infection.

PERSONAL PERSPECTIVE

Athletes and active people referred for evaluation of valvular abnormalities generally fall into 3 groups: those in whom the examination and additional studies reveal a physiological flow murmur; those with severe valvular disease or symptoms who require valve surgery; and those in whom the decision to proceed with repair or activity restriction is not clear. I find the most useful approach with the last group is to perform a careful history specifically eliciting information about competitive performance changes and subtle exercise intolerance. It is useful in this situation to have had some competitive athletic experience to understand symptoms that are a normal part of athletics. It is also extremely useful in valvular cases to retrieve old echocardiograms and to chart cardiac dimensions over time, since this often reveals progressive chamber enlargement. In most instances this indicates that surgery will be inevitable and that the only issue is when. When there is still doubt with the patient or the physician as to how or when to proceed, one rarely makes a mistake by waiting briefly and following the patient closely. Even in severe aortic stenosis the incidence of unheralded sudden death is rare although I do restrict athletic participation if severe aortic stenosis is possible. Oftentimes, a brief period of delay helps the patient, and even the physician, become more comfortable with the decision. In comparison, if there is no doubt that a valve lesion is severe and will require surgery, I encourage athletes to proceed with repair promptly to allow resumption of as active a lifestyle as possible.

Equally difficult is the decision as to whether patients should have a valve repair or replacement and with which prosthesis or technique. This decision is based on both the patient's wishes, the need for long-term anticoagulation, and, most importantly, on the skill of the surgeon. The physician should never hesitate to refer patients to other institutions when more complex surgery or newer techniques, such as the Ross Procedure, are most appropriate and yet not performed frequently locally.

ACKNOWLEDGMENTS

The author thanks Drs. Daniel Fram and Francis Kiernan who critiqued drafts of the manuscript and Dr. Anita Kelsey who reproduced the echocardiograms.

REFERENCES

1. Jokl E, Melzer L: Acute fatal non-traumatic collapse during work and sport. *MedSport* 5:5–18, 1971.
2. Maron BJ, Shirani J, Poliac LC, et al: Sudden death in young competitive athletes. Clinical, demographic, and pathological profiles. *JAMA* 276:199–204, 1996.
3. Van Camp SP, Bloor C, Mueller FO, et al: Nontraumatic sports death in high school and college athletes. *Med Sci Sports Exerc* 27:641–647, 1995.
4. Barry WH, Grossman W: Cardiac catheterization, in Braunwald E (ed): *Heart Disease: A Textbook of Cardiovascular Medicine.* Philadelphia, WB Saunders, 1980, p. 295.
5. Stewart BF, Siscovick D, Lind BK, et al: Clinical factors associated with calcific aortic valve disease. Cardiovascular Health Study. *J Am Coll Cardiol* 29:630–634, 1997.
6. Wilmshurst PT, Stevenson RN, Griffiths H, et al: A case-control investigation of the relation between hyperlipidaemia and calcific aortic valve stenosis. *Heart* 78:475–479, 1997.
7. Bonow RO, Carabello B, de Leon AC Jr, et al: Guidelines for the management of patients with valvular heart disease: Executive summary. A report of the American College of Cardiology/American Heart Association Task Force on Practice Guidelines (Committee on Management of Patients with Valvular Heart Disease). *Circulation* 98:1949–1984, 1998.
8. Braunwald E: The physical examination, in Braunwald E (ed): *Heart Disease: A Textbook of Cardiovascular Medicine.* vol. 1. Philadelphia, WB Saunders, 1980, p. 21.
9. Perloff JK: *The Clinical Recognition of Congenital Heart Disease.* Philadelphia, WB Saunders, 1970, p. 100.
10. Chatterjee K: Physical examination, in Topol E

(ed): *Textbook of Cardiovascular Medicine.* Philadelphia, Lippincott-Raven, 1998, pp. 307–308.

11. Herbert PN, Bernier DN, Cullinane EM, et al: High-density lipoprotein metabolism in runners and sedentary men. *JAMA* 252(8):1034–1037, 1984.

12. Douglas PS, Berman GO, O'Toole ML, et al: Prevalence of multivalvular regurgitation in athletes. *Am J Cardiol* 64:209–212, 1989.

13. Cheitlin MD, Douglas PS, Parmley WW: 26th Bethesda conference: Recommendations for determining eligibility for competition in athletes with cardiovascular abnormalities. Task Force 2: Acquired valvular heart disease. *J Am Coll Cardiol* 24, 1994, pp. 874–880.

14. Orsinelli DA, Aurigemma GP, Battista S, et al: Left ventricular hypertrophy and mortality after aortic valve replacement for aortic stenosis. A high risk subgroup identified by preoperative relative wall thickness. *J Am Coll Cardiol* 22: 1679–1683, 1993.

15. Barlow JB, Jankelow D: Prospective study of asymptomatic aortic stenosis. *Circulation* 97: 1651–1653, 1998.

16. Vongpatanasin W, Hillis LD, Lange RA: Prosthetic heart valves. *N Engl J Med* 335:407–416, 1996.

17. Doty DB: Aortic valve replacement with pulmonary autograft: The Ross Procedure. *Am Coll Card Curr J Rev* September/October 49–53, 1996.

18. Elkins RC, Knott-Craig CJ, Ward KE, et al: Pulmonary autograft in children: Realized growth potential. *Ann Thorac Surg* 57:1387–1393, 1994.

19. Potera C: A return to football after heart surgery. *Physic Sports Med* 25:16, 1997.

20. Tribouilloy CM, Enriquez-Sarano M, Schaff HV, et al: Impact of preoperative symptoms on survival after surgical correction of organic mitral regurgitation: Rationale for optimizing surgical indications. *Circulation* 99:400–405, 1999.

21. Kostuk WJ, Boughner DR, Barnett HJ, et al: Strokes: A complication of mitral-leaflet prolapse? *Lancet* 2:313–316, 1977.

22. Barnett HJ, Boughner DR, Taylor DW, et al: Further evidence relating mitral-valve prolapse to cerebral ischemic events. *N Engl J Med* 302: 139–144, 1980.

23. Marks AR, Choong CY, Sanfilippo AJ, et al: Identification of high-risk and low-risk subgroups of patients with mitral-valve prolapse. *N Engl J Med* 320:1031–1036, 1989.

24. Nishimura RA, McGoon MD, Shub C, et al: Echocardiographically documented mitral-valve prolapse. Long-term follow-up of 237 patients. *N Engl J Med* 313:1305–1309, 1985.

25. Maron BJ, Isner JM, McKenna WJ: 26th Bethesda conference: Recommendations for determining eligibility for competition in athletes with cardiovascular abnormalities. Task Force 3: Hypertrophic cardiomyopathy, myocarditis and other myopericardial diseases and mitral valve prolapse. *J Am Coll Cardiol* 24:880–885, 1994.

26. Graham Jr TP, Bricker JT, James FW, Strong WB: 26th Bethesda conference: Recommendations for determining eligibility for competition in athletes with cardiovascular abnormalities. Task Force 1: Congenital heart disease. *J Am Coll Cardiol* 24:867–873, 1994.

27. Stoddard MF, Prince CR, Dillon S, et al: Exercise-induced mitral regurgitation is a predictor of morbid events in subjects with mitral valve prolapse. *J Am Coll Cardiol* 25:693–699, 1995.

28. Dajani A, Taubert K, Ferrieri P, et al: Treatment of acute streptococcal pharyngitis and prevention of rheumatic fever: A statement for health professionals. Committee on Rheumatic Fever, Endocarditis, and Kawasaki Disease of the Council on Cardiovascular Disease in the Young, the American Heart Association. *Pediatrics* 96:758–764, 1995.

PART IV

EXERCISE AS ADJUNCTIVE THERAPY FOR PATIENTS WITH VASCULAR DISEASE

Chapter 15

EXERCISE FOR CHRONIC HEART FAILURE AND HEART TRANSPLANT PATIENTS

Randy W. Braith, Ph.D.

Chronic heart failure in the United States is now pandemic. Approximately 500,000 new cases of chronic heart failure are diagnosed each year and 70,000 of these patients qualify for heart transplantation. It is extremely important, therefore, to focus attention on interventions that may elicit significant decrements in morbidity and mortality in both patient populations. There is growing clinical consensus that stable, compensated patients with chronic heart failure respond favorably to exercise training. Exercise-trained patients with chronic heart failure not only "do better" through reduction in symptoms of chronic heart failure, but there is evidence that exercise may alter the clinical course of chronic heart failure.

Heart transplantation improves the survival rate for patients with severe symptoms of chronic heart failure and an ejection fraction of 20% or less. However, with dramatic improvements in immunosuppressive drug management, short-term survival is no longer the pivotal issue for most heart transplant recipients. Rather, a return to a functional lifestyle with good quality of life is now the desired procedural outcome. To achieve this outcome, aggressive exercise rehabilitation is essential. There is convincing evidence that exercise training is an effective adjunct therapy in postoperative management of patients with end-stage chronic heart failure who undergo orthotopic heart transplantation.

This chapter will explore advances in exercise physiology for both heart failure and heart transplantation patients. Included are reviews of the factors contributing to exercise intolerance in both patient populations and a summary of results from exercise rehabilitation studies in these patients. Current recommendations for exercise testing and exercise prescription are also provided.

PATIENTS WITH CHRONIC HEART FAILURE

Patients with chronic heart failure uniformly complain of fatigue and activity intolerance. Exercise tolerance, as assessed by peak oxygen consumption (Vo$_2$ peak), is a powerful predictor of survival in these patients (Fig. 15.1). Before the 1980s, patients with chronic heart failure were excluded from exercise rehabilitation programs because of concerns for safety. Previous treatment strategies maintained that rest was first-line treatment for all stages and forms of chronic heart failure, and patients were advised to restrict physical activity in order to reduce circulatory demands. In acute or unstable chronic heart failure, rest can increase renal blood flow, enhance urine output, and augment pharmacological diuresis.

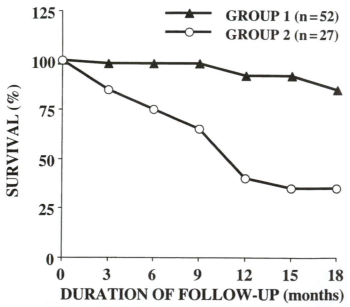

FIGURE 15.1. Survival curves for patients with heart failure with preserved exercise capacity (triangle, group 1) and those with markedly impaired exercise capacity (circle, group 2). Group 1: n = 52, age = 47 years, New York Heart Association (NYHA) class 3, Vo$_2$ peak = 19.0 ml/kg/min. Group 2: n = 27, age = 53 years, NYHA class 3, Vo$_2$ peak = 10.5 ml/kg/min. Adapted with permission from Mancini DM, Eisen H, Kussmaul W, et al: Value of peak exercise oxygen consumption for optimal timing of cardiac transplantation in ambulatory patients with heart failure. Circulation 83:778–786, 1991.

These changes improve hemodynamics and reduce ventricular volumes, both of which are beneficial in acute or unstable chronic heart failure. However, *prolonged* rest is neither necessary nor beneficial. In fact, similarity between physiological derangements of chronic heart failure and the changes seen with prolonged physical inactivity raises the possibility that deterioration of physical fitness may actually contribute to the secondary manifestations of chronic heart failure.

Over the past decade, exercise rehabilitation has been used increasingly, in conjunction with contemporary vasodilator drug therapy, to attain functional and symptomatic improvement in chronic heart failure. Aerobic exercise appears safe once patients with chronic heart failure have achieved clinical compensation. The risk of myocardial infarction or life-threatening arrhythmia in selected patients with chronic heart failure is probably not significantly higher with exercise than is the background level of risk conferred by their heart failure.

FACTORS CONTRIBUTING TO EXERCISE INTOLERANCE

IMPAIRED LEFT VENTRICULAR SYSTOLIC FUNCTION

Central hemodynamic abnormalities are, by definition, the primary pathophysiological features of chronic heart failure. Exercise tolerance, however, is not directly related to the degree of cardiac dysfunction. Left ventricular ejection fraction (LVEF) is important in assessing the extent of myocardial systolic dysfunction but is of little value in predicting an individual patient's ability to exercise.[1] Similarly, LVEF during exercise is not a sensitive index for determining the beneficial effects of exercise rehabilitation in chronic heart failure. Both resting and exercise LVEF are essentially unchanged in patients with chronic heart failure who successfully complete a program of endurance exercise training.[2,3] Thus, it is difficult to prove that the benefits of exercise rehabilitation programs for patients with chronic heart failure can be attributed to improved myocardial function. In fact, pharmacological augmentation of cardiac output through administration of dobutamine hydrochloride (Dobutrex) or dopamine hydrochloride (Dopastat, Intropin) does not immediately increase blood flow to exercising muscle. It also does not immediately elicit increases in V_{O_2} peak, clearly suggesting that forward cardiac output is not the singular factor contributing to exercise intolerance in chronic heart failure.

The weak relation between LVEF and exercise tolerance in chronic heart failure has stimulated interest in peripheral mechanisms to explain exercise intolerance. The heart and the periphery, however, are closely coupled, both in healthy adults and in patients with chronic heart failure.[4] A person's ability to use oxygen, measured as V_{O_2} peak, is closely related to maximal cardiac output; and cardiac output is related to exercise tolerance in patients with chronic heart failure (Fig. 15.2).

IMPAIRED LEFT VENTRICULAR DIASTOLIC FUNCTION

Patients with chronic heart failure with preserved left ventricular systolic function also have significant exercise intolerance. In these patients, abnormalities in left ventricular diastolic function prevent augmentation of stroke volume via the Frank Starling mechanism; the result is diminished cardiac output and severe exercise intolerance. One study reported that pulmonary wedge pressures were markedly elevated at peak exercise in these patients when compared with controls (26 vs. 7 mmHg) and V_{O_2} peak was reduced 48% primarily due to a 41% reduction in peak cardiac output.[5] Thus, in diastolic failure patients with restricted left ventricular filling, increased left ventricular filling pressure during exercise is not accompanied by increases in end-diastolic volume. A study found significant improvement in V_{O_2} peak after exercise training in patients with chronic heart failure with diastolic dysfunction caused by abnormal left ventricular relaxation, but patients with a restrictive pattern of diastolic dysfunction were unable to increase V_{O_2} peak.[6]

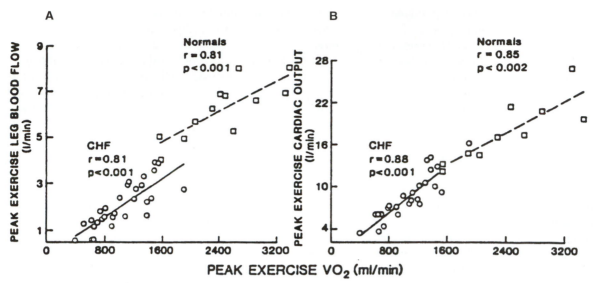

FIGURE 15.2. A. Relationship of Vo₂ peak to exercise leg blood flow in 30 patients with chronic heart failure (open circle) caused by systolic ventricular dysfunction versus 12 controls (open square): muscle blood flow is reduced with maintenance of arterial perfusion pressure. B. Relationship of Vo₂ peak to cardiac output. Adapted with permission from Sullivan MJ, Cobb FR: Central hemodynamic response to exercise in patients with chronic heart failure. Chest 101:340–346, 1992.

BAROREFLEX DESENSITIZATION AND SYMPATHETIC ACTIVATION

In the acute phase of low-output chronic heart failure, arterial and cardiopulmonary baroreflexes are activated to help maintain systemic blood pressure. However, sensitivity of both arterial and cardiopulmonary baroreceptors becomes diminished in chronic heart failure. The absence of baroreflex inhibitory input to medullary centers results in unrestrained sympathetic excitation. Sympathetic hyperactivation is observed at rest and during submaximal exercise.[7,8] Plasma norepinephrine levels at rest are two- to threefold higher in chronic heart failure patients than they are in healthy control patients. In addition, direct microneurographic recordings show dramatically increased levels of muscle sympathetic nerve activity both at rest and during exercise in patients with chronic heart failure. Patients with chronic heart failure become tachycardic with loss of heart rate variability, and peripheral vascular va-

sodilation is prevented by excessive sympathetic vasoconstrictor tone. The loss of baroreflex sensitivity and elevated levels of circulating norepinephrine are closely correlated with disease severity and overall survival.

ABNORMAL STIMULATION OF NEUROHORMONAL SYSTEMS

Neurohormonal mechanisms play a central role in the progression of chronic heart failure.[7,8] In acute heart failure, neurohormonal activation is a desirable compensatory mechanism that facilitates vasoconstriction and plasma volume expansion, which act to maintain forward cardiac output and systemic blood pressure. However, sustained neurohormonal arousal further complicates heart failure syndrome and is associated with poor long-term prognosis for those with chronic heart failure. The consequences of sustained neurohormonal activation are twofold: (a) Activation of the sympathetic nervous system, the renin-angiotensin-aldosterone system (RAAS), hypersecretion of pituitary arginine vasopressin (AVP), and release of cardiac natriuretic peptides (ANP) have adverse hemodynamic consequences in heart failure because they enhance vasoconstriction and promote fluid retention. (b) Prolonged neurohormonal activation exerts a direct deleterious effect on the heart, which is *independent* of the hemodynamic actions of these systems. High concentrations of angiotensin II (ANG II) induce necrosis of cardiac myocytes,[9] adversely influence matrix structure of myocardium,[10] increase sympathetic drive, and impair baroreceptor restraint on sympathetic drive.[11] Large multicenter clinical trials have provided compelling evidence that pharmacological suppression of neurohormonal activation, rather than direct stimulation of the failing myocardium, improves symptoms and survival in chronic heart failure.[12,13] These observations support the need for more therapeutic strategies directed at modulation of neurohormonal activation in chronic heart failure.

IMPAIRED VASODILATORY CAPACITY

Sympathetic stimulation and neurohormonal activation are potent sources of vasoconstriction in chronic heart failure. However, peripheral α-adrenergic blockade and angiotensin-converting enzyme (ACE) inhibitor therapy do not immediately restore vasodilating capacity in patients with chronic heart failure, indicating that intrinsic vascular abnormalities possibly contribute to impaired vasodilatory capacity. Currently, there are three mechanisms under investigation, all with long-time constants, which help explain the vasodilatory impairment seen in chronic heart failure:

1. Vascular stiffness, caused by increased sodium and water content within vascular tissue, may be responsible for up to one-third of vasodilatory impairment in chronic heart failure. Acute diuretic therapy improves muscle blood flow, but continued diuresis does not restore normal vasodilatory capacity, despite further reductions in fluid volume.

2. Chronic vascular deconditioning may also contribute to impaired vasodilatory capacity in patients with chronic heart failure. Immobilization of the forearm is known to reduce vasodilatory capacity, while unilateral forearm exercise training significantly improves vasodilatory capacity, but only in the trained arm.

3. There is now compelling evidence of endothelial dysfunction in both peripheral and coronary vessels in patients with chronic heart failure.[14,15] The consequence of endothelial dysfunction in patients with chronic heart failure is increased endothelin-1 and reduced nitric oxide (NO) production. L-arginine infusion (precursor of NO) significantly improves vasodilation in patients with chronic heart failure but not in control patients, presumably by increasing NO synthesis. In contrast, nitroprusside infusion (NO donor directly to smooth muscle) elicits normal vasodilation in patients with chronic heart failure, indicating that reduced vasodilatory capacity is due to a defect in NO synthesis rather than a defect in vascular smooth muscle.

SKELETAL MUSCLE ABNORMALITIES

Early speculative theories attributed exercise intolerance in patients with chronic heart failure to underperfusion of exercising muscle. However, it was subsequently demonstrated that increasing blood supply to skeletal muscle did not result in an immediate improvement in Vo_2 peak in these patients, suggesting that intrinsic intramuscular abnormalities exist that are unrelated to blood flow.[16] Indeed, studies have shown that reductions in skeletal muscle blood flow, skeletal muscle mass (13–15% reduction), aerobic enzyme activity, and an increased percentage of fast twitch type IIb fibers (more glycolytic, less fatigue resistant) in skeletal muscle all act in concert to induce early anaerobic metabolism during exercise.[17] Early onset of anaerobic metabolism, in turn, limits exercise tolerance in patients with chronic heart failure.[18] These findings have been confirmed by studies using ^{31}P magnetic reso-nance spectroscopy (^{31}P MRS), which revealed intrinsic intracellular abnormalities of skeletal muscle metabolism manifested by a greater mag-nitude (and increased rate) of phosphocreatine (PCr) depletion and a decreased pH in patients with chronic heart failure.[17,19]

Morphological data from biopsy studies cor-roborate that there is pronounced and selective at-rophy in highly oxidative, fatigue-resistant, type I muscle fibers resulting in a shift in fiber type dis-tribution toward the glycolytic, less fatigue-resist-ant, type II muscle fibers. One laboratory re-ported a significant correlation between the percent distribution of the 3 myosin heavy chain (MHC) isoforms in the gastrocnemius (namely MHC_1 = slow aerobic; MHC_{2a} = fast oxidative; MHC_{2b} = fast glycolytic), the severity of chronic heart failure, and VO_2 peak.[20]

PULMONARY ABNORMALITIES

Exertional dyspnea is a prominent symptom in chronic heart failure and a variety of abnormali-ties in pulmonary function are believed to be ex-acerbated by chronic heart failure. Traditionally, exertional dyspnea was attributed to exaggerated increases in left ventricular filling pressure and corresponding pulmonary capillary wedge pres-sure (PCWP); however, hemodynamic studies have failed to correlate dyspnea symptoms with measurements of PCWP.[21] Dyspnea in nonedema-tous chronic heart failure patients may be as much or more related to deconditioning and ab-normalities in the metabolism of exercising skele-tal muscle than to pulmonary congestion. In a group of patients with chronic heart failure, who were studied before and after exercise training, PCWP was unchanged by training, despite a 23% increase in VO_2 max and a reduction in dyspnea symptoms.[21]

Braith et al[22] performed spirometry and mea-sured pulmonary diffusion capacity in heart fail-ure patients immediately before and after cardiac transplantation to determine the impact of chronic heart failure on pulmonary function. Abnormalities on spirometry were completely re-versible with normalization of cardiovascular physiological processes after transplantation. The restrictive pulmonary defects are attributed to en-croachment by the enlarged heart. However, ab-normal pulmonary diffusing capacity observed in patients with chronic heart failure before trans-plantation was not resolved and persisted for at least 18 months (group mean) following trans-plantation, with or without restrictive or obstruc-tive pulmonary defects (Fig. 15.3).

Respiratory muscle fatigue also contributes to dyspnea in patients with chronic heart failure. A study using near-infrared spectroscopy to monitor accessory respiratory muscle perfusion found exercise-induced deoxygenation of accessory res-piratory muscles in patients with chronic heart failure, implying that decreased cardiac output during exercise results in deoxygenation of acces-sory respiratory muscles.[23]

RESPONSES TO EXERCISE TRAINING

PEAK OXYGEN CONSUMPTION
(VO_2 peak)

Training-induced improvements in VO_2 peak are a consistent finding in patients with chronic heart failure and range from 1.4 to 7 ml/kg/min. In their pioneering chronic heart failure training study, Sullivan et al[3] reported a 23% increase in VO_2 peak (16.8 vs. 20.6 ml/kg/min) in patients with chronic heart failure (LVEF 24 ± 10%) after 4 months of exercise training consisting of 4 h of monitored exercise per week. There were no changes in rest or exercise pulmonary wedge pressure, stroke volume, cardiac output, or LVEF. Researchers at the University of Florida reported a 25% increase in VO_2 peak in patients with chronic heart failure (New York Heart Association [NYHA], class II or III; LVEF 30%; age = 61 ± 7 years) who participated in a program of super-vised treadmill walking 3 days per week for 16 weeks at 40 to 70% of VO_2 peak[7] (Fig. 15.4).

Patients with chronic heart failure with < 40% LVEF and anginal symptoms on a treadmill test may not achieve exercise training-induced im-provements in VO_2 peak because the low anginal

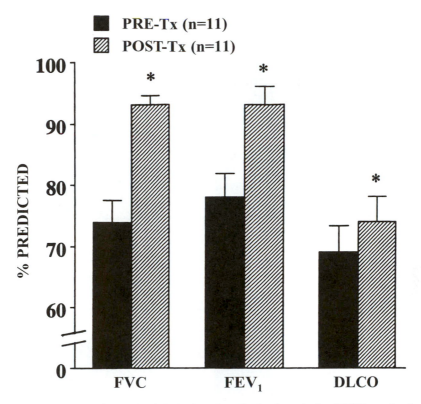

FIGURE 15.3. Forced vital capacity (FVC), forced expired volume in 1 s (FEV1), and pulmonary diffusing capacity (DLCO) in 11 patients before (solid bars) and after (hatched bars) cardiac transplantation. Values represent the mean plus or minus SEM. Significance: * $p < 0.05$. *Adapted with permission from Braith RW, Limacher MC, Leggett SH, et al: Exercise-induced hypoxemia in heart transplant recipients.* J Am Coll Cardiol *22:768–776, 1993.*

threshold could limit the exercise training intensity. However, patients whose LVEF is < 40% after a recent large myocardial infarction, but remain free of anginal symptoms, can safely engage in an exercise program and increase their $\dot{V}O_2$ peak.

MYOCARDIAL REMODELING

The influence of exercise training on myocardial wall thinning and the "remodeling" process in postmyocardial infarction patients generates considerable debate. For example, animal studies demonstrate further ventricular dilatation with training after experimentally induced infarc-

tions.[24] Similarly, an early nonrandomized controlled study reported a significant posttraining deterioration in LVEF and increase in left ventricular asynergy in patients with chronic heart failure with anterior myocardial infarction.[25] Subsequent studies, however, have not confirmed those findings.[3,26] Sullivan et al[3] reported no change in rest and exercise radionuclide measurements of LVEF, left ventricular end-diastolic volume, and left ventricular end-systolic volume in chronic heart failure patients after 4 to 6 months of exercise training. A multicenter randomized trial was designed to determine the effects of exercise on LV remodeling in patients recovering

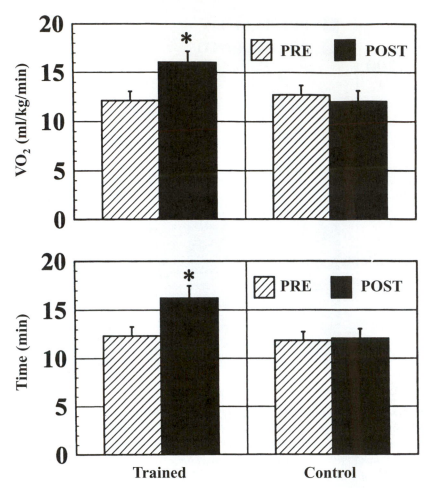

*FIGURE 15.4. Vo_2 peak and treadmill time to exhaustion in patients with heart failure before (hatched bars) and after (solid bars) 16 weeks of exercise training (trained, n = 10) or a control period (control, n = 9). Values represent the mean plus or minus the SEM. Significance: * p < 0.05. Reprinted with permission from the American College of Cardiology. Braith RW, Welsch MA, Feigenbaum MS, et al: Neuroendocrine activation in heart failure is modified by endurance exercise training.* J Am Coll Cardiol *34:1170–1175, 1999.*

from anterior myocardial infarction.[26] The 6 month training program consisted of aggressive stationary cycling and walking. Although patients with an LVEF of < 40% had greater ventricular enlargement before training, they did not have further enlargement or deterioration after training. Jette et al[27] used restriction (to anterior my-

ocardial infarctions), stratification (by LVEF < 30% and > 30%), and a controlled randomized design to overcome biases that have plagued most earlier exercise studies. Reliable and validated radionuclide ventriculography and echocardiography were used to assess left ventricular function at rest and during maximal exercise in the supine position before and after training. Training did not cause further deterioration in ventricular function. Dubach et al[28] used magnetic resonance imaging (MRI) before and after 8 weeks of high-intensity cardiac rehabilitation. Each patient's myocardium was measured in 80 segments and divided into anteroseptal and inferolateral areas, but the MRI detected no deleterious effects of exercise training on measures of supine resting left ventricular volume, function, or wall thickness regardless of infarct area. In aggregate, the experience to date indicates that selected patients with chronic heart failure without clinical complications can benefit from exercise training without having negative effects on left ventricular volume, function, or wall thickness.

BAROREFLEX AND SYMPATHETIC ACTIVATION

The mechanisms responsible for exercise-induced improvements in baroreflex sensitivity are not clearly understood. Investigators have studied all components of the reflex arc but specific mechanisms have not been identified because of the complexity of the neural circuitry. Nonetheless, markers of autonomic nervous system function in patients with chronic heart failure including resting heart rate, RR interval variability, whole-body radiolabeled norepinephrine spillover, and direct microneurography recordings show a significant shift away from sympathetic activity toward greater dominance of vagal parasympathetic tone after a program of exercise training. One study found a 30% improvement in baroreflex sensitivity in 70 patients with chronic heart failure following a program of exercise training.[29] Improved baroreceptor sensitivity was correlated with decreased sympathetic and neurohormonal activation and an increase in parasympathetic activity and heart rate variability. The clinical implication is that improved baroreflex function and vagal tone could diminish susceptibility to life-threatening arrhythmias in patients with chronic heart failure.

Two principal mechanisms are recognized in neurohormonal activation in patients with chronic

heart failure and both may be modulated by endurance exercise training. One mechanism contends that neuroendocrine hyperactivity in chronic heart failure is triggered by baroreflex dysfunction in association with a prolonged exposure to low cardiac output and reduced blood pressure. Sinoaortic and cardiac baroreceptors normally exert a tonic inhibitory influence on resting sympathetic activity, the kidney RAAS, and AVP pressure release.[30] In patients with chronic heart failure, tonic inhibitory baroreflexes are depressed and contribute to sympathetic excitation and elevated circulating neurohormone levels. An alternative but physiologically related mechanism for baroreflex and sympathetic activation in chronic heart failure is associated with the direct excitatory effects of circulating ANG II. Plasma ANG II levels initially become elevated due to renal underperfusion, the primary stimulus for ANG II production by the renal RAAS. Elevated ANG II, in turn, exerts excitatory effects at the level of the brain, ganglionic transmission, and at adrenergic nerve terminals.[31]

Baroreflex sensitivity, exercise capacity, and survival rate are all improved in patients with chronic heart failure by administration of ACE inhibitors.[11-13] In aggregate, the ACE inhibitor data suggest that ANG II plays an important role in the central integration of baroreflex information. Grassi et al[11] provided the first direct evidence, via muscle microneurography, that chronic ACE inhibitor treatment (i.e., diminished circulating ANG II) in chronic heart failure patients caused both a reduction in central sympathetic nerve traffic and an improved baroreceptor restraint on sympathetic traffic. Thus, a reduction in circulating ANG II levels achieved through exercise training may be one approach toward improving baroreflex control of sympathetic activity.

NEUROHUMORAL SYSTEMS

A study at the University of Florida was the first randomized controlled trial of intermediate-term exercise training to measure fluid regulatory hormone levels in patients with chronic heart failure.[7] Nineteen clinically stable coronary disease patients with chronic (> 4 months) symptoms of heart failure (NYHA II or III) were randomly assigned to a training group ($n = 10$; age = 61 ± 6; EF = 30 ± 6) or a control group ($n = 9$; age = 62 ± 7; EF = 29 ± 7). Exercise training consisted of supervised walking 3 times per week for 16 weeks at 40 to 70% of Vo_2 peak. Neurohormones were measured at rest and at Vo_2 peak before and after training. At study entry, values for ANG II, aldosterone, AVP, and ANP did not differ between groups (Fig. 15.5). After 16 weeks of training, all rest neurohormone levels were significantly reduced by approximately 30% in the exercise group, but remained unchanged in the control group.

Diminished neurohormonal activity in trained patients with chronic heart failure could be interpreted as a marker for improved cardiac pump function. Certainly, increased cardiac output would augment renal perfusion and thereby diminish the primary stimulus for activation of the kidney RAA system. However, results from previous chronic heart failure training studies do not reveal evidence of increased cardiac output. Improvements in Vo_2 peak are observed with no changes in rest or exercise measurements of left ventricular performance or central hemodynamics. Rather, the beneficial adaptations to endurance exercise training are attributed to peripheral mechanisms.

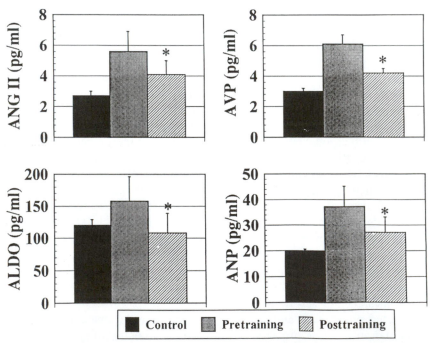

FIGURE 15.5. Rest plasma levels of angiotensin II (ANG II), aldosterone (ALDO), arginine vasopressin (AVP), and atrial natriuretic peptide (ANP) in age-matched untrained healthy controls (solid bars, n = 11) and heart failure patients (n = 10) before (shaded bars) and after (hatched bars) 16 weeks of exercise training. Values represent the mean plus or minus the SEM. Significance: * p < 0.05. Reprinted with permission from the American College of Cardiology. Braith RW, Welsch MA, Feigenbaum MS, et al: Neuroendocrine activation in heart failure is modified by endurance exercise training. J Am Coll Cardiol 34:1170–1175, 1999.

VASODILATORY CAPACITY

Studies have confirmed that the vascular endothelium must be considered a therapeutic target to reduce symptoms of chronic heart failure. Hornig et al[14] were the first to suggest that an exercise program can enhance vasodilatory capacity in patients with chronic heart failure. In this crossover trial, patients participated in 4 weeks of daily handgrip exercise at 70% of maximal voluntary contraction. High resolution ultrasound was used to measure radial artery diameter during reactive hyperemia (endothelium-dependent dilation) and during sodium nitroprusside infusion (endothelium-independent dilation). Exercise training restored flow-dependent vasodilatory capacity in chronic heart failure patients but enhanced vasodilation was specific to the region trained and was lost after 6 weeks of cessation of training. Their data suggested that exercise training induced biosynthesis of endothelial NO synthesis. In one report, Hambrecht et al[32] went a step further and demonstrated that exercise training improves both basal endothelial NO formation and agonist-mediated endothelium-dependent vasodilation of the skeletal muscle vasculature in patients with chronic heart failure. Twenty patients were randomized to a training group ($n = 10$; age = 54 ± 4 years; EF = $24 \pm 4\%$) or a control group ($n = 10$; age = 56 ± 3 years; EF = $23 \pm 3\%$). Exercise training consisted of 6 months of home-based bicycle ergometry performed twice daily (total of 40 min) 5 days per week at 70% of the heart rate at V_{O_2} peak. After exercise training, femoral artery blood flow improved 23% in response to 90 µg/min acetylcholine and the inhibiting effect of N^G-monomethyl-L-arginine (L-NMMA) increased by 174%, indicating that exercise increases basal NO formation in resistance vessels. In addition, the endothelium-dependent change in femoral blood flow was significantly ($p < 0.005$) correlated with V_{O_2} peak.

The importance of exercise training and endothelium-dependent vasodilation has also been documented in experimental models of heart failure. Expression of endothelial NO synthase (NOS) is reduced in a canine model of heart failure, but NOS was restored to normal after a 10-day exercise training program.[33] The expression of endothelial NOS is increased by shear stress in isolated endothelial cells. Thus, impaired endothelium-dependent vasodilation in chronic heart failure may be restored by repetitive increases in blood flow during exercise training, which cause intermittent enhanced shear stress and, consequently, increased expression and activity of endothelial NOS. These observations suggest that local mechanical forces play a key role in the beneficial effects of training. In addition to the regulation of endothelial NOS, other shear-dependent mechanisms may be involved as well; that is, shear stress upregulates the expression of superoxide dismutase, a radical-scavenging enzyme, but suppresses the expression and activity of ACE.[34]

SKELETAL MUSCLE METABOLISM

Studies in patients with chronic heart failure, using ^{31}P-NMR spectroscopy and in-magnet exercise protocols, reported significant improvement in metabolic capacity following exercise training. Muscle endurance was increased up to 260% without any change in muscle mass, limb blood flow, and cardiac output. Rather, improved exercise tolerance was attributed to reduced depletion of PCr, higher muscle pH at submaximal workloads, and more rapid resynthesis of PCr, which is an indicator of mitochondrial oxidative phosphorylation.[35]

Kluess et al,[19] in the longest randomized controlled exercise trial in patients with chronic heart failure to date, assessed muscle metabolism by ^{31}P-NMR spectroscopy in the medial head of the gastrocnemius before and after a 4-month walking program. The in-magnet exercise protocol consisted of repetitive plantar flexion at a low-intensity (25% of maximal voluntary contraction) and high-intensity (85%) workload. The results from this study show a marked reduction (19%) in the inorganic phosphate/PCr ratio (Pi/PCr) during the low-intensity exercise, and a significant decrease (30%) in intramuscular diprotonated inorganic phosphate (H_2PO_4) during the high-intensity exercise (Fig. 15.6). The 19% reduction in Pi/PCr during the low-intensity exercise protocol was thought to reflect an improved capacity of exercising muscle to produce adenosine triphosphate (ATP) from oxidative metabolic pathways. In addition, exercise training resulted in a significant improvement (28%) in PCr resynthesis following both the low- and high-intensity protocols, indicating improved recovery kinetics. In contrast, the skeletal muscle metabolic profile remained unchanged in the control group.

CLINICAL OUTCOMES

It was in the early 1990s that the first prospective controlled trials of exercise training in chronic heart failure were performed. Both home-based[2] and hospital-based[3,4] training studies have demonstrated that chronic exercise induces favorable clinical effects by significantly increasing Vo_2 peak, reducing sympathetic drive, improving endothelial function[14] and skeletal muscle metab-

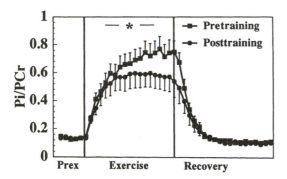

*FIGURE 15.6. The inorganic phosphate-phosphocreatine (Pi:PCr) ratio before, during, and immediately following low-intensity plantar flexion (25% maximal voluntary contraction) in heart failure patients (n = 14) before (squares) and after (circles) 16 weeks of exercise training. The Pi:PCr ratio, as determined by ^{31}P-nuclear magnetic resonance spectroscopy, is an index of skeletal muscle oxidative capacity. Values represent the mean plus or minus the SEM. Significance: * p < 0.05.*
Adapted with permission from Kluess HA, Welsch MA, Properzio AM, et al: Accelerated skeletal muscle recovery following exercise training in heart failure. Circulation 94(Suppl):I–192, 1996.

olism,[19] and suppressing neurohormonal overactivity.[7] However, the literature to date includes only approximately 500 to 600 patients with chronic heart failure who have participated in randomized trials of exercise training, and valuable long-term follow-up data are lacking. What is desperately needed is definitive information on the impact of this treatment on clinical outcomes. Thus, a critical question remains unanswered: Does exercise training have a beneficial effect on mortality or morbidity?

Belardinelli and colleagues[36] provided the first longitudinal data that argues that the benefits of long-term exercise training can translate into favorable clinical outcomes. The authors randomized 99 patients with moderate-to-severe chronic heart failure to supervised exercise rehabilitation or control for a period of 14 months. Subjects initially trained at 60% of Vo_2 peak 3 times per week for 8 weeks, then twice a week for 1 year. Changes were observed only in the training group. Both Vo_2 peak and thallium activity score improved ($p < 0.001$), 18 and 24%, respectively. Follow-up started after 14 months of exercise training, and patients were monitored for an average of 1214 ± 56 days (range, 1161 to 1268 days). Follow-up ended at the time of study closure or with an adverse event. Exercise training was associated with both lower total all-cause mortality (9 vs. 20 deaths; risk reduction −63%; 95% CI, 17 to 84%; $p < 0.01$) and hospital readmission for heart failure (5 vs. 14 admissions; risk reduction −71%; 95% CI, 11 to 88%; $p < 0.02$). While the results of this important study do not prove that exercise reduces mortality in patients with chronic heart failure (the study was not powered or designed to show these effects reliably), they do give encouragement that exercise training is a beneficial treatment in chronic heart failure.

SUMMARY OF RESPONSES TO EXERCISE

Exercise training increases functional capacity and improves symptoms in selected patients with compensated stable chronic heart failure and moderate-to-severe left ventricular systolic dysfunction. These favorable outcomes usually occur without deterioration in left ventricular function. Peripheral adaptations, particularly in skeletal muscle and peripheral circulation, appear to mediate the improvement in exercise tolerance rather than do adaptations in the cardiac musculature. Patients who have a combination of left ventricular dysfunction and residual myocardial ischemia, however, may not benefit from exercise training. Exercise training appears to optimize the symptomatic and functional benefits of ACE inhibitor therapy. The most consistent benefits occur with exercise training at least 3 times per week for 12 or more weeks. The duration of aerobic exercise training sessions can vary from 20 to 40 min, at an intensity of 50 to 85% of peak heart rate on the graded exercise test or 40 to 70% of Vo_2 peak.

DESIGNING AN EXERCISE PROGRAM

RISK STRATIFICATION AND PATIENT SCREENING

The American Heart Association (AHA), American College of Sports Medicine, American Association for Cardiovascular and Pulmonary Rehabilitation, and the Centers for Disease Control and Prevention have all published updated guidelines on exercise in clinical populations.[37] These organizations uniformly encourage stratification of individuals into risk categories prior to engaging in an exercise program. Using these risk strata, the AHA recommends that medically stable patients with chronic heart failure may participate in exercise training programs (Table 15.1). The majority of stable patients with chronic heart failure will be classified as Class C patients, but a significant number of patients with

TABLE 15.1.   AMERICAN HEART ASSOCIATION (AHA) RISK STRATIFICATION CRITERIA

AHA Classification	NYHA Class	Exercise Capacity	Angina/Ischemia and Clinical Characteristics	ECG Monitoring
A. Apparently healthy			Less than 40 years of age. Without symptoms, no major risk factors, and normal GXT.	No supervison or monitoring required.
B. Known stable coronary artery disease, low risk for vigorous exercise	1 or 2	5–6 METs	Free of ischemia or angina at rest or on the GXT. EF = 40 to 60%.	Monitored and supervised only during prescribed sessions (6 to 12 sessions). Light resistance training may be included in comprehensive rehabilitation programs.
C. Stable CV disease with low risk for vigorous exercise but unable to self-regulate activity	1 or 2	5–6 METs	Same disease states and clinical characteristics as Class B but without the ability to self-monitor exercise.	Medical supervision and ECG monitoring during prescribed sessions. Nonmedical supervision of other exercise sessions.
D. Moderate-to-high risk for cardiac complications during exercise	3	< 6 METs	Ischemia (4.0 mm ST depression) or angina during exercise. Two or more previous MIs. EF < 30%	Continuous ECG monitoring during rehabilitation until safety is established. Medical supervision during all exercise sessions until safety is established.
E. Unstable disease with activity restriction	3	< 6 METs	Unstable angina. Uncompensated heart failure. Uncontrollable arrhythmias.	No activity is recommended for conditioning purposes. Attention should be directed to restoring patient to Class D or higher.

ECG, electrocardiogram; GXT, graded exercise test; EF, ejection fraction; METs, metabolic equivalents; CV, cardiovascular; MIs, myocardial infarctions.

mild heart failure may be classified as Class B (i.e., an exercise capacity of 6 METs and LVEF of 40 to 60%) and be qualified to participate in comprehensive rehabilitation programs including light-to-moderate resistance training. Regardless of the classification, the exercise program should be individualized and medical supervision provided until safety is established.

Before starting an exercise program, patients with chronic heart failure must be in stable condition and fluid volume status should be controlled. Patients with chronic heart failure with an LVEF of < 30% should be carefully screened for ischemia. Pretraining evaluation with a symptom-limited bicycle or treadmill graded exercise test is essential. Only patients free of unstable or exercise-induced ventricular arrhythmias should be considered for exercise training. In addition, echocardiographic assessment of ventricular function and expired gas analysis for assessment of VO_2 peak are helpful in preparing exercise prescription guidelines concerning the frequency, intensity, duration, mode, and progression of the exercise program. The selection process is summarized in Figure 15.7.

INITIAL EXERCISE INTENSITY

The initial exercise intensity should be customized for each patient. Because many patients with chronic heart failure have marked exercise intolerance, it may be necessary to use an interval training approach. For example, we have employed initial training regimens that consisted of 2 to 6 min of low-level activities alternated with 1 to 2 min rest periods.[7] The frequency of training may be as much as 2 to 3 times a day during the early stages of the program, with symptoms and general fatigue serving as guidelines to determine frequency. Warm-up and cool-down periods should be longer than normal for observation of possible arrhythmias. Determination of appropriate exercise intensity for patients with chronic heart failure should be based on VO_2 peak rather than heart rate peak because the chronotropic response to exercise is frequently abnormal in patients with chronic heart failure.

A starting exercise intensity of 40 to 60% of VO_2 peak is recommended. Alternatively, the initial exercise intensity should be 10 beats below any significant symptoms including angina, exertional hypotension, dysrhythmias, and dyspnea. Continuous supervision may be necessary during the early stages of the exercise program for all patients with chronic heart failure, and frequent monitoring of blood pressure and echocardiographic responses should be used in patients with chronic heart failure at higher risk (AHA Class C). Rating of perceived exertion should range from 11 to 14 ("light" to "somewhat hard") on the 6 to 20 category Borg perceived exertion scale. Anginal symptoms should not exceed 2+ on the 0 to 4 angina scale ("moderate to bothersome") and exertional dyspnea should not exceed 2+ on the dyspnea scale ("mild, some difficulty").[37] Initially, full resuscitation equipment should be available.

EXERCISE PROGRAM PROGRESSION

The duration of exercise should be gradually increased to 30 min, as tolerated by the patient, at an intensity approximating 70 to 85% of peak heart rate on the graded exercise test or 40 to 60% of VO_2 peak. The most consistent benefits occur with exercise training at least 3 times per week for 12 or more weeks. In selected patients, after a prolonged period (6 to 12 weeks) of supervised exercise sessions without evidence of adverse events or arrhythmia, submaximal exercise may continue away from the supervised environment (i.e., home program). The choice of exercise should be activities that are predominantly cardiovascular in nature, such as walking and cycling. Current guidelines by the AHA and other exercise science organizations do not include recommendations for a resistance training component for patients with chronic heart failure. However, light-to-moderate resistance training could be integrated as part of a comprehensive rehabilitation program for low-risk (AHA Class B) patients with chronic heart failure who have successfully completed at least 6 to 12 weeks of cardiovascular exercise training without adverse events.

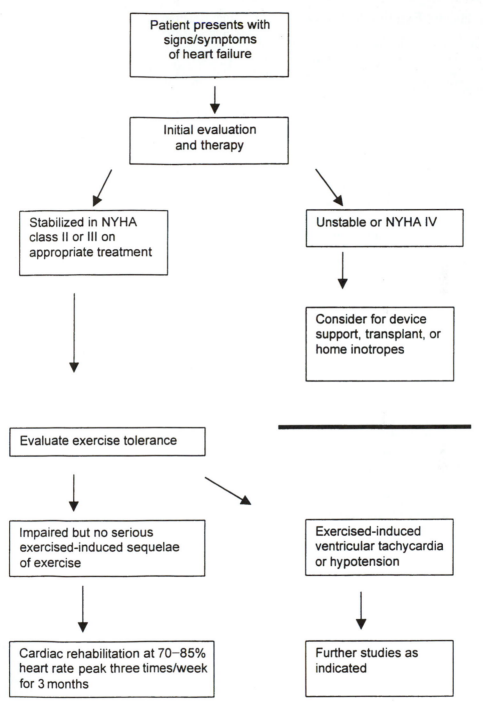

FIGURE 15.7. Screening of patients with chronic heart failure for cardiac rehabilitation.

CHRONIC HEART FAILURE SUMMARY

New standards and guidelines have been directed toward physicians and other health professionals who are involved in regular exercise testing and exercise training. For primary care physicians, who are increasingly using exercise testing, clinical competency requirements are available.[38]

Rehabilitation personnel must watch for symptoms of cardiac decompensation during exercise, including cough or dyspnea, hypotension, lightheadedness, cyanosis, angina, and arrhythmias. Patient's body weight should be recorded prior to exercise and daily pulmonary auscultation for rales and shortness of breath is recommended. Patients should avoid exercise immediately after eating or taking a vasodilator. Fluid and electrolyte balance is vital. Patients who have potassium or magnesium deficiency should take supplements to replenish electrolytes before embarking on an exercise program.

HEART TRANSPLANT RECIPIENTS

The second half of the chapter will review the unique exercise challenges presented by heart transplant recipients and summarize their adaptations to chronic exercise training. Most heart transplant recipients have suffered preoperatively from chronic debilitating cardiac illness. Many of them have had prolonged pretransplantation hospitalizations for inotropic support or a ventricular assist device. VO_2 peak and related cardiovascular parameters regress approximately 26% within the first 1 to 3 weeks of sustained bed rest.[38] Consequently, extremely poor aerobic capacity and cardiac cachexia are not unusual occurrences in heart transplant recipients who have required mechanical support or been confined to bed rest. Furthermore, heart transplant recipients must also contend with de novo exercise challenges conferred by chronic cardiac denervation and the multiple sequela resulting from immunosuppression therapy. Therefore, special emphasis in this section of the chapter is dedicated to the following 3 factors that determine exercise performance in this exotic patient population:

1. Altered anatomy and physiology of the transplanted heart
2. The effects of previous cardiac illness and supportive care
3. The effects of immunosuppressive drug therapy, most notably chronic glucocorticoid use

REINNERVATION OF THE TRANSPLANTED HUMAN HEART

The surgical denervation associated with orthotopic heart transplant and subsequent potential for reinnervation has been a focus of considerable interest among clinicians and physiologists. This question arises in part because models of surgical denervation have demonstrated functional and anatomic reinnervation in the majority of animals at 3 to 12 months after autotransplantation or allotransplantation. In contrast, evidence of reinnervation in human heart transplant recipients is much more equivocal and, if it does occur, the reinnervation is late after transplantation.

One justification for exploring the cardiovascular effects of cardiac denervation and reinnervation after transplantation is to better understand exercise responses in heart transplant recipients early and late after transplantation surgery. The presence or absence of reinnervation in the transplanted heart may determine the potential for improvement in exercise capacity late (> 1 year) after transplantation.

STRUCTURAL REINNERVATION

Early studies of structural (i.e., anatomical) reinnervation in heart transplant recipients directly measured myocardial catecholamine stores[39] and sympathetic nerve fibers per unit area[40] in routine right ventricular septal endomyocardial biopsy specimens. Results from those studies concluded that catecholamines were undetectable up to 5 years after transplantation and few neurons could be found in the transplanted heart up to 12 years after transplantation, suggesting that myocardial reinnervation was not likely to be restored in transplanted human hearts.

Subsequent investigations utilizing techniques that assess innervation in multiple regions of the heart, not simply the ventricular septum, have demonstrated that structural sympathetic reinnervation does occur after heart transplantation but it is heterogenous and region specific. For example, reinnervation of the sinus node does not necessarily imply that the ventricular septum (routine biopsy target) is also reinnervated. Alternatively, the heterogeneity of reinnervation could occur primarily in the ventricle away from the donor sinus node. Studies assessing cardiac sympathetic nerve reinnervation have used coronary tyramine infusion (causes release of norepinephrine from cardiac nerve terminals) and radiolabeled norepinephrine infusion (dilution method to determine release and reuptake of norepinephrine) to provide evidence for partial restoration of cardiac sympathetic nerve function. Wilson et al[41] were the first to find significant, albeit subnormal, cardiac release of norepinephrine in response to tyramine infusion in 39 of 50 patients ≥ 1 year after transplant. Subsequent physiological studies using positron emission tomography (PET)[42] and power spectrum analysis of RR intervals[43] also provided evidence of incomplete structural autonomic reinnervation of the transplanted human heart. Schwaiger et al[42] reported cardiac uptake of *C*-hydroxyephrine in patients > 2 years after transplantation. Predominant uptake was in the proximal anterior and septal walls, which is consistent with the normal cardiac reinnervation pattern that shows a high neuronal density at the base and progressively less density toward the apex. Using radioiodinated metaiodobenzylguanidine (MIBG) imaging, DeMarco et al[44] demonstrated significant uptake of this adrenergic false neurotransmitter in 48% of patients 1 to 2 years after transplantation, suggesting reinnervation late after transplantation. However, MIBG imaging failed to demonstrate reinnervation in patients < 6 months after transplantation.

Thus, evidence against the concept of structural reinnervation after transplantation is heavily based on histological studies of biopsy samples. However, biopsy samples taken from the right ventricular septal apex would be taken from the last site for reinnervation.[42] There appears to be enough evidence to suggest that structural sympathetic reinnervation does occur in the allograft of selected patients and the reinnervation pattern is heterogenous. Several lines of evidence argue that most patients studied late (generally > 1 year) after transplantation are not totally denervated and only heart transplant recipients studied very early after transplantation (within 3 to 4 months) can be considered totally denervated.

FUNCTIONAL REINNERVATION

The functional significance of partial anatomic reinnervation of the allograft after transplantation is not clearly understood. Few studies have carefully examined the relation between laboratory markers of reinnervation and improved chronotropic responsiveness and peak heart rate during physical exercise in heart transplant recipients. At present, there are conflicting data both supporting and refuting the functional significance of partial anatomic reinnervation in these patients.

EVIDENCE FOR FUNCTIONAL REINNERVATION

Evidence in support of functional reinnervation (i.e., improved kinetics of the heart rate response during exercise) is derived primarily from cross-sectional studies and exercise training studies. In a large cross-sectional study, Rudas et al[45] monitored heart rate responses during routine treadmill graded exercise testing (Bruce protocol) in 3 groups of heart transplant recipients: < 1 year (n = 14), 1 to 2 years (n = 20), and > 3 years (n = 18) after transplantation. Peak exercise heart rate values for the groups were 128 ± 22, 144 ± 17, and 161 ± 18, respectively. In addition to significantly greater heart rate, the tachycardic response at the onset of exercise and heart rate deceleration after exercise were improved in heart transplant recipients studied ≥ 3 years after transplantation.

Improved chronotropic responsiveness and increased peak heart rate are often reported in heart transplant recipients who participate in extensive endurance training. The first long-term endurance training study involving heart transplants ($n = 36$) reported a mean increase in peak heart rate of 13 $\pm$ 16 beats per minute after 2 years of a walk/jog program.[46] The most compliant heart transplant recipients in the study ($n = 8$), who were able to train at an average speed of 6.5 min/km, improved their Vo_2 peak by 51% and achieved a mean peak heart rate of 158 $\pm$ 12 beats per minute. Nevertheless, peak heart rate in both compliant and noncompliant heart transplant recipients was significantly ($p < 0.001$) lower than in age-matched normal subjects (148 $\pm$ 17 vs. 176 $\pm$ 13 beats per minute). Keteyian et al[47] found a mean increase in peak heart rate of 18 $\pm$ 4 beats per minute after 10 weeks of endurance training in 12 male heart transplant recipients (44 $\pm$ 3 years of age). Richard et al[48] reported that 14 enduranced-trained male heart transplant recipients (43 $\pm$ 12 years of age), who had trained for (36 $\pm$ 24 months) and participated in the 4-day 600-km Paris-to-La Plagne relay foot race, achieved 95% of predicted values for both peak heart rate and Vo_2 max during treadmill testing. In contrast to the preceding training studies, Kobashigawa and colleagues[49] conducted the only randomized study to date and observed comparable improvements in peak heart rate after 6 months of endurance training (+23%; $n = 14$) or control period (+27%; $n = 13$).

EVIDENCE AGAINST FUNCTIONAL REINNERVATION

Evidence against the concept of functional reinnervation after heart transplantation is provided in longitudinal studies that tracked sequential changes in exercise heart rate after transplantation. The influence of postsurgery time on peak exercise heart rate was studied by Mercier et al[50] in 9 untrained heart transplant recipients (52 $\pm$ 2 years of age). The authors administered serial graded exercise tests at 1, 3, 6, 9, and 12 months after transplantation. Peak heart rate increased at

each measurement period until 6 months posttransplantation and reached a plateau thereafter. Peak heart rate represented 58% of age-matched predicted values at 1 month, 69% at 3 months, 72% at 6 months, 75% at 9 months, and 71% at 12 months. Givertz et al[51] also tracked sequential changes in exercise heart rate response after transplantation. The authors studied 57 (45 $\pm$ 2 years of age) untrained heart transplant recipients at 1, 2, 3, 4, and 5 years after the procedure. No improvement in peak heart rate, chronotropic responsiveness, or Vo_2 peak were observed during treadmill graded exercise testing. These studies are consistent with a previous report of Mandak et al,[52] wherein 60 untrained patients performed 116 stress tests 0.5 to 60 months after transplantation with no improvements in peak heart rate observed after the first postoperative year. The investigators cited earlier all theorized that if anatomic reinnervation had functional consequences, higher exercise peak heart rate would have resulted over time. They concluded that lack of alteration in peak heart rate response over time suggests absence of functional reinnervation of the donor sinus node.

All of the preceding exercise studies share the same major limitation in that none of them included methodology to identify which heart transplants had evidence of reinnervation. The importance of this delineation was demonstrated by Ueberfuhr et al[53] who studied 34 heart transplant recipients during exercise testing and PET imaging using ^{11}C-hydroxyephedrine. Twenty patients had evidence of partial sympathetic reinnervation, but 14 patients did not have PET evidence of reinnervation. Patients with ^{11}C-hydroxyephedrine uptake had significantly greater peak heart rate (137 vs. 123) and higher Vo_2 peak (1676 vs. 1278 ml/min).

Unfortunately, the available exercise studies do not provide conclusive data supporting or refuting the occurrence of functional reinnervation after transplantation. The question of whether functional reinnervation occurs (in addition to anatomic reinnervation) in the transplanted human heart will require further investigation.

CENTRAL FACTORS CONTRIBUTING TO EXERCISE INTOLERANCE

HEART RATE

The transplanted heart exhibits unique characteristics that heavily influence exercise performance. Figure 15.8 illustrates typical resting and exercise responses of the transplanted heart. Resting heart rate is high in heart transplant recipients as compared to age-matched subjects, with rates approaching 100 beats per minute early after transplantation and diminishing somewhat to 80 to 90 beats per minute late after transplantation. The elevated resting heart rate appears to reflect the intrinsic depolarization rate of the sinoatrial node in the absence of parasympathetic innervation. Normal tachycardic responses at the onset of exercise are sluggish due to the loss of efferent sympathetic and parasympathetic innervation, and rate acceleration during exercise is nearly entirely dependent on the chronotropic effects of circulating catecholamines. Peak heart rate in untrained heart transplant recipients is markedly reduced, being only 70 to 80% of age-matched norms. Interestingly, peak heart rate in heart transplant recipients is frequently observed during recovery from graded exercise testing because circulating catecholamine levels reach their zenith early after termination of exercise. During recovery from exercise, heart rate decelerates very slowly due to high circulating catecholamine levels and the absence of parasympathetic inhibition.

Chronotropic incompetence is widely recognized as a major cause of exercise intolerance in many heart transplant recipients. The inability to mount an immediate tachycardic response during exercise and the restricted heart rate reserve (only 20 to 40 beats per minute in some patients) severely restricts exercise performance in heart transplant recipients.[54] Peak heart rate does increase with time after transplantation but most of the improvement occurs during the first postoperative year. Mercier et al[50] reported that peak heart rate was only 58% of age-matched norms at 1 month after transplantation and improved to 72% at 6 months, but no further increases were observed at 9 or 12 months. Mandak et al[52] and Givertz et al[51] performed serial assessment of exercise capacity for up to 5 years in large cohorts of heart transplant recipients ($n = 60$ and $n = 57$, respectively), and both studies concluded that no

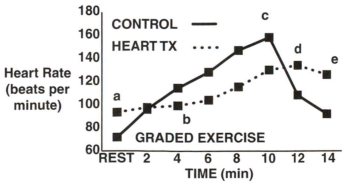

FIGURE 15.8. A representation of the typical evolution in heart rate responses before, during, and after exercise in heart transplant recipients when compared to normal age-matched control subjects: (a) Resting heart rate (HR) is elevated; (b) chronotropic response at initiation of exercise is sluggish; (c) peak heart rate is attenuated; (d) peak heart rate often occurs early in recovery after conclusion of exercise; and (e) deceleration of heart rate is prolonged.

significant improvements in peak heart rate occurred after the first year. In contrast, some heart transplant recipients who remain functionally denervated, but engage in strenuous long-term exercise training programs, are able to achieve peak heart rate values late after transplantation that approach age-matched norms.[48]

The critical importance of heart rate reserve in exercise performance has been illustrated in several studies. Kemp et al[55] reported that heart transplant recipients who could increase heart rate > 40% above resting values ($n = 34$) achieved a greater VO_2 peak and longer exercise duration than did heart transplant recipients unable to increase heart rate to this magnitude ($n = 34$). Richard et al[48] studied 14 heart transplant recipients who had maintained a demanding regimen of endurance training and had participated in competitive endurance athletic events. The significant finding was that highly trained heart transplant recipients achieved values for both peak heart rate (169 beats per minute) and VO_2 peak (39 ml/kg/min) that were 95% of age-matched norms. Braith et al[56] used a crossover design to explore the efficacy of rate-responsive cardiac pacemakers as a therapy for chronotropic incompetence. Eight stable heart transplant recipients (57 ± 12 years of age; 23 ± 9 months posttransplant), who had a pacemaker implanted at the time of transplantation, completed 2 maximal Naughton treadmill tests. During one of the treadmill tests, the pacemaker was programmed to be rate responsive but the other was not. Peak heart rate (+15%), VO_2 peak (+20%), and total treadmill time (+17%) were significantly improved by rate responsive pacing.

Exercise rehabilitation personnel must recognize that β-adrenergic antagonists contribute to chronotropic incompetence and have an exaggerated effect on exercise capacity and systolic blood pressure in heart transplant recipients. Leenen et al[57] evaluated the heart rate responses to cycle exercise in heart transplant recipients ($n = 7$) and patients with essential hypertension ($n = 8$) on placebo and beta blockers. Nonselective beta blockade (nadolol, 20 and 40 mg/day) decreased the peak exercise heart rate response by 60 and 70%, respectively, in heart transplant recipients, but only 10 and 20%, respectively, in the hypertensive group. Although oxygen consumption was not measured, beta blockade diminished total exercise time by approximately 2 min in the heart transplant group but had no effect in the hypertensive group.

CARDIAC OUTPUT

Cardiac output at rest is normal[46,58] or mildly reduced[54] in heart transplant recipients. Both left ventricular end-diastolic volume and stroke volume are reduced in heart transplant recipients at rest (20 to 40%), but the elevated resting heart rate serves to maintain cardiac index within a normal range (albeit low-normal). Left ventricular ejection fraction is also normal at rest and normal or near-normal during exercise.[54]

Peak exercise cardiac output is diminished by 30 to 40% in heart transplant recipients secondary to chronotropic incompetence and diastolic dysfunction.[54] The absence of sympathetic innervation appears to alter cardiac compliance, resulting in diastolic dysfunction and a leftward shift in the pressure-volume curve. Systolic function, in contrast, remains relatively normal after transplantation. Thus, despite normal contractile reserve and LVEF, the denervated heart becomes "stiff" and diastolic volume and stroke volume at peak exercise are only approximately 80% of that predicted.[54] Exercise training has not been shown to elicit changes in rest or peak exercise cardiac output.[46,59]

Despite chronotropic and inotropic limitations, however, heart transplant recipients are able to augment cardiac output during upright exercise but the mechanism differs from normally innervated persons. While immediate increases in heart rate augment cardiac output in the normal intact heart, augmentation of cardiac output in heart transplant recipients is achieved by increases in stroke volume (Fig. 15.9). Braith et al[58] demonstrated that heart transplant recipients augment stroke volume immediately (within 30 s) at the onset of exercise and achieve stroke volume

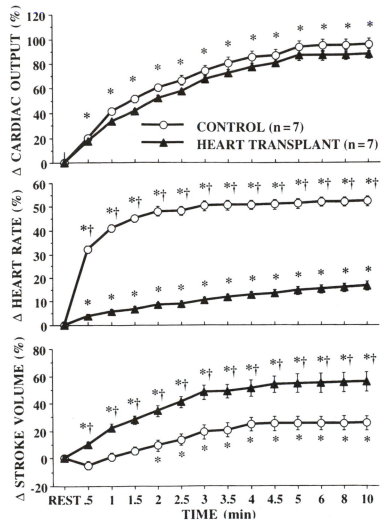

FIGURE 15.9. *Temporal pattern of relative changes (percent change from rest) in cardiac output, heart rate, and stroke volume during 10 min of constant load cycle exercise at 40% peak power output in heart transplant recipients and age-matched control subjects. Values are expressed as mean value ± SEM.* * p < 0.05 rest versus exercise. †p < 0.05 transplant versus control* **group.** *Reprinted with permission from the American College of Cardiology. Braith RW, Plunkett MB, Mills RM: Cardiac output responses during exercise in volume expanded heart transplant recipients.* Am J Cardiol *81:1152–1156, 1998.*

values that were 61% greater than resting baseline values. The adjustment in stroke volume was too rapid to be ascribed to elevated plasma catecholamines because norepinephrine levels did not increase above baseline values until nearly 4 min

after onset of exercise (Fig. 15.10). Rather, it is likely that an increase in venous return, facilitated by the "skeletal muscle pump," may offset the altered inotropic state and diastolic dysfunction of the denervated heart and permit acute augmenta-

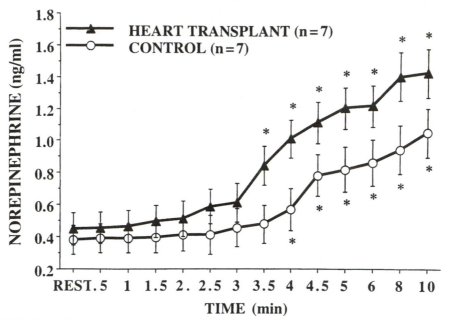

*FIGURE 15.10. Temporal pattern of absolute changes in plasma norepinephrine concentrations during 10 min of constant load cycle exercise at 40% of peak power output in heart transplant recipients and age-matched control subjects. Values are expressed as mean value ± SEM. * p < 0.05 rest versus exercise. Reprinted with permission from the American College of Cardiology. Braith RW, Plunkett MB, Mills RM: Cardiac output responses during exercise in volume expanded heart transplant recipients. Am J Cardiol 81:1152–1156, 1998.*

tion of stroke volume. Documentation of 12 to 14% expansion of blood volume in heart transplant recipients raises the possibility that volume expansion is a compensatory adaptation to cardiac denervation.[58,60] Indeed, heart transplant recipients may require an expanded blood volume to maintain cardiac output and blood pressure in the absence of efferent cardiac autonomic nerves.

HEMODYNAMICS

Intracardiac and pulmonary pressures are elevated in patients in end-stage chronic heart failure prior to transplantation. Transplantation improves the hemodynamic profile but right atrial pressure, pulmonary artery pressure (+40%), and PCWP (+30 to 35%)[54] remain elevated when compared to that of normal, suggesting that hemodynamic changes associated with heart failure may persist indefinitely. At peak exercise, PCWP

(25 to 50% greater than normal) and right atrial pressure (80 to 100% greater than normal) are significantly elevated in heart transplant recipients, even though absolute workload is substantially lower than in age-matched control patients.[54] Only one small study has assessed the effect of exercise training on central hemodynamics in heart transplant recipients ($n = 7$) and reported no changes in rest or exercise values for pulmonary artery pressure, PCWP, or right atrial pressure following 6 weeks of endurance exercise.[59]

The impact of elevated cardiac and pulmonary pressures on exercise tolerance is difficult to assess. However, postoperative elevation in pulmonary artery pressure was significantly correlated with exercise-induced hypoxemia in one study.[61] The investigators studied arterial blood gases and pH in heart transplant recipients ($n =$

10) during 10 min of constant-load cycle exercise at 70% of peak power output. Arterial oxygen pressure declined to < 80 mmHg in 5 patients and < 60 mmHg in 3 patients. None of the preoperative right heart catheterization variables were significantly correlated with exercise-induced hypoxemia. However, postoperative mean pulmonary artery pressure was significantly related to exercise-induced hypoxemia ($r = 0.71$; $p = 0.03$).[61]

DIASTOLIC FUNCTION

The consequence of cardiac diastolic dysfunction was also discussed earlier in the section on cardiac output. In brief, ventricular relaxation in heart transplant recipients does not occur as quickly as in normal age-matched control subjects. Left ventricular filling pressure, a measure of ventricular diastolic compliance, is elevated in heart transplant recipients both at rest and during exercise. Kao et al[54] reported that filling pressure decreased somewhat late after transplantation, but end-diastolic volume remained below normal and perpetuated diastolic dysfunction. The mechanism responsible for abnormal allograft compliance is unclear, but diastolic dysfunction may be another consequence of autonomic denervation and it has been demonstrated that β-adrenergic tone is, in part, responsible for regulation of diastolic filling in normal subjects.[35]

PULMONARY SPIROMETRY

The impact of preoperative chronic heart failure syndrome and postoperative immunosuppression regimens on pulmonary function in heart transplant recipients is incompletely understood. Patients in end-stage chronic heart failure (those without severe obstructive lung disease) have abnormal pulmonary diffusion capacity (DLCO) and diminished spirometric parameters including forced vital capacity (FVC), forced expiratory volume in 1 s (FEV_1), and total lung capacity (TLC).[61,62] However, most studies that performed serial pulmonary function tests in the same cohort of patients before and after heart transplantation report that abnormal spirometric parameters

are completely reversed with normalization of cardiovascular physiology and anatomy. In contrast, two studies[63,64] reported that mean values for FVC and FEV_1 did not change after heart transplantation. The explanation for these divergent findings is unclear but could be related to the incidence of established chronic obstructive pulmonary disease (COPD), rejection episodes, or severity of cytomegalovirus infection. Furthermore, it should be noted that values for both FVC and FEV_1 in the heart transplant patients studied by Egan et al[63] were within a normal range (approximately 80% of predicted) before transplantation.

The data support the conclusion that abnormal spirometry in heart transplant candidates can be attributed in large measure to chronic heart failure. A major part of the reduction in lung volumes is secondary to the space occupied by a large heart, but other factors such as pleural effusions and interstitial edema likely contribute to the reduction in lung volumes. Thus, in the absence of established COPD, spirometric parameters should not restrict exercise tolerance in most heart transplant recipients.

PULMONARY DIFFUSION

Numerous studies have shown that the abnormal DLCO observed in patients with chronic heart failure persists following heart transplantation, with or without restrictive or obstructive ventilatory defects.[61–64] However, few data are available concerning the impact of impaired DLCO on exercise capacity. Braith et al[61] collected serial arterial blood gases and found marked hypoxemia in 50% (5 of 10 subjects) of a small cohort of heart transplant recipients during 10 min of cycle ergometry at 70% of peak power output (Fig. 15.11). All subjects with exercise-induced hypoxemia ($n = 5$) had abnormal pulmonary diffusing capacity (< 70% of predicted). In 3 of the 5 heart transplant recipients who became hypoxemic, DLCO was diminished to approximately 50% of predicted. Ville et al[62] also measured arterial blood gases at maximal exercise in heart transplant recipients with normal ($n = 8$;

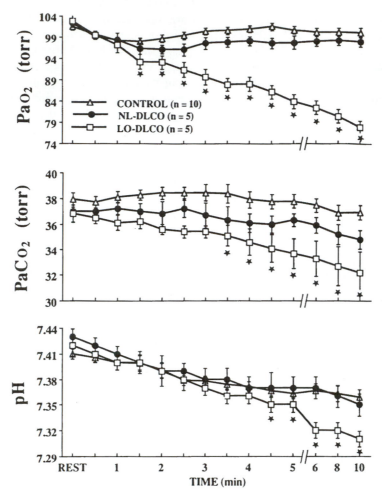

FIGURE 15.11. Temporal pattern of arterial oxygen pressure (Pao₂), arterial carbon dioxide pressure (Paco₂), and pH during 10 min of constant load cycle exercise at 70% of peak power output in patients with normal (NL-DLCO) and very low (LO-DLCO) pulmonary diffusion capacity and in normal age-matched control subjects. Values are expressed as mean value ± SEM. * p < 0.05 LO-DLCO versus control group and NL-DLCO during exercise. Reprinted with permission from the American College of Cardiology. Braith RW, Limacher MC, Mills RM, et al: Exercise-induced hypoxemia in heart transplant recipients. J Am Coll Cardiol 22:768–776, 1993.

DLCO 88% of norm) and abnormal (*n* = 9; DLCO 52% of norm) diffusing capacity. The two groups were closely matched with respect to age, spirometric parameters, postsurgery time, cyclosporine levels, ischemic time, and duration of chronic heart failure. Peak power, Vo₂ peak, peak oxygen pulse, and peak minute ventilation were all significantly greater in the group with normal DLCO. A strong correlation (*r* = 0.81) was found between DLCO and Vo₂ peak. Stepwise regression analysis revealed that DLCO explained 66% of the variance in Vo₂ peak in the heart transplant recipients. However, arterial oxygen partial pressure (Pao₂) remained within physiological limits, both at rest and at peak exercise. Squires et al[65] assessed arterial oxygen saturation (SaO_2) in a large ($n = 50$) group of heart transplant recipients undergoing symptom-limited treadmill testing. Only 4 subjects (8%) experienced exercise-induced desaturation (> 4%). Pulmonary diffusion capacity in subjects with exercise-induced desaturation (DLCO = 62% of predicted) was lower than it was in subjects that did not desaturate (DLCO = 69% of predicted).

The available evidence indicates that, while abnormal DLCO is prevalent in heart transplant recipients, exercise-induced hypoxemia is not a consistent finding and occurs only in those patients exhibiting the greatest deficits (approximately 50% of predicted) in DLCO. Thus, abnormal DLCO does not seem to be the main factor responsible for exercise intolerance in most heart transplant recipients.

PERIPHERAL FACTORS CONTRIBUTING TO EXERCISE INTOLERANCE

SKELETAL MUSCLE METABOLISM

Skeletal muscle myopathy associated with heart failure syndrome is characterized by muscle atrophy, decreased mitochondrial content, decreased oxidative enzymes, increased anaerobic enzymes, and a shift toward less fatigue-resistant type IIb fibers. These changes are not immediately resolved by heart transplantation and continue to contribute to exercise intolerance in heart transplant recipients. Indeed, a-VO_2 differences in heart transplant recipients at peak exercise are below normal and plasma lactate concentrations are above normal, suggesting metabolic insufficiency in skeletal muscle.[66]

Immunosuppression therapy, including both glucocorticoids and cyclosporine, further alters skeletal muscle metabolism after transplantation. Glucocorticoids promote muscle atrophy, particularly in type II fibers, by increasing the rate of protein catabolism and amino acid efflux while simultaneously decreasing the rate of protein synthesis.[67] Cyclosporine decreases oxidative enzymes in experimental animals and may further complicate the loss of oxidative capacity in heart transplant recipients.[68]

Several studies have attempted to track possible changes in skeletal muscle myopathy following cardiac transplantation. Bussieres et al[67] used a biopsy technique to study skeletal muscle in 14 heart transplant recipients before transplantation and at 3 and 12 months after transplantation. Consistent with other studies, they reported a predominance of type II fibers (66%) in patients with chronic heart failure before transplantation. At 3 and 12 months after transplantation, both glycolytic and oxidative enzyme activity were increased but no significant changes in fiber type were observed. Stratton et al[35] used a cross-sectional design and ^{31}P-NMR spectroscopy to assess metabolism in the forearm flexor digitorum superficialis muscle of subjects before transplantation ($n = 10$) and in patients < 6 months ($n = 9$) or > 6 months ($n = 8$) after transplantation. Phosphocreatine depletion remained significantly elevated and PCr resynthesis rate remained significantly diminished in heart transplant recipients studied late after transplantation (mean, 15 months), indicating a sustained emphasis on anaerobic bioenergetic pathways. In addition to fiber type and metabolic abnormalities, capillary density and capillary-fiber ratio in skeletal muscle remain significantly reduced below age-matched norms (24% and 27%, respectively) in heart transplant recipients late after transplantation.[68,69]

The available skeletal muscle research data in heart transplant recipients suggest that muscle metabolism is not normalized after restoration of forward cardiac output and remains abnormal in heart transplant recipients indefinitely after transplantation. However, all of the muscle metabolism studies to date were conducted with untrained heart transplant recipients and the patients were studied relatively early after transplantation. Thus, it is not known if a long-term program of endurance and/or resistance exercise training can normalize skeletal muscle metabolic responses to exercise, and this remains a fertile area for future research.

SKELETAL MUSCLE STRENGTH

As outlined earlier, diminished VO_2 peak is a consistent finding in heart transplant recipients and the mechanisms responsible for attenuated VO_2 peak include reduced cardiac index, depressed oxidative capacity of skeletal muscle, and impaired DLCO. However, muscle atrophy and weakness is a particularly important determinant of exercise capacity in heart transplant recipients. In fact, skeletal muscle weakness may preclude objective measurement of VO_2 peak in heart transplant recipients because treadmill and cycle ergometer testing devices place considerable demands on leg strength. Heart transplant recipients studied at the University of Florida consistently exhibit 1-repetition-maximum (RM) knee extension strength values (normalized for lean body mass) that are only 60 to 70% of values achieved by age-matched sedentary control subjects.[70]

Rather, knee extension strength (quadriceps) in heart transplant recipients ($n = 11$; 50 ± 14 years) is comparable to values achieved by untrained and sedentary 70- to 79-year-old subjects in this author's laboratory. More importantly, it has been shown that knee-extension strength is highly correlated ($r = 0.90$) with VO_2 peak in heart transplant recipients, when compared with normal control subjects ($r = 0.65$) (Fig. 15.12). These data can be interpreted as an indication that VO_2 peak in subjects with normal leg strength is restricted by cardiovascular function. In contrast, steroid-induced atrophy and weakness of leg muscles in heart transplant recipients may be a primary factor limiting aerobic power and optimal performance of the transplanted heart. It is reasonable to speculate that training-induced improvements in peak heart rate, VO_2 peak, and treadmill time to exhaustion in heart trans-

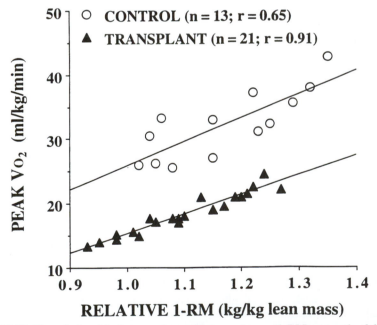

FIGURE 15.12. The relationship between 1 repetition maximum (1-RM) strength of the knee extensors, corrected for lean body mass and peak oxygen consumption (peak VO_2) in heart transplant recipients and age-matched normal control subjects. Reprinted from Braith RW, Limacher MC, Leggett SH, et al: Skeletal muscle strength in heart transplant recipients. J Heart Lung Transpl 12:1018–1023, 1993, with permission from Elsevier Science.

plant recipients are a function of increased leg strength.

PERIPHERAL CIRCULATION

Vasodilatory capacity is significantly impaired in patients with chronic heart failure, and inadequate regional blood flow to working muscle is one explanation for the lack of correlation between cardiac output and exercise tolerance. Cardiac transplantation, unfortunately, does not immediately restore vasodilatory capacity. Rather, peripheral vascular resistance remains elevated following transplantation. The pathophysiological mechanism appears to be a combination of residual factors from antecedent chronic heart failure[14] and de novo factors induced by immunosuppression with cyclosporine.[71,72]

Endothelium-independent vasodilation (response to NO donors), but not endothelium-dependent vasodilation (response to acetylcholine or hyperemia), is well-preserved in heart transplant recipients, indicating that reduced vasodilatory capacity results from a defect in NO synthesis or availability rather than a defect in vascular smooth muscle.[71] Cyclosporine-induced endothelial damage is implicated as a causal mechanism for inadequate NO production and availability.[14] Cyclosporine also alters the balance of other vasoactive substances by suppressing endothelial production of the potent vasodilator prostacyclin,[13,32] and by stimulating an increase in production of endothelin, a potent vasoconstrictor.[15,32]

Two studies have reported that vasodilatory capacity in heart transplant recipients is significantly correlated with exercise capacity. Andreassen et al[71] demonstrated that forearm vasodilatory responses to iontophoretically applied acetylcholine (i.e., endothelium-dependent responses) were significantly correlated ($r = 0.63$, $p < 0.05$) with Vo_2 peak in heart transplant recipients but not age-matched control subjects, suggesting that the endothelial defect in NO production contributes to exercise intolerance in these patients. Bussieres et al[72] reported significant correlations in heart transplant recipients ($n = 36$) between aerobic impairment and both peripheral vascular resistance at peak exercise ($r = 0.55$, $p < 0.002$) and peak a-Vo_2 difference ($r = -0.66$, $p < 0.002$). Exercise training in patients with chronic heart failure improves endothelial function and increases blood flow to working muscles, but it is not known if the same training benefits are possible in heart transplant recipients immunosuppressed with cyclosporine.

CONSEQUENCES OF GLUCOCORTICOID IMMUNOSUPPRESSION

Exogenous glucocorticoids (e.g., prednisone, methylprednisolone, Upjohn, Kalamazoo, MI) are part of the triple-drug immunosuppression regimen for most heart transplant recipients. After transplantation, glucocorticoid dose is tapered but continued indefinitely and episodes of acute graft rejection, as determined by routine surveillance endomyocardial biopsy, are treated with bolus glucocorticoids. Unfortunately, there are multiple sequela resulting from immunosuppression with glucocorticoids. Most notably, glucocorticoid-induced osteoporosis and skeletal muscle myopathy are major causes of morbidity after cardiac transplantation. Therefore, exercise rehabilitation of heart transplant recipients requires an understanding of the exercise challenges conferred by chronic glucocorticoid therapy.

GLUCOCORTICOID-INDUCED OSTEOPENIA

Osteopenia, defined as the loss of significant bone mineral density without fractures, occurs postoperatively in nearly 100% of heart transplant recipients. Trabecular or cancellous bone of the axial skeleton is lost more rapidly than cortical bone from the long bones of the appendicular skeleton. The lumbar vertebrae (trabecular bone) are particularly susceptible to osteopenia, with bone losses of 10 to 20% observed as early as 2 months after transplantation. Bone loss from the femoral neck is also dramatic, ranging from 20 to 40% below age-matched norms. In contrast, total-body bone mineral loss is approximately 2 to 3% at 2 months posttransplant.[73]

GLUCOCORTICOID-INDUCED OSTEOPOROSIS

Osteoporosis is defined as the loss of significant bone mineral density with accompanying fractures. The magnitude of this problem has been demonstrated by cross-sectional studies, which indicate that 30 to 50% of all subjects receiving long-term glucocorticoid therapy sustain osteoporotic fractures. In heart transplant recipients, there is radiologic evidence of long-bone fractures in up to 44% of patients early in the postoperative period.[74] More important clinically is the alarming prevalence (35%) of osteoporotic compression fractures in the lumbar vertebra in heart transplants.[75]

Resistance Exercise as Therapy for Osteoporosis.
Because osteoporotic fractures can be a crippling complication after transplantation, it is appropriate to implement effective prophylactic treatments to attenuate or prevent the excess bone loss. No preventative strategy for steroid-induced osteoporosis is generally accepted. Calcium supplementation, bisphosphonate agents, estrogenic and androgenic hormones, and calcitonin have all failed to prevent and/or reverse bone loss after heart transplantation.[73]

Braith et al[73] conducted the first prospective controlled study to determine the efficacy of resistance exercise training as a therapy for defective bone metabolism in heart transplant recipients. Sixteen ($n = 16$) consecutive male patients listed with the United Network for Organ Sharing (UNOS) as heart transplant candidates were recruited. The patients were randomly and prospectively assigned either to a training group that would participate in a program of resistance exercise after transplantation ($n = 8$, 56 ± 6 years of age; 21 ± 13 weeks UNOS list) or in a control group that would not perform resistance exercise ($n = 8$, 52 ± 10 years of age; 26 ± 17 weeks UNOS list). Changes in bone mineral density of the axial and appendicular skeleton were determined from bone scans (dual-energy x-ray absorptiometry [DXA]); Lunar Radiation, Madison, WI) performed before transplantation, 2 months

after transplantation, and after 3 and 6 months of a resistance training program or a control period. Resistance exercise training was initiated at 2 months after transplantation and consisted of 2 components: (a) lumbar extensor exercise 1 day per week on a MedX lumbar extension machine; and (b) upper and lower body resistance training 2 days per week using MedX variable resistance machines. Subjects used the greatest resistance possible to complete a single set consisting of 10 to 15 repetitions for each exercise. The last repetition was considered volitional failure. The specific resistance exercises are outlined in Table 15.2. The results of the study are presented in Figure 15.13. Dramatic regional bone demineralization occurred within 2 months after heart transplantation and was characterized by a rapid early phase and a plateau phase after approximately 5 months. Bone mineral density losses from compartments with trabecular bone, such as the lumbar spine, were proportionately greater than bone mineral density losses from regions

TABLE 15.2   REGIMEN FOR HEART TRANSPLANT RECIPIENTS[a]

1. Lumbar extension
2. Duo-decline chest press
3. Knee extension
4. Pullover
5. Knee flexion
6. Triceps extension
7. Biceps flexion
8. Shoulder press
9. Abdominals

[a] Heart transplant recipients performed this regimen of resistance exercises in order 2 times per week. Lumbar extension exercise was performed only 1 time per week. Subjects used the greatest resistance possible to complete a single set consisting of 10 to 15 repetitions for each exercise. We strived to have the subjects attain momentary volitional failure on the last repetion in each set. This regimen was effective as part of a strategy to prevent steroid-induced osteoporosis and steroid myopathy in heart transplant recipients.

Adapted from the CONSENSUS Trial Study Group of enalapril on mortality in severe congestive heart failure. Results of the Cooperative North Scandinavian Enalapril Survival Study (CONSENSUS). *N Engl J Med* 316:1429–1435, 1987; and the SOLVD Investigators. Effect on enalapril on survival in patients with reduced left ventricular ejection fraction and congestive heart failure. *N Engl J Med* 325:293–302, 1991.

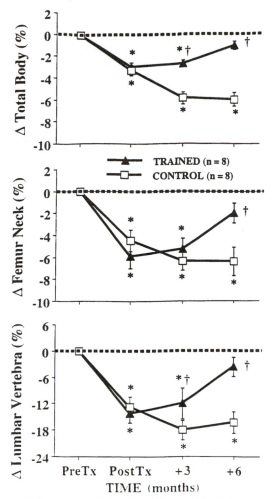

FIGURE 15.13. Changes in bone mineral density of the total body, femur neck, and lumbar vertebra at 2 months after heart transplantation (PostTx) and after 3 and 6 months of a resistance exercise program or a control period. Data are mean value ± SEM. * p < 0.05 versus pretransplantation (PreTx) value. †p < 0.05 trained group versus control group. *Reprinted with permission from the American College of Cardiology. Braith RW, Mills RM, Welsch MA, et al: Resistance exercise training restores bone mineral density in heart transplant recipients. J Am Coll Cardiol 28:1471–1477, 1996.*

with cortical bone, such as the femur neck. Bone mineral density losses in the lumbar vertebra were 12.2% and 14.9% in the control and training groups, respectively, at only 2 months after transplantation. The main finding of this study was that a 6-month program of variable resistance exercise was osteogenic and restored bone mineral density toward pretransplantation levels in heart transplant recipients despite continued immunosuppression with glucocorticoids. In contrast, regional bone mineral density in the control group did not indicate any statistically significant recovery toward preoperative levels by 8 months after transplantion.

GLUCOCORTICOID-INDUCED MYOPATHY

Muscle atrophy and weakness associated with exogenous glucocorticoid therapy are well documented.[76] Structural abnormalities in skeletal muscle include the decline of myofibrillar mass, mitochondrial volume, and decreased capillary number. The clinical presentation of steroid-induced muscle weakness is characterized by an insidious onset that is usually painless. The proximal muscles of the arms and legs are affected first, with the lower extremities demonstrating the earliest signs of weakness.

Quadriceps strength is markedly reduced in heart transplant recipients receiving glucocorticoids for immunosuppression. At the University of Florida, knee extension strength at 18 months after transplantation is approximately 70% of that achieved by age-matched untrained sedentary control subjects.[70] The difference cannot be explained by differences in lean body mass between the 2 groups. When strength is normalized for lean body mass, relative leg strength in heart transplant recipients is still only 73% of age-matched control values.

Resistance Exercise as Therapy for Myopathy. Despite the severity of steroid-induced skeletal muscle myopathy, few treatment strategies have been recommended for heart transplant recipients immunosuppressed with glucocorticoids. Pharmacologic therapies including growth hormone, potassium supplementation, and vitamin E have not proved valuable in amelioration of glucocorticoid-induced myopathy in these patients.

Braith et al[77] were the first to study the efficacy of progressive resistance training as a therapy to reduce or prevent the catabolic effects of glucocorticoids on skeletal muscle in heart transplant recipients. Fourteen male heart transplant recipients were randomly assigned to a resistance training group ($n = 7$) that trained for 6 months (54 ± 3 years of age) or a control group ($n = 7$) that did not participate in resistance training (51 ± 8 years of age). Fat mass and fat-free mass were assessed noninvasively using a Dual-Energy x-ray Ab-

sorptiometer (DXA) (Lunar Radiation, Madison, WI) before transplantation, 2 months after transplantation, and after 3 and 6 months of resistance training or control period. Upper and lower body strength was assessed: (a) an isometric lumbar extension strength test (MedX), (b) a dynamic 1-RM bilateral knee extension strength test (MedX), and (c) a dynamic 1-RM dual-decline chest press strength test (Nautilus, Independence, VA). Isometric lumbar extension strength was measured at 7 positions (72°, 60°, 48°, 36°, 24°, 12°, and 0° of lumbar flexion) through a 72° range-of-motion. The training regimen consisted of two components: (a) lumbar extensor training 1 day per week on a MedX lumbar extension machine, and (b) upper and lower body resistance training 2 days per week using Nautilus and MedX variable resistance machines. A single set consisting of 10 to 15 repetitions was completed for each exercise. The initial training weight represented 50% of 1-RM. The transplant recipients were not permitted to exceed 15 repetitions. Rather, when 15 repetitions were successfully achieved, the weight was increased by 5 to 10% at the next training session. Thus, the exercise prescription strived to have subjects use the greatest resistance possible to complete 15 repetitions, while avoiding a low-repetition and high-resistance regimen that could cause either skeletal or muscular injury in subjects at heightened risk due to catabolic steroid therapy. Fat-free mass decreased significantly (−3.4 and 4.3%, control and training groups, respectively) and fat mass increased dramatically (+7.3 and 8.3%) within 2 months after heart transplantation, while total body mass remained unchanged (Fig. 15.14). These Cushingoid alterations in body composition occurred concurrently with initiation of high-dose glucocorticoid administration (intravenous methylprednisolone and oral prednisone). The principal finding was that 6 months of resistance exercise could successfully reverse glucocorticoid-mediated muscle atrophy in clinically stable heart transplant recipients. Fat-free mass in the resistance training group was restored to pretransplantation levels after 3 months of exercise and

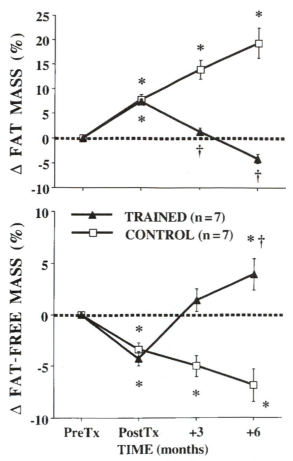

*FIGURE 15.14. Changes in fat mass (top panel) and fat-free mass at 2 months after heart transplantation, and after 3 and 6 months of a resistance exercise program or control period. Data are mean value ± SEM. * p < 0.05 versus pretransplantation (PreTx) value. †p < 0.05 trained group versus control group.* Adapted with permission from Braith RW, Welsch MA, Mills RM, et al: *Resistance exercise prevents glucocorticoid-induced myopathy in heart transplant recipients.* Med Sci Sports Exerc 30:483–489, 1998.

was increased to levels significantly greater than the pretransplantation baseline after 6 months (Fig. 15.14). In contrast, the control group experienced a progressive deterioration of fat-free mass that resulted in 7% reductions by 8 months after transplantation. When expressed in absolute terms, the control group lost 4 kg of fat-free mass (group mean) and gained 5.5 kg of fat mass. The resistance-trained group increased fat-free mass (+2.2 kg, group mean) and reduced fat mass

(−1.1 kg) during the study, indicating that a resistance exercise training program initiated early after heart transplantation attenuates the catabolic effects of glucocorticoids on skeletal muscle. Resistance exercise training also prevented the deterioration of skeletal muscle strength previously reported in patients receiving exogenous glucocorticoids at supraphysiological dosages. Some improvements in muscle strength were observed in the control group, which could be attributed to reversal of heart failure, the walking programs, or improved nutritional status. However, the magnitude of improvement in skeletal muscle strength in the training group was four- to sixfold greater than it was in the control group (Fig. 15.15).

SUMMARY OF ADAPTATIONS TO EXERCISE TRAINING

Resistance exercise training appears to be a safe modality for heart transplant recipients and is an effective countermeasure for steroid-induced osteoporosis and skeletal muscle myopathy when introduced early in the posttranplantation period. Exercise training also elicits a beneficial evolution of heart rate responsiveness during physical activity and significant increases in peak heart rate. These benefits are not seen in heart transplant recipients who do not participate in structured exercise training. However, the mechanisms responsible for improved peak heart

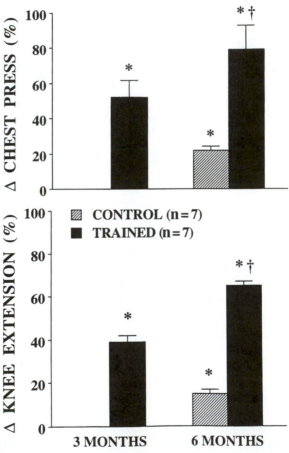

FIGURE 15.15. Changes in chest press strength (top panel) and bilateral knee extension strength after 3 and 6 months of a resistance exercise program or control period. Data are mean ± SEM. Control subjects did not train and were not tested at 3 months; * p < 0.05 versus post-transplantation baseline value. †p < 0.05 trained group versus control group. Adapted with permission from Braith RW, Welsch MA, Mills RM, et al: Resistance exercise prevents glucocorticoid-induced myopathy in heart transplant recipients. Med Sci Sports Exerc 30:483–489, 1998.

rate, $\dot{V}O_2$ peak, and total exercise time are not completely understood. There is evidence that metabolic and strength adaptations in skeletal muscle confer a "permissive" effect, allowing the transplanted human heart to approach optimal levels of function. Thus, increased exercise tolerance in heart transplant recipients may be related to skeletal muscle strength and aerobic bioenergetic capacity rather than to central adaptations or intrinsic cardiac mechanisms.

DESIGNING AN EXERCISE PROGRAM

Patients routinely stay in the surgical cardiac intensive care unit (CICU) for 5 to 7 days and are subsequently transferred to the cardiology floor for the remainder of the 10- to 14-day stay in the hospital. Thereafter, heart transplant recipients are usually discharged to local outpatient housing or home if the travel distance is short. Thus, outpatient aerobic exercise training programs can begin as early as the third postoperative week. Modalities for aerobic exercise can include walking, cycling, stair-stepping, arm ergometry, and calisthenics. Resistance training programs should not be initiated until 6 to 8 weeks after transplantation, thereby permitting time for sternum healing and glucocorticoid taper. Furthermore, resistance training should be discontinued during acute allograft rejection that requires enhanced glucocorticoid immunosuppression. The possibility of a coronary event is heightened during a serious rejection episode that requires bolus administration of glucocorticoids, and the catabolic influence of the glucocorticoids on bone and skeletal muscle supersedes the beneficial effects of exercise.

INITIAL EXERCISE INTENSITY AND PROGRESSSION

Traditional principles of exercise prescription, which are dependent on heart rate responses to determine exercise intensity, are not applicable in some cardiac denervated heart transplant recipients. Alternative methods to prescribe exercise intensity have proved to be adequate. Utilizing a rating of perceived exercise of 12 to 14, corresponding to 60 to 80% of target heart rate, improves $\dot{V}O_2$ peak by 29% in 10 weeks.[47] Moreover, the rating of perceived exercise of 12 to 14 accurately reflects the ventilatory threshold in heart transplant recipients.[78] Thus, setting initial exercise intensity at slightly below a rating of perceived exercise of 12 to 14 establishes an entry level of work rate. The rating of perceived exercise can subsequently be used to "fine tune" further adjustments and progressions in the intensity of exercise.

EXERCISE SAFETY PRECAUTIONS

Safety problems typically encountered with patients with coronary artery disease in cardiac rehabilitation programs are associated with cardiac work and myocardial ischemia. In contrast, heart transplant recipients are not limited by coronary underperfusion, provided they are free from acute rejection or allograft vascular disease. Rather, the rehabilitation staff must take special precautions to ensure adequate maintenance of systemic blood pressure. Approximately 25% of heart transplant recipients experience transient hypotension during resistance exercise, and this problem is exaggerated when the exercise requires lifting above the level of the heart (e.g., shoulder press). This hemodynamic problem is likely a consequence of autonomic sympathetic denervation. The denervated transplanted heart is almost entirely dependent on preload and the Frank-Starling mechanism for defending cardiac output and systemic blood pressure. The following maneuvers help sustain venous return and prevent blood pooling in patients who experience hypotension:

- Perform upper body exercises alternated with lower body exercises
- Symptomatic subjects walk 2 min between exercises or performed standing calf raises
- Conclude each resistance training session with a 5 min cool-down walk at low intensity on the treadmill

Subjects with bone mineral density deficits > 2 standard deviations from age-matched norms after transplantation are at great risk for fractures, and resistance training may be contraindicated. Heart transplant recipients participating in resistance exercise programs must be carefully managed with conservative initial resistances and gradual progressions in resistance loads.

SUMMARY

The era of exercise training as a treatment for chronic heart failure has begun. In the decade following the pioneering work from Duke University,[3,4] there has been a profusion of small predominantly single-center studies and a litany of impressive physiological benefits that can be achieved. There is growing clinical consensus that stable, compensated patients with chronic heart failure who engage in exercise training "do better" through reduction in secondary peripheral manifestations of chronic heart failure syndrome. Moreover, there is recent exciting evidence that exercise training may actually alter the clinical course of chronic heart failure. Much remains to be done, however, and many unanswered questions remain. For example, it is not known whether training effects in patients with chronic heart failure can be maintained over the long term, and it is not clearly established whether training is feasible outside of specialized research and clinical environments.

During the past 2 decades heart transplantation has evolved from a rarely performed experimental procedure to an accepted life-extending therapy for end-stage heart failure patients. However, with dramatic improvements in organ preservation, surgery, and immunosuppressive drug management, short-term survival is no longer the pivotal issue for most heart transplant recipients. Rather, a return to functional lifestyle with good quality of life is now the desired procedural outcome. To achieve this outcome, aggressive exercise rehabilitation is essential.

REFERENCES

1. Mancini DM, Eisen H, Kussmaul W, et al: Value of peak exercise oxygen consumption for optimal timing of cardiac transplantation in ambulatory patients with heart failure. *Circulation* 83:778–786, 1991.
2. Coats AJ, Adamopoulos S, Radaelli A, et al: Controlled trial of physical training in chronic heart failure: Exercise performance, hemodynamics, ventilation, and autonomic function. *Circulation* 85:2119–2131, 1992.
3. Sullivan MJ, Higginbotham MB, Cobb FR: Exercise training in patients with severe left ventricular dysfunction: Hemodynamic and metabolic effects. *Circulation* 78:506–515, 1988.
4. Sullivan MJ, Cobb FR: Central hemodynamic response to exercise in patients with chronic heart failure. *Chest* 101:340–346, 1992.
5. Kitzman DW, Higginbotham MB, Cobb FR, et al: Exercise intolerance in patients with heart failure and preserved left ventricular systolic function: Failure of the Frank-Starling mechanism. *J Am Coll Cardiol* 17:1065–1072,1991.
6. Belardinelli R, Georgiou D, Cianci G, et al: Exercise training improves left ventricular diastolic filling in patients with dilated cardiomyopathy: Clinical and prognostic implications. *Circulation* 91:2775–2784, 1995.
7. Braith RW, Welsch MA, Feigenbaum MS, et al: Neuroendocrine activation in heart failure is modified by endurance exercise training. *J Am Coll Cardiol* 1999: 34:1170–1175.
8. Cohn JN, Levine TB, Olivari MT, et al: Plasma norepinephrine as a guide to prognosis in patients with chronic congestive heart failure. *N Engl J Med* 311:819–823, 1984.
9. Tan LB, Jalil JE, Pick R, et al: Cardiac myocyte necrosis induced by angiotensin II. *Circ Res* 69:1185–1195, 1991.
10. Weber KT: Extracellular matrix remodeling in heart failure: A role for de novo angiotensin II generation. *Circulation* 96:4065–4082, 1997.
11. Grassi G, Cattaneo BM, Servavalle G, et al: Effects of chronic ACE inhibition on sympathetic nerve traffic and baroreflex control of the circulation. *Circulation* 96:1173–1179, 1997.
12. The CONSENSUS Trial Study Group. Effects of enalapril on mortality in severe congestive heart failure: Results of the Cooperative North

Scandinavian Enalapril Survival Study (CON-SENSUS). *N Engl J Med* 316:1429–1435, 1987.

13. The SOLVD Investigators. Effect of enalapril on survival in patients with reduced left ventricular ejection fraction and congestive heart failure. *N Engl J Med* 325:293–302, 1991.

14. Hornig B, Maier V, Drexler H: Physical training improves endothelial function in patients with chronic heart failure. *Circulation* 93:210–214, 1996.

15. Drexler H: Endothelial dysfunction: Clinical implications. *Prog Cardiovasc Dis* 39:287–324, 1997.

16. Drexler H, Reide U, Munzel T, et al: Alterations of skeletal muscle in chronic heart failure. *Circulation* 85:1751–1759, 1992.

17. Clark AL, Poole-Wilson PA, Coats AJ: Exercise limitation in chronic heart failure: Central role of the periphery. *J Am Coll Cardiol* 28:1092–1102, 1996.

18. Okita K, Yonezawa K, Nishijima H, et al: Skeletal muscle metabolism limits exercise capacity in patients with chronic heart failure. *Circulation* 98:1886–1891, 1998.

19. Kluess HA, Welsch MA, Properzio AM, et al: Accelerated skeletal muscle metabolic recovery following exercise training in heart failure. *Circulation* 94:I–192, 1996.

20. Vescovo G, Serafini F, Dalla Libera L, et al: Skeletal muscle myosin heavy chain composition in CHF: Correlation between the magnitude of the isoenzymatic shift, exercise capacity, and gas exchange measurements. *Am Heart J* 135:130–137, 1998.

21. Sullivan MJ, Higginbotham MB, Cobb FR: Exercise training in patients with chronic heart failure delays ventilatory anaerobic threshold and improves submaximal exercise performance. *Circulation* 79:324–329, 1989.

22. Braith RW, Limacher MC, Leggett SH, et al: Exercise-induced hypoxemia in heart transplant recipients. *J Am Coll Cardiol* 22:768–776, 1993.

23. Mancini DM, Henson D, LaManca J, et al: Respiratory muscle function and dyspnea in patients with chronic congestive heart failure. *Circulation* 86:909–918, 1992.

24. Gaudron P, Hu K, Schamberger R, et al: Effect of endurance training early or late after coronary artery occlusion on left ventricular remodeling, hemodynamics, and survival in rats with chronic transmural myocardial infarction. *Circulation* 89:402–412, 1994.

25. Jugdutt BI, Michorowski BL, Kappagoda CT: Exercise training after anterior Q wave myocardial infarction: Importance of regional left ventricular function and topography. *J Am Coll Cardiol* 12:362–372, 1988.

26. Giannuzzi P, Tavazzi L, Temporelli PL, et al: Long-term physical training and left ventricular remodeling after anterior myocardial infarction: Results of the Exercise in Anterior Myocardial Infarction (EAMI) trial. *J Am Coll Cardiol* 22:1821–1829, 1993.

27. Jette M, Heller R, Landry F, Blumchen G: Randomized 4-week program in patients with impaired left ventricular function. *Circulation* 84:1561–1567, 1991.

28. Dubach P, Myers J, Dziekan G, et al: Effect of exercise training on myocardial remodeling in patients with reduced left ventricular function after myocardial infarction. *Circulation* 95:2060–2067, 1997.

29. La Rovere MT, Mortara A, Specchia G, et al: Myocardial infarction and baroreflex sensitivity: Clincal studies. *J Ital Cardiol* 22:639–645, 1992.

30. Eckberg DL, Sleight P: Congestive heart failure, in Eckberg DL, Sleight P (eds.): *Human Baroreflexes in Health and Disease.* Oxford, UK, Clarendon Press, 1992, pp. 399–436.

31. Kaye DM, Lambert GW, Lefkovits J, et al: Neurochemical evidence of cardiac sympathetic activation and increased central nervous system norepinephrine turnover in severe congestive heart failure. *J Am Coll Cardiol* 23:570–578, 1994.

32. Hambrecht R, Fiehn E, Weigle C, et al: Regular physical exercise corrects endothelial dysfunction and improves exercise capacity in patients with chronic heart failure. *Circulation* 98:2709–2715, 1998.

33. Smith C, Sun D, Hoegler C, et al: Reduced gene expression of vascular endothelial NO synthase and cyclooxygenase-1 in heart failure. *Circ Res* 78:58–64, 1996.

34. Rieder M, Carmona R, Krieger J, et al: Suppression of angiotensin-converting-enzyme expression and activity by shear stress. *Circ Res* 80:312–319, 1997.

35. Stratton J, Dunn J, Adamopoulos S, et al: Training partially reverses skeletal muscle metabolic abnor-

malities during exercise in heart failure. *J Appl Physical* 76:1575–1582, 1994.

36. Belardinelli R, Georgiou D, Cianci G, et al: Randomized, controlled trial of long-term moderate exercise training in chronic heart failure: Effects on functional capacity, quality of life, and clinical outcome. *Circulation* 99:1173–1182, 1999.

37. ACSM Guidelines for exercise testing and prescription (5th ed.), Baltimore: Williams & Wilkins, 1995, pp. 98–100.

38. Braith RW, Mills RM: Exercise training in patients with congestive heart failure: How to achieve benefits safely. *Postgrad Med* 96:119–130, 1996.

39. Regitz V, Bossaller C, Strasser R, et al: Myocardial catecholamine content after heart transplantation. *Circulation* 82:620–623, 1990.

40. Rowan RA, Billingham ME: Myocardial innervation in long-term heart transplant survivors: A quantitative ultrastructural survey. *J Heart Transplant* 7:448–452, 1988.

41. Wilson RF, Christensen BV, Olivari MT, et al: Evidence for structural sympathetic reinnervation after orthotopic cardiac transplantation in humans. *Circulation* 83:1210–1220, 1991.

42. Schwaiger M, Hutchins GD, Kaiff V, et al: Evidence for regional catecholamine uptake and storage sites in the transplanted human heart by positron emission tomography. *J Clin Invest* 87:1681–1690, 1991.

43. Lord SW, Clayton RH, Mitchell L, et al: Sympathetic reinnervation and heart rate variability after cardiac transplantation. *Heart* 77:532–538, 1997.

44. DeMarco T, Dae M, Yuen-Green MS, et al: Iodine-123 metaiodobenzylguanidine scintigraphic assessment of the transplanted human heart: Evidence for late reinnervation. *J Am Coll Cardiol* 25:927–931, 1995.

45. Rudas L, Pflughelder PW, Menkis AH, et al: Evolution of heart rate responsiveness after orthotopic cardiac transplantation. *Am J Cardiol* 68:232–236, 1991.

46. Kavanagh T, Yacoub M, Mertens D, et al: Cardiorespiratory responses to exercise training after orthotopic cardiac transplantation. *Circulation* 77:162–171, 1988.

47. Keteyian S, Shepard R, Ehrman J, et al: Cardiovascular responses of heart transplant patients to exercise training. *J Appl Physiol* 70:2627–2631, 1991.

48. Richard R, Verdier JC, Duvallet A, et al: Chronotropic competence in endurance trained heart transplant recipients: Heart rate is not a limiting factor for exercise capacity. *J Am Coll Cardiol* 33:192–197, 1999.

49. Kobashigawa JA, Leaf DA, Lee N, et al: A controlled trial of exercise rehabilitation after heart transplantation. *N Engl J Med* 340:272–277, 1999.

50. Mercier J, Ville N, Wintrebert P, et al: Influence of post-surgery time after cardiac transplantation on exercise responses. *Med Sci Sports Exerc* 28:171–175, 1996.

51. Givertz MM, Hartley LH, Colucci WS: Long-term sequential changes in exercise capacity and chronotropic responsiveness after cardiac transplantation. *Circulation* 96:232–237, 1997.

52. Mandak J, Aaronson K, Mancini D: Serial assessment of exercise capacity after heart transplantation. *J Heart Lung Transplant* 14:468–478, 1995.

53. Ueberfuhr P, Ziegler S, Schwaiblmair M, et al: Functional significance of the sympathetic re-innervated orthotopically transplanted human heart. *Circulation* (Suppl I):I–291, 1996.

54. Kao AC, Vantrigt P, Shaeffer-Mccall GS, et al: Allograft diastolic dysfunction and chronotropic incompetence limit cardiac output response to exercise two to six years after heart transplantation. *J Heart Lung Transpl* 14:11–22, 1995.

55. Kemp DL, Jennison SH, Stelken AM, et al: Association of resting heart rate and chronotropic response. *Am J Cardiol* 75:751–752, 1995.

56. Braith RW, Clapp L, Mills RM, et al: Rate responsive cardiac pacing increases exercise capacity in heart transplant recipients. *Med Sci Sports Exerc* 31(Suppl):339, 1999.

57. Leenen FH, Davies RA, Fourney A: Role of cardiac B_2-receptors in cardiac responses to exercise in cardiac transplant patients. *Circulation* 91:685–690, 1995.

58. Braith RW, Plunkett MB, Mills RM: Cardiac output responses during exercise in volume expanded heart transplant recipients. *Am J Cardiol* 81:1–5, 1998.

59. Geny B, Saini J, Mettauer B, et al: Effect of short-term endurance training on exercise capacity, hemodynamics and atrial natriuretic peptide secretion in heart transplant recipients. *Eur J Appl Physiol* 73:259–266, 1996.

60. Braith RW, Mills RM, Wilcox CS, et al: Fluid homeostasis after heart transplantation: The role of

cardiac denervation. *J Heart Lung Transpl* 15:872–880, 1996.

61. Braith RW, Limacher MC, Mills RM, et al: Exercise-induced hypoxemia in heart transplant recipients. *J Am Coll Cardiol* 22:768–776, 1993.

62. Ville N, Mercier J, Varray A, et al: Exercise tolerance in heart transplant patients with altered pulmonary diffusion capacity. *Med Sci Sports Exerc* 30:339–344, 1998.

63. Egan JJ, Kalra S, Yonan N, et al: Pulmonary diffusion abnormalities in heart transplant recipients. *Chest* 104:1085–1089, 1993.

64. Ohar J, Osterloh J, Ahmed N, Miller L: Diffusing capacity decreases after heart transplantation. *Chest* 103:857–861, 1993.

65. Squires RW, Hoffman CJ, James GA, et al: Arterial oxygen saturation during graded exercise testing after cardiac transplantation. *J Cardiopul Rehabil* 18:348, 1998.

66. Mettauer B, Lampert E, Pefitjean P, et al: Persistent exercise intolerance following cardiac transplantation despite normal oxygen transport. *Int J Sports Med* 17:277–286, 1996.

67. Bussieres LM, Pflugfelder PW, Taylor AW, et al: Changes in skeletal muscle morphology and biochemistry after cardiac transplantation. *Am J Cardiol* 79:630–634, 1997.

68. Biring M, Fournier M, Ross D, et al: Cellular adaptations of skeletal muscle to cyclosporine. *J Appl Physiol* 84:1967–1975, 1998.

69. Lampert E, Oyono-Enguelld S, Mettauer B, et al: Short endurance training improves lactate removal in patients with heart transplants. *Med Sci Sports Exerc* 28:801–807, 1996.

70. Braith RW, Limacher MC, Leggett SH, et al: Skeletal muscle strength in heart transplant recipients. *J Heart Lung Transplant* 12:1018–1023, 1993.

71. Andreassen AK, Gullestad L, Holm T, et al: Endothelium-dependent vasodilation of the skin microcirculation in heart transplant recipients. *Clin Transplantation* 12:324–332, 1998.

72. Bussieres LM, Pflughelder PW, Menkes AH, et al: Basis for aerobic impairment in patients after heart transplantation. *J Heart Lung Transpl* 14:1073–1080, 1995.

73. Braith RW, Mills RM, Welsch MA, et al: Resistance exercise training restores bone mineral density in heart transplant recipients. *J Am Coll Cardiol* 28:1471–1477, 1996.

74. Rich GM, Mudge GH, Laffel GL, et al: Cyclosporine A and prednisone associated osteoporosis in heart transplant recipients. *J Heart Lung Transpl* 11:950–958, 1992.

75. Shane E, Rivas MD, Silvergerg SJ, et al: Osteoporosis after cardiac transplantation. *Am J Med* 94:257–264, 1993.

76. Hickson RC, Marone JR: Exercise and inhibition of glucocorticoid-induced muscle atrophy. *Exerc Sport Sci Rev* 21:135–167, 1993.

77. Braith RW, Welsch MA, Mills RM, et al: Resistance exercise prevents glucocorticoid-induced myopathy in heart transplant recipients. *Med Sci Sports Exerc* 30:483–489, 1998.

78. Brubaker P, Berry MJ, Brozena SC, et al: Relationship of lactate and ventilatory thresholds in cardiac transplant patients. *Med Sci Sport Exerc* 25:191–196, 1993.

Chapter 16

EXERCISE FOR PATIENTS WITH CORONARY ARTERY AND/OR CORONARY HEART DISEASE

Paul D. Thompson, M.D.

The adage that there is rarely anything new in medicine, just the rediscovery of prior knowledge, is not usually applicable to cardiology, which has seen enormous gains in treatment strategies over the last several decades. This adage does apply, however, to the use of exercise training for patients with coronary artery disease. In 1772, Heberden, the English physician who described angina pectoris, remarked that he had "little or nothing to advance. . ." for the treatment of angina but did know of one patient "who set himself a task of sawing wood for half an hour every day and was nearly cured."[1] The benefit of exercise for patients with heart disease continues to be rediscovered, and the use of exercise training with more impaired patient groups, such as those with congestive heart failure, continues to expand. Nevertheless, despite its documented benefits, exercise training continues to be underutilized in the patient population with coronary artery disease. Less than 15% of eligible patients with coronary artery disease are referred to exercise-based cardiac rehabilitation programs,[2] and the duration of the standard exercise program for patients with coronary artery disease is rarely more than 3 months.

Exercise training for patients with coronary artery disease is generally referred to as cardiac rehabilitation, but exercise is really only 1 component of what I refer to as "postdischarge intensive cardiac care." The length of hospital stay for patients with coronary artery disease after acute myocardial infarction (MI) has decreased remarkably from several weeks in the late 1960s to several days in the late 1990s. These changes have occurred because of increased awareness of the deleterious effects of bed rest and because of the use of thrombolytic therapy and primary angioplasty as standard treatment for acute MI. Similar reductions in length of stay have occurred for patients with unstable angina pectoris and for patients after coronary bypass surgery. With this decrease in hospitalization has come the need for clinicians to focus more of their intensive care of cardiac patients in the outpatient setting.

There are 3 main goals to any postdischarge intensive cardiac care program. They are: to maintain or improve the patient's functional capacity, to improve the patient's quality of life, and to prevent recurrent cardiac events. Exercise training is a critical part of such a rehabilitative and secondary prevention program. Other critical elements of postdischarge intensive cardiac care include aggressive dietary and pharmacologic treatment of serum lipids, smoking cessation, the routine use of antiplatelet agents such as aspirin, the selective use of other anticoagulants such as coumadin, the use of β-adrenergic blocking agents, and the use of angiotensin converting enzyme (ACE) inhibitors in patients with reduced left ventricular ejection fraction.[3]

Most cardiac rehabilitation programs now include counseling and education to ensure that patients with coronary artery disease receive all aspects of postdischarge intensive cardiac care. The present chapter will focus on the role of exercise training in this treatment paradigm.

DEFINITION OF TERMS: CORONARY ARTERY DISEASE VERSUS CORONARY HEART DISEASE

The terms used to describe cardiac patients require clarification. *Coronary artery disease* refers to any abnormality of the coronary arteries. The predominant cause of coronary artery disease is atherosclerosis, but other conditions such as vasculitis, anomalous coronary artery origin or course, and coronary artery aneurysms from prior vasculitis can cause coronary artery disease. *Coronary heart disease* is often used interchangeably with coronary artery disease. Coronary heart disease, however, more correctly refers to myocardial dysfunction produced by coronary artery disease, either as a result of MI or chronic ischemia. Not all patients with coronary artery disease have cardiac myocardial disease or coronary heart disease, but all coronary heart disease patients have coronary artery disease as the proximate cause of their myocardial dysfunction.

REVIEW OF EXERCISE PHYSIOLOGY IN HEALTHY SUBJECTS

Maximal functional capacity during dynamic exercise using large muscle groups is limited by the cardiovascular system's ability to deliver, and the peripheral musculature's ability to use, oxygen. An individual's maximum capacity to utilize oxygen is defined as the person's maximal oxygen uptake, or Vo_2 max. It is measured during such dynamic exercise challenges as cycling or treadmill exercise. Vo_2 max is expressed either as liters of oxygen per minute or "normalized" for body weight as milliliters of oxygen per minute per kilogram of body weight. Vo_2 max is the product of maximal cardiac output and the maximal arteriovenous O_2 difference (AV O_2 diff).[4] Maximal cardiac output is itself the product of peak heart rate and maximal stroke volume. The AV O_2 diff is determined by the arterial O_2 content, the muscles' ability to extract O_2, and the circulatory system's ability to redirect arterial blood from nonexercising tissue to exercising muscle. Change in any of the components of this system can affect maximal exercise capacity, including changes in maximum cardiac output, hemoglobin concentration, the ability to fully oxygenate the red blood cells, the capacity to shunt blood to exercising muscle, and the ability of muscles to extract the available oxygen.

There are clear differences among individuals in their exercise skill and efficiency, which affects the amount of oxygen required to perform a physical task. Nevertheless, within a range determined by variations in efficiency, a specific physical task requires approximately the same oxygen uptake even when performed by different individuals. The O_2 consumption required by a physical task is referred to as the external work rate,[5] and as mentioned previously, identical external work rates require roughly similar oxygen uptakes among different individuals. The external work rate also determines the cardiac output response to the exercise task. In general, a 1 L increase in O_2 consumption produces a 6 L increase in cardiac output.[6] The external work rate is also referred to as the absolute work rate, or the absolute V_{O_2}. The relative work rate refers to the percent of an individual's V_{O_2} max that is required for that person to perform a certain physical task. In other words, relative work rate is the required V_{O_2} relative to the individual's maximum. Individuals differ in their maximal exercise capacity primarily because maximal cardiac output varies among individuals. Because of differences in individual exercise capacity, the same physical task usually requires approximately the same absolute work rate for different individuals, but often requires markedly different relative work rates.

Identical external work rates can produce markedly different myocardial O_2 demand. Myocardial O_2 demand has been referred to as the internal work rate.[5] Myocardial oxygen demand increases with increasing heart rate and systolic blood pressure.[7] Indeed the product of heart rate and systolic blood pressure is referred to as the rate pressure product or double product and is used clinically to estimate the myocardial

oxygen demand of exertion.[7] Both heart rate and systolic blood pressure increase linearly with the relative work rate. Consequently, identical external work rates can produce markedly different internal work rates or myocardial O_2 demands depending on the individual's V_{O_2} max. The implication of this observation is that a physical task requires less myocardial oxygen supply for an individual with a high V_{O_2} max than that same task requires for a less fit individual.

In contrast to skeletal muscle, the myocardium is never really at rest, so that myocardial oxygen demand without physical activity is already high and the myocardium extracts 70 to 80% of the available arterial O_2 at "rest." The increased myocardial O_2 needs of physical exercise, therefore, must be met primarily by augmented coronary blood flow. Consequently, identical external workloads can produce markedly different internal workloads and coronary blood flows depending on the exercise capacity of the individual.

V_{O_2} max is an excellent measure of exercise capacity because it is highly reproducible in the absence of any change in the factors determining V_{O_2}.[8] Nevertheless, maximal exercise capacity and even V_{O_2} can underestimate an individual's ability to perform sustained submaximal exercise. Since few tasks are performed at maximum exercise capacity, this is a critical shortcoming of measuring only V_{O_2} max when assessing a patient's effort tolerance, although among sedentary individuals there is a general correlation between maximal capacity and the ability to sustain submaximal effort.

PHYSIOLOGY OF EXERCISE IN PATIENTS WITH CORONARY ARTERY DISEASE

A physically inactive lifestyle[9] and low exercise capacity[10] are important risk factors for coronary artery disease. Nevertheless, patients with only coronary artery disease and no concomitant coronary heart disease often have exercise capacity that is within the average range for their age and sex. Such patients may be those who have had an MI aborted by thrombolytic therapy or primary coronary angioplasty and sustained no permanent myocardial injury. In contrast to patients with only coronary artery disease, patients with coronary heart disease generally demonstrate reduced maximal exercise capacity with the magnitude of the reduction dependant on the severity of the existing myocardial damage and the limits such damage places on the ability to increase cardiac output. Patients with angina pectoris may also have no detectable myocardial damage, but limited exercise capacity because of exercise-limiting discomfort. Patients with asymptomatic myocardial ischemia are often limited by exercise dyspnea produced by a reduction in stroke volume attending the exercise-induced ischemia.

Patients with classic angina pectoris experience exercise-induced chest discomfort at a highly reproducible internal workload or rate pressure product. This anginal threshold corresponds to the point where myocardial oxygen demand cannot be adequately supplied by coronary flow because of the coronary lesion. Many patients do not experience classic angina, however, and have considerable variation in the internal workload that produces symptoms. Much of this variation is probably due to coronary artery vasomotion, since it is now clear that the coronary arteries are not fixed conduits but can alter their internal diameter in response to various stimuli. Exercise produces arterial dilatation in normal coronary arteries, but can induce vasoconstriction in atherosclerotic coronary segments.[11] Time of day also appears to affect the angina threshold. The amount of coronary artery dilatation in response to nitroglycerin is greater in the morning than it is in the evening[12] suggesting that coronary arteries are more constricted in the morning. In addition to changes in blood flow produced by vasomotion, other factors such as ventricular volume can also influence the anginal threshold. The internal workload at the onset of angina is lower during supine than during upright exercise, for example, because ventricular volume is larger in the supine exercise.[13]

EFFECT OF EXERCISE TRAINING ON EXERCISE PERFORMANCE IN PATIENTS WITH CORONARY ARTERY DISEASE

Exercise training increases Vo_2 max in healthy subjects by increasing both maximal stroke volume and the maximal AV O_2 diff. Approximately one-half of the increase in Vo_2 max is due to increases in stroke volume and one-half is due to the change in AV O_2 diff.[8] The magnitude of the change varies among subjects. Increases in Vo_2 max are greater with increasing duration and intensity of the exercise training program, whereas increases in Vo_2 max are less in more fit and older individuals. The magnitude of the increase in Vo_2 max in healthy subjects after training studies of 3 to 12 months duration is approximately 20%.[14] This increase in absolute work capacity means that the same external workload after training represents less of the individual's relative workload. Since exercise-induced increases in heart rate and systolic blood pressure are related to the relative, as opposed to the absolute, exercise workload, the same external workload after training elicits smaller increments in heart rate and blood pressure. Since heart rate and systolic blood pressure determine myocardial oxygen needs or the internal workload, the same external workload elicits markedly different internal workloads depending on the fitness and Vo_2 max of the exercising individual.

Similar adaptations to exercise training occur in patients with coronary artery disease and coronary heart disease. The average increase in Vo_2 max in published studies of exercise training in patients with coronary artery disease ranges from 11 to 56%.[15] The relative contribution of increases in stroke volume and AV O_2 diff to the increase in exercise capacity vary among individuals depending on the severity of their coronary heart disease and length of training. Patients with severely injured myocardium may only be able to augment the AV O_2 diff and therefore achieve an attenuated increase in maximal exercise capacity.

Patients with angina pectoris provide the clearest example of the physiological adaptations that occur in patients with coronary artery disease with exercise training. The increase in stroke volume with exercise training means that the same absolute external workload, which determines cardiac output, can be performed at a lower heart rate than before training. The lower heart rate requires less myocardial oxygen supply and coronary blood flow. Consequently, the same task can be performed after exercise training with a delayed onset of angina (Fig. 16.1). In many studies of exercise training for patients with angina pectoris, angina continues to occur at the same rate pressure product although exercise capacity at the onset of angina is higher.[16,17] Other studies, however, have clearly demonstrated increases in the rate pressure product at the onset of angina.[18,19] It is unlikely that this ostensible improvement in myocardial oxygen supply after short-term exercise training is related to reductions in the coronary artery lesion or to collateral artery development and most likely that it is related to changes in vasomotor tone. In a classic early study, Sim

and Neill noted an increase in exercise performance and in the rate pressure product at the onset of exercise-induced angina after only 13 weeks of exercise training.[19] There was no change in the double product at the onset of angina during cardiac pacing, however, suggesting that the improvement in coronary flow was not structural, but was related to the coronary artery response to exercise. The authors, in what is now a clairvoyant statement, suggested that exercise training may reduce coronary artery vasoconstriction during exercise. Other studies assessing the effect of exercise on ST-segment depression[20] or on myocardial perfusion images[21] have also suggested improvements in myocardial oxygen supply. Several animal studies using aortic ring preparations[22,23] and human studies using brachial artery flow as a surrogate marker of coronary function[24] have documented that exercise training increases arterial vasodilatory capacity.

Such possible vasomotion effects make exercise an effective adjunctive therapy for angina pa-

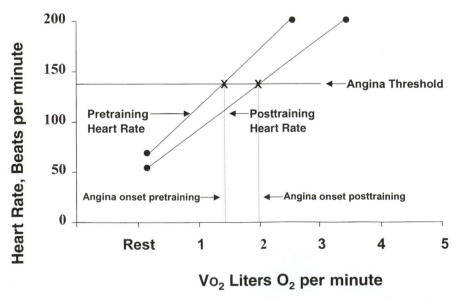

FIGURE 16.1. *This represents the changes in exercise tolerance and the onset of ischemia in a patient with angina pectoris. T_1 and T_2 are the heart rate versus oxygen uptake (VO_2) response lines before and after exercise training. After training, the patient can achieve a higher VO_2 level at a similar angina heart rate because of training-induced reductions in exercise heart rate.*

tients who are not candidates for revascularization. For example, among 18 patients with coronary artery disease whose exercise performance was limited by angina, only 7 continued to be limited by angina after only 12 weeks of an exercise training program.[25] Similar although less dramatic results have been reported by other authors.[20]

Assessment of only maximal effort capacity can underestimate many of the benefits of exercise function on daily activities, since few real-life tasks require maximal effort. Exercise training also had dramatic effects on submaximal working capacity in patients with coronary artery disease and coronary heart disease although this parameter has rarely been examined. Ades et al measured time to exhaustion in 45 cardiac patients aged 62 to 82 years.[26] Time to exhaustion was measured by treadmill walking at a workload requiring 80% of the individual's pretraining V_{O_2} max. Time to exhaustion increased 37% with exercise training. Whereas only 10 of 45 patients could complete the 45-min exercise session before training, 33 of 45 could do so after 3 months of exercise. The increase in V_{O_2} max in contrast was only 16%.

There is controversy over whether one can predict which patients are most likely to improve their effort tolerance with exercise training.[27] Fioretti et al found no significant relation between baseline exercise capacity and the change in exercise tolerance after 3 months of exercise training in post-MI patients.[28] Others noted less improvement in exercise performance with 3 months of training in patients with pretraining exercise-induced ischemia even though exercise performance at baseline was similar in the ischemic and nonischemic groups.[25] Among patients, all of whom had exercise-induced angina pectoris at baseline, we noted the greatest improvement in the workload at the onset of angina among those whose angina occurred at a rate pressure product above 20,000 before training.[17] Others have suggested that a leisure time physical energy expenditure above 1400 kcal daily is required to improve exercise tolerance in patients with coronary

artery disease.[20] Such discordant results prohibit definitive decisions as to which patients with coronary artery disease will or will not improve their effort tolerance with exercise training.

Many of the adaptations produced by exercise training are related to changes in the exercised skeletal muscle. These changes include increased capillary density, increased mitochondrial size and function, and increased muscle strength. These local muscle-specific adaptations plus early observations that much of the increase in exercise performance in patients with coronary artery disease after exercise training was mediated by increased AV O_2 diff[29] led to the separation of exercise training effects into "central" or cardiac adaptations and "peripheral" or muscle-specific changes. This separation seems arbitrary because of the close integration of peripheral and cardiac muscle function. Skeletal muscle is richly endowed with afferent nerves that help regulate the cardiovascular response to exercise.[4] Also, both healthy subjects[30] and patients with coronary artery disease[16,17] demonstrate enhanced exercise performance with both trained and untrained limbs after exercise training. For example, we[17] and others[16] have demonstrated increased work capacity at the onset of angina when subjects trained by leg cycling performed arm ergometry and visa versa. Furthermore, local peripheral decreases in vascular resistance may contribute to the "central" increase in cardiac output during exercise.[31] Consequently, it is probably more accurate to refer to "muscle-specific" and "generalized" exercise training effects rather than to "central" and "peripheral" adaptations.

EFFECTS OF EXERCISE TRAINING ON CORONARY ARTERY COLLATERALS AND STENOSES

Although there is increasingly strong evidence that exercise training can reduce the coronary artery vasoconstrictor response to exercise and thereby increase coronary artery flow, there is no conclusive evidence that exercise training can increase coronary collateral flow in patients with coronary artery disease or reduce the severity of stenotic lesions. A series of coronary angiographic studies from the 1970s failed to demonstrate collateral vessel development after 3 to 13 months of exercise training.[19,32–35] These early studies were hampered by poor resolution of the available angiographic imaging systems, but this author is unaware of studies that have reexamined this issue. More recent studies have examined the effect of exercise training on coronary artery stenoses using quantitative angiography. Most of these studies include exercise as one component of an intensive lifestyle or medical intervention.

The Lifestyle Heart Trial[36] is generally regarded as a test of low-fat diets but included multiple interventions. In this study, patients were randomized to lifestyle ($n = 53$) or control ($n = 43$) groups. Only 28 treatment and 20 control subjects agreed to participate. One control and 6 intervention subjects failed to have usable repeat angiograms including 1 intervention subject who died exercising, leaving results for only 22 treated and 19 control subjects. Intervention subjects also spent 3 h a week exercising. Coronary angiography was performed before and after a year of intervention.

The average diameter stenosis decreased from $40.0 \pm 16.9\%$ to $37.8 \pm 16.5\%$ in the treatment group and increased from $42.7 \pm 15.5\%$ to $46.1 \pm 18.5\%$ in the control group. The frequency of angina also decreased 91% in the experimental group, but exercise testing results were not reported. These improvements have generally been ascribed to the lifestyle program, which included a low-fat diet, social support sessions, stress management, and exercise, but we have speculated that the reduction in angina pectoris could have been produced by the exercise training component.[37]

The Stanford Coronary Risk Intervention Project (SCRIP)[38] randomly assigned patients with documented coronary atherosclerosis to a risk reduction program ($n = 145$) or to usual care ($n = 155$). The risk reduction program was individualized to include dietary and drug blood-lipid

management, home-based exercise training, weight loss, and smoking cessation. Coronary angiography was performed at baseline and at 4 years. Of the 300 randomized subjects, 82% had comparable angiograms at follow-up. The yearly rate of lesion progression was 47% lower in the risk reduction group. There were 44 hospitalizations for cardiac events in the control and only 25 hospitalizations in the intervention group giving a rate ratio of 0.61 and 95% confidence limits of 0.4 to 0.9. Although average low-density lipoprotein (LDL) cholesterol (−22%), high-density lipoprotein (HDL) cholesterol (+12%), and triglycerides (−20%) showed beneficial changes with the intervention, change in treadmill exercise performance (+20%) was the single best predictor of the change in minimal luminal diameter over the course of the study.

A trial in Heidelberg, Germany, randomized 45 patients with coronary artery disease to an intervention and 43 subjects to a usual care group.[20] Coronary angiograms were performed before and after a year of the trial. The control group spent 1 week, and the intervention group 3, on a metabolic ward at the start of the study for dietary instruction. Thirty minutes of daily exercise was recommended for both groups. The intervention group also engaged in two 60-min supervised exercise sessions weekly. Leisure time caloric expenditure was measured before and after the trial.

Only 29 of the intervention subjects and 33 of the control group completed the study. VO_2 max increased 7% in the exercise group and decreased 1% in controls. The ventilatory threshold, or the point at which respiratory rate becomes nonlinear because of excess CO_2 production formed by the buffering of lactic acid by bicarbonate, increased 14% in the intervention group and decreased 8% in the controls. Coronary artery stenoses for the intervention and control groups, respectively, regressed in 28 versus 6%, progressed in 10 versus 45%, and were unchanged in 62 versus 49%. These differences were highly significant. The best predictors of change in coronary artery lesions were exercise energy expenditure and change in LDL cholesterol. The authors estimated from their data that in order to change cardiorespiratory fitness, patients with coronary artery disease would need to expend 1400 kcal weekly whereas 1533 kcal and 2200 kcal per week would be required to stabilize or regress coronary lesions.

Unfortunately, these and similar studies are seriously flawed because it is impossible to be certain whether increases in fitness[38] or exercise energy expenditure[20] are measures of fitness or surrogate measures of adherence to other changes such as low-cholesterol diets. It is reassuring that these fitness measures are the strongest predictors of change in coronary lesion stenosis, but not sufficient to conclude that the exercise training alone is the mediator.

An additional problem with all trials using angiography as an endpoint is that they may underestimate changes in atherosclerotic plaque burden. Coronary arteries enlarge as atherosclerosis develops in an attempt to preserve the original lumen.[39] Indeed, approximately 30 to 40% of the original lumen has been replaced by atherosclerosis even before minimal amounts of plaque are visible on angiography.[40] An angiographic stenosis of 50% can represent a lesion of 75% of the original lumen and 89% of the cross-sectional diameter because the artery has enlarged and remodeled to accommodate the plaque.[40] It is also possible that egress of cholesterol from an atherosclerotic plaque does not alter the angiographically determined stenosis because of contraction of the adventitia. This may be an explanation as to why aggressive cholesterol reduction is associated with only minimal changes in the coronary lumen as visualized by angiography. A better way to assess coronary plaque burden would be with intravascular ultrasound imaging.

Another failing of two of these angiography studies[20,36] is that they fail to measure the most important cardiac endpoint, the incidence of cardiac events. It is now clear that most acute cardiac events such as MI and sudden cardiac death in asymptomatic persons are related to rupture of so-called "vulnerable plaques."[41] Angiographic trials such as the Familial Atherosclerotic Treatment Study, or FATS, note, at most, only a 3% difference in coronary stenosis between a control group and groups treated with lipid-lowering drugs, but there is a statistically significant reduction in the number of cardiac events.[42] Similarly although the SCRIPS trial showed marked differences in the rate of lesion progression, the absolute difference in change of % stenosis between the groups was quite small. Nevertheless, there was a significant reduction in cardiac admissions.[38] Such results suggest that interventions such as lipid-lowering medications can stabilize coronary plaques and render them less vulnerable to rupture without producing large changes in the coronary artery lumen. Consequently, studies of any intervention, including exercise training, should be judged on their ability to reduce the sequelae of coronary artery disease and not on their effect on "lumenology" alone.

EFFECTS OF EXERCISE TRAINING ON SURVIVAL IN PATIENTS WITH CORONARY ARTERY DISEASE

There is suggestive evidence that exercise training can reduce cardiac events in patients with coronary artery disease, although this evidence is not definitive. No single study has been sufficiently powered to address this issue. This is in contrast to pharmacologic interventions that have been studied in several large trials of patients with coronary artery disease. Unfortunately, there is no group with sufficient financial motivation to test directly the hypothesis that exercise training reduces subsequent MI or cardiac death in patients with coronary artery disease.

O'Connor et al addressed this issue of small sample sizes by performing a meta-analysis of randomized, controlled, exercise-based cardiac rehabilitation trials for post-MI patients.[43] These authors reviewed 36 studies and selected 22 for inclusion. Studies were excluded if they failed to contribute usable data, did not randomize patients individually, followed patients for less than a year after the intervention, or included patients with coronary artery disease who had not suffered an MI. The randomization methods varied among the studies. Most studies randomized patients 1 to 3 months after the infarct, but some patients were randomized as long as 36 months later. Follow-up also varied from 1 to 5 years, but two-thirds of the studies presented at least 3 years of follow-up. The sample included a total of 2310 patients randomized to rehabilitation and 2244 controls, but was heavily weighted toward middle-aged males. Most trials excluded patients older than 65 or 70 years. Two trials excluded patients over age 55 and 1 trial restricted patients to ages 40 to 55. Only 3% of the sample were women. All of the studies included exercise-based cardiac rehabilitation, but most studies included other interventions such as smoking cessation and dietary instruction; only 7 studies used exercise training as the only intervention.

At 1 year of follow-up, the % change in total mortality (and the 95% confidence limits) were −23 (−41 to +1%), at 2 years they were −26 (−41 to −8%), and at 3 years −20 (−34 to −4%), in favor of the rehabilitation group. Confidence limits that do not include 0 signify a statistically significant effect, so that these results demonstrate a reduction in total mortality of 20 to 26% in favor of the rehabilitation programs. This reduction was statistically significant in all but the first year. The % reduction in total mortality was similar for the exercise-only studies (−19, −40 to +10%) and for those studies that included interventions other than exercise (−21, −38 to +1%), but in neither group was the reduction statistically significant. Most deaths in post-MI patients are related to cardiovascular causes, so it is not surprising that cardiovascular deaths were 22% lower during the 3 years examined. This was statistically significant only during the third year. Sudden death in the first year after randomization was 37% lower (−39 to −3%). This reduction was not statistically significant for years 2 (−24, −46 to +3%) and 3 (−8, −31 to +23%). Fatal MIs were also 33% lower during year 1, 27% lower during year 2, and 25% lower during year 3, and all of these reductions were statistically significant. Interest-

ingly, there was no reduction in nonfatal reinfarctions that were slightly, but nonsignificantly higher by 9, 10, and 9% during years 1 to 3, respectively.

This well-conducted meta-analysis provides strong support for the use of exercise-based cardiac rehabilitation, but has multiple limitations. Only post-MI patients were examined, so the results may not be applicable to other types of patients with coronary artery disease and coronary heart disease. Subjects were primarily middle-aged males, and the study cannot address whether exercise is beneficial for women and elderly patients. Both of these groups comprise a growing percentage of the cardiac population. The studies were all performed between 1960 and 1984 and may not be reproducible in the present medical environment. At present, fewer "post-MI" patients are left with myocardial damage because of the more frequent use of reperfusion therapies such as thrombolytic therapy or primary angioplasty. Similarly, fewer post-MI patients have residual ischemia because of aggressive bypass surgery and angioplasty. Also, several of the physiological effects of exercise training are achievable by pharmacological means. β-adrenergic blocking agents reduce resting and exercise heart rates, and a variety of medications produce peripheral vasodilatation. Consequently, if some of the benefits of exercise training observed in the meta-analysis were due to reductions of ischemia, the present prevalence of fewer MI patients with residual ischemia would reduce an exercise training effect. This uncertainty will likely persist because there is no financial support for a definite trial of the effects of exercise training in patients with coronary artery disease.

As noted earlier, sudden death was 37% lower than normal during the first year after randomization. This raises important questions as to how this effect was achieved. Exercise training reduces the incidence of ventricular fibrillation during ischemia in animal models, and the reduction correlates with increases in parasympathetic tone.[44,45] This suggests that the exercise program itself may have reduced sudden death. Alternatively, exercise can provoke malignant ventricular arrhythmias and the reduction in sudden death only during the first year of rehabilitation may be due to the availability of defibrillators and trained personnel to resuscitate victims of exercise-related ventricular fibrillation. This raises the possibility that benefits observed for this study of supervised exercise training may not accrue to patients with coronary artery disease who are participating in unsupervised or home programs.

The reduction in fatal infarctions without a reduction in recurrent nonfatal events also suggests that exercise training may represent a form of ischemic preconditioning. *Ischemic preconditioning* refers to the observation primarily in animal models that brief periods of ischemia before coronary occlusion can reduce subsequent infarct size.[46] Ischemic preconditioning is of growing importance in cardiology since it is widely recognized as second only to early reperfusion as a mechanism to protect the myocardium against ischemic injury.[46] This effect is observable in 2 time periods: immediately after the temporary ischemia indicating an acute adaptation, and 24 to 72 h after the ischemia implying the production of such possible protein mediators as heat shock proteins, superoxide dismutase, nitric oxide synthase, and protein kinase C.[46] One possible clinical correlate of ischemic preconditioning is the observation that angina within 48 h before a subsequent MI reduces the severity of the event as measured by peak creatinine kinase, left ventricular dysfunction, ventricular fibrillation, hospital death, and congestive heart failure.[47] There is evidence that the benefits of preinfarction angina before an MI do not occur in patients over the age of 65 years.[47]

Exercise has been suggested as a form of ischemic preconditioning that helps lessen the effects of subsequent ischemia.[48] Interestingly, exposing the heart to endogenous or exogenous norepinephrine or other catecholamines produces changes similar to ischemic preconditioning.[49] There are 3 implications from the possibility that some of the benefits of exercise in patients with coronary artery disease are mediated by ischemic

preconditioning. First, the exercise must be frequent and sustained over time because the ischemic preconditioning is transient. Second, the benefits might only accrue to patients who have exercise-induced ischemia since only in such patients would exercise induce ischemia with the resultant adaptations. Third, in the absence of ischemia, the exercise may have to be sufficiently intense to increase circulating catecholamines to elicit the preconditioning effect.

COST-EFFECTIVENESS OF EXERCISE-BASED CARDIAC REHABILITATION

The survival benefit from the preceding meta-analysis has been used to estimate the cost-effectiveness of cardiac rehabilitation. Ades et al compared medical expenses in 589 patients after MI or bypass surgery who were ($n = 230$) or did not ($n = 350$) referred to a cardiac exercise program.[50] Patients participating in the rehabilitation program had fewer hospital admissions and shorter hospital stays than those who did not, resulting in a savings of $739 per patient per year. Using these results, the 20% reduction in mortality demonstrated by the meta-analysis after year 3 and an average life expectancy of 15.4 years based on the Duke Database, the authors estimated a value for cardiac rehabilitation of $4950 per year of life saved based on 1995 dollars.[51] This analysis did not include direct and indirect nonmedical costs, which should have improved the value of cardiac rehabilitation. The analysis also assumed that there was no additional value to rehabilitation participation after the approximately 20% risk reduction in year 3. Nevertheless, these calculated benefits compare favorably with other accepted interventions such as thrombolytic therapy, coronary bypass surgery, and lipid-lowering medications. All of the same limitations of the meta-analysis, however, apply to this analysis as well because the same data and assumptions were used.

Much of the cost saving observed with cardiac rehabilitation participation appears to be related to frequent contact with the rehabilitation professional staff. Patients with coronary artery disease are repetitively admonished while hospitalized to monitor themselves for chest discomfort and to report such symptoms if they persist. Among patients in supervised rehabilitation programs, these symptoms can be related to the staff and evaluated. The exercise session itself can be used as a modified stress test to evaluate the symptoms further and to appropriately triage the patient. Patients for whom this service is not available often come to the emergency room or seek other care prompted more by concern than discomfort. Once in the emergency room or with a physician unaware of their status, they are often admitted with attendant costs.

This effect seems much more strongly related to staff contact than to the exercise component of the program. Bondestam et al compared the use of medical care in elderly patients after MI who were or were not referred to a cardiac rehabilitation program.[52] All of the participants in cardiac rehabilitation received individual counseling in their home and at a local health center, but only 21% participated in a moderate intensity, facility-based exercise program. Patients in the rehabilitation program had a lower incidence of emergency room visits and rehospitalization at 3 and 12 months after the infarct. Emergency room visits were generally justified among the participants in the rehabilitation program, but among the patients who were not in the rehabilitation program such visits were often prompted by what the authors called "vague" symptoms.

RISKS OF EXERCISE TRAINING IN PATIENTS WITH CORONARY ARTERY DISEASE

The primary risks of exercise training are rare and include cardiac arrest (1 event for every 112,000 patient hours of participation), MI (1 event for every 294,000 patient hours), and death (1 event for every 784,000 patient-hours).[53] Assuming that each patient exercises 3 h per week for 12 weeks, these incidence figures suggest that there should be 1 cardiac arrest per year for every 2871 participating patients, 1 MI per year for every 7538, and 1 death per year for every 20,102. In supervised programs approximately 85% of patients suffering a cardiac arrest are successfully resuscitated.[53] Nevertheless, the risks of exercise during vigorous cardiac rehabilitation are real and of concern. In several published studies involving vigorous rehabilitation, sudden death did occur. For example in the Lifestyle Heart Trial,[36] it is often overlooked that one of the intervention participants died during exercise. The authors state that this subject was "overexercising." Similarly in the Heidelberg study, there were 3 cardiac arrests, 2 in the intervention group and 1 in the control group.[20] One of the arrests in the intervention group was successfully treated with prompt cardioversion and he was said to have exceeded his training heart rate by 30% prior to the arrest. Despite these disclaimers,[20,36] such events highlight the potential risks of vigorous exercise.

I recognize the benefits of therapeutic exercise training for patients with coronary artery disease and the low risk of participating in supervised exercise programs, but am cautious about permitting patients with diagnosed coronary artery disease to compete in vigorous athletics. Vigorous exercise clearly increases the risk of cardiac arrest and MI in patients with coronary artery disease.[54,55] Patients with diagnosed coronary artery disease and coronary heart disease should be encouraged to participate in cardiac rehabilitation programs and also to exercise moderately in unsupervised settings. Such patients should be discouraged from competing in athletic events where their ability to restrict their competitive instincts might be compromised. This is often a problem since many athletes with coronary artery disease are competitive by nature and feel a loss of self-worth when their athletic participation is curtailed.

There has been debate as to whether exercise training accelerates the deterioration of left ventricular function in patients with anterior wall MI and reduced left ventricular function. This concern was initiated by Jugdutt et al who examined the effect of 12 weeks of exercise training on left ventricular size and function in 13 patients after Q-wave anterior wall MI and 24 nonrandomized, matched control patients.[56] Left ventricular function, before and after training, was assessed by 2-dimensional echocardiograms. The exercise training program started 15 weeks after the MI and was atypical. Training was based on the Canadian Air Force Exercise Program and required 11 min of daily exercise split between calisthenics and a stationary run. After the 12 weeks of training, the training group and control group were subdivided into two additional groups depending on whether or not their functional status had remained constant or deteriorated during the study. Among the exercise trainers, the group whose functional status decreased had greater pretraining left ventricular asynergy, which progressed with training. This group also experienced a decrease in left ventricular ejection fraction with training. The authors suggested that exercise training worsened left ventricular function in anterior wall MI patients and that the deterioration may be related to incomplete healing of the infarction.

This report initiated considerable concern in the cardiac rehabilitation community since it is widely appreciated that deteriorating left ventricular function is a poor prognostic sign. Fortunately, the concern has not been confirmed by subsequent studies. Giannuzzi et al[57] randomly assigned patients with Q-wave infarction to 6 months of exercise training ($n = 39$) or control ($n = 38$). Of the subjects, 78% had suffered an anterior wall MI so the results are directly applicable to the concerns raised by Jugdutt et al.[56] The exercise training program was intense. Patients exercised under supervision for 30 min thrice weekly for 2 months on bicycle ergometers at 80% of their predetermined maximal heart rate. They then continued the same program at home but added a brisk 30 min daily walk and continued this program for an additional 4 months.

Left ventricular volumes appeared to expand only in the control subjects perhaps to compen-

sate for the reduced left ventricular function. Left ventricular end-diastolic volume increased 5%, end-systolic volume increased 8%, and regional dilatation 21% in the control subjects, but was unchanged in the exercise trained group. Left ventricular ejection fraction increased from 34 ± 5% to 38 ± 8% in the trainers ($p < 0.01$), but was unchanged in the control subjects (34 ± 5% to 33 ± 7%). In contrast to the results of Judgutt et al,[56] the absence of left ventricular dilatation and the increase in ejection fraction in the training group suggest that vigorous exercise training may increase left ventricular contractility and actually prevent deterioration in left ventricular function. Also in contrast to Judgutt et al's study, the majority of patients were receiving both β-adrenergic blocking agents and ACE inhibitors suggesting that exercise training contributes to improved left ventricular function despite maximal medical therapy. The authors raise the possibility that prolonged exercise training may enhance the effects of ACE inhibition perhaps by a vasodilatory effect.

PRACTICAL ASPECTS OF EXERCISE TRAINING PROGRAMS FOR PATIENTS WITH CORONARY ARTERY DISEASE

Cardiac rehabilitation is usually divided into 4 stages. Phase 1 refers to in-patient rehabilitation, which has been abandoned by most centers because of the short duration of most hospital stays and evidence that such programs do not improve predischarge exercise performance.[58] Phase 2 refers to the first 12 weeks of rehabilitation after a cardiac event or interventional procedure. Some insurers occasionally extend this duration to 24 weeks for certain indications. Phase 3 refers to patients who have completed the initial 12 to 24 weeks but elect to remain in a supervised setting often without insurance coverage and on a self-pay basis. Phase 4 refers to cardiac rehabilitation performed away from an organized rehabilitation program in sites such as a local fitness facility.

Most exercise-based cardiac rehabilitation programs have a similar structure and exercise training schedule. Most, but not all, programs require a baseline exercise stress test to determine maximal exercise heart rate, to document baseline exercise performance, and to exclude significant cardiac ischemia. Other programs do not require such testing if the patient has recently undergone a revascularization procedure and use symptoms and rating of perceived exertion as a guide for exercise training intensity. Exercise training starts as soon as possible after the myocardial infarction or interventional procedure. Our program tries to start patients after an uncomplicated MI or angioplasty within a week of discharge and patients after uncomplicated coronary bypass graft surgery within 3 weeks of discharge. Characteristically, exercise training is performed thrice weekly for 20 to 40 min a session at 70 to 85% of the baseline maximal heart rate and is continued for 12 or more weeks. Patients with exercise-induced ischemia or angina are exercised below their ischemic threshold in most programs although we prefer to exercise patients in a supervised program to the onset of angina or to the predetermined ischemic rate pressure product. We also use sublingual or spray nitroglycerin liberally in order to increase the tolerated exercise intensity. This approach is based on the unsubstantiated belief that inducing ischemia may induce coronary artery adaptations or ischemic preconditioning, whereas less intense exercise would not. This possibility is also supported by the observation that patients with claudication appear to obtain the most benefit for exercise therapy if they walk to the onset of discomfort. Such an approach is not routinely recommended for at-home exercise training and the distinction must be clear to the patients. We do allow some patients with stable angina pectoris to exercise to the onset of pain during unsupervised sessions, but restrict patients with silent exercise-induced ischemia to an intensity below their ischemic rate pressure product in order to avoid prolonged asymptomatic ischemia. Most cardiac rehabilitation programs also include education and counseling sessions, although there is little data to support the utility of these educational activities.

Cardiac rehabilitation programs before the 1990s generally prohibited resistance exercise training because of misguided concerns that such exercise would inappropriately increase systolic blood pressure and produce cardiac complications.[59] At present, almost all rehabilitation programs include some strength training component involving large muscle groups to enable patients to more adequately meet the demands of daily household tasks. Common exercises included in such strength training programs include modified push-ups, biceps curls, military presses, bench presses, quadriceps extensions, hamstring curls, and bent knee sit-ups.[59]

Insurers generally require that patients participating in rehabilitation programs have electrocardiographic monitoring during the exercise sessions. There is little support for such monitoring except for the early observation that cardiac complications appeared to be less in programs providing this service.[53] Nevertheless, such monitoring is standard in all programs because of Medicare's and other insurance providers' requirements for reimbursement. The usual ratio of personnel to participants is 1 to 5 during phase 2 and 1 to 8 during phase 3 rehabilitation.

PERSONAL PERSPECTIVE

I feel strongly that exercise-based cardiac rehabilitation is underutilized in contemporary cardiology. Exercise training is one of the few nonsurgical interventions that can make patients feel better physically and mentally, yet only approximately 15% of eligible patients are referred to programs.[2] The reasons for this low referral rate are unclear, but I suspect that many physicians are uncomfortable with exercise and do not personally know its benefits. I also feel that many patients with stable angina pectoris, which occurs at a high rate pressure product and who have only 1- or 2-vessel disease, can be as well treated with a trial of therapeutic exercise as with prompt angioplasty. Patients who worsen or do not improve with aggressive medical treatment, including an exercise program, can then be referred for interventional therapy.

My personal bias is that most cardiac rehabilitation

programs do not exercise patients vigorously enough to obtain the maximal benefits of therapeutic exercise. There has been an increasing emphasis on moderate exercise for both the public and for cardiac patients.[60] Such an approach is clearly justified on a public health basis, but may reduce the benefits of exercise training in patients with coronary artery disease. Many of the effects of exercise appear to be related to reduced sensitivity to adrenergic stimulation. These sort of adaptations may require repeated exposure to adrenergic stimuli, which does not occur unless the exercise is at least moderately intense. I should emphasize that the vigorous aspects of exercise training should be restricted to supervised programs because there is no doubt that vigorous exercise does increase the risk of cardiac events.

There is at present great interest in reducing the cost of cardiac rehabilitation by using home-based programs and such devices as heart rhythm telephone monitoring. Home-based programs for low-risk patients can produce increases in VO_2 max that are similar to those obtained in the supervised setting.[61] Such programs are also described as safe because no complications have occurred, but given the rarity of exercise complications in supervised programs[53] considerably more experience is required before the safety of home-based programs will have been adequately addressed. I believe that many of the cardiovascular adaptations to exercise training in patients with coronary artery disease require vigorous training. Consequently, I prefer that at least the initial training be performed in a supervised setting and that home exercise be restricted to moderate exercise. I also suspect that much of the cost saving observed with cardiac rehabilitation participation is related to frequent interaction with the rehabilitation professional staff. Staff support and reassurance is not as readily available to home participants. In addition, participants in home rehabilitation do not obtain the group support that is often an important part of patients adjusting to their disease.

There are important benefits to exercise for patients with coronary artery disease. The issue as to whether patients participate in home-based or facility-based exercise is less important than their participation in some structured program. The best approach for most clinical issues is a flexible approach depending on the individual patient's circumstances. Patients who live too far from an exercise facility to participate easily should be instructed in a home-based program. Patients who

are exceptionally anxious about their condition are often best served by a supervised program.

I also believe that many of the current practices in cardiac rehabilitation are based more on economics than on clinical care principles. There is little compelling reason to perform electrocardiographic monitoring on all patients at all exercise sessions and yet this is routinely done because it is required for most medical reimbursements. Similarly, most cardiac rehabilitation programs last 12 weeks because insurance coverage ends at this point. This is sufficient to induce an exercise training response, but more substantial gains probably occur with more prolonged training. Also, little of the initial exercise training benefit persists if the patient subsequently becomes inactive. I would prefer a reimbursement approach that encourages both providers and patients to develop long-term exercise programs for patients with coronary artery disease. I recommend that all participants in cardiac rehabilitation enter into a maintenance program. Indeed the goal of present cardiac rehabilitation programs should be to provide patients with the skills to maintain a lifelong exercise program.

Finally, I believe that exercise-based cardiac rehabilitation should be critically reevaluated in a randomized control clinical trial modeled after the meta-analysis.[43] This meta-analysis suggested a 20% reduction in mortality 3 years after the program. The rehabilitation intervention was sufficiently robust so that only 4554 patients were required to demonstrate this effect. This reduction compares favorably with other accepted interventions for cardiac patients. For example, the Scandinavian Simvastatin Survival Study randomized 4444 patients with coronary artery disease to simvastatin or a placebo and documented a 30% reduction in total mortality with Simvastatin after only an average of 5.4 years.[62] Similarly, the Cholesterol and Recurrent Events (CARE) trial randomized 4159 patients with coronary artery disease to pravastatin or a placebo and documented a 24% reduction in cardiac events after a mean average of only 5 years.[63] The 20% mortality reduction with cardiac rehabilitation[43] is especially impressive given that the formal exercise intervention lasted only 2 to 6 months, that follow-up was only for 3 years, and that patients exercised on their own, if at all, for most of this time. It is not clear whether cardiac rehabilitation will be as successful in contemporary medical care, but it may be even more successful if exercise training is maintained indefinitely for the patient. At any point, a definitive trial that is appropriately powered is needed to determine if long-term cardiac rehabilitation is as valuable as present evidence suggests.

REFERENCES

1. Heberden W: Commentary on the history and cure of disease, in Willius FA, Keys TE (ed.): *Cardiac Classics.* CV Mosby, St. Louis: 1941, p. 224.
2. Balady GJ, Fletcher BJ, Froelicher ES, et al: Cardiac Rehabilitation Programs: A statement for healthcare professionals from the American Heart Association. *Circulation* 90:1602–1610, 1994.
3. Ryan TJ, Antman EM, Brooks NH, et al: 1999 update: ACC/AHA guidelines for the management of patients with acute myocardial infarction: Executive summary and recommendations: A report of the American College of Cardiology/American Heart Association task force on practice guidelines. *Circulation* 100:1016–1030, 1999.
4. Mitchell JH, Victor RG: Neural control of the cardiovascular system: Insights from muscle sympathetic nerve recordings in humans. *Med Sci Sports Exerc* 10(Suppl):S60–S69, 1996.
5. Amsterdam EA, Hughes JL, DeMaria AN, et al: Indirect assessment of myocardial oxygen consumption in the evaluation of mechanisms and therapy of angina pectoris. *Am J Cardiol* 33: 737–743, 1974.
6. Wilmore JH, Costill DL: *Physiology of Sport and Exercise.* Champaign, ll, Human Kinetics, 1994, p. 180.
7. Gobel FL, Nelson RR, Jorgensen CR, et al: The rate-pressure product as an index of myocardial oxygen consumption during exercise in patients with angina pectoris. *Circulation* 57:549–556, 1978.
8. Mitchell JH, Blomqvist G: Maximal oxygen uptake. *N Engl J Med* 284:1018–1022, 1971.
9. Powell KE, Thompson PD, Caspersen CJ, et al: Physical activity and the incidence of coronary heart disease. *Ann Rev Pub Health* 8:253–287, 1987.
10. Blair SN, Kampert JB, Kohl HW 3rd, et al: Influences of cardiorespiratory fitness and other precursors on cardiovascular disease and all-cause mortality in men and women. *JAMA* 276:205–210, 1996.
11. Gordon JB, Ganz P, Nabel EG, et al: Atherosclerosis influences the vasomotor response of epicardial coronary arteries to exercise. *J Clin Invest* 83:1946–1952, 1989.
12. Yasue H, Omote S, Takizawa A, et al: Circadian variation of exercise capacity in patients with Prinzmetal's variant angina: Role of exercise-induced coronary arterial spasm. *Circulation* 59: 938–948, 1979.
13. Bygdeman S, Wahren J: Influence of body position on the anginal threshold during leg exercise. *Eur J Clin Invest* 4:201–206, 1974.
14. Brooks G, Fahey TD, White TP: Exercise physiology: Human bioenergetics and its applications. Mountain View, California, Mayfield Publishing Company, 1996, pp. 281–299.
15. Thompson PD: The benefits and risks of exercise training in patients with chronic coronary artery disease. *JAMA* 259:1537–1540, 1998.
16. Clausen JP, Trap-Jensen J: Heart rate and arterial blood pressure during exercise in patients with angina pectoris. Effects of training and of nitroglycerin. *Circulation* 53:436–442, 1976.
17. Thompson PD, Cullinane E, Lazarus B, et al: Effect of exercise training on the untrained limb exercise performance of men with angina pectoris. *Am J Cardiol* 48:844–850, 1981.
18. Redwood DR, Rosin DR, Epstein SE: Circulatory and symptomatic effects of physical training in patients with coronary artery disease and angina pectoris. *N Engl J Med* 286:959–965, 1972.
19. Sim DN, Neill WA: Investigation of the physiological basis for increased exercise threshold for angina pectoris after physical conditioning. *J Clin Invest* 54:763–770, 1974.
20. Hambrecht R, Niebauer J, Marburger C, et al: Various intensities of leisure time physical activity in patients with coronary artery disease: Effects on cardiorespiratory fitness and progression of coronary atherosclerotic lesions. *J Am Coll Cardiol* 22(2):468–477, 1993.
21. Froelicher V, Jensen D, Genter F, et al: A randomized trial of exercise training in patients with coronary heart disease. *JAMA* 252:1291–1297, 1984.
22. Gaukler HM, Dicarlo SE, Stallone JN: Acute exercise attenuates phenylephrine-induced contraction of rabbit isolated aortic rings. *Med Sci Sports Exerc* 24:1102–1107, 1992.
23. Chen H, Li HT, Chen CC: Physical conditioning decreases norepinephrine-induced vasoconstric-

tion in rabbits: Possible roles of norepinephrine-evoked endothelium-derived relaxing factor. *Circulation* 90:970–975, 1994.

24. Higashi Y, Sasaki S, Kurisu S, et al: Regular aerobic exercise augments endothelium-dependent vascular relaxation in normotensive as well as hypertensive subjects. *Circulation* 100:1194–1202, 1999.

25. Ades PA, Grunvald MH, Weiss RM, et al: Usefulness of myocardial ischemia as predictor of training effect in cardiac rehabilitation after acute myocardial infarction or coronary artery bypass grafting. *Am J Cardiol* 63:1032–1036, 1989.

26. Ades PA, Waldmann ML, Poehlman ET, et al: Exercise conditioning in older coronary patients: Submaximal lactate response and endurance capacity. *Circulation* 88:572–577, 1993.

27. Myers J, Froehlicher VF: Predicting outcome in cardiac rehabilitation. *J Am Coll Cardiol* 15: 983–985, 1990.

28. Fioretti P, Simoons ML, Zwiers G, et al: Value of predischarge data for the prediction of exercise capacity after cardiac rehabilitation in patients with recent myocardial infarction. *Eur Heart J* 8:330–338, 1987.

29. Detry J-MR, Rousseau M, Vandenbroucke G, et al: Increased arteriovenous oxygen difference after physical training in coronary heart disease. *Circulation* 44:109–118, 1971.

30. Lewis S, Thompson P, Areskog N-H, et al: Transfer effects of endurance training to exercise with untrained limbs. *Eur J Appl Physiol* 44: 25–34, 1980.

31. Rowell LB: *Human Circulation Regulation during Physical Stress.* New York, Oxford University Press, 1986.

32. Nolewajka AJ, Kostuk WJ, Rechnitzer PA, et al: Exercise and human collateralization: An angiographic and scintigraphic assessment. *Circulation* 60:114–121, 1979.

33. Conner JF, LaCamera F, Swanick EJ, et al: Effects of exercise on coronary collateralization-angiographic studies of six patients in a supervised exercise program. *Med Sci Sports Exerc* 8:145–151, 1976.

34. Ferguson RJ, Petitclerc R, Choquette G, et al: Effect of physical training on treadmill exercise capacity, collateral circulation and progression of coronary disease. *Am J Cardiol* 34:764–769, 1974.

35. Kennedy CC, Spiekerman RE, Lindsay MI, et al:

One-year graduated exercise program for men with angina pectoris. *Mayo Clin Proc* 51:231–236, 1976.

36. Ornish D, Brown SE, Scherwitz LW, et al: Can lifestyle changes reverse coronary heart disease? The Lifestyle Heart Trial. *Lancet* 336:129–133, 1990.

37. Thompson PD: More on low-fat diets. *N Engl J Med* 338:1623–1624, 1998.

38. Haskell WL, Alderman EL, Fair JM, et al: Effects of intensive multiple risk factor reduction on coronary atherosclerosis and clinical cardiac events in men and women with coronary artery disease: The Stanford coronary risk intervention project (SCRIP). *Circulation* 89:975–990, 1994.

39. Glagov S, Weisenberg E, Zarins CK, et al: Compensatory enlargement of human atherosclerotic coronary arteries. *N Engl J Med* 316:1371–1375, 1987.

40. Birnbaum Y, Fishbein MC, Luo H, et al: Regional remodeling of atherosclerotic arteries: A major determinant of clinical manifestations of disease. *J Am Coll Cardiol* 30:1149–1164, 1997.

41. Fuster V, Badimon L, Badimon JJ, et al: The pathogenesis of coronary artery disease and the acute coronary syndromes (1). *N Engl J Med* 326:242–250, 1992.

42. Brown BG, Zhao XQ, Sacco DE, et al: Lipid lowering and plaque regression: New insights into prevention of plaque disruption and clinical events in coronary disease. *Circulation* 87:1781–1791, 1993.

43. O'Connor GT, Buring JE, Yusuf S, et al: An overview of randomized trials of rehabilitation with exercise after myocardial infarction. *Circulation* 80:234–244, 1989.

44. Kent KM, Smith ER, Redwood DR, et al: Electrical stability of acutely ischemic myocardium. *Circulation* 47:291–298, 1973.

45. Billman GE, Schwartz PJ, Stone HL: The effects of daily exercise on susceptibility to sudden cardiac death. *Circulation* 69:1182–1189, 1984.

46. Kloner RA, Bolli R, Marban E, et al: Participants, medical and cellular implications of stunning, hibernation, and preconditioning: An NHLBI workshop. *Circulation* 97:1848–1867, 1998.

47. Abete P, Ferrara N, Cacciatore F, et al: Angina-induced protection against myocardial infarction in adult and elderly patients: A loss of preconditioning mechanism in the aging heart? *J Am Coll Cardiol* 30:947–954, 1997.

48. Maybaum S, Ilan M, Mogilevsky J, et al: Improvement in ischemic parameters during repeated exercise testing: A possible model for myocardial preconditioning. *Am J Cardiol* 78:1087–1091, 1996.

49. Bankwala Z, Hale SL, Kloner RA: Alpha-adrenoceptor stimulation with exogenous norepinephrine or release of endogenous catecholamines mimics ischemic preconditioning. *Circulation* 90:1023–1028, 1994.

50. Ades PA, Huand G, Weaver SO: Cardiac rehabilitation participation predicts lower rehospitalization costs. *Am Heart J* 123:916–921, 1992.

51. Ades PA, Pashkow FJ, Nestor JR: Cost-effectiveness of cardiac rehabilitation after myocardial infarction. *J Cardiopul Rehabil* 17:222–231, 1997.

52. Bondestam E, Breikss A, Hartford M: Effects of early rehabilitation on consumption of medical care during the first year after acute myocardial infarction in patients > or = 65 years of age. *Am J Cardiol* 75(12):767–771, 1995.

53. Van Camp SP, Peterson RA: Cardiovascular complications of outpatient cardiac rehabilitation programs. *JAMA* 256:1160–1163, 1986.

54. Giri S, Thompson PD, Kiernan FJ, et al: Clinical and angiographic characteristics of exertion-related acute myocardial infarction. *JAMA* 282:1731–1736, 1999.

55. Thompson PD, Funk E, Carleton RA, et al: Incidence of death during jogging in Rhode Island from 1975 through 1980. *JAMA* 247:2535–2538, 1982.

56. Jugdutt BI, Michorowski BL, Kappagoda CT: Exercise training after anterior Q wave myocardial infarction: Importance of regional left ventricular function and topography. *J Am Coll Cardiol* 12:362–372, 1988.

57. Giannuzzi P, Temporelli L, Corra U, et al: Attenuation of unfavorable remodeling by exercise training in postinfarction patients with left ventricular dysfunction: Results of the exercise in left ventricular dysfunction (ELVD) trial. *Circulation* 96:1790–1797, 1997.

58. Sivarajan ES, Bruce RA, Almes MJ, et al: In-hospital exercise after myocardial infarction does not improve treadmill performance. *N Engl J Med* 305:357–362, 1981.

59. Ghilarducci LE, Holly RG, Amsterdam EA: Effects of high resistance training in coronary artery disease. *Am J Cardiol* 64:866–870, 1989.

60. Pate RR, Pratt M, Blair SN, et al: Physical activity and public health. A recommendation from the Centers for Disease Control and Prevention and the American College of Sports Medicine. *JAMA* 273:402–407, 1995.

61. Miller NH, Haskell WL, Berra K, et al: Home versus group exercise training for increasing functional capacity after myocardial infarction. *Circulation* 70:645–649, 1984.

62. Scandinavian Simvastatin Survival Study Group, Randomised trial of cholesterol lowering in 4444 patients with coronary heart disease: The Scandinavian Simvastatin survival study (4S). *Lancet* 344:1383–1389, 1994.

63. Sacks FM, Pfeffer MA, Moye LA, et al: The effect of pravastatin on coronary events after myocardial infarction in patients with average cholesterol levels. *N Engl J Med* 335:1001–1009, 1996.

Chapter 17

EXERCISE TRAINING FOR PATIENTS WITH PERIPHERAL ARTERIAL DISEASE

Andrew W. Gardner, Ph.D.

Cardiac diseases were the first leading cause of death in 1990 and cerebrovascular diseases were the fourth,[1] making atherosclerotic cardiovascular disease the most significant health problem in the United States. Atherosclerosis in the arteries of the lower extremities, termed *peripheral arterial disease (PAD),* is also an important medical concern because of a high prevalence of concomitant coronary and cerebral artery disease,[2] and because ischemic pain in the leg musculature (intermittent claudication) severely limits the performance of daily physical activities. The majority of research on PAD comes from the discipline of vascular surgery, but the contributions in exercise physiology are growing because of studies documenting the effectiveness of exercise rehabilitation in many of these patients. The synergistic collaboration between vas-

Dr. Gardner is supported by a Special Emphasis Research Career Award from the National Institute on Aging (NIA) (K01-AG-00657), and by a Claude D. Pepper Older American Independence Center (OAIC) from NIA (P60-AG12583).

371

cular surgeons and exercise clinicians is important for the clinical management of patients with PAD. This is true because the primary goal for the vascular surgeon is to improve circulation and limb viability, whereas the primary concern of the exercise clinician is to regain function that was lost through years of physical inactivity secondary to intermittent claudication. This chapter will concentrate on the definition and classification of PAD, evaluation of patients with PAD, exercise rehabilitation programs for patients with PAD, and pharmacologic and revascularization interventions for patients with PAD.

DEFINITION AND CLASSIFICATION OF PERIPHERAL ARTERIAL DISEASE

Peripheral arterial disease occurs from lesions in the abdominal aorta, iliac, femoral, popliteal, and tibial arteries. Blood flow distal to the arterial lesions is reduced, which ultimately has a negative impact on ambulation and functional independence of elderly patients with PAD. The hallmark clinical measure for detecting PAD is the ankle-brachial index (ABI), or the ratio of systolic blood pressure measured in the ankle and in the arm.[3] In patients with PAD, the reduction in leg blood flow results in a low ankle pressure and a low ABI value. The defined prevalence of PAD is highly dependent on the ABI cutpoint used to detect inadequate peripheral circulation. The definition of an abnormal ABI has ranged between < 0.80 to < 0.97,[4-7] with ≤ 0.90 accepted as the reference standard.[8] The normal ABI is ≥ 1.00 because systolic pressure increases the further the pressure is measured from the central aorta. Values between 0.91 and 1.00 represent borderline PAD.[8] The prevalence of PAD is 16% in the general population above 55 years of age when an ABI value of ≤ 0.90 is used as the definition of PAD.[8]

In the early stages of PAD development, the reduction in blood flow does not produce noticeable symptoms. This is defined as stage I or asymptomatic PAD, according to the Fontaine

classification system (Table 17.1).[9] As PAD progresses, ischemic pain in the leg musculature occurs when patients walk, and is classified as stage II (intermittent claudication). Stage II patients can be further classified as having mild intermittent claudication (distance to onset of pain > 200 m) or severe intermittent claudication (distance to onset of pain < 200 m). In more advanced stages of disease, blood flow is reduced to such an extent that pain is experienced even at rest (stage III, rest pain). Further progression of the disease leads to ischemic ulcerations on the lower extremities and gangrene (stage IV, gangrene/tissue loss). Patients with stage III or stage IV PAD have critical leg ischemia in which the ischemic process endangers part or all of the lower extremity. These patients are candidates for surgical or percutaneous revascularization procedures.

Exercise rehabilitation programs are indicated for patients with stage I and stage II PAD, and in revascularized patients who have significant hemodynamic improvements but who remain functionally dependent due to the extreme deconditioning that occurs with critical leg ischemia. These patients can benefit greatly from exercise rehabilitation, medication therapy, and atherosclerotic risk factor reduction. It should be noted that patients with asymptomatic PAD (stage I), if they are identified, also are excellent candidates for exercise rehabilitation to prevent the onset of symptoms and to improve functional capacity be-

TABLE 17.1. FONTAINE CLASSIFICATION OF PERIPHERAL ARTERIAL DISEASE

Stage	Symptoms
I	Asymptomatic
II	Intermittent claudication
IIa	distance to onset of pain > 200 m
IIb	distance to onset of pain < 200 m
III	Rest pain
IV	Gangrene, tissue loss

Adapted with permission from Pentecost MJ, Crigai MH, Dorros G, et al: Guidelines for peripheral percutaneous transluminal angioplasty of the abdominal aorta and lower extremity vessels. *Circulation* 89:511, 1994.

fore the atherosclerotic process interferes with walking ability. Consequently, the focus of the remainder of this chapter will center on the evaluation and treatment of patients with Fontaine stage I and stage II PAD.

EVALUATION OF PATIENTS WITH PERIPHERAL ARTERIAL DISEASE

The main effect that PAD has on acute exercise is the development of claudication pain in the leg musculature due to insufficient blood flow. As a result, claudication and peripheral hemodynamic measurements obtained from a treadmill test are the primary criteria to assess the functional limitations imposed by PAD.[10] The specific claudication variables that are measured include the distances (or times) to onset and to maximal claudication pain. Peripheral hemodynamic measurements are obtained in conjunction with claudication measurements to provide a more objective assessment of disease severity. The most accepted variable is the ankle systolic blood pressure measured before and after the treadmill test, which is used to calculate ABI values.

The primary objective of a treadmill test for patients with PAD is to obtain reliable measures of (a) the rate of claudication pain development, (b) the peripheral hemodynamic responses to exercise, and (c) the presence of coexisting coronary heart disease. The test should be a progressive test with gradual increments in grade. By having a test with small increases in exercise intensity, claudication distances of patients can be stratified according to disease severity. Highly reliable treadmill protocols for patients with PAD utilize a constant walking speed of 2 mi/h at 0% grade, with gradual increases in grade of either 2.0% every 2 min or 3.5% every 3 min.[11,12] Typical distances to onset of pain and to maximal pain are approximately 170 m and 360 m, respectively.[13] These protocols also are effective in documenting the inadequacy of the circulation in the lower extremities with exercise, since the ABI typically drops from a resting value of 0.6 to ap-

proximately 0.2 immediately following the treadmill test.[11] Serial measurements of ABI following exercise should be done for 5 to 15 min to establish the time course of recovery to the resting baseline value. Gas exchange measures during the treadmill test show that patients with PAD with intermittent claudication have peak oxygen consumption values in the range of 12 to 15 ml/kg/min,[14] which is approximately 50% of age-matched control subjects. Favorable changes following interventions such as exercise rehabilitation, medication therapy, or surgery should include greater walking distances to the onset of claudication pain and to maximal pain, an increase in peak oxygen consumption, and possibly a blunted drop in ABI and a faster recovery of ABI to the resting baseline value.

Claudication distances and ABI are the most common measurements obtained in patients with intermittent claudication because the literature has primarily taken a vascular perspective on this population. However, further contributions to the literature concerning the improvement in function of patients with PAD following exercise rehabilitation may be best accomplished in the future by taking a more gerontological perspective that goes beyond the measurement of claudication distances and ABI. Since the typical profile of a patient with PAD is that of an elderly person with chronic ambulatory disability, the decline in physical functioning with aging may be accelerated in this population due to the extreme deconditioning brought about from the disease process. Consequently, performance on a 6-min walk test as well as measures of gait, walking economy (i.e., efficiency), balance, flexibility, and lower extremity strength may be worse in patients with PAD than in age-matched controls, and should improve after a program of exercise rehabilitation. However, little information is available on these measures in the PAD population.[15–17]

In addition to the previously mentioned laboratory measures of physical function, assessment of patient-perceived ambulatory function and health-related quality of life should be measured with the Walking Impairment Questionnaire (WIQ)[18] and the Medical Outcomes Survery Short-Form 36 (MOS SF-36) item questionnaire,[19] respectively. These questionnaires are becoming standard assessments in patients with PAD to quantify the impact of intermittent claudication on performing activities of daily living. In addition to the WIQ and MOS SF-36 questionnaires, monitoring the physical activity levels of patients with PAD in the community setting provides a more accurate assessment of the daily limitations imposed by intermittent claudication. Free-living daily physical activity can be measured by an accelerometer as it quantifies movement over an extended period of time. The daily physical activity measured in this manner is approximately 33% lower in patients with PAD than it is in subjects who do not have PAD of similar age, and it decreases in claudicants with worsening disease.[20] Thus, patients with PAD with intermittent claudication are at the extreme low end of the physical activity spectrum.

EXERCISE REHABILITATION PROGRAMS

IMPROVEMENTS IN CLAUDICATION MEASUREMENTS

Significant improvements in claudication pain occur following exercise rehabilitation. A meta-analysis[21] of 21 exercise rehabilitation studies[22–42] reported between 1966 and 1993 demonstrates that the average distance walked to onset of claudication increased 179% from 126 ± 57 m (mean $\pm$ standard deviation) to 351 ± 189 m following rehabilitation, and the average distance walked to maximal claudication pain increased 122% from 326 ± 148 m to 723 ± 592 m.

POTENTIAL MECHANISMS FOR THE IMPROVEMENT IN CLAUDICATION MEASUREMENTS

Numerous mechanisms have been proposed to explain the improvement in walking distance following exercise rehabilitation. These mechanisms include an increased blood flow[23,32,41,43] to the exercising leg musculature due to a greater collateral network, a more favorable redistribution of blood flow,[42,44] greater utilization of oxygen[45] due to a higher concentration of oxidative enzymes,[26] improved hemorrheological properties of the blood,[22] decreased reliance upon anaerobic metabolism,[40,45] and an improvement in the efficiency of walking.[46,47] It may be that no single mechanism is responsible for the improvement in walking distances with exercise rehabilitation, but several factors contribute. Improvements in psychosocial attitude due to accomplishments that are achieved during exercise rehabilitation may further enhance this effect.

To address the peripheral hemodynamic mechanism, a number of studies have assessed calf blood flow and ABI both before and after a program of exercise. On average, calf blood flow under resting and maximal conditions increases by approximately 19%[26–29,32,33,35–37,42,45,48–51] and ABI increases by approximately 7%[30,34–37,40,43,44,50–52] following exercise rehabilitation. Only a few studies have examined the change in redistribution of peripheral blood flow, blood viscosity, leg arteriovenous oxygen difference, concentration of oxidative enzymes, and efficiency of walking. Consequently, the changes in these variables following exercise rehabilitation are not well established in patients with PAD. Since the magnitude of increases in calf blood flow (19%) and ABI (7%) are much smaller than the increases in the walking distances to onset (179%) and to maximal (122%) claudication pain,[21] either small changes in peripheral blood flow yield exponential improvements in claudication pain symptoms, or the other mechanisms mentioned earlier also contribute to the improved walking distances.

EXERCISE PROGRAM COMPONENTS PREDICTING IMPROVED CLAUDICATION MEASUREMENTS

Although the average increase in walking distances is substantial in the preceding studies, these studies also show considerable variability.

For example, the increased distance to onset of pain ranges from 72 and 746%, and the increased distance to maximal pain ranges from 61 and 739%.[21] Differences in the components of exercise programs (e.g., intensity, duration, and frequency of exercise sessions) may largely account for these widely divergent responses. Although the previous exercise programs are generally effective in the treatment of intermittent claudication, none of the studies compared different components of exercise to determine an optimal exercise rehabilitation program.

Because no experimental study can systematically examine the effects of all of the components of an exercise rehabilitation program, this author examined existing studies using meta-analytic techniques to identify the most important exercise training components for optimally improving claudication pain distances. Six of the following components were examined: (a) frequency of exercise (sessions per week); (b) duration of exercise (minutes per session); (c) mode of exercise (walking vs. a combination of exercises); (d) length of the program (weeks); (e) claudication pain endpoint used in the program (onset vs. near maximal pain); and (f) level of supervision (supervised vs. supervised plus home-based exercise). All of these components, except for the level of supervision, had a significant effect on the change in the claudication distances. Programs exercising patients during training to near-maximal claudication pain were more effective than programs exercising patients to only the onset of pain (Fig. 17.1). Furthermore, programs consisting of high exercise duration, high frequency, great program length (Fig. 17.2), and walking as the only mode of exercise (Fig. 17.3) were more effective than programs consisting of low exercise duration, low frequency, short program length, and having patients train by a combination of exercise modes. The addition of home exercise to supplement the amount of exercise performed in a supervised setting did not result in additional ambulatory benefit.

Of the 5 components that had an effect on the change in the claudication distances, only 3 were

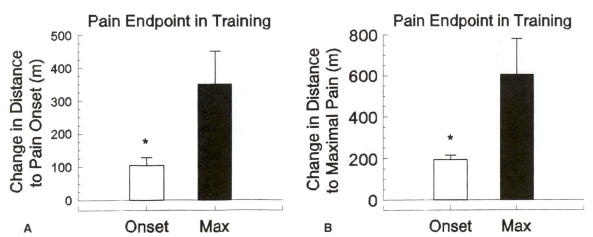

FIGURES 17.1 A and B. *The effect of the claudication pain endpoint used during training sessions on changes in claudication pain distances from 21 studies.[21] Onset: studies where patients exercised to onset of claudication. Max: studies where patients exercised to near-maximal claudication. Values are means ± standard errors of the change in the pain-free (A) and maximal pain (B) distances after adjusting for 5 other program components. * Significantly lower than Max group (p < 0.01). Adapted with permission from Gardner AW, Poehlman ET: Exercise rehabilitation programs for the treatment of claudication pain: A meta-analysis. JAMA 274:975, 1995.*

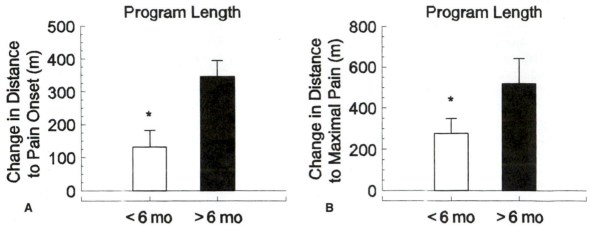

*FIGURES 17.2 A and B. The effect of the length of the exercise program on changes in claudication pain distances from 21 studies.[21] < 6 mo: studies that had patients exercise less than 6 months; > 6 mo: studies that had patients exercise at least 6 months. Values are means ± standard errors of the change in the pain-free (A) and maximal pain (B) distances after adjusting for 5 other program components. * Significantly lower than > 6 mo group (p < 0.01). Adapted with permission from Gardner AW, Poehlman ET: Exercise rehabilitation programs for the treatment of claudication pain: A meta-analysis. JAMA 274:975, 1995.*

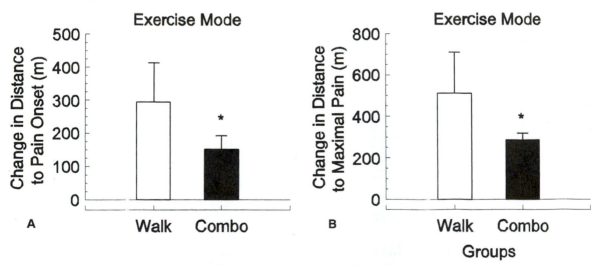

*FIGURES 17.3 A and B. The effect of exercise training mode on changes in claudication pain distances from 21 studies. Walk: studies that had patients train solely by walking; Combo: studies that had patients train using a combination of exercises. Values are means ± standard errors of the change in the pain-free (A) and maximal pain (B) distances after adjusting for 5 other program components. * Significantly lower than Walk group (p < 0.05). Adapted with permission from Gardner AW, Poehlman ET: Exercise rehabilitation programs for the treatment of claudication pain: A meta-analysis. JAMA 274:975, 1995.*

found to have an independent effect through multivariate analyses. These components were walking to near-maximal claudication pain during training, walking for long duration, and using walking as the sole training modality.[21] The combination of these components explained nearly 90% of the variance in the increase in the walking distances following exercise rehabilitation.[21] Although the duration and frequency of the exercise sessions are not independent predictors of the change in claudication pain times, programs should have the patients walk for at least 30 min per session and for at least 3 sessions per week, as these amounts were more beneficial than programs using a low exercise duration and frequency. Finally, it should be noted that the appropriate exercise intensity to use during training could not be determined at this time because no study has addressed this issue. There is a common misconception that walking beyond the onset of pain to near maximal pain is an increase in intensity when, in fact, it is merely an increase in duration. The rate of work performed while walking, regardless of the duration, is the important consideration when evaluating exercise intensity. Since heart rate is commonly used as a means to adjust the intensity of exercise, a conservative recommendation for claudicants who are beginning rehabilitation is to walk at an appropriate speed and grade on a treadmill to elicit an intensity of approximately 50% of their heart rate reserve, and to gradually increase the intensity to 70 to 80% by completion of the program. Recommendations for an exercise program for patients with PAD are summarized in Table 17.2.

PHARMACOLOGIC AND REVASCULARIZATION INTERVENTIONS

In addition to exercise rehabilitation, pharmacologic and revascularization interventions are other options to treat intermittent claudication. Pharmacologic therapy for intermittent claudication in the United States is limited to pentoxifylline and cilostazol. Pentoxifylline, which has a hemorrhe-

TABLE 17.2.   RECOMMENDED EXERCISE PROGRAM FOR PATIENTS WITH PERIPHERAL ARTERIAL DISEASE

Exercise Component	Comment
Frequency	3 Exercise sessions per week
Intensity	Progression from 50% of peak exercise capacity to 80% by the end of the program
Duration	Progression from 15 min of exercise per session to more than 30 min by the end of the program
Mode	Walking, nonweight-bearing tasks (e.g., bicycling) may be used for warming up and cooling down
Type of Exercise	Intermittent walking to near-maximal claudication pain
Program Length	At least 6 months

ologic effect by improving the flexibility of red blood cell membranes and by reducing platelet aggregration, was first studied in the United States in 1982.[53] It was found to increase the distance to onset of claudication pain by 45% and the distance to maximal pain by 32% following 24 weeks of treatment. These were significantly greater changes than the 23 and 20% increases seen with placebo treatment. Although this initial study demonstrated the efficacy of pentoxyifylline, its usefulness in treating intermittent claudication has been questioned.[54] Cilostazol is a new medication with more potent vasodilatory and antiplatelet activity than aspirin.[55] Cilostazol was found to increase the distances to onset by 40% and to maximal claudication pain by 42%, which were significantly greater than the 1% (for onset) and −14% (for maximal claudication pain) changes seen with placebo treatment.[56] These studies suggest that pharmacologic intervention may be used to treat intermittent claudication in a large percentage of patients. However, exercise rehabilitation results in far greater increases in walking distances in patients who are capable and motivated to walk on a regular basis.

Revascularization is another treatment option for patients with intermittent claudication. Percutaneous transluminal angioplasty (PTA) is suitable for patients whose symptoms are not severe enough to justify arterial reconstructive surgery.[57] Percutaneous transluminal angioplasty was directly compared to that of exercise rehabilitation for increasing walking distances. Three months following PTA the distances to onset and to maximal claudication pain increased by more than 100%, but these gains had diminished to approximately 60% at 1 year follow-up.[57] In contrast, the exercise group had gradual and progressive improvements throughout the study, as the distance to onset of claudication pain increased by more than 300% by the end of the year and the distance to maximal pain increased by more than 400%.[57] In patients with more severe intermittent claudication who underwent arterial reconstruction, the distances to onset increased by 376% and to maximal claudication pain by 173% at 1 year follow-up.[58] Patients who exercised during the 1-year study increased their walking distances by 179 and 151%, while a group who had arterial reconstruction followed by exercise rehabilitation had the greatest improvements as their walking distances increased by 699 and 263%. These studies suggest that exercise is superior to PTA for increasing walking distances in patients with mild-to-moderate claudication, and exercise rehabilitation provides an additive effect to arterial reconstruction for increasing walking distances in patients with severe claudication.

SUMMARY

Peripheral arterial disease is a significant health concern in the elderly population, and it will continue to increase in future years. Nonsurgical management, including atherosclerotic risk factor management and exercise rehabilitation, is indicated to modify risk factors and improve ambulatory ability of patients with asymptomatic PAD and patients with intermittent claudication. Patients with more severe PAD typically require revascularization. Exercise rehabilitation is a highly effective, conservative treatment to improve ambulation in patients with intermittent claudication, as the average increase in distances to onset is 179% and to maximal claudication pain is 122%. Pharmacologic therapy, PTA, and arterial reconstruction are other potential treatment options to increase walking distances. The effectiveness of intervention has primarily been evaluated by increases in walking distances to onset and to maximal claudication pain during a treadmill test. Future research should also focus on other functional outcomes that may be more representative of everyday activities in geriatric populations such as submaximal exercise performance, walking economy, balance, flexibility, and lower extremity strength. It is also not clear if improved walking ability translates into an overall increase in physical activity and enhanced quality of life. Until these measures are obtained, the full benefit of exercise rehabilitation for patients with PAD is likely to be underestimated.

REFERENCES

1. U.S. Health trends. *J NIH Res* 4:95, 1992.
2. Kannel WB: Some lessons in cardiovascular epidemiology from Framingham. *Am J Cardiol* 37: 269, 1976.
3. Carter SA: Clinical measurement of systolic pressures in limbs with arterial occlusive disease. *JAMA* 207:1869, 1969.
4. Criqui MH, Fronek A, Barrett-Connor E, et al: The prevalence of peripheral arterial disease in a defined population. *Circulation* 71:510, 1985.
5. Hiatt WR, Marshall JA, Baxter J, et al: Diagnostic methods for peripheral arterial disease in the San Luis Valley Diabetes Study. *J Clin Epidemiol* 43:597, 1990.
6. Carter SA: Indirect systolic pressures and pulse waves in arterial occlusive disease of the lower extremities. *Circulation* 37:624, 1968.
7. Ouriel K, McDonnell AE, Metz CE, et al: A critical evaluation of stress testing in the diagnosis of peripheral vascular disease. *Surgery* 91:686, 1982.
8. Weitz JI, Byrne J, Clagett P, et al: Diagnosis and treatment of chronic arterial insufficiency of the lower extremities: A critical review. *Circulation* 94:3026, 1996.
9. Pentecost MJ, Criqui MH, Dorros G, et al:

Guidelines for peripheral percutaneous transluminal angioplasty of the abdominal aorta and lower extremity vessels. *Circulation* 89:511, 1994.

10. Hiatt WR, Hirsch AT, Regensteiner JG, et al: Clinical trials for claudication: Assessment of exercise performance, functional status, and clinical end points. *Circulation* 92:614, 1995.

11. Gardner AW, Skinner JS, Cantwell BW, et al: Progressive versus single-stage treadmill tests for evaluation of claudication. *Med Sci Sports Exerc* 23:402, 1991.

12. Hiatt WR, Nawaz D, Regensteiner JG, et al: The evaluation of exercise performance in patients with peripheral vascular disease. *J Cardiopul Rehabil* 12:525, 1988.

13. Gardner AW, Ricci MR, Pilcher DB, et al: Practical equations to predict claudication pain distances from a graded treadmill test. *Vasc Med* 1:91, 1996.

14. Gardner AW: The effect of cigarette smoking on exercise capacity in patients with intermittent claudication. *Vasc Med* 1:181, 1996.

15. Montgomery PS, Gardner AW: The clinical utility of a 6-minute walk test in peripheral arterial occlusive disease patients. *J Am Geriatr Soc* 46:706, 1998.

16. Hiatt WR, Wolfel EE, Meier RH, et al: Superiority of treadmill walking exercise versus strength training for patients with peripheral arterial disease. *Circulation* 90:1866, 1994.

17. Scherer SA, Bainbridge S, Hiatt WR, et al: Gait characteristics of patients with claudication. *Arch Phys Med Rehab* 79:529, 1998.

18. Regensteiner JG, Steiner JF, Panzer RL, et al: Evaluation of walking impairment by questionnaire in patients with peripheral arterial disease. *J Vasc Med Biol* 2:142, 1990.

19. Ware JE, Sherbourne CD: The MOS 36-item short-form health survey (SF-36). *Med Care* 30:473, 1992.

20. Sieminski DJ, Gardner AW: The relationship between daily physical activity and the severity of peripheral arterial occlusive disease. *Vasc Med* 2:286, 1997.

21. Gardner AW, Poehlman ET: Exercise rehabilitation programs for the treatment of claudication pain: A meta-analysis. *JAMA* 274:975, 1995.

22. Ernst EEW, Matrai A: Intermittent claudication, exercise, and blood rheology. *Circulation* 76:1110, 1987.

23. Alpert JS, Larsen A, Lassen NA: Exercise and intermittent claudication: Blood flow in the calf muscle during walking studied by the Xenon-133 clearance method. *Circulation* 39:353, 1969.

24. Carter SA, Hamel ER, Paterson JM, et al: Walking ability and ankle systolic pressures: Observations in patients with intermittent claudication in a short-term walking exercise program. *J Vasc Surg* 10:642, 1989.

25. Clifford PC, Davies PW, Hayne JA, et al: Intermittent claudication: Is a supervised exercise class worth while? *Br Med J* 281:1503, 1980.

26. Dahllof AG, Bjorntorp P, Holm J, et al: Metabolic activity of skeletal muscle in patients with peripheral arterial insufficiency: Effect of physical training. *Eur J Clin Invest* 4:9, 1974.

27. Dahllof AG, Holm J, Schersten T, et al: Peripheral arterial insufficiency: Effect of physical training on walking tolerance, calf blood flow, and blood flow resistance. *Scand J Rehab Med* 8:19, 1976.

28. Ekroth R, Dahllof AG, Gundevall B, et al: Physical training of patients with intermittent claudication: Indications, methods, and results. *Surgery* 84:640, 1978.

29. Ericsson B, Haeger K, Lindell SE: Effect of physical training on intermittent claudication. *Angiology* 21:188, 1970.

30. Feinberg RL, Gregory RT, Wheeler JR, et al: The ischemic window: A method for the objective quantitation of the training effect in exercise therapy for intermittent claudication. *J Vasc Surg* 16:244, 1992.

31. Holm J, Dahllof AG, Bjorntorp P, et al: Enzyme studies in muscles of patients with intermittent claudication: Effect of training. *Scand J Clin Lab Invest* 31(Suppl 128):201, 1973.

32. Jonason T, Ringqvist I: Effect of training on the post-exercise ankle blood pressure reaction in patients with intermittent claudication. *Clin Physiol* 7:63, 1987.

33. Larsen OA, Lassen NA: Effect of daily muscular exercise in patients with intermittent claudication. *Lancet* 2:1093, 1966.

34. Lepantalo M, Sundberg S, Gordin A: The effects of physical training and flunarizine on walking capacity in intermittent claudication. *Scand J Rehab Med* 16:159, 1984.

35. Lundgren F, Dahllof AG, Schersten T, et al: Muscle enzyme adaptation in patients with peripheral arterial insufficiency: Spontaneous adaptation,

effect of different treatments and consequences on walking performance. *Clin Sci* 77:485, 1989.

36. Mannarino E, Pasqualini L, Menna M, et al: Effects of physical training on peripheral vascular disease: A controlled study. *Angiology* 40:5, 1989.

37. Mannarino E, Pasqualini L, Innocente S, et al: Physical training and antiplatelet treatment in Stage II peripheral arterial occlusive disease: Alone or combined? *Angiology* 42:513, 1991.

38. Rosetzsky A, Struckmann J, Mathiesen FR: Minimal walking distance following exercise treatment in patients with arterial occlusive disease. *Ann Chir Gynecol* 74:261, 1985.

39. Rosfors S, Bygdeman S, Arnetz BB, et al: Long term neuroendocrine and metabolic effects of physical training in intermittent claudication. *Scand J Rehab Med* 21:7, 1989.

40. Ruell PA, Imperial ES, Bonar FJ, et al: Intermittent claudication: The effect of physical training on walking tolerance and venous lactate concentration. *Eur J Appl Physiol* 52:420, 1984.

41. Skinner JS, Strandness DE Jr: Exercise and intermittent claudication: II. Effect of physical training. *Circulation* 36:23, 1967.

42. Zetterquist S: The effect of active training on the nutritive blood flow in exercising ischemic legs. *Scand J Lab Invest* 25:101, 1970.

43. Hall JA, Barnard RJ: The effects of an intensive 26-day program of diet and exercise on patients with peripheral vascular disease. *J Cardiac Rehabil* 2:569, 1982.

44. Jonason T, Ringqvist I: Prediction of the effect of training on the walking tolerance in patients with intermittent claudication. *Scand J Rehab Med* 19:47, 1987.

45. Sorlie D, Myhre K: Effects of physical training in intermittent claudication. *Scand J Clin Lab Invest* 38:217, 1978.

46. Ernst E: Physical exercise for peripheral vascular disease: A review. *Vasa* 16:227, 1987.

47. Womack CJ, Sieminski DJ, Katzel LI, et al: Improved walking economy in patients with peripheral arterial occlusive disease. *Med Sci Sports Exerc* 29:1286, 1997.

48. Jonason T, Ringqvist I, Oman-Rydberg A: Home-training of patients with intermittent claudication. *Scand J Rehab Med* 13:137, 1981.

49. Fitzgerald DE, Keates JS, MacMillan D: Angiographic and plethysmographic assessment of graduated physical exercise in the treatment of chronic occlusive arterial disease of the leg. *Angiology* 22:99, 1971.

50. Hiatt WR, Regensteiner JG, Hargarten ME, et al: Benefit of exercise conditioning for patients with peripheral arterial disease. *Circulation* 81:602, 1990.

51. Lundgren F, Dahllof AG, Lundholm K, et al: Intermittent claudication—Surgical reconstruction or physical training? A prospective randomized trial of treatment efficiency. *Ann Surg* 209:346, 1989.

52. Williams LR, Ekers MA, Collins PS, et al: Vascular rehabilitation: Benefits of a structured exercise/risk modification program. *J Vasc Surg* 14: 320, 1991.

53. Porter JM, Cutler BS, Lee BY, et al: Pentoxifylline efficacy in the treatment of intermittent claudication: Multicenter controlled double-blind trial with objective assessment of chronic occlusive arterial disease patients. *Am Heart J* 104:66, 1982.

54. Isner J: Redefining intervention. *Circulation* 88: 1534, 1993.

55. Money SR, Herd JA, Isaacsohn JL, et al: Effect of cilostazol on walking distances in patients with intermittent claudication caused by peripheral vascular disease. *J Vasc Surg* 27:267, 1998.

56. Dawson DL, Cutler BS, Meissner MH, et al: Cilostazol has beneficial effects in treatment of intermittent claudication: Results from a multicenter, randomized, prospective, double-blind trial. *Circulation* 98:678, 1998.

57. Creasy TS, McMillan PJ, Fletcher EWL, et al: Is percutaneous transluminal angioplasty better than exercise for claudication? Preliminary results from a prospective randomised trial. *Eur J Vasc Surg* 4:135, 1990.

58. Lundgren F, Dahllof AG, Lundholm K, et al: Intermittent claudication—surgical reconstruction or physical training? *Ann Surg* 209:346, 1989.

PART V

EXERCISE IN PREVENTING CARDIAC DISEASE

Chapter 18

THE ROLE OF PHYSICAL ACTIVITY IN THE PREVENTION OF CORONARY ARTERY DISEASE

I-Min Lee, M.B.B.S., Sc.D.   *Ralph S. Paffenbarger, Jr., M.D., Dr.P.H.*

Despite dramatic declines in the mortality rate for coronary heart disease over the past quarter of a century, it remains the leading cause of death in the United States and most western countries.[1] In 1996, coronary artery disease was responsible for approximately 476,000 of the over 2 million deaths in the United States, or about 1 out of every 4.9 deaths.[2] It is a leading cause of death not only among men, but also women. While heart disease rates are much higher in comparably aged men than in premenopausal women, after menopause, heart disease rates increase substantially in women, so that women account for approximately one-half of all coronary heart disease deaths that occur each year in the United States.[3]

Many risk factors for coronary heart disease have been identified over the years. Among the modifiable characteristics widely accepted to increase risk of coronary heart disease are cigarette smoking, high blood pressure, dyslipidemia, obesity, diabetes, and physical inactivity.[2] With regard to this last risk factor, the idea that physical activity is beneficial for health is not new. Ancient

China, circa 2500 B.C., has perhaps the earliest records of organized exercise for health promotion by Hua T'o.[4] The ancient Greek physicians, Hippocrates, Plato, and Galen, believed that physical activity was important in maintaining well-being and was useful for treating disease and disability.[4] Even in ancient times, the issue of optimal intensity of physical activity was debated: Hippocrates and Galen eschewed the excess training of the professional athlete in their day, favoring, instead, more moderate physical activity.[5] In eighteenth century Italy, Ramazzini observed the well-being of foot messengers ("runners"), as contrasted to the ill-health of sedentary workers, such as cobblers and tailors, and attributed this difference in health to their different occupational activity.[6]

This chapter will focus on physical inactivity as a risk factor for coronary heart disease. First, potential mechanisms through which physical activity might decrease risk of coronary heart disease will be discussed. Then, epidemiologic studies investigating the association between physical activity and coronary heart disease risk will be reviewed to evaluate the evidence for a protective role of physical activity. Next, how much, what intensity, and how long physical activity should be carried out in order to reap coronary heart disease benefits will be examined. Finally, a brief discussion on the potential hazard of sudden death following exercise is included.

POTENTIAL MECHANISMS FOR DECREASED RISK OF CORONARY HEART DISEASE THROUGH PHYSICAL ACTIVITY

Physical activity has been postulated to reduce the risk of developing coronary heart disease through many different mechanisms. It may do so via a direct action on the heart: Physical activity increases myocardial oxygen supply, decreases oxygen demand, and improves myocardial contraction and its electrical stability.[7] This reduced oxygen demand and myocardial work is reflected

in lowered heart rate and blood pressure at rest and a general reduction in sympathetic tone. Physical activity also increases the diameter and dilating capacity of coronary arteries, increases collateral artery formation, and reduces rates of progression of coronary artery atherosclerosis.[8–10] Additionally, high levels of activity are associated with low systolic and diastolic blood pressure, high levels of high-density lipoproteins, and perhaps low levels of low-density lipoproteins (LDL), as well as increased insulin sensitivity and glucose tolerance.[11–17] Other likely mechanisms include a reduced tendency for platelet aggregation and increased fibrinolytic activity, possibly the consequence of lower levels of PAI-1.[18,19] Preliminary data suggest that physical activity also may be associated with decreased levels of homocysteine, a risk factor for coronary heart disease.[20] Finally, physically active individuals are less likely to be overweight, another factor associated with increased coronary heart disease risk.[21] All of these potential mechanisms, alone or in combination, can reduce the risk of developing coronary heart disease.

EPIDEMIOLOGIC STUDIES OF PHYSICAL ACTIVITY OR PHYSICAL FITNESS AND RISK OF CORONARY HEART DISEASE

Many studies have examined the association between physical activity or physical fitness and risk of developing coronary heart disease. Powell et al in 1987 conducted a qualitative review of all articles published in the English language that had sufficient information to calculate the relative risks of coronary heart disease associated with different levels of physical activity.[22] Analyzing the 43 studies that satisfied these criteria, the authors observed that the data consistently supported an inverse association between physical activity and coronary heart disease risk, and that this inverse association was more pronounced in the better-designed studies. In 1990, Berlin and Colditz expanded on this qualitative review to estimate quantitatively the increased risk associated with being sedentary.[23] In their meta-analysis, they concluded that those who were sedentary had about a twofold increased risk of developing coronary heart disease or dying from coronary heart disease, as compared with those who were active.

In these reviews, most of the studies were conducted in men; only 12% of the studies in the meta-analysis included women. However, more recently published studies have tended to include women (see later); these studies indicate that physical activity is associated with decreased risk of coronary heart disease in women as well.

The following paragraphs review several studies of physical activity or physical fitness and risk of coronary heart disease that are representative of other studies on this topic, in order to provide more detail regarding individual study design and findings. This review is not intended to be exhaustive; instead, it is an arbitrary selection of studies intended to reflect the many other studies in the field.

STUDY OF BRITISH CIVIL SERVANTS

Some of the earliest observations demonstrating an inverse association between physical activity and coronary heart disease risk were made by Morris and colleagues in London.[24–26] These observations have been made among bus drivers and conductors, postal workers, and civil servants.

In one of their later studies, investigators prospectively followed a cohort of 9376 male British civil servants, who were aged 45 to 64 years and free of coronary heart disease, for an average of 9.3 years.[26] These men were involved in sedentary jobs and, thus, obtained most of their physical activity during their leisure time. Men often were habitual gardeners, do-it-yourself handymen, and less often involved in recreational sports after work or on holidays. At study entry in 1976, investigators queried subjects, via mailed questionnaires, about the different activities in which they had engaged over the previous 4 weeks, as well as the frequency of participation.

Information regarding health habits and medical history also was obtained. Investigators then categorized men according to their frequency of participation in vigorous recreational sports and their frequency of participation in nonvigorous sports. Sports defined as vigorous tended to demand at least 7.5 kcal/min or 6 times the resting metabolic rate (METs), while less intense sports were considered nonvigorous. Some 17.5% of men reported vigorous sports play, while twice that proportion reported nonvigorous sports play. During follow-up, 474 men developed coronary heart disease.

With increasing frequency of participation in vigorous sports, coronary heart disease incidence rates declined (Table 18.1). These differences persisted after accounting for smoking habits, body mass index, and personal and family medical history. However, dietary data were unavailable and could not be accounted for. In contrast, no association was noted with increasing frequency of nonvigorous sports play. Furthermore, higher amounts of energy expended in all activities other than vigorous sports play were unrelated to coronary heart disease incidence rates. In addition, investigators observed that in order for physical activity to be beneficial, the exercise had to be current, not historical in nature. Coronary heart disease incidence rates were similarly high among men who played no vigorous sports at study entry in 1976, regardless of whether they had played vigorous sports previously. Among men who reported no vigorous sports play at study entry, coronary heart disease incidence rates were 5.9 per 1000 person years in those who also had never previously engaged in vigorous sports play. This rate was similar to the rates for men who had previously played sports up to 25, 30, or 40 years of age (5.1, 5.1, and 6.5 per 1000, respectively), or past 40 years of age (5.2 per 1000). This was in contrast to a rate of 2.1 per 1000 among men who engaged in vigorous sports play at least 8 times in the previous 4 weeks before study entry, regardless of whether they had played such sports previously.

This study is one of the few specifically de-

TABLE 18.1. AGE-ADJUSTED INCIDENCE RATES AND RELATIVE RISKS OF CORONARY HEART DISEASE IN MEN ACCORDING TO PHYSICAL ACTIVITY: STUDY OF BRITISH CIVIL SERVANTS

Physical Activity (episodes in previous 4 weeks)	No. of Events	Incidence Rate (per 1000)	Relative Risk
Vigorous sports			
None	413	5.8	1.00 (referent)
1–3	37	4.5	0.78
4–7	17	4.1	0.71
≥ 8	7	2.1	0.36
			$p < 0.005$
Nonvigorous sports			
None	310	5.4	1.00 (referent)
1–3	85	5.9	1.09
4–7	52	5.9	1.09
8–11	19	3.5	0.65
≥ 12	8	6.8	1.26
			$p > 0.05$

Adapted with permission from Morris JN, Clayton DG, Everitt MG, et al: Exercise in leisure-time: Coronary attack and death rates. *Br Heart J* 63:325–334, 1990.

signed to investigate the relation between physical activity and coronary heart disease risk; thus, detailed information on physical activity (type, intensity, and frequency) was collected. This information allowed investigators to address the question of intensity of physical activity, showing that vigorous intensity activity was necessary for coronary heart disease risk reduction. Additionally, the study also evaluated physical activity at different ages and showed that contemporary, but not historical, physical activity was associated with decreased coronary heart disease risk.

THE HARVARD ALUMNI HEALTH STUDY

Paffenbarger and colleagues have made a series of observations regarding physical activity and risk of developing coronary heart disease in a cohort of male alumni who had matriculated as undergraduates at Harvard University between 1916 and 1950.[27–29] Physical activity was assessed at multiple points in time: during college tenure, and seriatim beginning in 1962, when men were middle-aged.

In one of their earlier reports, investigators followed 16,936 Harvard alumni, who were aged 35 to 74 years and free of coronary heart disease,

from 1962 or 1966 (1962/1966) until 1972.[27] On the baseline questionnaire mailed in 1962/1966, men were asked about the number of flights of stairs climbed daily, the number of city blocks walked daily, the types of sports or recreational activities engaged in, and the time spent on each of these sports and recreational activities. While investigators did not inquire specifically about occupational activity, alumni were unlikely to have expended much energy on the job apart from walking and climbing stairs. Additionally, data on health habits and medical history also were obtained. Investigators quantified physical activity thus: Walking 7 city blocks rated 56 kcal, while climbing 7 flights of stairs rated 28 kcal. Sports and recreational activities were classified as light (requiring 5 kcal/min of energy expenditure or 4 METs), vigorous (10 kcal/min or 8 METs), or mixed (7.5 kcal/min or 6 METs). Investigators then summed kilocalories per week from blocks walked, flights climbed, and sports or recreational activities carried out to obtain an index of weekly energy expenditure. Physical activity then was related to incidence of first heart attack occurring between 1962/1966 and 1972, with 572 such events observed.

Table 18.2 shows that the age-adjusted inci-

TABLE 18.2. AGE-ADJUSTED INCIDENCE RATES AND RELATIVE RISKS OF FIRST HEART ATTACK IN MEN ACCORDING TO PHYSICAL ACTIVITY: THE HARVARD ALUMNI HEALTH STUDY

Physical Activity (kcal per week)	Number of Events	Incidence Rate (per 10,000)	Relative Risk
< 2,000	307	57.9	1.64
≥ 2,000	122	35.3	1.00 (referent)
			$p < 0.001$

Adapted with permission from Paffenbarger RS Jr, Wing AL, Hyde RT: Physical activity as an index of heart attack risk in college alumni. *Am J Epidemiol* 108:161–175, 1978.

dence rate of first heart attack among alumni expending < 2000 kcal per week was 1.64 times higher than those expending ≥ 2000 kcal per week. A higher risk among the more sedentary was consistently observed in alumni of different ages, whether cigarette smokers or not, those with lower or higher blood pressures, those lean and not-so-lean, and those experiencing early parental mortality and those who did not. As in the previous study, investigators noted that only contemporary physical activity was beneficial. Men who were varsity athletes but who were no longer physically active in 1962/1966 (< 500 kcal per week) experienced far higher rates of first heart attack (92.7 per 10,000 person years) than those who were not active during their college days, but who were physically active (≥ 2000 kcal per week) in 1962/1966 (33.3 per 10,000).

To clarify the role of intensity of physical activity in preventing coronary heart disease, investigators later conducted a more detailed scrutiny of the intensity of physical activities carried out by these Harvard men.[30,31] This later study involved 17,321 healthy men, aged 30 to 79 years at baseline, 1962/1966. Physical activity was assessed in 1962/1966 and again in 1977. The energy expended on walking and stair climbing was estimated as described previously. For sports and recreational activities, investigators assigned a multiple of resting metabolic rate (MET score) to every activity. The energy expended on each activity was estimated by multiplying its MET score with body weight in kilograms and hours per week of participation. Investigators then summed kilocalories per week from blocks walked, flights climbed, and activities carried out to provide an

index of total energy expenditure per week. They further divided total energy expenditure into 2 components: that derived from vigorous (≥ 6 METs) and nonvigorous activities (< 6 METs). Because walking speed was not ascertained in 1962/1966 and 1977, all walking was deemed nonvigorous, while stair climbing was considered vigorous. Men then were classified into 5 categories each of vigorous and nonvigorous energy expenditure, using the same cutpoints: < 150, 150–399, 400–749, 750–1,499 and ≥ 1500 kcal per week. During follow-up from 1962/1966 through 1988, 465 men died from coronary heart disease.

In relating physical activity assessed in 1962/1966 and updated in 1977 to coronary heart disease mortality, investigators found that vigorous, but not nonvigorous, activity significantly predicted decreased risk in the 22–26 year follow-up through 1988. The relative risks for coronary heart disease mortality, adjusted for age, cigarette smoking, hypertension, diabetes mellitus, body mass index, and early parental death, associated with the 5 categories of vigorous energy expenditure were 1.00 (referent), 0.94, 0.77, 0.89, and 0.68, respectively; *p,* trend = 0.02. For nonvigorous energy expenditure, the corresponding relative risks were 1.00, 1.15, 1.10, 1.12, and 0.89, respectively; *p,* trend = 0.24. Analyses of the 2 kinds of energy expenditure were mutually adjusted. In analyses, diet was not adjusted for since detailed dietary data were not collected at baseline or 1977. For the subset of alumni who provided dietary information in 1988, estimated intake of total calories increased with increasing total, vigorous, and nonvigorous energy expenditure in 1962/1966. However, the percentage consumed as fat or saturated fat did not vary across activity categories. Thus, confounding by fat intake was unlikely, assuming that later diet was indicative of earlier habits.

As with the British Civil Servants Study, the Harvard Alumni Health Study is one of the few studies specifically designed to investigate physical activity in relation to incidence of chronic diseases, including coronary heart disease. As such, the detailed information on and multiple assessments of physical activity allowed investigators to examine questions regarding quantity, intensity, and timing of physical activity. The data corroborate findings from the British Civil Servants Study, showing that vigorous intensity physical activity, conducted contemporaneously, was needed to reduce risk of coronary heart disease.

THE ALAMEDA COUNTY STUDY

The Alameda County Study is a prospective cohort study of the predictors of mortality among a random sample of 6928 adult residents of Alameda County, California. In this study, Kaplan and colleagues were interested in whether factors associated with increased mortality risk among older men and women were the same as those for younger individuals.[32] While coronary heart disease mortality was not specifically examined, presumably, a large proportion of the deaths would have been due to cardiovascular causes, as is typical in the United States.

In this analysis, study subjects were restricted to 4174 men and women who were aged 38 years or older at baseline in 1965, so that these individuals would be aged at least 55 years at the end of the 17-year follow-up.[32] Subjects completed a questionnaire on demographic, behavioral, social, and psychological characteristics in 1965. Physical activity was assessed based on frequency and presumed intensity of leisure-time participation in active sports, swimming, long walks, physical exercise, gardening, and hunting and fishing. Based on these data, investigators

classified men and women as inactive or active. During follow-up, 1219 men and women died.

After adjusting for age, self-reported health status and factors predictive of mortality in this cohort (cigarette smoking, alcohol intake, weight-for-height, hours of sleep, regular breakfast, and snacking), physical inactivity was a significant predictor of mortality among men and women of all ages, even including the old (Table 18.3). Indeed, when crude survival curves were plotted by age group over the 17 years, the differential in mortality between inactive and active subjects was more marked in the oldest than the youngest age group. An important contribution of this study is that it showed an inverse association between physical activity and mortality, even among old individuals.

THE MULTIPLE RISK FACTOR INTERVENTION TRIAL (MRFIT)

The MRFIT was a randomized, multicenter primary prevention trial designed to test whether multifactor intervention could reduce coronary heart disease mortality in men, aged 35 to 57 years, who were at high risk for this disease because of their cigarette habit, diastolic blood pressure, and serum cholesterol. Of the 12,866 men

TABLE 18.3. RELATIVE RISKS[a] OF MORTALITY IN MEN AND WOMEN BY PHYSICAL ACTIVITY AND AGE GROUP: THE ALAMEDA COUNTY STUDY

Age group (years)	Relative Risk (95% Confidence Interval), Inactive vs. Active
38–49	1.48 (1.08–2.02)
50–59	1.27 (0.97–1.66)
60–69	1.38 (1.09–1.75)
≥ 70	1.37 (1.09–1.72)

[a] Adjusted for age, self-reported health status, cigarette smoking, alcohol intake, weight-for-height, hours of sleep, regular breakfast, and snacking.

Adapted with permission from Kaplan GA, Seeman TE, Cohen RD, et al: Mortality among the elderly in the Alameda County Study: Behavioral and demographic risk factors. *Am J Public Health* 77:307–312, 1987.

enrolled in the cohort, all were free of clinical coronary heart disease at baseline, 1973 to 1976.

In the first report on physical activity and risk of coronary heart disease, Leon and colleagues followed 12,138 men with acceptable data on physical activity for an average of 7 years.[33] Physical activity was assessed in 1973 to 1976 using the Minnesota Leisure-Time Physical Activity Questionnaire. Men were queried regarding the frequency and duration of participation in 62 individual physical activities over the past year. These activities were considered light (requiring 2 to 4 kcal/min of energy expenditure or about 1.5 to 3 METs), moderate (4.5 to 5.5 kcal/min or about 3.5 to 4.5 METs), or heavy ($\geq$ 6.0 kcal/min or about 5 METs). Investigators estimated leisure-time physical activity for each person, in minutes per day, as well as in kilocalories expended per day. Based on these data, men were classified into thirds: the least active third having a mean of 15 min of leisure-time physical activity per day at a cost of 74 kcal; the middle third, 47 min and 224 kcal per day; the most active third, 3,134 min and 638 kcal per day. Subjects in this study expended energy mainly on light and moderate activities; on average, only 19% of total daily energy expenditure was spent on heavy activities. During follow-up, 781 nonfatal and fatal coronary heart disease events were observed.

Table 18.4 presents the findings from this study. With increasing energy expenditure, risk of fatal and nonfatal coronary heart disease declined. Findings were adjusted for differences in age, treatment assignment, cigarette smoking, diastolic blood pressure, and blood cholesterol.

While this study was not specifically designed to address research questions on physical activity, the information collected was nevertheless detailed, allowing investigators to show that even moderate intensity physical activity was inversely related to coronary heart disease risk.

THE BRITISH REGIONAL HEART STUDY

The British Regional Heart Study is a prospective study of cardiovascular disease among 7735 men aged 40 to 59 years, randomly chosen from general medical practices in 24 British communities representative of the socioeconomic distribution of men in that country.

In this report on physical activity and coronary heart disease risk,[34] 7630 men who provided information on physical activity were studied: 5714 men without and 1916 men with preexisting coronary heart disease. Using interview techniques, histories of leisure-time physical activities (regular walking or cycling, recreational activity, and sporting activity) and other health habits were obtained. Based on the frequency and intensity of physical activities in which men engaged, Shaper and Wannamethee used a complex classification scheme to categorize men into 6 ordinal groups, where 9% of the men were considered inactive, 31% occasionally active, 23% lightly active, 16% moderately active, 15% moderately

TABLE 18.4. AGE-ADJUSTED INCIDENCE RATES AND RELATIVE RISKS[a] OF CORONARY HEART DISEASE IN MEN ACCORDING TO PHYSICAL ACTIVITY: THE MULTIPLE RISK FACTOR INTERVENTION TRIAL

Physical Activity (thirds)	Number of Events	Incidence Rate (per 1000)	Relative Risk (95% Confidence Interval)
1 (least active)	286	71.8	1.00 (referent)
2	260	63.5	0.90 (0.76–1.06)
3	235	58.0	0.83 (0.70–0.99)

[a] Adjusted for age, treatment assignment, cigarette smoking, diastolic blood pressure, and blood cholesterol.

Adapted with permission from Leon AS, Connett J, Jacobs DR Jr, et al: Leisure-time physical activity levels and risk of coronary heart disease and death: The Multiple Risk Factor Intervention Trial. *JAMA* 258:2388–2395, 1987.

vigorous, and 7% vigorous.[34] During 8 years of follow-up, 480 men suffered at least 1 major heart attack; 242 men without and 238 men with preexisting coronary heart disease.

Among men free from preexisting coronary heart disease, rates of first heart attack declined with increasing physical activity until the moderately vigorous category; the rates for moderate or moderately vigorous men being less than one-half the rates of those for inactive men (Table 18.5). Vigorously active men experienced higher rates, roughly similar to those for men classified as occasionally or lightly active, although this finding was based on a small group of men. These analyses were not adjusted for dietary differences, but age, social class, body mass index, cigarette smoking, systolic blood pressure, total and high-density lipoprotein (HDL) cholesterol, forced expiratory volume in time interval t (FEV_1), complaints of breathlessness, and heart rate were accounted for. Among men with preexisting coronary heart disease, rates of heart attack generally declined with increasing physical activity levels, with no upturn in rates observed among the most vigorous category.

The findings among men without preexisting coronary heart disease are in contrast to most other studies that have observed coronary heart disease risk to decline progressively with higher levels of physical activity. The reasons for the observation of similar rates of first heart attack among men occasionally or lightly active and those vigorously active, instead of lower rates among the latter group, remain unclear.

THE IOWA WOMEN'S HEALTH STUDY

The Iowa Women's Health Study is a large prospective study of 41,836 postmenopausal women, who were aged 55 to 69 years in 1985. Subjects were recruited from a random sample of women in these ages, holding a valid Iowa driver's license.

In this analysis of physical activity and cardiovascular disease mortality, Kushi and colleagues included 40,417 women with information on physical activity and cigarette smoking habit at study entry.[35] In 1986, women completed a baseline questionnaire on physical activity and other health habits. Physical activity was assessed using two questions asking about the frequency of participation in moderate activity (e.g., bowling, golf, light sports or physical exercise, gardening, or taking long walks) and the frequency of participation in vigorous activity (e.g., jogging, racket sports, swimming, aerobics, or strenuous sports). In analyses, women were categorized into three levels of a physical activity index: those who reported participation in vigorous activities at least twice a week, or participation in moderate activi-

TABLE 18.5.   RELATIVE RISKS[a] OF CORONARY HEART DISEASE ACCORDING TO PHYSICAL ACTIVITY AMONG MEN FREE OF PREEXISTING CORONARY HEART DISEASE: THE BRITISH REGIONAL HEART STUDY

Physical Activity Index	Number of Events	Relative Risk (95% Confidence Interval)
Inactive	30	1.0 (referent)
Occasional	86	0.9 (0.5–1.3)
Light	65	0.9 (0.6–1.4)
Moderate	24	0.5 (0.2–0.8)
Moderately vigorous	20	0.5 (0.3–0.9)
Vigorous	17	0.9 (0.5–1.8)

[a] Adjusted for age, social class, body mass index, cigarette smoking, systolic blood pressure, total and high-density lipoprotein, cholesterol, FEV_1, complaints of breathlessness, and heart rate.

Adapted with permission from Shaper AG, Wannamethee G, Weatherall R: Physical activity and ischaemic heart disease in middle-aged British men. *Br Heart J* 66:384–394, 1991.

ties at least 4 times a week were classified as having high activity. Those engaged in vigorous activities once a week or moderate activities 1 to 4 times a week were labeled as the medium activity category. All other women were deemed as having low activity. In separate analyses, investigators also examined cardiovascular mortality rates according to frequency of participation in moderate and vigorous activities. During 7 years of follow-up, 739 women died from cardiovascular disease.

Among all women, all-cause mortality rates declined with increasing levels of the physical activity index. When analyzing cause-specific mortality, investigators restricted their analyses to 32,763 women who were free of coronary heart disease and cancer at baseline and who had survived at least 3 years into the study. This was done in order to minimize potential bias from women who may have decreased their physical activity at baseline because of ill health, whether overt or undiagnosed. The assumption made is that those with undiagnosed disease would likely die early during follow-up. Table 18.6 shows that the most active group of women had almost one-half the cardiovascular mortality rate of the least active group. When investigators examined cardiovascular mortality rates according to frequency of participation in moderate activities, a significant inverse association was seen (p, trend = 0.003). Women who engaged in moderate activities ≥ 4 times a week had a 47% lower risk than

those who did so rarely or never. For vigorous activities, the gradient was even more marked: Those who participated in vigorous activities ≥ 4 times a week had an 80% lower risk than those who did so rarely or never. However, the trend of declining cardiovascular mortality rates with higher frequency of participation in vigorous activity was only of marginal significance (p, trend = 0.09), since few women participated in such activities with any regularity. These analyses took into account differences in age, educational level, marital status, body mass index, waist-to-hip ratio, cigarette smoking, alcohol intake, diet, reproductive variables, and use of estrogen replacement.

This study provides an important contribution to the literature regarding physical activity and coronary heart disease risk. Many previous studies had investigated only men; this study showed similar inverse associations between physical activity and cardiovascular disease risk in women as well. Furthermore, while physical activity was assessed using only a few simple questions, dietary assessment was detailed. Investigators showed that even after taking dietary differences into account, the inverse association persisted.

THE FINNISH TWIN COHORT STUDY

The Finnish Twin Cohort comprises all same-sex twins born in Finland before 1958, with both cotwins alive in 1967. For this analysis of physi-

TABLE 18.6.   RELATIVE RISKS^a OF CARDIOVASCULAR DISEASE MORTALITY ACCORDING TO PHYSICAL ACTIVITY AMONG WOMEN FREE OF CORONARY HEART DISEASE AND CANCER AT BASELINE AND WHO SURVIVED 3 YEARS FROM BASELINE: THE IOWA WOMEN'S HEALTH STUDY

Physical Activity Index	Number of Events	Relative Risk (95% Confidence Interval)
Low	151	1.00 (referent)
Medium	65	0.86 (0.63–1.17)
High	42	0.55 (0.38–0.81)
		p, trend = 0.002

^{a} Adjusted for age, educational level, marital status, body mass index, waist-to-hip ratio, cigarette smoking, alcohol intake, diet, reproductive variables, and use of estrogen replacement.

Adapted with permission from Kushi LH, Fee RM, Folsom AR, et al: Physical activity and mortality in postmenopausal women. *JAMA* 277:1287–1292, 1997.

cal activity and mortality, Kujala and colleagues enrolled 7925 men and 7977 women, who were aged 25 to 64 years in 1976 and who were free of coronary heart disease, cancer, and chronic obstructive pulmonary disease.[36] Additionally, subjects provided information regarding their physical activity. This was ascertained via questionnaires at baseline in 1976, where subjects were queried regarding their leisure-time physical activities; the frequency, duration, and intensity of these activities; as well as other health habits. Investigators classified subjects into 3 categories of physical activity: sedentary, occasional exercisers, or conditioning exercisers. Sedentary subjects were those who did not report any leisure-time physical activity. Conditioning exercisers were those who declared exercising at least 6 times a month, for an average of at least 30 min each session, with an intensity corresponding to vigorous walking or jogging. All others were deemed occasional exercisers. The distribution of men and women in the different exercise categories were sedentary, 15% of men and 17% of women; occasional exercisers, 69% of men and 78% of women; and conditioning exercisers, 16% of men and 5% of women. During follow-up from 1977 to 1994, 1253 subjects died. Investigators did not specifically analyze mortality from coronary heart disease. However, coronary heart disease was the most common cause of death, accounting for 319 of the deaths.

In the total cohort, physical activity was inversely related to all-cause mortality. The relative risks for dying during follow-up, adjusted for age, occupation, cigarette smoking, and alcohol consumption were 1.00 (referent) for those sedentary, 0.80 (95% confidence interval 0.69–0.91) among occasional exercisers, and 0.76 (0.59–0.98) among conditioning exercisers; *p*, trend = 0.002. When analysis was restricted only to the 434 same-sex twin pairs discordant for death, a similar trend was observed (Table 18.7). This was seen for male twins (relative risks 1.00, 0.76, and 0.62, respectively), as well as female twins (relative risks 1.00, 0.66, and 0.24, respectively). Findings among twins of both sexes were only of

borderline significance (Table 18.7), a likely consequence of the small numbers. These analyses included both monozygotic, as well as dizygotic, twins, since there were too few of the former to analyze separately. Among the 120 monozygotic twins who were discordant for death during follow-up, only 1 twin-pair was discordant in their exercise habit; the sedentary twin died during follow-up while the conditioning exerciser cotwin survived.

The Finnish Twin Study is the first study where investigators attempted to take genetic factors into account when examining the relation between physical activity and mortality. These data provide some evidence arguing for a causal relation between higher levels of physical activity and greater longevity, as opposed to a selective genetic process that confers an individual with both the capability for high levels of physical activity, as well as low coronary heart disease risk.

THE AEROBICS CENTER LONGITUDINAL STUDY

The studies described earlier all have examined physical activity. In the Aerobics Center Longitudinal Study, Blair and colleagues investigated physical fitness, rather than physical activity. Physical activity and physical fitness are two

TABLE 18.7.   RELATIVE RISKS[a] OF MORTALITY AMONG MALE AND FEMALE SAME-SEX TWIN PAIRS DISCORDANT FOR DEATH: THE FINNISH TWIN COHORT STUDY

Physical Activity	Relative Risk (95% Confidence Interval)
Sedentary	1.00 (referent)
Occasional exercisers	0.73 (0.50–1.07)
Conditioning exercisers	0.56 (0.29–1.11)
	p, trend = 0.06

[a] Adjusted for age, occupation, cigarette smoking, and alcohol intake.

Adapted with permission from Kujala UM, Kaprio J, Sarna S, et al: Relationship of leisure-time physical activity and mortality: The Finnish Twin Cohort. *JAMA* 279:440–444, 1998.

interrelated measures, with physical activity being an optional behavior and physical fitness a physiological condition.[37] Regular physical activity can improve physiological fitness over time, while physiological fitness limits the amount of physical activity that may be performed. Thus, physical activity and physical fitness each may act independently to influence risk of coronary heart disease.

The Aerobics Center Longitudinal Study is the largest epidemiologic investigation of physical fitness to date.[38] Investigators enrolled 10,244 men and 3210 women, aged 20 to 60+ years, who received a preventive medical examination between 1970 and 1981 at the Cooper Institute for Aerobics Research in Dallas, Texas. Subjects were predominantly white and of middle-to-upper socioeconomic status. As part of their medical examination, men and women underwent a maximal treadmill exercise test. Investigators used total treadmill test time, specific for each sex and age group, to classify subjects into fifths of physical fitness. They then followed subjects for an average of over 8 years, during which 240 men and 43 women died. Of these deaths, 66 in men and 7 in women were due to cardiovascular causes.

There was a strong inverse association between fitness level and age-adjusted all-cause mortality rates in men. Although the number of deaths was small, the pattern appeared similar in women. The inverse associations persisted after

additional adjustment for cigarette smoking, systolic blood pressure, serum cholesterol, serum glucose, body mass index, and parental history of coronary heart disease. Furthermore, investigators noted the inverse association between physical fitness and all-cause mortality to hold within categories of each of these risk factors. With regard to cardiovascular mortality, while the small number of cardiovascular deaths in either sex preclude a definitive conclusion, similar findings were observed (Table 18.8). The difference in cardiovascular mortality rates between subjects in the extremes of physical fitness appeared more pronounced for women than men.

This study is one of the few specifically designed to examine the relation of physical fitness with various health outcomes. Further, it provides an important contribution in showing that physical fitness is associated with greater longevity in women, as well as men. Previous studies generally had not included women.

THE LIPID RESEARCH CLINICS MORTALITY FOLLOW-UP STUDY

The original purpose of the Lipid Research Clinics Prevalence Study, conducted between 1972 and 1976, was to describe the lipid profile of men and women in North America. Participating subjects were recruited at 10 different centers and examined up to 2 times. Subsequently, the

TABLE 18.8. AGE-ADJUSTED RATES AND RELATIVE RISKS OF CARDIOVASCULAR DISEASE MORTALITY IN MEN AND WOMEN ACCORDING TO PHYSICAL FITNESS: THE AEROBICS CENTER LONGITUDINAL STUDY

Physical Fitness (fifths)	Mortality Rates (per 10,000)	Relative Risk (95% Confidence Interval)
Men		
1 (least fit)	24.6	1.00 (referent)
2 and 3	7.8	0.32
4 and 5	3.1	0.13
Women		
1	7.4	1.00 (referent)
2 and 3	2.9	0.39
4 and 5	0.8	0.11

Adapted with permission from Blair SN, Kohl HW III, Paffenbarger RS Jr, et al: Physical fitness and all-cause mortality: A perspective study of healthy men and women. *JAMA* 262:2395–2401, 1989.

Lipid Research Clinics Mortality Follow-up Study was initiated to examine the relation between factors ascertained at the second visit and mortality among participants aged ≥ 30 years.

In this study of physical fitness, Ekelund and colleagues enrolled 3106 healthy white men, aged 30 to 69 years at baseline, with valid exercise test data.[39] Women were excluded because the small number of deaths precluded meaningful analyses. Physical fitness was assessed using a submaximal treadmill exercise test, according to a modified Bruce protocol. Men then were classified into fourths of physical fitness, according to heart rate at stage 2 of the exercise test. During an average follow-up of 8.5 years, 45 deaths from cardiovascular disease occurred among the men.

With higher levels of physical fitness, crude death rates from cardiovascular disease declined (Table 18.9). There was a more than eightfold difference in cardiovascular mortality rates between the least and most fit men. When coronary heart disease mortality rates were examined, a similar pattern was observed, with a more than sixfold difference in coronary heart disease mortality rates between men in the extreme categories of physical fitness. Findings were similar when analyses took into account age, cigarette smoking, systolic blood pressure, and HDL and LDL cholesterol.

TABLE 18.9.   RATES AND RELATIVE RISKS OF CARDIOVASCULAR DISEASE MORTALITY IN MEN ACCORDING TO PHYSICAL FITNESS: THE LIPID RESEARCH CLINICS MORTALITY FOLLOW-UP STUDY

Physical Fitness (fourths)	Mortality Rates (per 100)	Relative Risk
1 (least fit)	221	8.5
2	156	6.0
3	130	5.0
4	26	1.0 (referent)

Adapted with permission from Ekelund L-G, Haskell WL, Johnson JL, et al: Physical fitness as a predictor of cardiovascular mortality in asymptomatic North American men: The Lipid Research Clinics Mortality Follow-Up Study. *N Engl J Med* 319:1379–1384, 1988.

Investigators then made further attempts to clarify that the lower cardiovascular mortality rates among men who were more fit was valid and not the result of bias due to men with subclinical illness. They examined plots of cumulative mortality from cardiovascular disease, adjusted for the variables listed earlier, according to fourths of physical fitness. Over the 8.5 years of follow-up, the curves for the least and most fit men continued to diverge, suggesting that the benefit of physical fitness was unlikely to be artifactual, resulting from early mortality among men with subclinical illness who were unfit.

WEIGHT OF THE EPIDEMIOLOGIC EVIDENCE

All of the epidemiologic studies that have examined the association between physical activity or physical fitness and risk of coronary heart disease have been observational studies. The preceding studies are representative of the many other studies in the field. The majority of studies have observed lower risk of coronary heart disease among persons with higher levels of physical activity or physical fitness. In a meta-analysis conducted by Berlin and Colditz, investigators reported about a twofold difference in risk between those active and those sedentary.[23] Studies of physical fitness, as exemplified by the Aerobics Center Longitudinal Study and the Lipid Research Clinics Mortality Follow-up Study earlier, suggest that the difference in coronary heart disease risk between those most fit and those least fit may be even more pronounced.

However, observational epidemiologic studies cannot presume cause and effect.[40] The strength of evidence from such studies is weaker than that from randomized clinical trials. It is highly improbable that randomized clinical trials examining the relation between physical activity and coronary heart disease risk will ever be conducted, because of cost constraints and the unfeasibility of maintaining high compliance with physical activity over the long term. Instead, randomized clinical trials examining the association between physical activity and risk factors for coronary heart disease, such as blood pressure[11,41,42] or lipid profile,[12,13,41,42] have been conducted. Such randomized trials have shown that physical activity is capable of improving risk factors for coronary heart disease. The assumption made is that improvements in risk factors will translate to a lower risk of coronary heart disease. However, this assumption does not always hold true;[43] therefore, it is important to evaluate observational studies where the association between physical activity or physical fitness and coronary heart disease risk is directly assessed.

Based on data from such observational studies then, can it be concluded that high levels of either activity or fitness cause low risk of coronary heart disease to result? One issue of concern is bias. Bias resulting from incomplete follow-up is unlikely, since all the studies reviewed earlier had good follow-up of subjects. Another concern is that findings might reflect a selective process (such as a genetic predisposition) that renders an individual capable of high levels of physical activity or fitness, in addition to favoring him or her with low coronary heart disease risk. Data from the Finnish Twin Cohort Study, where matched pairs of dizygotic twins were analyzed,[36] makes this bias less likely. Unfortunately, the study did not have sufficient pairs of monozygotic twins for analyses; had similar findings been observed among monozygotic twins, this would have provided an even stronger argument against such a selection bias. A third bias to consider is that subjects might self-select themselves into the low spectrum of physical activity due to occult coronary heart disease. This would result in an artifactual observation of high coronary heart disease rates among those with little physical activity (and, hence, low physical fitness). With longer follow-up, however, the impact of this bias would be diluted as those with occult disease likely would be diagnosed soon after the start of the study. Follow-up in the studies reviewed earlier generally has been long, making such a bias less likely. Moreover, in the Lipid Research Clinics Mortality Follow-up Study,[39] when cumulative cardiovascular disease mortality rates were plotted as a function of time, the curves for the least and most fit men continued to diverge over time. This suggests that the benefit of physical fitness was unlikely to be artifactual, resulting from early cardiovascular disease mortality among men with subclinical illness who were unfit.

In observational epidemiologic studies, another threat to the validity of findings is confounding. Individuals who exercise or are physically fit likely differ with respect to other health habits. Perhaps it is these other health habits, and not physical activity, that is responsible for the low coronary heart disease rates observed among those physically active. In the studies described earlier, investigators have attempted to control for confounding by various other predictors of coronary heart disease risk,[2,44] including age, cigarette habit, alcohol consumption, body mass index, reproductive variables, family history of coronary heart disease, diet, blood pressure, lipid profile, in analyses. Even after accounting for these other factors, an inverse association between physical activity or physical fitness and coronary heart disease risk has persisted.

Thus, bias and confounding are unlikely to explain the findings of observational studies in this field. Biologically, the observations are very plausible since physical activity, as discussed earlier, favorably influences a whole host of physiological parameters that affect risk of developing coronary heart disease. Based on the data from epidemiologic studies, it is concluded that the association between high levels of physical activity or physical fitness and decreased coronary heart disease risk is likely to be causal in nature.

AMOUNT, INTENSITY, AND DURATION OF PHYSICAL ACTIVITY REQUIRED TO PREVENT CORONARY HEART DISEASE

While the epidemiologic evidence is clear regarding an inverse association between physical activity or physical fitness and coronary heart disease risk, details regarding this association are less clear. Debate continues regarding the optimal amount, intensity, and duration of physical activity for prevention of coronary heart disease. What has fueled this debate is the development of a new recommendation for physical activity in 1995 that calls for the accumulation of at least 30 min of moderate intensity physical activity on most days of the week.[45] Moderate intensity activities would be those requiring 3 to 6 METs, or the equivalent of brisk walking at 3 to 4 mi/h for most healthy adults. Previous recommendations typically prescribed vigorous exercise, for at least 20 min continuously, at least 3 times a week.[46] Vigorous exercise gets the heart rate up and causes sweating; such activities generally require 6 METs or greater and would include activities such as jogging or running. Therefore, the new recommendation differs from previous recommendations in 2 ways: a concession to moderate intensity activity, as opposed to the prior requirement for vigorous exercise, and an allowance for the accumulation of short bouts of activity, as contrasted to the earlier necessitation for one continuous, long session.

With regard to the amount of physical activity required for decreased coronary heart disease risk, very few studies have tried to quantify this. In the Harvard Alumni Health Study described earlier,[27] heart attack rates declined progressively, beginning at 500 to 999 kcal per week. Beyond 2000 kcal per week, it appeared that the benefit began to plateau. Thus, the new physical activity recommendation, which would expend energy on the order of 1000 kcal per week, is likely to be sufficient to decrease coronary heart disease risk, at least with regard to the amount of energy expenditure.

What is more contentious is how intense should physical activity be, and how long each episode of physical activity should last. Randomized trials have compared an intervention of lifestyle physical activity with an intervention of structured exercise.[41–42] The lifestyle physical activity intervention promoted the new physical activity recommendation, emphasizing moderate intensity activity and accumulation of short bouts

of activity. The structured exercise intervention promoted previous exercise recommendations, where vigorous exercise in a longer, continuous session was emphasized (e.g., aerobics classes). These trials showed that lifestyle physical activity was sufficient to improve physical fitness, blood pressure, lipid profile, and body weight. However, observational epidemiologic studies that have examined the outcome of coronary heart disease itself have been less clear in their findings. While many studies have examined the association between physical activity and coronary heart disease risk,[22,23] relatively few have investigated the kinds and intensities of activities associated with benefits for coronary heart disease. Of those that have, the data are about evenly divided between studies that have observed vigorous intensity physical activity to be necessary,[25,26,31,47,48] and studies that have found that even moderate intensity activity is sufficient[33–35,49–51] for benefit.

Several explanations are possible for the lack of consistent findings regarding intensity of physical activity and coronary heart disease risk. First, the studies enrolled different populations for investigation: Some of the studies were conducted in men, others in women. Subjects also belonged to different age groups and likely had different basal levels of physical fitness. Perhaps populations with lower levels of fitness might benefit with moderate intensity activity, while populations with higher levels of fitness might need more vigorous activity for benefit. So the different findings might reflect the fact that the populations studied were not homogenous. Second, these studies all asked subjects to recall their physical activities. Vigorous activities, such as running, probably are recalled more accurately than moderate activities such as gardening or dancing. Perhaps the studies that observed no association with moderate activities were merely reflecting the imprecision with which such activities were recalled. Finally, there currently is no uniform scheme for classifying the intensity of activities. A particular activity may have been classified as moderate in one study, vigorous in another. Furthermore, all the studies assessed intensity on an absolute level. For example, brisk walking usually is assigned an intensity level of 4 METs, or moderate intensity, regardless of how fit the subject might be. For an older (say, 70+), unfit person, this might actually represent a vigorous, relative effort, while for a young, fit marathon runner, this might only be a light, relative effort. For these reasons, therefore, different studies might have come to different conclusions regarding the intensity of physical activity required to reduce coronary heart disease risk.

With regard to the duration of physical activity that is optimal, several clinical trials have investigated exercise of different durations in relation to risk factors for coronary heart disease. The 2 trials described earlier that tested lifestyle physical activity against structured exercise[41,42] did not provide data regarding actual durations per episode of physical activity. Presumably, subjects assigned to the former group would likely accumulate short bouts of activity, while those assigned to the latter group would likely incline toward exercising in a continuous, long session. As mentioned, the lifestyle physical activity group also did achieve improvements in physical fitness, blood pressure, lipid profile, and body weight. In another experiment, Ebisu reported that young men running 6 miles a day, whether in 1, 2, or 3 bouts, experienced similar increases in physical fitness after 10 weeks, while HDL-cholesterol levels increased most in the 3-bout group.[52] DeBusk et al observed that physical fitness improved after 8 weeks among middle-aged men who jogged 30 min a day, whether in a 1 or 2 bouts, although the former improved more.[53] However, no study has examined duration per exercise episode in relation to risk of developing coronary heart disease itself.

CARDIOVASCULAR HAZARDS WITH PHYSICAL ACTIVITY

Sudden unexpected cardiac death can occur occasionally during or shortly after an acute bout of exercise, and more commonly than during sedentary periods.[54,55] This is discussed more fully in other chapters. Here, this chapter will briefly describe 2 studies where heavy physical exertion was shown to precipitate nonfatal myocardial infarction (MI), especially in subjects who are habitually sedentary. While both studies highlight the potential for cardiovascular hazards from vigorous physical activity, they also demonstrate the benefits associated with habitual physical activity.

Mittelman and colleagues interviewed 1228 patients with MI as to the time, kind, and intensity of physical activities carried out in the 26 h before onset of the infarction.[56] Investigators compared the frequencies of patients reporting physical activity at an intensity level of ≥ 6 METs during each of the 26 h. The risk of MI that accompanied such vigorous exertion in the hour prior to the onset of MI was 5.6 times (95% confidence interval, 2.7–12.8) the risk that accompanied heavy exertion > 1 h and up to 26 h prior to the onset, suggesting a triggering effect from such vigorous exercise. Additionally, an inverse graded effect of risk was observed with number of times the men habitually exercised each week. The relative risks associated with physical activity of ≥ 6 METs in the hour prior to onset of MI were 107 (95% confidence interval, 67–171) and 2.4 (1.5–3.7), respectively, among men and women who habitually engaged in vigorous exercise less than once per week and ≥ 5 times per week. These data suggest that individuals who habitually exercise vigorously have both a low overall risk of MI, and a low risk that any infarction they do sustain would be precipitated by heavy physical exertion.

Similar findings were observed in a study conducted by Willich and colleagues in Augsburg, Germany.[57] Interviews with 1194 patients with MI and an equal number of control subjects from the general population revealed that 7.1% of patients were exerting themselves at a level of 6 or more METs at the onset of infarction, as compared with 3.9% of controls at the corresponding time. Thus, the relative risk of precipitating an MI by vigorous physical exertion of ≥ 6 METs was 2.1 (95% confidence interval, 1.1–3.6), which was a lesser magnitude than that observed in the previous study. As with the previous study, those who exercised regularly had a lower risk of MI than those who did not. The relative risks associated with physical activity of $\geq$ 6 METs at the onset of MI were 6.9 (95% confidence interval, 4.1–12.2) and 1.3 (0.8–2.2), respectively, among men and women who regularly exercised < 4 and $\geq$ 4 times per week, providing further support for the hypothesis of a protective effect from habitual physical activity.

SUMMARY AND CONCLUSIONS

Coronary heart disease is a leading cause of mortality among both men and women in the United States, as well as in other western countries. In 1996, 1 out of every 4.9 deaths in the United States was caused by coronary heart disease, or a total of some 476,000 deaths.[2] Over the years, researchers have identified many risk factors for this disease.[2,44] An important risk factor is physical inactivity because it impacts a whole host of other physiological variables that adversely influence heart disease risk. Epidemiologic studies consistently show that high levels of physical activity or physical fitness are associated with low risk of coronary heart disease.[22,23] Men and women who are sedentary have about twice the risk of developing coronary heart disease, compared with those who are active. The differential in risk between those least and most physically fit appears to be even greater.

Therefore, it is very unfortunate that Americans are an extremely sedentary lot. National data from the Behavioral Risk Factor Surveillance Survey indicate that about 30% of men and women do not engage in any physical activity at all during their leisure time.[21] This proportion has not changed much over the years. If adults who do no physical activity, as well as those who do engage in physical activity but only on an irregular basis, are counted the proportion jumps to an alarming 60%.[58] Physical inactivity is, therefore, a public health problem. Clinicians and other health professionals should aggressively promote physical activity.

When promoting physical activity, what specifically should be advocated? How much physical activity, at what intensity, and for what duration should activity be carried out in order to gain benefit for coronary heart disease risk? There is no consensus regarding these issues, even though the principle that physical activity reduces coronary heart disease risk is widely accepted. A physical activity recommendation from the Centers for Disease Control and Prevention and the American College of Sports Medicine has called for the accumulation of at least 30 min of moderate intensity physical activity over most days of the week.[45] This contrasts with previous physical activity prescriptions, which generally require vigorous intensity exercise to be carried out for at least 20 min continuously, 3 times a week.[46]

When trying to promote physical activity to sedentary individuals, moderate intensity activity is likely to be more attainable and sustainable than vigorous intensity exercise.[59] There is sufficient evidence to indicate that moderate intensity physical activity can improve risk factors for coronary heart disease, such as blood pressure and lipid profile.[11–13,41,42] With vigorous activity, greater benefits are realized, especially with regard to lipid profile and insulin sensitivity.[14–17] Studies that have examined the outcome of coronary heart disease itself, rather than risk factors, have been less clear. Several studies have shown that moderate intensity activity is beneficial.[33–35,49–51] Vigorous activity, in comparison, clearly is associated with decreased heart disease risk.[25,26,31,47,48]

Few data are available regarding optimal duration of an episode of physical activity. These preliminary data suggest that even accumulated, short bouts of physical activity may be associated with improvements in coronary heart disease risk factors.[41,42,52,53] No study, however, has examined the association of different durations of an exercise episode with coronary heart disease risk itself.

What message then should be imparted? In

these authors' opinion, moderate intensity activity, of at least 10 to 15 min duration, should be promoted to those recalcitrant to exercise, because this is more realistic than asking such individuals to exercise vigorously. Such physical activity is likely to be beneficial with regard to coronary heart disease risk factors and may also reduce coronary heart disease risk. However, vigorous activity of 20 min or longer should receive no less emphasis as a health promotion message among those for whom such activity is not medically contraindicated. In today's fast-paced world where time is a precious commodity, one-half h of vigorous activity expends as much energy as moderate activity carried out for twice or three times as long.

PERSONAL PERSPECTIVE

Physical activity clearly is associated with decreased risk of coronary heart disease. The benefit associated with a habitually active lifestyle is of approximately the same magnitude as the benefit associated with not smoking, maintaining normal blood pressure, normal cholesterol levels or normal glucose tolerance, or not being overweight. Americans, who are highly sedentary, need to become physically more active. While the research community does not yet have all the answers to questions regarding optimal amount, intensity, frequency, and duration of physical activity, this should not serve as an excuse for postponing physical activity. Current guidelines that recommend at least 30 min of moderate intensity physical activity on most days of the week would be a good starting point for those sedentary. When previously sedentary individuals can adopt this regimen comfortably, they should strive for the goal of more vigorous exercise, provided there are no contraindications.

REFERENCES

1. Ventura SJ, Anderson RN, Smith BL, et al: *Births and Deaths: Preliminary Data for 1997. National Vital Statistics Reports*: vol 47, no.4. Hyattsville, MD: National Center for Health Statistics, 1998.
2. American Heart Association: *1999 Heart and Stroke Statistical Update.* Dallas, TX: American Heart Association, 1998.
3. Rich-Edwards JW, Manson JE, Hennekens CH, et al: The primary prevention of coronary heart disease in women. *N Engl J Med* 332:1758–1766, 1995.
4. Lyons AS, Petrucelli RJ: *Medicine: An Illustrated History.* New York: Harry N. Abrams Inc., 1978, pp. 130, 195–203.
5. Robinson RS: *Sources for the History of Greek Athletics.* Chicago, IL: Ares Publishers, Inc., 1955, pp. 191–197.
6. Ramazzini B: *DeMorbis Artificum Diatriba.* (The Latin text of 1713 revised with translation and notes by Wright WC. *Diseases of Workers.* Chicago: University of Chicago Press, 1940, pp. 281–285, 295–301.)
7. Saltin B: Cardiovascular and pulmonary adaptation to physical activity, in Bouchard C, Shephard RJ, Stephens T, et al (eds.): *Exercise, Fitness, and Health: A Consensus of Current Knowledge.* Champaign, IL: Human Kinetics Books, 1990, pp. 187–203.
8. Fuster V, Badimon L, Badimon JJ, et al: The pathogenesis of coronary artery disease and the acute coronary syndromes. *N Engl J Med* 326: 242–250, 310–318, 1992.
9. Hambrecht R, Niebauer J, Marburger C, et al: Various intensities of leisure time physical activity in patients with coronary artery disease: Effects on cardiorespiratory fitness and progression of coronary atherosclerotic lesions. *J Am Coll Cardiol* 22: 468–477, 1993.
10. Kramsch DM, Aspen AJ, Abramowitz BM, et al: Reduction of coronary atherosclerosis by moderate conditioning exercise in monkeys on an atherogenic diet. *N Engl J Med* 305:1483–1489, 1981.
11. Hagberg JM, Brown MD: Does exercise training play a role in the treatment of essential hypertension? *J Cardiovasc Risk* 2:296–302, 1995.
12. Wood PD, Stefanick ML, Williams PT, et al: The effects on plasma lipoproteins of a prudent weight-reducing diet, with or without exercise, in overweight men and women. *N Engl J Med* 325: 461–466, 1991.
13. Stefanick ML, Mackey S, Sheehan M, et al: Effects of diet and exercise in men and post-menopausal women with low levels of HDL cholesterol and high levels of LDL cholesterol. *N Engl J Med* 339:12–20, 1998.

14. Williams PT: High-density lipoprotein cholesterol and other risk factors for coronary heart disease in female runners. *N Engl J Med* 334:1298–1303, 1996.

15. Williams PT: Relationship of distance run per week to coronary heart disease risk factors in 8283 male runners: The National Runners' Health Study. *Arch Intern Med* 157:191–198, 1997.

16. Mayer-Davis EJ, D'Agostino R Jr, Karter AJ, et al: Intensity and amount of physical activity in relation to insulin sensitivity: The Insulin Resistance Atherosclerosis Study. *JAMA* 279:666–674, 1998.

17. Holloszy JO, Schultz J, Kusnierkiewicz J, et al: Effects of exercise on glucose tolerance and insulin resistance. *Acta Med Scand* 711(Suppl):55–65, 1986.

18. Kestin AS, Ellis PA, Barnard MR, et al: Effect of strenuous exercise on platelet activation state and reactivity. *Circulation* 88:1502–1511, 1993.

19. Szymanski LM, Pate RR, Durstine JL: Effects of maximal exercise and venous occlusion on fibrinolytic activity in physically active and inactive men. *J Appl Physiol* 77:2305–2310, 1994.

20. Nygard O, Vollset SE, Refsum H, et al: Total plasma homocysteine and cardiovascular risk profile: The Hordaland Homocysteine Study. *JAMA* 274:1526–1533, 1995.

21. US Department of Health and Human Services: *Physical Activity and Health: A Report of the Surgeon General.* Atlanta, GA: US Department of Health and Human Services, Centers for Disease Control and Prevention, National Center for Chronic Disease Prevention and Health Promotion, 1996, pp. 133–135, 175–207.

22. Powell KE, Thompson PD, Caspersen CJ, et al: Physical activity and the incidence of coronary heart disease. *Ann Rev Public Health* 8:253–287, 1987.

23. Berlin JA, Colditz GA: A meta-analysis of physical activity in the prevention of coronary heart disease. *Am J Epidemiol* 132:612–628, 1990.

24. Morris JN, Heady JA, Raffle PAB, et al: Coronary heart disease and physical activity of work. *Lancet* 2:1053–1057, 1111–1120, 1953.

25. Morris JN, Everitt MG, Pollard R, et al: Vigorous exercise in leisure-time: Protection against coronary heart disease. *Lancet* 2:1207–1210, 1980.

26. Morris JN, Clayton DG, Everitt MG, et al: Exercise in leisure-time: Coronary attack and death rates. *Br Heart J* 63:325–334, 1990.

27. Paffenbarger RS Jr, Wing AL, Hyde RT: Physical activity as an index of heart attack risk in college alumni. *Am J Epidemiol* 108:161–175, 1978.

28. Paffenbarger RS Jr, Hyde RT, Wing AL, et al: Physical activity, all-cause mortality, and longevity of college alumni. *N Engl J Med* 314:605–613, 1986.

29. Paffenbarger RS Jr, Hyde RT, Wing AL, et al: The association of changes in physical-activity level and other lifestyle characteristics with mortality among men. *N Engl J Med* 328:538–545, 1993.

30. Lee I-M, Hsieh C-c, Paffenbarger RS Jr: Exercise intensity and longevity in men: The Harvard Alumni Health Study. *JAMA* 273:1179–1184, 1995.

31. Lee I-M, Paffenbarger RS Jr: Is vigorous physical activity necessary to reduce the risk of cardiovascular disease? in Leon AS (ed.): *Physical Activity and Cardiovascular Health: A National Consensus.* Champaign, IL: Human Kinetics Publishers, 1997 pp. 67–75.

32. Kaplan GA, Seeman TE, Cohen RD, et al: Mortality among the elderly in the Alameda County Study: Behavioral and demographic risk factors. *Am J Public Health* 77:307–312, 1987.

33. Leon AS, Connett J, Jacobs DR Jr, et al: Leisure-time physical activity levels and risk of coronary heart disease and death: The Multiple Risk Factor Intervention Trial. *JAMA* 258:2388–2395, 1987.

34. Shaper AG, Wannamethee G, Weatherall R: Physical activity and ischaemic heart disease in middle-aged British men. *Br Heart J* 66:384–394, 1991.

35. Kushi LH, Fee RM, Folsom AR, et al: Physical activity and mortality in postmenopausal women. *JAMA* 277:1287–1292, 1997.

36. Kujala UM, Kaprio J, Sarna S, et al: Relationship of leisure-time physical activity and mortality: The Finnish Twin Cohort. *JAMA* 279:440–444, 1998.

37. Caspersen CJ, Powell KE, Christenson GM: Physical activity, exercise, and physical fitness: Definitions and distinctions for health-related research. *Public Health Rep* 100:126–131, 1985.

38. Blair SN, Kohl HW III, Paffenbarger RS Jr, et al: Physical fitness and all-cause mortality: A prospective study of healthy men and women. *JAMA* 262:2395–2401, 1989.

39. Ekelund L-G, Haskell WL, Johnson JL, et al: Physical fitness as a predictor of cardiovascular mortality in asymptomatic North American men:

The Lipid Research Clinics Mortality Follow-up Study. *N Engl J Med* 319:1379–1384, 1988.

40. Smith GD, Phillips AN, Neaton JD: Smoking as "independent" risk factor for suicide: Illustration of an artifact from observational epidemiology? *Lancet* 340:709–712, 1992.

41. Dunn AL, Marcus BH, Kampert JB, et al: Comparison of lifestyle and structured interventions to increase physical activity and cardiorespiratory fitness: A randomized trial. *JAMA* 281: 327–334, 1999.

42. Andersen RE, Wadden TA, Bartlett SJ, et al: Effects of lifestyle activity vs. structured aerobic exercise in obese women: A randomized trial. *JAMA* 281:335–340, 1999.

43. Hulley S, Grady D, Bush T, et al for the Heart and Estrogen/Progestin Replacement Study (HERS) Research Group: Randomized trial of estrogen plus progestin for secondary prevention of coronary heart disease in postmenopausal women. *JAMA* 280:605–613, 1998.

44. Manson JE, Ridker PM, Gaziano JM, et al (eds.): *Prevention of Myocardial Infarction.* New York: Oxford University Press, 1996.

45. Pate RR, Pratt M, Blair SN, et al: Physical activity and public health: A recommendation from the Centers for Disease Control and Prevention and the American College of Sports Medicine. *JAMA* 273:402–407, 1995.

46. American College of Sports Medicine: *Guidelines for Graded Exercise Testing and Exercise Prescription,* 3rd ed. Philadelphia: Lea & Febiger, 1985, pp. 31–52.

47. Slattery ML, Jacobs DR, Nichaman MZ: Leisure time physical activity and coronary heart disease death: The US Railroad Study. *Circulation* 79: 304–311, 1989.

48. Lakka TA, Venalainen JM, Rauramaa R, et al: Relation of leisure-time physical activity and cardiorespiratory fitness to the risk of acute myocardial infarction in men. *N Engl J Med* 330:1549–1554, 1994.

49. Magnus K, Matroos A, Strackee J: Walking, cycling, or gardening, with or without seasonal interruption, in relation to acute coronary events. *Am J Epidemiol* 110:724–733, 1979.

50. Haapanen N, Miilunpalo S, Vuori I, et al: Characteristics of leisure time physical activity associated with decreased risk of premature all-cause and cardiovascular disease mortality in middle-aged men. *Am J Epidemiol* 143:870–880, 1996.

51. Hakim AA, Petrovitch H, Burchfiel CM, et al: Effects of walking on mortality among nonsmoking retired men. *N Engl J Med* 338:94–99, 1998.

52. Ebisu T: Splitting the distance of endurance running: On cardiovascular endurance and blood lipids. *Jpn J Phys Educ* 30:37–43, 1985.

53. DeBusk RF, Stenestrand U, Sheehan M, et al: Training effects of long versus short bouts of exercise in healthy subjects. *Am J Cardiol* 65:1010–1013, 1990.

54. Thompson PD, Funk EJ, Carleton RA, et al: Incidence of death during jogging in Rhode Island from 1975 through 1980. *JAMA* 247:2535–2538, 1982.

55. Siscovick DS, Weiss NS, Fletcher RH, et al: The incidence of primary cardiac arrest during vigorous exercise. *N Engl J Med* 311:874–877, 1984.

56. Mittelman MA, Maclure M, Tofler GH, et al: Triggering of acute myocardial infarction by heavy physical exertion: Protection against triggering by regular exertion. *N Engl J Med* 329:1677–1683, 1993.

57. Willich SN, Lewis M, Löwel H, et al: Physical exertion as a trigger of acute myocardial infarction. *N Engl J Med* 329:1684–1690, 1993.

58. Anonymous. Prevalence of sedentary lifestyle: Behavioral Risk Factor Surveillance System, United States, 1991. *MMWR* 1993, 42:576–579.

59. Hillsdon M, Thorogood M: A systematic review of physical activity promotion strategies. *Br J Sports Med* 30:84–89, 1996.

Chapter 19

EXERCISE IN THE PREVENTION AND TREATMENT OF HYPERTENSION

Jirayos Chintanadilok, M.D.   *David T. Lowenthal, M.D., Ph.D.*

Hypertension is defined by the Fifth Report of the Joint National Committee (JNC-V) as blood pressure greater or equal to 140/90 mmHg with or without the current use of antihypertensive medication.[1] Based on provisional data from the Third National Health and Nutrition Examination Survey conducted during 1988 through 1991, approximately 50 million Americans are hypertensive.[1] The clinical diagnosis of hypertension is based on the persistent presence of high blood pressure on at least 3 occasions. The degree of hypertension relates to the target organ damage. Individuals who have blood pressure that is more than 160/95 have an annual incidence rate one- to threefold times higher for coronary artery disease, congestive heart failure, intermittent claudication, and stroke than they do when compared to normotensive persons.[2] Also, exercise capacity is reduced by 30% compared to age-matched normotensives.[3]

Antihypertensive medications are effective in lowering blood pressure, but their associated side-effects are inevitable, especially in the elderly. Nonetheless, medication can also decrease the risk of heart failure, hypertensive renal failure, stroke, and coronary heart disease. The cost-benefit and risk-benefit of mild hypertension has been studied for decades. Adverse drug effects are common, yet the benefits of antihypertensive medications outweigh the risks. Nonpotassium-sparing diuretics can increase the risk of hypokalemia and sudden death and change glucose tolerance and lipid profiles,[4,5] yet their effectiveness in normalizing blood pressure has been known for 40 years. Thus, nonpharmacological interventions have been recommended as an initial approach for mild-to-moderate hypertension with ongoing follow-up according to the JNC-VI.[6]

The evidence upon which the JNC-VI bases its recommendations for physical activity are the 1996 report from the Centers for Disease Control and Prevention as well as other individual research reports.[6] Data show that regular aerobic physical activity (i.e., brisk walking), performed with moderate intensity (40–60% of maximum oxygen consumption) 30 to 40 min on most days of the week, can safely lower blood pressure. The intensity can generally be increased without an extensive medical evaluation as long as symptoms of overt cardiac, neurologic, and musculoskeletal diseases are not provoked by walking. Conversely, individuals with normal blood pressure and a sedentary lifestyle have a 20 to 30% higher risk of developing hypertension than they would if they exercised.[7]

Physicians should strongly encourage all people to increase physical activity, especially for hypertensive patients, since it may lower blood pressure or decrease the use of antihypertensive medications. This chapter will review the rationale for using exercise as a treatment and prevention for hypertension, and how an exercise prescription can be individualized for hypertensive patients.

PATHOPHYSIOLOGY OF HYPERTENSION

Hypertension is clinically divided into two categories: primary and secondary hypertension. It is important to differentiate between them because secondary hypertension should be treated appropriately either by medical or surgical interventions, depending on the etiology (shown in Fig. 19.1). The most common cause of secondary hypertension is renovascular disease. Additional causes are pheochromocytoma, primary aldosteronism, oral contraceptive pills, coarctation of the aorta, and sleep apnea syndrome. The clinician should search for secondary causes of hypertension when hypertension is severe or refractory despite high doses of multiple antihypertensive medications; the blood pressure rises acutely in previously stable patients; the age of onset is less than 20 years old or older than 70 years old; there is a localized abdominal bruit; the serum creatinine rises acutely after initiation of angiotensin-converting enzyme (ACE)-inhibitors; or there is

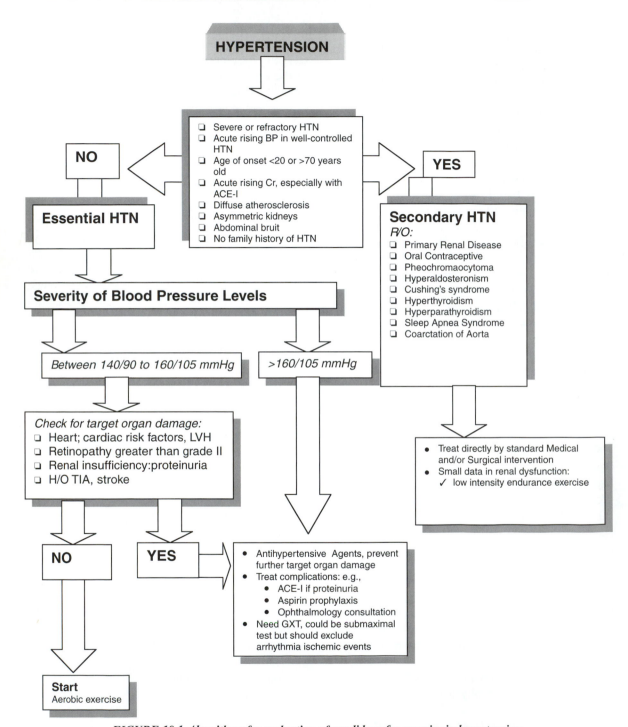

FIGURE 19.1. Algorithms for evaluation of candidacy for exercise in hypertension.

evidence of diffuse atherosclerosis. Only 5% of sustained hypertensive patients have a secondary cause for hypertension and the rest have primary hypertension. The causes for primary hypertension in the adolescent, young adult, middle-aged adult, and elderly are multifactorial (Fig.19.2), yet the common denominator is presumably genetic. This is supported by the common clinical observation of clustering of hypertension in certain families.

HEMODYNAMIC CHANGES

Blood pressure is the product of cardiac output and systemic vascular resistance. The hemodynamic variables can be equated as the following:

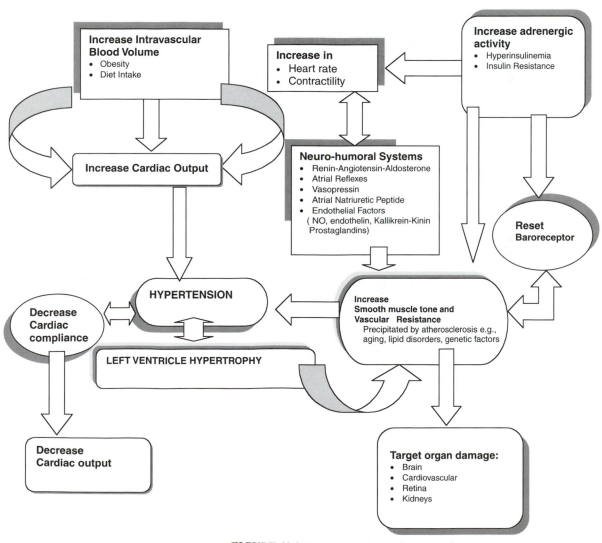

FIGURE 19.2. Pathophysiology of hypertension.

Blood Pressure (BP) = Cardiac Output (CO) × Total Peripheral Resistance (TPR), or Systemic Vascular Resistance (SVR)

These variables change depending on age and other comorbid events. They also vary with the stage or severity of hypertension. Early hypertension is characterized by high cardiac output produced by increased heart rate and stroke volume that is part of a more general activation of the sympathetic nervous system. Total peripheral resistance may be normal or slightly increased.[8] In a meta-analysis comparison of normotensive and essential hypertensive subjects, Fagard et al showed that cardiac output was not elevated in the hypertensives, except in young patients with mild blood pressure elevation.[9] The high cardiac output in the adolescent hypertensive is due to a high level of adrenergic activity. There are two factors that result in high cardiac output hypertension: peripheral factors (increased tissue demands or hypervolemia) and cardiac stimulation factors (adrenergic hyperactivity or hypokalemia combined with hypercalcemia). Cardiac output in the chronic established phase of hypertension is reduced to normal or below by reduced ventricular compliance, along with elevated systemic vascular resistance due to arteriolar narrowing.[10]

The obese person, with or without hypertension, has an increase in cardiac output, supported by a rise in stroke volume with no change in heart rate in response to elevated metabolic requirements. The essential hypertensive, nonobese patient has a normal cardiac output with high total peripheral resistance and a contracted intravascular volume. The obese, hypertensive patient has elevations in both cardiac output and total peripheral resistance.[11] These findings result in an extensive rise in left ventricular stroke work which enhances the cardiac risk especially for congestive heart failure.[12]

Because of the previously described hemodynamic characteristics and other contributing factors to support the disease hypertension, the physician must not only individualize the antihypertensive drug therapy, but also individualize nonpharmacologic approaches as well.

EPIDEMIOLOGIC EVIDENCE LINKING LOWER BLOOD PRESSURE AND PHYSICAL ACTIVITY

PHYSICAL ACTIVITY: GENERAL PRINCIPLES

Regular physical activity has a protective effect against cardiovascular disease and all-cause mortality.[13] Physical activity, also, increases longevity.[14] On the contrary, physical inactivity increases the relative risk of developing coronary artery disease to as high as that of hypertension, hypercholesterolemia, and smoking.[15]

PHYSICAL ACTIVITY: IN HYPERTENSION

HYPERTENSION AND LESS PHYSICAL ACTIVITY

Physical inactivity is an independent risk factor for hypertension, regardless of age, body mass index, and fasting plasma insulin levels.[7,16,17] Blood pressure is inversely related to the level of habitual physical activity.[18] In a study of 6039 healthy normotensive men and women followed for 1 to 12 years, those individuals with low levels of physical fitness at the initial examination had a 1.52 greater relative risk of developing hypertension than did those with high levels of activity. Conversely, interventions that included exercise can lower the risk for developing hypertension by 50%.[7]

MORE ACTIVITY, LESS HYPERTENSION

There are associations between physical activity, physical fitness, and blood pressure levels among children and adolescents, which suggests that an early start of the physical activity in childhood may reduce the risk of future hypertension.[19] A review of cross-sectional studies in children, evaluating physical fitness, physical activity and blood pressure, as well as longitudinal dynamic training studies in young adults below the age of 30, indicate that blood pressure is inversely related to leisure time physical activity.[20–22] Young men up to 40 years of age who engaged in regular physical activity had a 30% lower chance of developing hypertension than more sedentary individuals.[17] These findings are useful for preventive medicine. Primary prevention by lifestyle modifications including an increase in physical activity provides an attractive opportunity to interrupt and prevent the high cost of treating hypertension and its complications.

COMBINED EFFECT OF PHYSICAL INACTIVITY AND OTHER FACTORS: WEIGHT GAIN

The prospective studies by Paffenbarger et al studied patterns of physical activity and other characteristics that might deter hypertension or delay all-cause mortality among 5463 University of Pennsylvania alumni and 14,998 Harvard male alumni.[23] The data revealed that an energy expenditure of less than 500 kcal per week, high body mass index, weight gain since college, and parental hypertension were independent risk factors for hypertension. Moderately vigorous exercise > 4.5 METs per day), such as swimming, tennis, squash, jogging, or running, was associated with a 23% lower risk of death and lower blood pressure. Thus, blood pressure control may require both exercise and dietary regimens to maintain a balanced energy intake and output.[23]

DYNAMIC OR AEROBIC EXERCISE AND THE BLOOD PRESSURE RESPONSE

ACUTE DYNAMIC EXERCISE AND THE BLOOD PRESSURE RESPONSE

Blood pressure rises during dynamic or aerobic exercise (e.g., running and cycling), and the rate of rise is related to intensity and level of training. Systolic blood pressure starts to rise at the beginning of exercise, continues rising in a linear relationship with higher workload, and reaches the peak at the end of the exercise or maximal workload. In a retrospective study of 7863 male and 2406 female apparently healthy subjects, Daida et al reported that maximal blood pressure was 210 mmHg for the ages of 20 to 29 years and increased to 234 mmHg for ages of 70 to 79 years in men. Men had higher maximal blood pressure than women at the same age by 20 to 30 mmHg.[24] The increase in systolic blood pressure of 50 to 70 mmHg at peak exercise shows no significant difference between treadmill and bicycle exercise.[25,26] The exercise-induced increase of systolic blood pressure in borderline or definite hypertensive persons, in whom target organ damage is limited to World Health Organization (WHO) stages I or II, is roughly parallel to the changes in normotensive persons. The maximal blood pressure at peak exercise in hypertensive subjects is higher than it is in normotensive subjects due to the higher starting levels, in both treadmill or bicycle exercise. These findings suggest that blood pressure is reset in hypertensive subjects and maintained at higher levels throughout the spectrum of activity from rest-to-peak exercise than it would be in normotensives.[27] The differences in blood pressure between normotensive and hypertensive individuals are related to systemic vascular resistance because there are no differences in cardiac output, and those who have the highest blood pressure at rest have the highest vascular resistance during exercise.[28]

The blood pressure measurement and types of exercise cause different changes in diastolic blood pressure during exercise. During treadmill exercise, diastolic blood pressure slightly decreases 4 to 8 mmHg or no change occurs. Diastolic blood pressure tends to increase ranging from 12 to 50 mmHg during bicycle exercise.[25] This is related to greater resistance to the exercising skeletal muscle than is encountered with running. During a step exercise, using intraarterial blood pressure measurement, systolic blood pressure increases 47 to 64 mmHg and diastolic blood pressure increases 32 to 36 mmHg.[29]

PREDICTION OF HYPERTENSION AND CARDIOVASCULAR EVENTS AND MORTALITY BY EXERCISE TESTING

Several prospective studies suggest that an excessive or an exaggerated increase in blood pressure during an exercise test in normotensive healthy individuals may be a marker of future sustained hypertension. The cause of the exaggerated blood pressure response may be due to a failure to reduce total peripheral resistance adequately during exercise, as a result of initial structural vascular change.[28] The Framingham Offspring Study showed that an exaggerated response to exercise (systolic blood pressure ≥ 210 mmHg in men and ≥ 190 mmHg in women) increased the risk of hypertension fourfold.[30] But in the CARDIA study, the risk was increased only 1.51-fold in white subjects and 1.61-fold in black subjects.[31] The difference may be due to subject age in the two studies. The Framingham subjects were mainly at mid-life, which may suggest that an exaggerated response is higher at middle age than it is in young adulthood.[29,30] Both normotensive[31] and borderline hypertensive[32,33] subjects with elevated exercise blood pressure have a higher mean 24-h blood pressure than do subjects with normal exercise blood pressure. After 1 year of aerobic exercise, hypertensive patients with an exaggerated blood pressure response did not have a significant change in systolic and diastolic blood pressure during submaximal exercise.[34] The association between the excessively elevated systolic blood pressure and risk of cardiovascular event rates and mortality is uncertain due to discrepancies in standardized and accurate measurements of maximal blood pressure and the different initial workload. These data are very important in the hypertensive subject who wants to continue strenuous exercise, since the repetitive blood pressure peaks triggered by physical activity may impact chronic end-organ damage or cardiovascular events. This however is teleological and not proven. No convincing evidence at present indicates that the blood pressure level during steady-state endurance exercise can be predicted by the maximal blood pressure attained during a short-lasting incremental effort in young borderline hypertensive subjects.[35]

CHRONIC EFFECT OF EXERCISE ON HYPERTENSION

Exercise training lowers both systolic and diastolic blood pressure approximately 5 to 10 mmHg in mild-to-moderate essential hypertension and probably in more severe controlled hypertension as well.[36] A meta-analysis by Fagard of 36 controlled intervention studies reported that the average net hypotensive effect of exercise was a reduction of 3 mmHg systolic and 3 mmHg diastolic pressure (3/3 mmHg) in normotensive subjects, 6/7 mmHg in borderline hypertensive subjects, and 10/8 mmHg in hypertensive patients.[37] Most of these exercise intervention studies in hypertensive patients are limited by sample sizes. The reports from other meta-analyses also demonstrate that aerobic exercise training reduces resting systolic and diastolic blood pressure (Table 19.1).[37–42] The randomized trials tend to have smaller reductions in blood pressure than nonrandomized studies. The efficacy of exercise in reducing blood pressure is multifactorial and related to genetic and environmental factors. The minimal available data did not show any effect of gender, but Asians and Pacific Islanders may be more responsive than Caucasians.[43] A very well-designed study by Nelson et al studied patients with untreated hypertension in a 3-phase crossover design: a continuation of sedentary habits, and 2 levels of graded exercise on a bicycle ergometer.[44] The most active training program of 45 min per day for 4 weeks had the highest reduction in blood pressure of 16/11 mmHg, independent of changes in body weight or sodium secretion.[44] In a randomized controlled study by Jessup et al, 16 weeks of aerobic training showed lowered mean 24-h ambulatory systolic blood pressure by 7.9 mmHg and diastolic blood pressure by 3.6 mmHg in healthy older adults as well as an increase in V_{O_2} max.[45] Age is not a limiting factor since the effect of exercise training on low-

TABLE 19.1.   THE LOWERING BLOOD PRESSURE EFFECT OF EXERCISE (META-ANALYSIS STUDIES)

Author	Characteristics	Numbers of Studies	Control Group Resting Blood Pressure mmHg		Exercise Group Resting Blood Pressure mmHg	
			SBP	DBP	SBP	DBP
Fagard, 1993	Age 16–72 years old Mostly men 4–68 weeks training WHO classification 27 Normotensive groups 7 Borderline groups 7 Hypertensive groups Endurance training	36 publications 48 experimental groups	−5.3	−4.8	Normotensive: −3.2 Borderline: −6.2 Hypertensive: −9.9	Normotensive: −3.1 Borderline: −6.8 Hypertensive: −7.6
Kelly, 1994	Age 29–72 years old Hypertensive (mild-to-moderate) 44% had one or more patients using antihypertensive drugs Mostly men (40–100%) 10–37 weeks training, 3–4 days/week Vo_2 max 50–77% 30–65 min per session Type: walking, jogging, cycling	30 studies 9 randomized control studies 39 exercise groups 12 control groups	−3 ± 4	−3 ± 4	−7 ± 5	−6 ± 2
Hagberg, 1995	Age 15–70 years old Normotensive vs. hypertensive Mostly men 4–52 weeks duration of study Endurance training	47 studies Average blood pressure > 140	NA	NA	−10.8 (−19 in a small subset, women subjects)	−8.2 (−14 in a small subset, women subjects)
Halbert, 1997	Age 20–87 years old Mostly men Combine aerobic programs Vo_2 max 30–87% Hypertensive and normotensive 4–52 weeks duration of study Mostly low quality control of selection bias	29 studies 1533 subjects 2 resistance trials 1 combined trial	NA	NA	−4.7	−3.1
Kelly, 1997	Age 20–72 years old Normotensive and borderline or stage 1 hypertensive Mostly men Dynamic resistance exercise 8–26 wks training, 1–3 sets of 5–25 Reps and rest 15–216 seconds, 3 days/week Nautilus, Universal, free weights	259 subjects 9 exercise groups 9 control groups Only 3 studies in Hypertensive patients	NA	NA	−4.55 ± 5.69 by calculated Δ3[a]	−3.72 ± 3.46 by calculated Δ3[a]

[a] Δ3 or treatment effect = difference in change of blood pressure before and after training between control groups and exercise groups.

SBP, systolic blood pressure; DBP, diastolic blood pressure, WHO, World Health Organization.

Adapted with permission from Manolio TA, Burke GL, Savage PJ, et al: Exercise blood pressure response and 5-year risk of elevated blood pressure in a cohort of young adults: The CARDIA study. *Am J Hypertens* 7:234–241, 1994; Fragola PV, Romitelli S, Moretti A, et al: Precursors of established hypertension in borderline hypertensives. A two-year follow-up. *Int J Cardiol* 39:113–119, 1993; Polonia J, Martins L, Bravo-Faria A, et al: Higher left ventricle mass in normotensives with exaggerated blood pressure response to exercise associated with higher ambulatory blood pressure load and sympathetic activity. *Eur Heart J* 13:S30–S36, 1992; Attina DA, Giuliano G, Arcangeli G, et al: Effects of one year of physical training on borderline hypertension: An evaluation by bicycle ergometer exercise testing. *J Cardiovasc Pharmacol* 8(Suppl 5):S145–S147, 1986; Palatini P: Exaggerated blood pressure response to exercise: Pathophysiologic mechanisms and clinical relevance. *J Sports Med Phys Fitness* 38:1–9, 1998; Kokkinos PF, Narayan P, Colleran JA, et al: Effects of regular exercise on blood pressure and left ventricular hypertrophy in African-American men with severe hypertension. *N Engl J Med* 333:1462–1467, 1995.

ering blood pressure also occurs in the elderly.[45,46,47,136]

BENEFIT OF LOWERING BLOOD PRESSURE WITH EXERCISE TRAINING

Although the blood pressure reduction from exercise is small, it may have significant effects on the incidence of stroke and coronary heart diseases. Antihypertensive medications can reduce diastolic blood pressure by 5 to 6 mmHg and death rate from stroke by 42% and from coronary heart diseases by 14%.[48] The risk of cardiovascular events is reduced in hypertensive subjects performing physical activity at low levels of intensity. There is a greater effect on blood pressure reduction with moderate exercise and protection against coronary disease, but this benefit is lost in subjects performing vigorous sports.[49,50] Low intensity exercise can decrease the blood pressure response to stress, blunt daytime blood pressure peaks and reduce variability and, thus, attenuate the response of the blood pressure to stressful situations, an independent contribution to subsequent target organ damage.

Acute and chronic aerobic exercise can improve cardiac function. Pescatello et al reported that postexercise hypotension after an acute bout of dynamic exercise was associated with a reduced 24-h average blood pressure and myocardial wall stress, resulting in a decrease in left ventricular mass.[51] Baglivo et al reported that endurance training 3 days per week can reduce blood pressure and left ventricular mass.[52] A study of black men with severe hypertension indicated that, after 16 weeks of regular aerobic exercise, blood pressure was lower, left ventricular wall thickness was reduced,[36] and substantial reductions in the doses of medication were achieved.

Endurance training in individuals on antihypertensive medications can lower their blood pressure significantly and may eliminate or reduce the need for antihypertensive medications.[53–55] It may help inhibit increases in blood pressure associated with normal aging.

EFFECT OF TRAINING ON EXERCISE TOLERANCE AND MAXIMAL BLOOD PRESSURE DURING EXERCISE

The exercise tolerance or capacity in hypertensive individuals is reduced by 30% compared with age-matched controls.[56,57] This can be reversed by exercise training.[45,58] Unlike the resting blood pressure, the maximal blood pressure during exercise is not reduced, but in fact is increased parallel to exercise tolerance and higher fitness levels in the individuals. Tanaka et al demonstrated that maximal systolic blood pressure and maximal oxygen uptake are higher in endurance-trained subjects (225 vs. 204 mmHg) during submaximal and maximal exercise.[58] The results confirmed previous studies that showed an increase of maximal systolic blood pressure approximately 6 to 20 mmHg with higher exercise capacity after endurance training of approximately 20 weeks duration.[59,60] It appears that the increase in maximal systolic blood pressure in trained subjects and untrained subjects occurs via different hemodynamic mechanisms. In untrained subjects, an increased total peripheral resistance is the most likely mechanism for the rise in blood pressure with exercise. Trained subjects had increases in cardiac output and stroke volume to support the rise in systolic pressure. Hypertensive people have a shift of the cardiac function curve (stroke volume vs. mean wedge pressure) to the right in the absence of heart failure. The stroke volume drops after reaching a peak at submaximal workload because of diastolic dysfunction at a higher heart rate.[61] This effect is exaggerated in the patients with higher blood pressure who have lower stroke volume and higher pulmonary wedge pressure at rest, during exercise and at the peak of exercise.[62] In hypertensive people, the higher maximal blood pressure after training is probably due to an increase in cardiac output and improved left ventricular function.[58] The concept of endurance training improving exercise tolerance or capacity is widely accepted, however, the data on blood pressure response to exercise training is inconsistent.[63,64] Braun et al[64] demonstrated that the fitness level was a significant predictor of diastolic blood pressure response and that high fitness levels were associated with low diastolic pressure. The systolic blood pressure had the same trend and the rate of the systolic blood pressure rise was slower in the high fitness group than it was in the sedentary group.

EFFECT OF STATIC EXERCISE OR STRENGTH TRAINING ON HYPERTENSION

ACUTE STATIC EXERCISE AND THE BLOOD PRESSURE RESPONSE

Static or resistance exercise is designed to improve strength. The term *strength training* is generally used in clinical practice and refers to this type of exercise. It has both acute and chronic effects on cardiovascular hemodynamics, especially blood pressure. Acute static exercise increases both systolic and diastolic blood pressure in either normotensive or hypertensive subjects by reflex increases in cardiac output with minimal or no change in vascular resistance.[65,66] The effects of acute static exercise on blood pressure have been studied extensively in weightlifting subjects. MacDougall et al[67] recorded systolic and diastolic blood pressure and found that they increased rapidly to extremely high values during the concentric contraction phase for each lift and declined with the eccentric contraction. The greatest peak pressures occurred during the double-leg press where the mean value for the group was 320/250 mmHg, with pressures in one subject exceeding 480/350 mmHg. Peak pressures with the single-arm curl exercise reached a mean group value of 255/190 mmHg when repetitions were discontinued by fatigue or exhaustion. The mechanisms for the rise in pressure could be due to increased intrathoracic pressure from the Valsalva maneuver during heavy weightlifts, pressor reflexes originating from tendons stretching, and the mechanical compression of the arteries by the contracting muscles.[67,68] The intraabdominal pressure is simultaneously increased, and this is immediately transmitted to the cerebrospinal fluid through the intervertebral foramina; thus, the actual transmural pressure across cerebral vessels is reduced and protects the cerebral vessels from acute damage. Thus, weightlifters can tolerate great elevations of blood pressure without stroke during their lifetime.[68] Early recruitment of type II fibers activates sympathetic reflexes, which result in an increased heart rate and cardiac output with little or no effect on stroke volume and total peripheral resistance.[69]

The magnitude of the blood pressure response (maximal minus rest) is proportional to the intensity of muscle contraction, the size of muscle mass used in contraction, and the duration of exercise.[70] But the relation between blood pressure and the size of muscle mass is inconsistent. MacDougall et al recorded brachial artery pressure in 31 healthy males and found that weightlifting at the same relative intensity produced similar increases in blood pressure, regardless of individual differences in muscle size or strength.[71] The degree of voluntary effort is the major determinant of the blood pressure response, rather than the resistance mode or the type (concentric, eccentric, or isometric) of muscle action. Repetitive resistance exercise (e.g., a set of repetitions to failure in weightlifting) tends to produce greater pressure elevations than isolated, single maximal effort actions.[72]

The concern about acute change of cardiac function has been studied extensively as well. There are little or no changes in left ventricular function during handgrip maintained at 30 to 50% of maximum voluntary contraction.[73] Left ventricular function declines initially during the contraction phase, but then is restored by the Frank-Starling mechanism. In the relaxation phase, left ventricular function increases with the rapid fall in blood pressure.[66]

During heavy weightlifting with a Valsalva maneuver, the blood pressure response is extremely exaggerated but may be dramatically reduced when the exercise is performed with an open glottis or slow exhalation. Narloch and Brandstater[74] studied blood pressure responses in 10 males performing double-leg press sets at 85%

and 100% of maximum with closed glottis (i.e., Valsalva) and slow exhalation during concentric contraction. The mean blood pressure at 100% maximum with Valsalva was 311/284 mmHg compared to that of slow exhalation when the mean blood pressure was 198/175 mmHg. This breathing technique may help to prevent cardiovascular complications in hypertensive patients.

CAN RESISTANCE EXERCISE BE A MODALITY FOR THE TREATMENT OF HYPERTENSION?

PROS

Strength training is not a widely acceptable modality for the treatment of hypertension. Moderate strength training blunts the acute blood pressure response to static exercise and induces either no effect[75] or a modest fall[42,76,77] in resting blood pressure in both normotensive and hypertensive subjects. The emerging evidence from studies supports the beneficial effect of this exercise in different populations, but there are fewer studies of strength training than there are of dynamic exercise training in hypertensive subjects. For example, a controlled study in normotensive subjects who performed hand grip contractions at 30 to 50% of maximal voluntary contraction for 3 to 5 days per week for 5 to 8 weeks reduced resting systolic blood pressure 10 mmHg and diastolic blood pressure 15 mmHg.[76] Hurley et al observed no significant change in resting systolic blood pressure in normotensive subjects after 16 weeks of resistive strength training. Diastolic blood pressure was reduced by 5 mmHg but only when measured in the supine position.[77]

Strength training for 5 to 8 weeks reduced systolic blood pressure 16 to 42 mmHg and diastolic blood pressure 2 to 24 mmHg in hypertensive elderly patients, but no control group was included.[78] Free-weight training for 5 months reduced resting systolic blood pressure 4 mmHg in adolescent hypertensive subjects who had previously completed an aerobic training program.[79]

The combination of dynamic and resistance exercise such as circuit weight training can lower resting systolic and diastolic blood pressure 4.5 and 3.8 mmHg, respectively, in both normotensive and hypertensive subjects. Three studies in the meta-analysis by Kelly[42] (Table 19.1) were done in hypertensive subjects. However, the results are impressive and comparable in magnitude to the effects of aerobic exercise. Consequently, circuit weight training alone or combined with running and jogging can decrease blood pressure and is an acceptable mode for lowering blood pressure.

A controlled study of circuit weight training alone for 9 weeks in borderline hypertensive subjects showed a decrease in diastolic blood pressure of 5 mmHg, but systolic blood pressure did not change. Total lifted weight increased by 57%, along with 12 to 53% increase in strength.[80] Training was performed 3 times per week, doing 3 sets of 20 to 25 repetitions on a 10-station circuit using the large muscle groups, and at 40% of repetition maximum for intensity. The resistance was set between 40 and 50% of maximum capacity to avoid excessive increases in blood pressure. In hypertensive patients, exercise training should start with 1 set of 8 to 10 repetitions per specific exercise.[81]

These preliminary studies demonstrate that supervised strength training programs, particularly circuit training, have acceptable hemodynamic responses and safe clinical limits and can reduce blood pressure in hypertensive patients despite the inherent potential to acutely elevate blood pressure. It is possible that antihypertensive medications may blunt the acute rise in blood pressure during a single bout of exercise. For example, Lowenthal et al[82–84] reported that antihypertensive medications, which lower resting blood pressure, can also blunt the rise in blood pressure during handgrip. In studies using prazosin, verapamil, nifedipine, atenolol, and propranolol, the absolute increase in blood pressure with handgrip was the same as before treatment, but the peak exercise blood pressure was lower because of the lower resting blood pressure. Grossman et al have shown similar results with fosinopril.[85] Such results suggest that effective antihypertensive treatment reduces the concern that weight training will acutely produce an extreme hypertensive response in hypertensive subjects.

CONS

Hypertensive patients, most often, are told to refrain from strength training to avoid an acute increase in blood pressure, but there is no direct evidence that strength training is associated with increased morbidity or mortality. A study in genetic hypertensive rats with systolic blood pressure at least 200 mmHg, who performed isometric hanging exercises for 16 weeks, did not have more cerebrovascular lesions or higher resting pressures.[86] There are rare case reports of weightlifting leading to aortic dissection in hypertensive and normotensive patients who had cystic degenerative disease.[87] Weightlifting also can lead to life-threatening cardiac arrhythmias or syncope due to rapid hypotensive episodes with or without bradycardia.[88]

There is also concern that static exercise can result in concentric myocardial hypertrophy without changes in left ventricular function. The magnitude of physiological hypertrophy is similar in normotensive and mildly hypertensive subjects[54,89,90] suggesting that the myocardial changes are not magnified by concomitant hypertension. However, an abrupt elevation of blood pressure induced by weightlifting can increase myocardial oxygen consumption, which may jeopardize ischemic myocardial tissue. Therefore, heavy-resistance training requiring high voluntary effort is generally not recommended in hypertensive patients. Furthermore, even moderate weight training at 40 to 60% of the 1 repetition maximum should be postponed until resting blood pressure is under control.

POSTEXERCISE HYPOTENSIVE EFFECT

At the end of a single bout of dynamic exercise in both normotensive and hypertensive individuals, resting blood pressure is often lower or normalized. This effect is referred to as "postexercise

hypotension." This effect has been documented in experimental investigations done in both human and spontaneously hypertensive rats.[91–97] It occurs in response to dynamic exercise (e.g., walking, running, cycling, and swimming) at intensities between 40 to 70% of maximal oxygen consumption, as well as after exercise to exhaustion. Strength training using an intensity of 70% of 1-repetition maximum can also cause this effect.[92] The exercise duration required to induce acute hypotension has varied from 3 to 60 min, yet it can occur even after a single bout of exercise in habitually sedentary subjects. Hypertensive individuals have greater acute reductions in systolic and diastolic blood pressure than normotensive individuals (18–20 vs. 8–10 and 7–9 vs. 3–5 mmHg, respectively).[93,94] Rueckert et al[95] demonstrated that the postexercise hypotension is biphasic. Initially, there is a drop in both total and regional vascular resistance, followed by a drop in cardiac output with total peripheral resistance at or above preexercise levels. Acute changes in postexercise heart rate and cardiac output, however, have been inconsistent and may be influenced by exercise intensity or the initial hemodynamic state of the subjects. Sustained decreases in limb (forearm and calf) or regional vascular and total peripheral resistance have been more consistent. These findings suggest that vasodilatation in skeletal muscle and other arterial beds may contribute to postexercise hypotension. Possible mechanisms include a reduction in sympathetic nerve discharge, vascular responsiveness to α-adrenergic-receptor-medicated stimulation, group III somatic afferent activation, altered baroreceptor reflex circulatory control, and activation of endogenous opioid and serotoninergic systems.[93]

The postexercise hypotensive response has sufficient magnitude to be considered clinically significant, even though its effect lasts only a few hours. The hypotensive effect disappears once subjects leave the test site and go about their normal activities.[95] This result confirms the previous controlled study by Somers et al, using the same moderate intensity dynamic exercise.[96] Overall, duration of this effect has varied from 1 to 13 h, but postexercise hypotension has been consistently documented for 2 to 3 h. Postexercise hypotension alone is unlikely to mediate the reduction in blood pressure that occurs with dynamic exercise training because of the small magnitude and brief duration of this effect. Nevertheless, this phenomenon may contribute to the beneficial effects of exercise on cardiovascular risk and it is possible that the cumulative effect of repetitive single bouts of exercise may contribute to the blood pressure reduction produced by "exercise training."[95]

TIME COURSE AND MECHANISMS OF THE ANTIHYPERTENSIVE ACTION OF EXERCISE

All of the studies of the mechanisms and time-course of the antihypertensive action of exercise have focused more on dynamic exercise than on static exercise because of consistent data on the hypotensive effect of dynamic exercise. Meredith et al examined the time-course of changes in hemodynamics in 10 normotensive individuals who performed 40 min of bicycle exercise at 60 to 70% of maximum work.[97] They found that a significant fall in blood pressure occurred at the third training bout or at the beginning of the second week, and no further reduction occurred beyond the fourth bout of exercise.[97] In most studies, blood pressure is reduced early (3 weeks to 3 months) after the initiation of moderate intensity-exercise training in both normotensive and hypertensive individuals, and no further reductions occur after 3 months.[98] The blood pressure lowering effect of exercise training is evident only as long as a regular endurance exercise training program is maintained[46,96] and blood pressure rises gradually toward the baseline for 1 to 2 weeks after cessation of exercise.

There are several hemodynamic changes of exercise training that might be associated with the antihypertensive effect of exercise. Whole blood and plasma volume expand, yet there is a de-creased heart rate and systemic vascular resistance after training, probably because of a simultaneous decrease in sympathetic activity. Grassi et al used direct recording of postganglionic muscle sympathetic nerve activity from the peroneal nerve to demonstrate that the blood pressure reduction induced by exercise was mediated by neural sympathetic mechanisms.[99] There is also a correlation between blood pressure and norepinephrine levels used as a marker of sympathetic activity.[100] In a small randomized controlled study, Urata et al demonstrated a progressive reduction of plasma norepinephrine levels during 10 weeks of bicycle exercise training in hypertensive subjects.[101] Since blood pressure decreased before a decrease in plasma norepinephrine levels in this study, it is likely that some factor other than sympathetic activity is responsible for the initial fall in blood pressure with exercise training. A fall of blood pressure before the decrease in plasma norepinephrine raises the question of some factors other than suppression of sympathetic activity, which must influence the initial fall of blood pressure. One of the possible factors is resetting of the operating point and a reduction in the gain of the arterial baroreceptor reflex accompanied by lower sympathetic nerve traffic.[102]

The other possible mechanisms include ameliorating of the hyperinsulinemic state, lowering plasma renin, increasing natriuretic hormones (atrial natriuretic peptides, endogenous ouabain-like substance), releasing vasodilatory mediators, increasing plasma prostaglandin E and s-taurine,[103] and reducing catecholamine biosynthesis by altering gene regulation for tyrosine hydroxylase activity.[103]

PROBLEMS WITH EPIDEMIOLOGY AND INTERVENTION STUDIES

The reported beneficial effects of physical activity on the development of hypertension and coronary heart disease have been based primarily on epidemiological studies. Studies that examine the effect of exercise on blood pressure have at least one major flaw, for example, lack of randomization and a valid control group, varying definitions for hypertension and levels of physical activity, blood pressure measurement methods, and the presence of cointerventions (i.e., diet, medications). In spite of these design problems, increased physical activity consistently is associated with, or produces, lower blood pressure. There is minimal definitive evidence to support the conclusion that exercise cannot lower blood pressure. For example, in a randomized controlled study, Blumenthal et al demonstrated that there was no difference in the blood pressure lowering effect between trained and untrained hypertensive individuals, and blood pressure decreased in all groups.[104] Blood pressure measurement can be inaccurate due to either "white coat" effect or technical errors. The "white coat" effect refers to the observation that some individuals have higher pressures in physicians' offices or when measured by physicians than at home or measured by non-physician personnel. The 24-h ambulatory blood pressure measurement (ABPM) is used mainly for ascertainment of the usual level of blood pressure (i.e., to circumvent the white coat effect), and may be more predictive of target organ damage than is an isolated resting measurement.[105,106] Unfortunately, only a few exercise studies have used APBM as reviewed by Fagard.[43] The results showed that exercise reduces the daytime diastolic blood pressure but only in individuals with higher baseline diastolic blood pressure. Similarly, the daytime systolic blood pressure did not decrease in subjects with baseline systolic blood pressure below 140 mmHg. The nighttime blood pressure also did not change except in one study that combined regular vigorous exercise with caloric intake restriction in hypertensive patients whose diastolic blood pressure was reduced by 5 mmHg.[107] These observations may be explained by low sympathetic activity during sleep and suggest that sympathetic withdrawal contributes to the antihypertensive effect of exercise training. Exercise training can lower resting blood pressure in habitually sedentary people, but there are several studies to support the notion that there is no

additional blood pressure lowering effect of exercise in already active people. For example, among expeditioners to Antarctica who were active in summer and sedentary in winter, a study of the physical training effect on blood pressure using ABPM showed that blood pressure was lower during the working day in winter (17/5 mmHg) than in the summer.[52] Ambulatory blood pressure measurement also demonstrated that the blood pressure in the fit state (average 136/81) is lower than in the unfit state (average 141/89).[108] Seals and Reiling reported a decrease in average daytime blood pressure from 142 to 135 mmHg after 12 months of training, but reported no change in ambulatory pressure after the first 6-month period when subjects had exercised at a lower intensity.[109]

The average daytime 24-h ambulatory blood pressure reflects the combined effect of mental and physical stress and is lower than that based on the random resting office blood pressure.[110] The variability recorded by ABPM may explain the inconsistency and smaller reduction in blood pressure compared to the resting blood pressure measurement. Systolic and diastolic load (the percentage of pressures > 140/90 mmHg during daytime hours and > 120/80 mmHg during sleep) may be more sensitive than average systolic and diastolic blood pressure for detection of 24-h ABPM changes with exercise training. Wallace et al found that there was no significant decrease in average blood pressure with exercise training even though systolic and diastolic load decreased 20 to 25% from 6 am to 10 pm.[111]

NONPHARMACOLOGIC APPROACHES TO BLOOD PRESSURE REDUCTION

The data from the randomized controlled trial, The Hypertension Detection and Follow-up Program (HDFP), indicated that pharmacologic management of hypertension reduces mortality in hypertensive patients.[112] The study also strongly supports suggestions that those with mild hypertension should have their cardiovascular risk assessed individually and should be treated with anti-hypertensive medications based on a composite of factors and not merely on blood pressure. Some patients with mild hypertension are at low risk to develop cardiovascular diseases and can be safely spared antihypertensive medications. Thus, the benefit from treatment of mild hypertension with antihypertensive medications is debatable. Hoes et al suggested that treatment has no benefit when the risk of all-cause death is 3% over 5 years and may increase mortality when the risk is lower.[113,114] Hypertensive patients are likely to have additional atherosclerotic risk factors.[115] The Framingham study reported that the association of hypercholesterolemia, glucose intolerance, cigarette smoking, and systolic hypertension has additive effects on the incidence of coronary heart disease at different levels of blood pressure.[116] Antihypertensive medications are more effective in lowering the blood pressure (-15 mmHg) than nonpharmacologic treatments (-5 mmHg).[117] The definitive outcome of the treatment, however, of mild-to-moderate hypertension has not been fully satisfied since the coronary mortality and morbidity reduction with treatment is not the same degree as seen in cerebrovascular disease. Hypertensive patients may not lower their risk to that of persons with normal blood pressure even if adequately treated. One of the possible reasons is that the atherosclerotic process is irreversible. Furthermore, some antihypertensive medications may have negative effects on other risk factors for atherosclerosis, such as the increase in plasma lipids with diuretics and propranolol. Antihypertensive medications also have medical and financial side effects.[6] The Multiple Risk Factor Intervention Trial reported that the cardiovascular disease mortality was not greatly affected even though systolic blood pressure was reduced by 20% unless the cholesterol level was reduced concomitantly.[118]

The prevention of coronary heart disease among hypertensive patients requires a combination of nonpharmacologic treatments with the aim to decrease atherosclerosis. These lifestyle interventions include weight loss, physical exercise, lowering of dietary salt intake, reduction of stress, and lowering of alcohol consumption. Currently, aerobic exercise and diet-induced weight loss have emerged as the most effective and physiologically desirable approaches.[119] A multicenter randomized clinical trial, known as the Trial of Hypertension Prevention study (TOHP), indicated that an average weight loss of 5 to 6 kg, produced by mild-to-moderate physical exercise of 3 to 6 METs for 2 to 3 days a week and a reduction in caloric intake, reduced both systolic and diastolic blood pressure an average of 3.5 mmHg in both men and women.[120] A randomized trial by Gordon et al indicates that the antihypertensive effects of exercise training and diet-induced weight loss are not additive and both have comparable effects on blood pressure reduction of 10 to 12 mmHg.[121]

The role of exercise in treating high blood pressure is well established. Exercise not only reduces the blood pressure level, but also low-density lipoprotein cholesterol, insulin resistance, and glucose intolerance, and often is associated with a reduction in body weight.[122,123] All currently available guidelines (i.e., JNC-VI and the World Hypertension League) recommend exercise as an adjunctive nonpharmacologic intervention in mild hypertension and antihypertensive medications in more severe hypertension. The guidelines from JNC-VI for initiating drug therapy should be followed once nonpharmacologic approaches have been adhered to for 6 to 12 months in low-risk patients. Physicians should give a detailed exercise prescription and provide regular encouragement and follow-up to improve compliance and motivation.

HOW TO PRESCRIBE EXERCISE TRAINING TO PATIENTS

PATIENT SELECTION AND EVALUATION

All controlled hypertensive patients should participate in exercise training (Table 19.2). Exercise can be used with other nonpharmacologic interventions and without antihypertensive medications in uncomplicated mild-to-moderate hyper-

TABLE 19.2. INDIVIDUALIZED EXERCISE PRESCRIPTIONS

	Adolescent Hypertension	Obese Hypertension	Diabetic Hypertension	Adult Onset Hypertension	Elderly Hypertension
Patient Selection and Evaluation	• Borderline-to-mild hypertension • Antihypertensive medication to reduce baseline resting pressure • Switch to an endurance sport, heavy-resistance sports are contraindicated	• Borderline-to-mild hypertension • Look for associated diseases: DM, ischemic heart disease, peripheral vascular disease • Weight loss is the first priority • Walking program as tolerated to lose some weight before testing	• Borderline-to-mild hypertension • Exclude silent MI • Look for associated diseases; lipid disorders, retinopathy, peripheral neuropathy, peripheral vascular disease, renal insufficiency, depressed LV function • Control blood glucose • Medication and diet modification to avoid hypoglycemia from exercise	• Borderline-to-mild hypertension • Adjuvant therapy in postmenopausal women (e.g., hormone replacement)	• Borderline-to-mild hypertension • Fall precautions • Check for the musculoskeletal diseases: osteoarthritis, osteoporosis, herniated disc, fractures • Associated and underlying diseases, especially neurological, cardovascular diseases
Exercise Testing and Monitoring	• GXT with Bruce protocol to gauge the magnitude of the BP response during exercise and rate of recovery	• GXT with a modified Naughton protocol	• GXT with a modified Naughton protocol • Rule out asymptomatic ischemic heart disease • Radionuclear imaging if needed	• No risk factors, begin with walking exercise program without a maximal GXT • GXT with a modified Naughton protocol	• GXT with a modified Naughton protocol
Type (Mode)	• Aerobic activities: jogging, biking, swimming • Circuit weight training	• Aerobic, low-impact activities; walking until weight has dropped by 10–15% then biking, step-climbing, swimming, treadmill walking	• Aerobic, low-impact activities; walking, biking, swimming	• Aerobic activities: jogging, if over 40 years old should have low-impact exercise: walking, swimming, biking	• Aerobic, low-impact activities; walking, biking, swimming, T'ai chi
Frequency	• 6–7 Days per week	• 5 Days per week (minimum)	• 5 Days per week (minimum)	• 5 Days per week (minimum)	• 3–5 Days per week (minimum)
Intensity	• Up to 85% of maximum HRR or 85% of maximal heart rate	• Start at 50–60% maximum HRR and slowly increase to 70%: within 6 weeks, 85% HRR or from 50–90% of maximal heart rate	• Start at 50–60 maximum HRR and slowly increase to 70%: within 6 weeks, 85% HRR or from 50–90% of maximal heart rate	• Start at 50–60% maximum HRR and slowly increase to 70%: within 6 weeks, 85% HRR or from 50–90% of maximal heart rate	• Start at 50–60% maximum HRR and slowly increase to 70%: within 6 weeks, 85% HRR or from 50–90% of maximal heart rate
Duration	• 45–60 min per day	• 20–30 min per day of continuous activity for first 3 weeks then • 30–45 min per day for next 4–6 weeks and 60 min per day as maintenance	• 20–30 min per day of continuous activity for first 3 weeks then • 30–45 min per day for next 4–6 weeks and 60 min per day as maintenance	• 20–30 min per day of continuous activity for first 3 weeks then • 30–45 min per day for next 4–6 weeks and 60 min per day as maintenance	• Duration depends on intensity of the activity: lower intensity for longer periods, can start with 20–30 min per day of continuous activity for first 3 weeks then • 30–45 min per day for next 4–6 weeks and 60 min per day as maintenance

DM, diabetes mellitus; MI, myocardial infarction; LV, left ventricular; GXT, graded exercise test; HRR, heart resting rate.

tensive patients. Patients with cardiovascular complications (i.e., target organ damage, diabetes, or those who are elderly) need antihypertensive medications.[6] Moderately obese patients need aggressive weight reduction as a top priority combined with a walking program before more vigorous and intense exercise training. The patients with blood pressure that is higher than 180/105 should add endurance exercise training to their treatment regimen only after blood pressure is controlled by antihypertensive medications. The exercise may reduce blood pressure further, decrease antihypertensive medications, and attenuate the risk for premature mortality.

Some patients with end-stage renal disease can benefit from exercise training. Boyce et al found improvement in functional aerobic capacity, muscular strength, and a reduction in blood pressure of up to 20 mmHg after 4 months of exercise training in patients with predialysis chronic renal failure. Cessation of exercise resulted in detraining effects reflected by an increase in blood pressure within 2 months.[124] Similar results were seen in hemodialysis patients with chronic renal failure but to a greater extent than in individuals with essential hypertension. Exercise substantially reduced the required doses of antihypertensive medications.[125,126] Patients with unilateral renovascular disease with controlled blood pressure can exercise without further damage to the kidneys. Using exercise renography, exercise-mediated functional disturbances characterized by a low filtration fraction exist in hypertensive patients. Hypertensive patients with normal exercise renograms did not have the exercise-mediated abnormal clearance pattern. Similar results were observed in the control population of essential hypertensive patients, 65% of whom developed a functional disturbance.[127] Finally, Jessup et al have shown that elderly healthy persons can endure 4 months of exercise training with no decrement in renal function.[128]

Initially, the pretraining assessment requires a focused clinical evaluation. The history should address significant coronary artery disease, syncope or near-syncope (due to hypertrophic car-

diomyopathy, valvular heart disease, or arrhythmias), premature coronary artery disease or sudden death in family members, or conditions that might limit exercise capability. The physical examination should emphasize the cardiovascular and musculoskeletal systems. A resting electrocardiogram (ECG) is recommended for all hypertensive patients, whether or not they want to start an exercise program.

EXERCISE TESTING AND MONITORING

The role of exercise testing is not settled. Most patients require only a good clinical evaluation. The potential complication of exercise—sudden cardiac death—is the most worrisome, but the absolute risk is very minimal. The most common cause of sudden cardiac death during exercise in young persons aged ≤ 30 is hypertrophic cardiomyopathy, whereas the most common cause in older persons is coronary artery disease. Both diseases can be associated with hypertension and can be detected by careful history taking, physical examination, resting ECG, and an echocardiogram.

The American College of Sports Medicine recommends that exercise testing should not be used as a screening test to identify those at high risk for developing hypertension as a result of an exaggerated exercise blood pressure response. But information from available exercise tests does provide some indication of risk stratification for the patient with the blood pressure response above the 85th percentile and the necessity for appropriate lifestyle modification to decrease the risk of hypertension.[129]

A graded exercise stress test (GXT) can be performed to gauge the magnitude of the blood pressure response during exercise and rate of recovery, as well as the provocation of arrhythmias during the GXT and recovery. It is often recommended for adults over the age of 40 years who plan to begin an exercise training program. Most patients with mild hypertension and no other risk factors for cardiovascular diseases can start a walking exercise program without a maximal GXT.

Moderate-to-severe hypertensive patients with evidence of left ventricular hypertrophy from an ECG should be thoroughly evaluated with a GXT and probably myocardial radionuclide imaging.[129] Diabetic hypertensive patients should be evaluated carefully by exercise testing because of high incidence of silent myocardial infarction.

A treadmill GXT should use protocols that maintain a constant walking speed for accurate blood pressure measurement during the exercise.[130] A young healthy person would tolerate a standard Bruce protocol, but in the elderly or sedentary persons with or without comorbidities a modified Naughton protocol is preferred.[129] Submaximal exercise testing to monitor blood pressure and heart rate response may be used for exercise training prescriptions in patients who are at low risk for cardiovascular disease.

TYPE

AEROBIC: WALK, RUN, OR SWIM

Endurance exercise is the preferred exercise modality in hypertensive patients. Current recommendations suggest the modes of training. The blood pressure response to dynamic (aerobic) exercise varies from sport to sport. Most studies have employed walking, running, or cycling as activity modes that have been incorporated within daily lifestyles. Walking or running do not cause a sustained increase in blood pressure and possibly are the most suitable endurance exercises for hypertensive patients. Some showed higher blood pressure levels with swimming than with running at comparable heart rates but had smaller cardiopulmonary effects. A study by Tanaka et al demonstrated that moderate swimming training with 30- to 45-min-sessions, 3 days per week, can lower systolic, but not diastolic, blood pressure at rest. These changes were independent of the alterations in body weight and dietary intake. Swimming can be an alternative exercise in patients with obesity, exercise-induced asthma, or orthopedic injuries.[131] Vigorous sprints and rowing are activities requiring rhythmical muscle contractions performed with very high muscular force and are unsuitable for hypertensive patients. Downhill skiing can also elevate blood pressure. Mountain sports (e.g., cross-country skiing and climbing) may increase the risk of hypoxia-related activation of the sympathetic nervous system from a decreased partial pressure of oxygen as well as from cold, which may exaggerate an elevated blood pressure response.[132]

T'AI CHI

T'ai chi, a 1000-year-old martial art, is a low-impact exercise that combines low velocity rhythmic movements with changes in direction, plane, and center of balance. It is simple and does not require any special equipment such as a gym or changing shoes or clothing, and it is well tolerated by sedentary older persons. A randomized trial by Young et al reported that a program of T'ai chi reduced blood pressure to an extent similar to that produced by moderate intensity aerobic exercise; however, there was no change in maximal aerobic capacity with T'ai chi and fewer other changes in measures of physical activity. T'ai chi exercise, in this study, consisted of 13 movements, performed twice per week in 1-h group classes led by a certified instructor.[133] Even though T'ai chi is well known and accepted widely in the Eastern countries, there is no large-scale randomized controlled clinical trial documenting its cardiovascular effects.

INTENSITY AND FREQUENCY

LOW-TO-MODERATE INTENSITIES ARE ENOUGH

There are no specific guidelines in exercise management of hypertension regarding intensity and frequency. Nevertheless, there is insufficient evidence to justify the role of high intensity exercise ($> 70\%$ Vo_2 max) in lowering blood pressure.[41] Low-to-moderate intensity endurance exercise training at 40 to 70% Vo_2 max may be as, or more, efficacious than high intensity in lowering blood pressure in hypertensive subjects.[133] Based on the intervention studies and a consensus statement by the World Hypertension League, hypertensive patients should exercise at an intensity of 50 to 85% maximum oxygen uptake for 20 to 60 min, 3 to 5 days per week. Alternatively, the exercise heart rate can be used and should be in the range of 50 to 70% of its predicted maximum (predicted maximum heart rate = 220 − age in years). The lower intensity requires longer duration. Exercise at 60 to 70% of maximum work capacity, 3 days per week of 45 min per session for 1 month, has the same hypotensive effect as exercise at 47% maximum work capacity, 3 days per week of 60 min, for 2.5 months.[134–137] Low intensity (about 50% maximum oxygen consumption) is also more beneficial than the high level in the response to stressful stimulus. The level of exercise must be enough to accomplish a conditioning effect, usually achieved by 3 or 4 periods of exercise each week at 60 to 70% of maximal heart rate for 30 to 45 min.

DURATION

Exercise training programs longer than 10 weeks appear to reduce systolic blood pressure by 1 to 2 mmHg and diastolic blood pressure by 2 to 2.5 mmHg more than shorter duration programs.[40] No further blood pressure reduction after 3 months of training is generally seen with rare exceptions.[87,137] The duration of exercise should be at least 1 to 3 months to reach the stable stage and training should be maintained indefinitely because the hypotensive effect of exercise training persists only as long as a regular endurance exercise training program is maintained.

DRUG-TREATMENT OF HYPERTENSION FOR THE ACTIVE PERSON AND THE ATHLETE

OVERVIEW FOR CLINICIANS WHO ADDRESS DRUG TREATMENT IN THEIR ACTIVE PATIENTS

There is no "best" medication for the active hypertensive person. The physician should individualize the choice of medication based on lone hypertension or hypertension in association with

which disease the patient has, for example, stable coronary artery disease, hyperlipidemia, left ventricular hypertrophy, diabetes mellitus, prostatism, chronic obstructive lung disease, or chronic renal failure.

The lone active hypertensive patient regardless of age could take a thiazide diuretic, 12.5 to 25 mg daily, with potassium supplementation. Diuretics are effective and inexpensive. They are useful in postmenopausal women with hypertension and osteoporosis because thiazides decrease urinary calcium loss. All of the other classes of antihypertensive drugs are effective in controlling blood pressure, yet they are expensive and can be used as monotherapy for the lone, active hypertensive patient. Patients who need to take a beta blocker can gradually train through the blunted cardiovascular response to aerobic exercise. Beta blockers are effective in controlling blood pressure and are inexpensive.

Patients with other diseases associated with hypertension would need more specific treatment. For example, in coronary artery disease, the hypertensive patient would benefit from either a calcium entry blocker or a beta blocker; a diabetic patient would need an ACE inhibitor (ACE-I); a patient who coughs while on an ACE-I yet who has left ventricular hypertrophy should take an angiotensin II receptor blocker; an active elderly hypertensive male with prostatism would achieve blood pressure control and relief from outlet obstruction with a peripheral alpha blocker (i.e., terazosin, doxazosin). If these drugs cause the active person to be dizzy and develop orthostatic hypotension, the alpha-blocker tamsulosin can be given with any other low-dosage antihypertensive drug. Specific issues in each class of antihypertensives for the active patient follows.

INTERACTIONS BETWEEN EXERCISE AND ANTIHYPERTENSIVE MEDICATIONS IN DYSLIPIDEMIAS

Some antihypertensive medications can alter the lipid profile. Diuretics and beta blockers, especially the nonselective beta blockers, can increase triglycerides and very-low-density lipoprotein cholesterol by 10 to 30% and reduce high-density lipoprotein cholesterol by 6 to 25%. Peripheral α-1 inhibitors and calcium channel blockers have a positive effect on lipid profiles. Angiotensin-converting enzyme inhibitors and angiotensin II receptor blockers seem to have a neutral effect.[138] A double-blind randomized control study by Keleman comparing diltiazem, propranolol, and a placebo in middle-aged men receiving circuit weight and endurance training 3 times a week for 10 weeks showed that the baseline blood pressure fell in all groups including the placebo group after training. Exercise alone lowered plasma total and low-density lipoprotein cholesterol concentrations in all groups, but high-density lipoprotein increased only in the placebo and diltiazem groups. High-density lipoprotein concentration in the propranolol group was decreased despite regular exercise. The authors concluded beta blockers interfere with the beneficial effects of exercise on serum lipids whereas calcium channel blockers may enhance the exercise effect.[55]

EFFECTS OF ANTIHYPERTENSIVE THERAPY ON EXERCISE PERFORMANCE

The goals of hypertensive treatment in athletes and other physically active people is to control the blood pressure without interfering with actual exercise performance or performance surrogates such as the increases in heart rate, stroke index, and cardiac index during exertion. There are no absolute contraindications to the use of any of the drug classes in active hypertensive patients although certain classes of drugs are preferred, or are better tolerated.

DIURETICS

Diuretics limit the plasma volume expansion that is needed for aerobic training.[139] Thiazides cause a fall in blood pressure during exercise by decreasing peripheral resistance and plasma volume. Long-term use of thiazides does not cause a reduction in cardiac output. The effects of loop-

blocking drugs such as furosemide on exercise have not been well studied but these are infrequently used for blood pressure control because of their short duration of action.

The most worrisome yet manageable problem with diuretics for active individuals is hypokalemia. Potassium regulates and maintains skeletal muscle blood flow. In hypokalemic states, muscle blood flow decreases. During exercise and hypokalemia, skeletal muscle necrosis may occur resulting in rhabdomyolysis and acute renal failure. To ensure against potassium loss, patients taking diuretics should receive potassium supplements. Thus, diuretics result in a moderate decrease in the blood pressure response to exercise and, with adequate potassium supplementation, should not provoke any drug-related risks during physical activity in the young[140] and old.

β-ADRENERGIC BLOCKING DRUGS

Beta blockers, unlike ACE-I and calcium channel blockers, blunt exercise-mediated increases in heart rate and cardiac output and may reduce exercise performance. The blunting of the hemodynamic response to exercise is more profound with nonselective beta blockade (i.e., propranolol), and is greater with chronic administration than with acute dosing.[141,142] Nevertheless, training intensity can be estimated using a scale of perceived exertion in subjects on beta blockers.[143,144]

In a comparison of propranolol, metoprolol, and placebo in graded exercise tests, heart rate, systolic blood pressure, and Vo_2 max were reduced at maximum exertion, although there were no major changes in the anaerobic threshold. These exercise effects were dose related. There was no difference between the placebo and 40 mg/day of propranolol administration, whereas 160 and 320 mg/day significantly reduced the heart rate response and Vo_2 max.[144,145] Beta blockers may cause exertional fatigue and elevated serum potassium concentrations during exercise to levels greater than those seen with exercise alone, but clinical consequences in exercise are remote.[142] In patients with bronchospasm as a component of their chronic lung disease, beta blockers of any category should be avoided. Exercise-induced asthma should be managed with cromolyn sodium, and selective beta blockers, if indicated, can be used cautiously.

Virtually all studies regarding the effects of beta blockers on exercise and how exercise alters the pharmacodynamics and kinetics of these drugs have been done in relatively young people.[144] In healthy elderly volunteers who performed 4 months of dynamic exercise training there were no changes in kinetic or protein-binding characteristics of propranolol.[145]

VASODILATORS

α-ADRENERGIC BLOCKING DRUGS

The α-adrenergic blockers prazosin, terazosin, and doxazosin do not suppress cardiac output or exercise capacity[139] and are excellent choices for use in athletes and active patients. Prazosin decreases mean arterial blood pressure and total peripheral resistance at rest and with dynamic work. In contrast to hydralazine, prazosin blunts any reflex increase in heart rate or pressor response during isometric exercise.[83]

CALCIUM CHANNEL BLOCKERS

In normal, active persons, verapamil, diltiazem, and nifedipine exert adequate control on blood pressure during exercise. A mild blunting of the diastolic blood pressure response to handgrip was observed with verapamil.[82] In hypertensive patients, verapamil and nifedipine reduce systolic and diastolic blood pressure during exercise, perhaps owing to a reduction in systemic vascular resistance.[146,147] There is no change in serum potassium levels when comparing verapamil and nifedipine to placebo during isometric exercise.[82]

Therefore, calcium antagonists are of value for hypertensive patients who exercise. These medications are beneficial for patients who are not good candidates for beta blockers including those with bronchospastic pulmonary disease, insulin-dependent diabetes mellitus and those in whom beta blockers induce fatigue or are contraindicated.

ANGIOTENSIN-CONVERTING ENZYME INHIBITORS

ACE-I reduces systolic and diastolic blood pressure during exercise.[148] Early studies with the angiotensin II partial antagonist, saralasin, also has the same effect.[149] In the absence of diabetes mellitus, ACE-I does not influence the microalbuminuria observed with prolonged vigorous physical activity. Elevated serum potassium from ACE-I and exercise does not result in clinical consequences because catecholamine action is not blunted by ACE-I, thereby allowing potassium to move intracellularly. This is in contrast to beta blockers, which block the action of catecholamines to drive potassium back into the cell.

The overall responses to dynamic and static activities are not impaired with these drugs or angiotensin II receptor blockers, losartan and valsartan.[150]

CENTRAL ALPHA AGONISTS

Methyldopa in mildly hypertensive patients may decrease the blood pressure response to exercise but does not alter the heart rate response to exercise.[151,152] Clonidine reduces both blood pressure and heart rate during exercise and produces an acute vagally mediated decrease in cardiac output that does not persist with chronic use.[153,154]

Transdermal clonidine patches are superior to oral atenolol in improving aerobic conditioning in a group of relatively young mild hypertensive patients.[155]

Clonidine and methyldopa do not augment the changes in serum potassium, renin, and aldosterone that are normally observed in exercising healthy persons[156] or in persons taking beta blockers.[144]

SUMMARY

Hypertension is a common disease in the United States. Even mild-to-moderate elevations in blood pressure dramatically increase an individual's risk for developing left ventricular hypertrophy, stroke, and renal disease. Antihypertensive medications can reduce blood pressure, but side effects and cost have led to a search for alternatives such as nonpharmacologic interventions. JNC-VI reported on the benefit of using risk stratification as part of the treatment strategy. This report strongly encourages lifestyle modification to prevent high blood pressure, as definitive therapy for some and as adjunctive therapy for all hypertensive patients.

Physical inactivity increases the risk of hypertension. Physical activity in the control and prevention of hypertension among adults has so many advantages that physicians should not hesitate to recommend exercise for hypertensive management. Aerobic exercise or endurance training is the exercise of choice for hypertensive patients. Some studies showed that aerobic exercise can reduce blood pressure in approximately 75% of mild hypertensive patients. Low and moderate intensity exercise of 40 to 70% Vo_2 max appears to lower systolic and diastolic blood pressure with an average reduction of 10 mmHg. From a public health perspective and compared to more vigorous exercise, such exercise intensities may have more benefit with better adherence and lower musculoskeletal and cardiovascular risks. Emerging modes such as circuit weight training and T'ai chi are of potential benefit but have not been adequately studied.

The blood pressure lowering effect of aerobic exercise occurs early in the exercise program but disappears abruptly with detraining. Hypertensive subjects have more reduction in blood pressure than normotensive subjects. Antihypertensive medications such as diuretics and beta blockers can interfere with the exercise performance but ACE-I, alpha blockers, and calcium channel blockers do not interfere with exercise performance and are well tolerated by athletes and active individuals.

Exercise alone can reduce blood pressure. Nevertheless, a combination of nonpharmacologic interventions such as exercise and weight loss may provide sufficient benefit to decrease cardiovascular risks independent of drug treatment.

REFERENCES

1. The Fifth Report of the Joint National Committee on detection, evaluation, and treatment of high blood pressure. *Arch Intern Med* 153: 154–183, 1993.
2. Kannel WB, Doyle AM, Ostfeld AM, et al: Original resources for primary prevention of atherosclerotic diseases. *Circulation* 70:157A–205A, 1984.
3. Lim PO, MacFadyen RJ, Clarkson PB, et al: Impaired exercise tolerance in hypertensive patients. *Ann Intern Med* 124:41–55, 1996.
4. Hoes AW, Grobbee DE, Lubsen J: Diuretics, beta-blockers, and the risk for sudden cardiac death in hypertensive patients. *Ann Intern Med* 123:481–487, 1995.
5. Stolk RP, Hoes AW, Pols HA, et al: Insulin, hypertension and antihypertensive drugs in elderly patients: The Rotterdam Study. *J Hypertens* 14:237–242, 1996.
6. The Sixth Report of the Joint National Committee on Prevention, Detection, Evaluation and Treatment of High Blood Pressure. *Arch Intern Med* 157:2413–2445, 1997.
7. Blair SN, Goodyear NN, Gibbons LW, et al: Physical fitness and incidence of hypertension in healthy normotensive men and women. *JAMA* 252: 487–490, 1984.
8. Lund-Johansen P: Hemodynamic in the hypertension. *Acta Med Scand* 181:1–10, 1967.
9. Fagard R, Staessen J, Amery A: *Hemodynamic Aspects of Human Essential Hypertension,* in Zanchetti A, Mancia G (eds.): *Handbook of Hypertension: Pathophysiology of Hypertension,* vol. 17. Amsterdam, Elsevier Science B.V., 1997, pp. 213–240.
10. Fouad-Tarazi FM: Hypertension hemodynamics. *Med Clin North Am* 81:1131–1145, 1997.
11. Rocchini AP: Cardiovascular regulation in obesity-induced hypertension (Review). *Hypertension* 19(Suppl 1):156–160, 1992.
12. Hubert HB, Feinleib M, Menamacre PM, et al: Obesity as an independent risk factor for cardiovascular disease: A 26 year follow up of participants in the Framingham heart study. *Circulation* 67:968–977, 1983.

13. Blair SN, Kohl III HW, Paffenbarger RS, et al: Physical fitness and all-cause mortality: A prospective study of healthy men and women. *JAMA* 262:2395–2401, 1989.

14. Paffenbarger RS, Hyde RT, Wing AL, et al: Physical activity, all-cause mortality, and longevity of college alumni. *N Engl J Med* 314:650–663, 1986.

15. Powell KE, Thomson PH, Caspersen CJ, et al: Physical activity and incidence of coronary heart disease. *Ann Rev Public Health* 8:253–287, 1987.

16. Reaven PD, Barrett-Connor E, Edelstein S: Relation between leisure-time physical activity and blood pressure in older women. *Circulation* 83:559–565, 1991.

17. Paffenbarger RS Jr, Wing AL, Hyde RT, et al: Physical activity and incidence of hypertension in college alumni. *Am J Epidemiol* 117:245–257, 1983.

18. Montoye HJ, Metzer HL, Keller JB: Habitual activity and blood pressure. *Med Sci Sports* 4:175–181, 1972.

19. Fraser GE, Phillips RL, Harris R: Physical fitness and blood pressure in school children. *Circulation* 67:405–412, 1983.

20. Hofman A, Walter HS, Corinelly PA, et al: Blood pressure and physical fitness in children. *Hypertension* 9:188–191, 1988.

21. Sallis JF, Patterson TL, Buono MJ, et al: Relation of cardiovascular fitness and physical activity to cardiovascular disease risk factors in children and adults. *Am J Epidemiol* 127:933–951, 1988.

22. Hansen HS, Froberg K, Nielsen JR, et al: Physical fitness, physical activity and blood pressure in children. *Ann Clin Res* 20(Suppl 48):S68–S70, 1988.

23. Paffenbarger RS Jr: Physical activity and hypertension: An epidemiological view. *Ann Med* 23:319–327, 1991.

24. Daida H, Allison TG, Squires RW, et al: Peak exercise blood pressure stratified by age and gender in apparently health subjects. *Mayo Cin Proc* 71:445–452, 1996.

25. Radice M, Alli C, Avanzini F, et al: Role of blood pressure response to provocative tests in the prediction of hypertension in adolescents. *Eur Heart J* 6:490–496, 1985.

26. Franz IW: Ergometry in the assessment of arterial hypertension. *Cardiology* 72:147–159, 1985.

27. Palatini P: Exaggerated blood pressure response to exercise: Pathophysiologic mechanisms and clinical relevance. *J Sports Med Phys Fitness* 38:1–9, 1998.

28. Fagard R, Amery A: Exercise and hypertension, in Largah JH, Brenner BM (eds.): *Hypertension: Pathophysiology, Diagnosis, and Management,* 2nd ed. New York: Raven Press, 1995, pp. 2669–2681.

29. Palatini P, Pessina AC, Ardigo A, et al: Blood pressure response to pressor tests in patients with labile and established hypertension, before and after atenolol treatment. *Boll Soc Ital Cardiol* 22:1477–1484, 1977.

30. Singh JP, Larson MG, Manolio TA: Blood pressure response during treadmill testing as a risk factor for new-onset hypertension. The Framingham heart study. *Circulation* 99:1831–1836, 1999.

31. Manolio TA, Burke GL, Savage PJ, et al: Exercise blood pressure response and 5-year risk of elevated blood pressure in a cohort of young adults: The CARDIA study. *Am J Hypertens* 7:234–241, 1994.

32. Fragola PV, Romitelli S, Moretti A, et al: Precursors of established hypertension in borderline hypertensives: A two-year follow-up. *Int J Cardiol* 39:113–119, 1993.

33. Polonia J, Martins L, Bravo-Faria A, et al: Higher left ventricle mass in normotensives with exaggerated blood pressure response to exercise associated with higher ambulatory blood pressure load and sympathetic activity. *Eur Heart J* 13:S30–S36, 1992.

34. Attina DA, Giuliano G, Arcangeli G, et al: Effects of one year of physical training on borderline hypertension: An evaluation by bicycle ergometer exercise testing. *J Cardiovasc Pharmacol* 8(Suppl 5):S145–S147, 1986.

35. Palatini P: Exaggerated blood pressure response to exercise: Pathophysiologic mechanisms and clinical relevance. *J Sports Med Phys Fitness* 38:1–9, 1998.

36. Kokkinos PF, Narayan P, Colleran JA, et al: Effects of regular exercise on blood pressure and left ventricular hypertrophy in African-American men with severe hypertension. *N Engl J Med* 333:1462–1467, 1995.

37. Fagard RH: Physical fitness and blood pressure. *J Hypertens* 11(Suppl 5):S47–S52, 1993.

38. Arroll B, Beaglehole R: Does physical activity lower blood pressure? A critical review of the

clinical trials. *J Clin Epidemiol* 45:439–447, 1992.

39. Kelley G, McClellan P: Antihypertensive effects of aerobic exercise: A brief meta-analysis review of randomized controlled trials. *Am J Hypertens* 7:115–119, 1994.

40. Hagberg JM, Brown MD: Does exercise training play a role in the treatment of essential hypertension? *J Cardiovasc Risk* 2:296–302, 1995.

41. Halbert JA, Silagy CA, Finucane P, et al: The effectiveness of exercise training in lowering blood pressure: A meta-analysis of randomized controlled trials of 4 weeks or longer. *J Hum Hypertens* 11:641–649, 1997.

42. Kelly G: Dynamic resistance exercise and resting blood pressure in adults: A meta-analysis. *J Appl Physiol* 82:1559–1565, 1997.

43. Fagard RH: Exercise in blood pressure control. *J Hypertension* 13:1223–1227, 1995.

44. Nelson L, Jennings GL, Esler MD, et al: Effect of changing levels of physical activity on blood-pressure and in essential hypertension. *Lancet* 2:473–476, 1986.

45. Jessup JV, Lowenthal DT, Pollock ML, et al: The effects of endurance exercise training on ambulatory blood pressure in normotensive older adults. *Geriatr Nephr Urol* 8:103–109, 1998.

46. Coconie CC, Graves JE, Pollock ML, et al: Effect of exercise training on BP in 70-to-79-year-old men and women. *Med Sci Sports Exerc* 23:505–511, 1991.

47. Hagberg JM, Montain SJ, Martin WH, et al: Effect of exercise training on 60-69-year old persons with essential hypertension. *Am J Cardiol* 64:348–353, 1989.

48. Collins R, Peto R, MacMahon S, et al: Blood pressure, stroke and coronary heart disease. Part 2: Short-term reductions in blood pressure; overview of randomized drug trials in their epidemiological context. *Lancet* 335:765–774, 1990.

49. Shaper AGE, Wannamethee G, Walker M: Physical activity, hypertension and risk of heart attack in men without evidence of ischemic heart disease. *J Hum Hypertens* 8:3–10, 1994.

50. Blair SN, Kohl HW, Barlow CE, et al: Physical fitness and all-cause mortality in hypertensive men. *Ann Med* 23:307–312, 1991.

51. Pescatello LS, Falkenham A, Leach Jr CN, et al: Short-term effect of dynamic exercise on arterial blood pressure. *Circulation* 83:1557–1561, 1991.

52. Baglivo HP, Fabreques H, Burrieza RC, et al: Effect of moderate physical training on left ventricular mass in mild hypertensive persons. *Hypertension* 15:(S1)1153–1156, 1990.

53. Rogers MW, Probst MM, Gruber JJ, et al: Differential effects of exercise training intensity on blood pressure and cardiovascular responses to stress in borderline hypertensive humans. *J Hypertens* 14:1369–1375, 1996.

54. Cade R: Effect of aerobic exercise training on patients with systemic arterial hypertension. *Am J Med* 77:785–790, 1984.

55. Kelemen MH: Exercise training combined with antihypertensive drug therapy: Effects on lipids, blood pressure, and left ventricular mass. *JAMA* 263:2766–2771, 1990.

56. Lim PO, MacFadyen RJ, Clarkson PBM, et al: Impaired exercise tolerance in hypertensive patients. *Ann Intern Med* 124:41–55, 1996.

57. Sawada S, Tanaka H, Funakoshi M, et al: Five year prospective study on blood pressure and maximal oxygen uptake. *Clin Exp Pharmacol Physiol* 20:483–487, 1993.

58. Tanaka H, Basset DR Jr, Turner MJ: Exaggerated blood pressure response to maximal exercise in endurance-trained individuals. *Am J Hypertens* 9:1099–1103, 1996.

59. Ekblom B, Astrand PO, Saltin B, et al: Effect of training on circulatory response to exercise. *J Appl Physiol* 24:518–528, 1968.

60. Stratton JR, Levy WC, Cerqueira MD, et al: Cardiovascular responses to exercise: Effects of aging and exercise training in healthy men. *Circulation* 89:1648–1655, 1994.

61. Tubau JF, Szlachnic J, Braun S, et al: Impaired left ventricular functional reserve in hypertensive patients with left ventricular hypertrophy. *Hypertension* 14:1–10, 1989.

62. Fagard R, Staessen J, Amery A: Maximal aerobic power in essential hypertension. *J Hypertens* 6:859–865, 1988.

63. Steinhaus LA, Dustman RE, Ruhling RO, et al: Cardiorespiratory fitness of young and older active and sedentary men. *Br J Sports Med* 22:163–166, 1988.

64. Braun LT, Potempa K, Holm K, et al: The role of catecholamines, age, and fitness on blood pressure reactivity to dynamic exercise in patients with essential hypertension. *Heart Lung* 23:404–412, 1994.

65. Chaney RH, Arndt S: Predictability of blood pressure response to isometric stress. *Am J Cardiol* 51:787–790, 1983.

66. Sullivan J, Hanson P, Rahdo PS, et al: Continuous measurement of left ventricular performance during and after maximal isometric deadlift exercise. *Circulation* 85:1406–1413, 1992.

67. MacDougall JD, Tuxen D, Sale G, et al: Arterial blood pressure response to heavy resistance exercise. *J Appl Physiol* 58:785–790, 1985.

68. Palatini P: Exercise haemodynamics in the normotensive and the hypertensive subjects. *Clin Sci* 87:275–287, 1994.

69. Mitchell JH, Reardon WC, Mclosky I: Reflex effects on circulation and respiration from contracting skeletal muscle. *Am J Physiol* 233:H374–H378, 1977.

70. Seals DR, Washburn RA, Hanson PG, et al: Increased cardiovascular response to static contraction of larger muscle groups. *J Appl Physiol* 54:434–437, 1983.

71. MacDougall JD, McKelvie RS, Moroz DE, et al: Factors affecting blood pressure during heavy weight lifting and static contractions. *J Appl Physiol* 73:1590–1597, 1992.

72. Sale DG, Moroz DE, McKelvie RS, et al: Comparison of blood pressure response to isokinetic and weight-lifting exercise. *Eur J Appl Physiol* 67:115–120, 1993.

73. Ben-Ari E, Gentile R, Feigenbaum H, et al: Left ventricular dynamics during strenuous isometric exercise in marathon runners, weight lifters and healthy sedentary men: Comparative echocardiographic study. *Cardiology* 82:75–80, 1993.

74. Narloch JA, Brandstater ME: Influence of breathing technique on arterial blood pressure during heavy weight lifting. *Arch Phys Med Rehabil* 76:457–462, 1995.

75. Van Hoof R, Macor F, Lijnen P, et al: Effect of strength training on blood pressure measured in various conditions in sedentary men. *Int J Sports Med* 17(6):415–422, 1996.

76. Wiley RL, Dunn CL, Cox RH, et al: Isometric exercise training lowers resting blood pressure. *Med Sci Sports Exerc* 24:749–754, 1992.

77. Hurley BF, Hagberg JM, Goldberg AP, et al: Resistive training can reduce coronary risk factors without altering Vo$_2$ max or percent body fat. *Med Sci Sports Exerc* 20:150–154, 1988.

78. Kiveloff B, Huber O: Brief maximal isometric exercise in hypertension. *J Am Geriatr Soc* 19:1006–1012, 1971.

79. Hagberg JM, Ehsani AA, Goldring D, et al: Effect of weight training on blood pressure and haemodynamics in hypertensive adolescents. *J Pediatr* 104:147–151, 1984.

80. Harris KA, Holly RG: Physiological responses to circuit weight training in borderline hypertensive subjects. *Med Sci Sports Exerc* 19:246–252, 1987.

81. Tipton CM: Exercise, training, and hypertension. *Exerc Sports Sci Rev* 12:245–306, 1984.

82. Stein DT, Lowenthal DT, Porter S, et al: Effects of nifedipine and verapamil on isometric and dynamic exercise in normal subjects. *Am J Cardiol* 54:386–389, 1984.

83. Lowenthal DT, Dickerman D, Saris SD, et al: The effect of pharmacologic interaction on central and peripheral alpha-receptors and pressor response to static exercise. *Ann Sports Med* 1:100–104, 1983.

84. Lowenthal DT, Powers SK, Pollock ML, et al: Interactions of β-blockade and exercise: Implications and applications for the elderly. *Am J Geri Card* 1:42–57, 1992.

85. Grossman E, Messerli FH, Oren S, et al: Disparate cardiovascular response to stress tests during isradipine and fosinopril therapy. *Am J Cardiol* 72:574–579, 1993.

86. Tipton CM, Edwards JG, Pepin EB, et al: Response of hypertensive rats to acute and chronic conditions of static exercise. *Am J Physiol* 254:H592–H598, 1988.

87. De Virgilio C, Nelson RJ, Milliken J, et al: Ascending aortic dissection in weight lifters with cystic medial degeneration. *Ann Thorac Surg* 49:638–642, 1990.

88. Palatini P: Blood pressure behaviour during physical activity. *Sports Med* 5:353–374, 1988.

89. Effron MB: Effects of resistive training on left ventricular function. *Med Sci Sports Exerc* 21:694–697, 1988.

90. Fleck SJ: Cardiovascular adaptations of resistance training. *Med Sci Sports Exerc* 20:S146–S151, 1988.

91. Overton JM, Joyner MJ, Tipton CM: Reductions in blood pressure after acute exercise by hypertensive rats. *J Appl Physiol* 64:748–752, 1988.

92. Hill DW, Collins MA, Cureton KJ, et al: Blood

pressure response after weight training exercise. *J Appl Sport Sci Res* 3:44–47, 1989.

93. Kenney MJ, Seals DR: Postexercise hypotension: Key features, mechanisms and clinical significance. *Hypertension* 22:653–664, 1993.

94. Kaufman FL, Hughson RL, Schaman JP: Effect of exercise on recovery blood pressure in normotensive and hypertensive subjects. *Med Sci Sports Exerc* 19:17–20, 1987.

95. Rueckert PA, Slane PR, Lillis DL, et al: Hemodynamic patterns and duration of post-dynamic exercise hypotension in hypertensive humans. *Med Sci Sports Exerc* 28:24–32, 1996.

96. Somers VK, Conway J, Coats A, et al: Postexercise hypotension is not sustained in normal and hypertensive humans. *Hypertension* 18:211–215, 1991.

97. Meredith IT, Jennings GL, Esler MD, et al: Timecourse of the antihypertensive and autonomic effects of regular endurance exercise in human subjects. *J Hypertens* 8:859–866, 1990.

98. American College of Sports Medicine Position Stand. Physical activity, physical fitness and hypertension. *Med Sci Sports Exerc* 25(10):I–X, 1993.

99. Grassi G, Seravalle G, Calhoun D, et al: Physical exercise in essential hypertension. *Chest* 101 (Suppl 5):312S–314S, 1992.

100. Duncan JJ, Farr JE, Upton SJ, et al: The effect of aerobic exercise on plasma catecholamine and blood pressure in patients with mild essential hypertension. *JAMA* 254:2609–2613, 1985.

101. Urata H, Tanabe Y, Kiyonaga A, et al: Antihypertensive and volume-depleting effects of mild exercise on essential hypertension. *Hypertension* 9:245–252, 1987.

102. Chandler MP, Rodenbaugh DW, Dicarlo SE: Arterial baroreflex resetting mediates postexercise reductions in arterial pressure and heart rate. *Am J Physiol* 275(Heart Circ. Physiol.44):H1627–H1634, 1998.

103. Tümer N, Hale C, Lawler J, et al: Modulation of tyrosine hydroxylase gene expression in the rat adrenal gland by exercise: Effects of age. *Brain Res Mol Brain Res* 14:51–56, 1992.

104. Blumenthal JA, Siegel WC, Appelbaum M: Failure of exercise to reduce blood pressure in patients with mild hypertension. Results of a randomized controlled trial. *JAMA* 266:2098–2104, 1991.

105. Frattola A, Parati G, Cuspidi C, et al: Prognostic value of 24-hour blood pressure variability. *J Hypertens* 11:1133–1137, 1993.

106. Parati G, Pomidossi G, Albini F, et al: Relationship of 24-hour blood pressure variability. *J Hypertens* 5:93–98, 1987.

107. Marceau M, Kouame N, Lacourciere Y, et al: Effects of different training intensities on 24 hour blood pressure in hypertensive subjects. *Circulation* 88:2803–2811, 1993.

108. Somers VK, Conway J, Jonston J: Effects of endurance training on baroreflex sensitivity and blood pressure in borderline hypertension. *Lancet* 337:1363–1368, 1991.

109. Seals DR, Reiling MJ: Effect of regular exercise on 24-hour arterial pressure in older hypertensive humans. *Hypertension* 18:583–592, 1991.

110. Palatini P, Granjero G, Mormino F, et al: Relation between physical training and ambulatory blood pressure in stage 1 hypertensive subjects. Results of the HARVEST trial. *Circulation* 90:2870–2876, 1994.

111. Wallace JP, Bogle PG, King BA, et al: A comparison of 24-h average blood pressures and blood pressure load following exercise. *Am J Hypertens* 10:728–734, 1997.

112. The Hypertension Detection and Follow-up Program Cooperative Group. Five-year findings of the hypertension detection and follow-up program. *JAMA* 242:2562–2571, 1979.

113. Hoes AW, Grobbee DE, Lubson J: Does drug treatment improve survival reconciling the trials in mild-to-moderate hypertension. *J Hypertens* 13:805–811, 1995.

114. Egger M, Davey Smith G: Risks and benefits of treating mild hypertension: A misleading meta-analysis? *J Hypertension* 13:813–815, 1995.

115. Pierdomenico SD, Costantini F, Bucci A, et al: Blunted nocturnal fall in blood pressure and oxidative stress in men and women with essential hypertension. *Am J Hypertension* 12:356–363, 1999.

116. Kannel WB: Hypertension: Relationship with other risk factors. *Drugs* 109:581–585, 1986.

117. Ebrahim S, Smith GD: Lowering blood pressure: A systematic review of sustained effects of non-pharmacological interventions. *J Pub Health Med* 20:441–448, 1998.

118. Multiple Risk Factor Intervention Trial Research Group. Multiple Risk Factor Intervention Trial:

Risk factor changes and mortality results. *JAMA* 248:1456–1470, 1982.

119. Gordon NF, Scott CB, Wilkinson WJ, et al: Exercise and mild essential hypertension: Recommendations for adults. *Sports Med* 10:390–404, 1990.

120. TOPH Collaborative Research Group: The effects of nonpharmacologic interventions on blood pressure of persons with high normal levels. *JAMA* 267:1213–1220, 1992.

121. Gordon NF, Scott CB, Levine BD: Comparison of single versus multiple lifestyle interventions: Are the antihypertensive effects of exercise training and diet-induced weight loss additive? *Am J Cardiol* 79:763–767, 1997.

122. Wood PD, Haskell WL, Blair SN, et al: Increased exercise level and plasma lipoprotein concentrations: A one-year, randomized, controlled study in sedentary, middle-aged men. *Metabolism* 32:31–33, 1983.

123. Ramsey LE, Yeo WW, Chadwick IG, et al: Non-pharmacological therapy of hypertension. *Br Med Bull* 50:494–499, 1994.

124. Boyce ML, Robergs RA, Avasthi PS, et al: Exercise training by individuals with predialysis renal failure: Cardiorespiratory endurance, hypertension, and renal function. *Am J Kidney Dis* 30:180–192, 1997.

125. Painter PL, Nelson-Worrel N, Hill MM, et al: Effects of exercise training during hemodialysis. *Nephron* 43:87–92, 1986.

126. Hagberg JM, Goldring D, Ehsani AA, et al: Exercise training improves hypertension in hemodialysis patients. *Am J Nephrol* 3:209–212, 1983.

127. Clorius JH, Mandelbaum A, Hupp T, et al: Exercise activates renal dysfunction in hypertension. *Am J Hypertens* 9:653–661, 1996.

128. Jessup JV, Lowenthal DT, Pollock ML, et al: Exercise training in older men and women: Effects on cardiovascular and renal function. *Geriatr Nephr Urol* 6:27–34, 1996.

129. American College of Sports Medicine. *Guidelines for Exercise Testing and Prescription,* 4th ed. Philadelphia: Lea & Febiger, 1990, pp. 1–10.

130. Schauer J, Hanson P: Usefulness of a branching treadmill protocol for evaluation of cardiac functional capacity. *Am J Cardiol* 60:1371–1377, 1987.

131. Tanaka H, Bassett Jr DR, Howley ET, et al: Swimming training lowers the resting blood pressure in individuals with hypertension. *J Hypertens* 15:651–657, 1997.

132. Palatini P: Exercise haemodynamics. *Clin Sci* 87:275–287, 1994.

133. Young DR, Appel LJ, Jee S, et al: The effects of aerobic exercise and T'ai Chi on blood pressure in older people: Results of a randomized trial. *J Am Geriatr Soc* 47:277–282, 1999.

134. World Hypertension League: Physical exercise in the management of hypertension: A consensus statement by the World Hypertension League. *J Hypertens* 9:282–287, 1991.

135. McMurray RG, Ainsworth BE, Harrell JS, et al: Is physical activity or aerobic power more influential on reducing cardiovascular disease risk factors? *Med Sci Sports Exerc* 10:1521–1529, 1998.

136. Bouchard C: Genetics of aerobic power and capacity, in Malina RM, Bouchard C (eds.): *Sports and Human Genetics,* Champaign, IL: Human Kinetics Publishers, 1985, pp. 59–81.

137. Braith RW, Pollock ML, Lowenthal DT, et al: Moderate- and high-intensity exercise lowers blood pressure in normotensive subjects 60 to 79 years of age. *Am J Cardiol* 73:1124–1128, 1994.

138. Krone W, Nagele H: Effects of antihypertensives on plasma lipids and lipoprotein metabolism. *Am Heart J* 116:1729–1734, 1988.

139. Nadel ER, Fortney SM, Wenger CB: Effect of hydration state of circulatory and thermal regulations. *J Appl Physiol* 49:715–721, 1980.

140. Falkner B, Onesti G, Lowenthal DT, et al: Effectiveness of centrally acting drugs and diuretics in adolescent hypertension. *Clin Pharmacol Ther* 32:577–583, 1982.

141. Gullestad L, Hallen J, Medbo JI, et al: The effect of acute vs chronic treatment with beta-adrenoceptor blockade on exercise performance, haemodynamic and metabolic parameters in healthy men and women. *Br J Clin Pharmacol* 41:57–67, 1996.

142. Van Baak MA: Beta-adrenoceptor blockade and exercise. An update. *Sports Med* 5:209–225, 1988.

143. Eston R, Connolly D: The use of ratings of perceived exertion for exercise prescription in patients receiving β-blocker therapy. *Sports Med* 21:176–190, 1996.

144. Pollock M, Lowenthal DT, Foster C, et al: Acute and chronic responses in patients treated with beta blockers. *J Cardiopul Rehabil* 11:132–144, 1991.

145. Panton LB, Guillen GJ, Williams L, et al: The lack of effect of aerobic exercise training on propranolol pharmacokinetics in young and elderly adults. *J Clin Pharmacol* 35:885–894, 1995.

146. Subramanian B, Bowles MF, Davies AB, et al: Combined therapy with verapamil and propanolol in chronic stable angina. *Am J Cardiol* 49:125–132, 1982.

147. Moskowitz RM, Piccini PA, Nacarelli G, et al: Nifedipine therapy for stable angina pectoris: Preliminary results of effects on angina frequency and treadmill exercise response. *Am J Cardiol* 44:811–816, 1979.

148. Paran E, Neumann L, Cristal N, et al: Response to mental and physical stress before and during adrenoreceptor blocker and angiotensin converting enzyme inhibitor treatment in essential hypertension. *Am J Cardiol* 68:1362–1366, 1991.

149. Fagard R, Amery A, Reybrouck T, et al: Effects of angiotension antagonism on hemodynamics, renin and catecholamines during exercise. *J Appl Physiol* 43:440–444, 1977.

150. Lang R, Elkayam U, Yellen L, et al: Comparative effects of losartan and enalapril on exercise capacity and clinical status in patients with heart failure: The Losartan Pilot Exercise Study Investigators. *J Am Coll Cardiol* 30:982–991, 1997.

151. Sannerstedt R, Varnaskes E, Werko L: Hemodynamic effects of methyldopa (Aldomet) at rest and during exercise in patients with arterial hypertension. *Acta Med Scand* 171:75–82, 1962.

152. Rosenthal L, Affrime MB, Lowenthal DT: Biochemical and pharmacodynamic responses to single and multiple dose methyldopa and propranolol during physical activity. *Clin Pharmacol Ther* 32:701–710, 1982.

153. Lund-Johansen P: Hemodynamic changes at rest and during exercise in long-term clonidine therapy of essential hypertension. *Acta Med Scand* 195:111–117, 1974.

154. Lowenthal DT, Affrime MB, Rosenthal L, et al: Dynamic and biochemical responses to single and repeated doses of clonidine during dynamic physical activity. *Clin Pharmacol Ther* 32:18–24, 1982.

155. Davies SF, Graif JL, Husebye D, et al: Comparative effects of transdermal clonidine and oral atenolol on acute exercise performance and response to aerobic conditioning in subjects with hypertension. *Arch Intern Med* 149:1551–1556, 1989.

156. Lowenthal DT, Affrime MB, Falkner B, et al: Potassium disposition and neuroendocrine effects of propanolol, methyldopa and clonidine during dynamic exercise. *Clin Exp Hypertens* 4:1895–1911, 1982.

Chapter 20

EXERCISE AND DIABETES

Bret H. Goodpaster, Ph.D.   *David E. Kelley, M.D.*

Exercise can play a key role in the treatment of diabetes mellitus, for both type 1 (insulin-dependent) and type 2 (non-insulin-dependent) diabetes mellitus. It has been recognized for many years, and indeed centuries, that exercise can help restore toward normal metabolism in diabetes. In part spurred by the interest in understanding "insulin resistance" within skeletal muscle, there has also been a renewed interest in understanding the physiological and biochemical mechanisms by which exercise improves glucose metabolism in patients with diabetes mellitus or those at risk for developing diabetes. One of the purposes of this chapter is to review these interesting findings. It is of practical value for health care professionals to be knowledgeable about these physiological data as this information can help practitioners formulate a rational approach to exercise prescriptions for patients with diabetes, while anticipating the adjustments of diet and medications that are often needed.

While the positive role of exercise for patients with an established diagnosis of diabetes has been recognized for many years, recent epidemio-

430

logic findings emphasize the valuable contribution that exercise can have in the prevention of diabetes. This is an extremely important public health issue. Both in the United States and around the world, the incidence and prevalence of type 2 diabetes continue to rise. Educating practitioners and, in turn, the public about the health benefits of exercise and articulating the amount and type of physical activity that are needed to achieve these benefits should be a principal goal for the coming years.

OVERVIEW OF DIABETES MELLITUS

Diabetes mellitus is a prevalent disease, especially among the elderly. Approximately 6% of the total U.S. population and 10% of people over age 65 has diabetes mellitus.[1] There are several types of diabetes mellitus. Type 1 diabetes mellitus, previously termed *insulin-dependent* diabetes mellitus (IDDM) or *juvenile-onset,* accounts for approximately 10% of patients with diabetes in the United States. Nearly 90% of the individuals with diabetes mellitus have type 2 diabetes, previously termed *non-insulin-dependent* or *adult-onset* diabetes mellitus. Gestational diabetes mellitus, as the name would imply, develops during pregnancy and has a pathophysiology similar in many respects to type 2 diabetes mellitus. A small percentage of patients have "secondary" diabetes mellitus, which arises as a consequence of other illnesses such as surgical removal of the pancreas, or hemachromatosis.

The diagnostic criteria for diabetes mellitus have been modified. Diabetes mellitus is diagnosed based on one or more of the following criteria: (a) 2 values for fasting plasma glucose (FPG) > 126 mg/dl; (b) 2 random plasma glucose determinations that are > 200 mg/dl; or (c) plasma glucose > 200 mg/dl 2 h following ingestion of 75 g of glucose. The main modification of diagnostic criteria was to lower the value for fasting plasma glucose from 140 mg/dl to the new diagnostic level of 126 mg/dl, and this change was precipitated by the recognition that perhaps as many as one-half of all patients with type 2 diabetes mellitus are undiagnosed. Various data indicated that one means to improve recognition of this diagnosis is to revise the fasting glucose threshold.

PATHOPHYSIOLOGY OF TYPE 1 DIABETES MELLITUS

The pathogenesis of type 1 and type 2 diabetes differ. Type 1 diabetes is caused by an autoimmune destruction of the insulin-producing cells of the pancreas. Age of onset of IDDM is most common during childhood or in young adults, but the onset of IDDM can be at any age. Because of the destruction of insulin-producing cells, patients with type 1 diabetes have an absolute need for insulin therapy. In the absence of insulin replacement, patients with IDDM will develop extreme hyperglycemia and a metabolic acidosis caused by excess production of ketones, derived from excess breakdown of fat due to the absence of insulin. Diabetic ketoacidosis (DKA) is a medical emergency.

Because of the reliance on administration of exogenous insulin, a chief clinical issue in managing exercise is to coordinate the timing of exercise in relation to the timing and dose of injected insulin. On the one hand, vigorous exercise in the absence of sufficient insulin can aggravate hyperglycemia and might even precipitate the onset of DKA. More commonly, on the other hand, exercise during periods of elevated plasma insulin can precipitate symptomatic hypoglycemia. Thus, practitioners need to carefully consider the pharmacokinetics of insulin in advising patients with type 1 diabetes about exercise, and this issue is discussed more fully in a later part of this chapter.

PATHOPHYSIOLOGY OF TYPE 2 DIABETES MELLITUS

Type 2 diabetes mellitus is by far the most common form of diabetes in the United States, accounting for nearly 90% of all patients with diabetes. The incidence of type 2 diabetes increases each decade of aging and while it was previously thought that type 2 diabetes mellitus was nearly always a disease of adults, there is an alarming increase in the incidence of type 2 diabetes mellitus among young adults and adolescents, usually in those who are obese. A family history of type 2 diabetes is common and obesity is a major risk factor. Type 2 diabetes is regarded as a metabolic disorder tied to modern lifestyles of stress, excess calorie intake (particularly fat), and inadequate physical activity.

From a metabolic perspective, the pathogenesis of type 2 diabetes entails insulin resistance within peripheral tissues, elevated rates of hepatic glucose production, and an impaired capacity for insulin secretion. The increase of hepatic glucose production is the prime determinant of the level of fasting hyperglycemia. Impaired insulin secretion is a key determinant of the severity of postprandial hyperglycemia. The defect in insulin secretion is generally progressive and is one of the prime determinants of the typical need to evolve more complex medical regimens. Often, with long duration of type 2 diabetes, exogenous insulin injections can be needed. The third defect of metabolism in type 2 diabetes is insulin resistance. Skeletal muscle and adipose tissue are the two principal tissues responsible for insulin resistance. It is now recognized that insulin resistance can precede the onset of overt diabetes by decades and is a major risk for the development of diabetes.

Exercise can have a major effect to ameliorate insulin resistance and, accordingly, the concept of insulin resistance should be defined. Insulin is the principal hormone mediating the signals for fuel storage and anabolic processes in general. Accordingly, insulin resistance can potentially be defined in reference to many metabolic pathways. By far, however, insulin resistance is most typically used to denote impaired glucose utilization and, more specifically, impaired rates of glucose metabolism within skeletal muscle. In relation to the mechanisms of insulin resistance, defects have been identified in insulin signaling, within the transport of glucose into muscle, and in the formation of glycogen within muscle. Another aspect of insulin resistance is a blunting of the usual effect of insulin to stimulate a modest increase of blood flow within skeletal muscle. Increasingly, impairments in the pattern of fatty acid utilization by skeletal muscle, leading to the accumulation of triglyceride within skeletal muscle, are being defined with respect to insulin resistance.

With respect to adipose tissue, a key manifestation of insulin resistance is a blunted suppression of lipolysis. Ordinarily, lipolysis is sensitive to inhibition by insulin, and, in insulin resistance, plasma fatty acids tend to remain elevated. The elevations of fatty acids may aggravate the defects in glucose metabolism through "substrate competition."[2] With respect to the liver, insulin resistance is manifest as a decreased suppression of the insulin suppression of hepatic glucose production.

INSULIN-RESISTANT SYNDROME

Within the past decade, the term *insulin resistance* has been expanded beyond the consideration of specific impairments in insulin signaling and pathways of glucose metabolism. The term *insulin resistance* is also commonly used to denote a metabolic syndrome characterized by the clustering of essential hypertension, dyslipidemia, type 2 diabetes and impaired glucose tolerance, and an upper body pattern of fat distribution. A sedentary lifestyle is among the factors considered to increase the risk of developing the insulin-resistant syndrome and, conversely, exercise is regarded as one of the key behavioral changes that can prevent or reverse the insulin resistant or metabolic syndrome.[3–5]

EPIDEMIOLOGIC STUDIES OF EXERCISE AND DIABETES MELLITUS

There are strong epidemiologic data that a program of regular exercise can reduce the risk for developing type 2 diabetes mellitus.[6–10] Large-scale prospective studies have provided compelling evidence that regular exercise reduces the incidence of type 2 diabetes.[7–10] These studies followed individuals who were without diabetes at the start of the period of observation and then undertook to identify whether the level of usual physical activity influenced the later development of the disease. Helmrich et al[7] found that among 5990 University of Pennsylvania male alumni, increased physical activity was associated with a reduction in the incidence of diabetes. As shown in Figure 20.1, the benefit of exercise was particularly strong in those men who were at the highest risk for developing the disease (defined by a body mass index of > 25, a history of hypertension, or a parental history of diabetes).[7] Manson et al[9] found that among 21,271 male physicians, the incidence of type 2 diabetes was reduced in association with increased physical activity levels after adjusting for age and body mass index (Fig. 20.2). In a similar study by this group,[8] the incidence of diabetes was determined in 87,253 female nurses during an 8-year follow-up. Women participating in vigorous exercise at least once per week had a reduced age and body mass index-adjusted risk for developing diabetes. These studies suggest that the most favorable effects of physical activity in the prevention of diabetes appear to be strongest in those who are at highest risk, and in those who are the most sedentary, though recent weight gain will lessen the protective effect of exercise.[7]

Perhaps the most powerful epidemiologic evidence that exercise reduces the incidence of diabetes comes from intervention studies in which efforts are made to either delay or prevent the development of the disease. These studies, however, are difficult to execute because they are costly

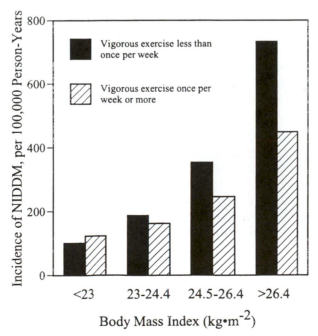

FIGURE 20.1. Age-adjusted incidence rates of type 2 diabetes mellitus according to frequency of vigorous exercise, presented by body mass index quartile. *Adapted with permission from Helmrich SP, Ragland DR, Leung RW, et al: Physical activity and reduced occurrence of non-insulin-dependent diabetes mellitus.* N Engl J Med *325:147–152, 1991. Copyright © 1991 Massachusetts Medical Society. All rights reserved.*

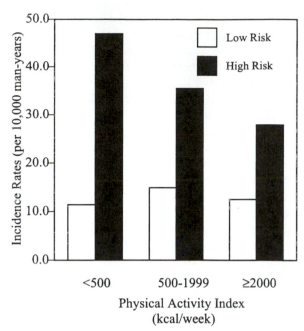

FIGURE 20.2. Age-adjusted incidence rates of type 2 diabetes mellitus among 5990 men according to low-risk and high-risk subgroups and physical activity. High-risk men (n = 2634) had at least 1 or more of the following risk factors: body mass index > 25, a history of hypertension, or a history of diabetes. Adapted with permission from Manson JE, Nathan DM, Krolewski AS, et al: A prospective study of exercise and incidence of diabetes among U.S. male physicians. JAMA *268(1):63–67, 1992 Copyright 1992. American Medical Association.*

and labor intensive, and there are often insufficient controls on the amount and intensity of the exercised performed. In a randomized controlled study conducted in Da Qing, China, 577 individuals with impaired glucose tolerance were identified after screening a population of more than 110,660 men and women and randomized into diet only, exercise only, exercise plus diet, or control groups. The exercise intervention lowered the risk of conversion to type 2 diabetes during the ensuing 6 years.[10] Positive effects were also observed for diet alone, or in combination with exercise. Similar results have been obtained during a 6-year intervention of exercise and diet in Swedish patients with early-stage type 2 diabetes or impaired glucose tolerance.[11] Unfortunately, within a trial of this size and design, it is difficult to clearly ascertain the amount of exercise actu-

ally performed or the extent of crossover between arms of treatment. Nevertheless, these data do suggest the potential effectiveness of lifestyle interventions of exercise and diet to lessen the risk of type 2 diabetes mellitus among individuals with impaired glucose tolerance. Furthermore, data from the Malmo preventive trial in men with impaired glucose tolerance indicate favorable effects on mortality rates among those engaged in long-term interventions of diet and physical activity.[11] Taken together, these data from large-scale epidemiologic studies provides overwhelming evidence that increased physical activity prevents or delays the onset of type 2 diabetes mellitus. Moreover, it appears that physical activity may confer the greatest benefit in individuals at the highest risk for developing type 2 diabetes mellitus.

ACUTE EFFECTS OF EXERCISE ON GLUCOSE METABOLISM IN HEALTH AND IN DIABETES

SUBSTRATE UTILIZATION DURING EXERCISE

During physical activity, energy expenditure by skeletal muscle increases substantially. The increase in energy production is supported by an increased utilization of plasma glucose and plasma fatty acids and by utilization of glycogen and triglyceride stored within skeletal muscle. The intensity and duration of exercise are key determinants of the proportions of carbohydrate versus lipid, and of the relative role of plasma substrates versus mobilization of muscle glycogen and triglyceride. Several excellent research studies and review articles delineate these effects.[12–17] Briefly, for exercise of low intensity such as walking, particularly if sustained for long intervals, the predominate substrate that is oxidized is lipid, and this is primarily supported by an increased use of plasma fatty acids. There is relatively little depletion of muscle glycogen during low intensity exercise. At the other extreme, during brief, high intensity exercise, there is a predominant use of glycogen and plasma glucose.

The most complex admixture of substrates occurs during moderate intensity exercise. During moderate intensity exercise there is an increased utilization of plasma glucose. Rates of systemic glucose utilization increase approximately three- to fourfold above basal rates. In those without diabetes, there is close matching of hepatic glucose production to the increased rates of glucose utilization by skeletal muscle, and plasma glucose levels remain stable. There is also an enhanced rate of lipolysis and lipid oxidation. Both duration of exercise and the underlying fitness of the individual are determinants of the relative oxidation of lipid versus carbohydrate, with longer duration of exercise and higher fitness favoring increased reliance on lipid oxidation. In addition, there is use of muscle glycogen and triglyceride and, with increased duration of exercise and increased fitness, there appears to be a great reliance on the use of muscle triglyceride.

GLUCOSE METABOLISM DURING EXERCISE IN DIABETES

These principles of substrate metabolism are of relevance to diabetes. First, diabetes is associated with hyperglycemia, often with elevated plasma-free fatty acids, diminished muscle glycogen, and, at least in obese patients with type 2 diabetes mellitus, increased muscle content of triglyceride.[18] Moreover, as previously described, skeletal muscle manifests marked insulin resistance in type 2 diabetes. Therefore, it would seem reasonable to postulate that patterns of substrate metabolism during exercise in patients with diabetes might be considerably altered (as compared to those without diabetes), as is well-described to occur during resting insulin-stimulated conditions. Yet, findings indicate that patterns of substrate utilization during exercise, perhaps somewhat surprisingly, are in most respects more similar than dissimilar to the patterns of substrate use by skeletal muscle during exercise in individuals without diabetes.[19,20]

One of the effects of exercise in patients with diabetes is that it lowers plasma glucose, and this is of course desirable, provided the fall is not great enough to produce symptomatic hypoglycemia. How much glucose lowering is typically achieved? In patients with type 2 diabetes mellitus, moderate intensity exercise of approximately 45 to 60 min duration has been shown to lower plasma glucose by approximately 20 to 40 mg/dl.[19–21] These research studies involved diabetic patients who were treated by diet alone. None of the participants developed hypoglycemia; in fact all remained with elevated plasma glucose despite the exercise-induced reductions of hyperglycemia. It is reasonable to anticipate potentially greater decreases in blood glucose when patients are using pharmacologic agents, such as sulfonylurea drugs or insulin. Indeed, many patients treated with these agents experience mild-to-moderate symptoms of hypoglycemia during exercise. Less information has been published concerning plasma glucose lowering during exercise when patients are treated with insulin-sensitizing agents such as metformin or a thiazolidinedione (e.g., troglitazone, rosiglitazone, and pioglitazone). Though these agents do not induce hypoglycemia when used as monotherapy, the effects with concomitant exercise have not been systematically described.

The mechanisms that account for lowering of plasma glucose in patients with diabetes during exercise have been examined. In those without diabetes, rates of increased glucose utilization by skeletal muscle are counterbalanced by increased rates of glucose production from the liver. The increase in glucose production, as well as an increased production of fatty acids during exercise is related to a relatively small but essential decline in circulating insulin levels, as well as increments in counterregulatory hormones (e.g., catecholamines, growth hormone, and glucagon). Clearly, in view of a decline in plasma glucose levels in patients with diabetes during exercise there is an imbalance of these two processes in favor of a net increase in glucose utilization. Earlier studies in patients with type 2 diabetes attributed the decline in plasma glucose during exercise chiefly to a blunted increase of glucose production by the liver.[22] However, several studies offer an alternative explanation.

An investigation by Colberg et al[20] employed isotope dilution methods as well as respiratory gas exchange to examine the flux and oxidation of substrates. They found that the overall oxidation of glucose and lipids was similar among subjects with type 2 diabetes in comparison with lean and obese subjects without diabetes when they exercised at moderate intensity (45% Vo_2 max) using cycle ergometry. However, the utilization of plasma glucose was actually greater in type 2 diabetes, while the utilization of muscle glycogen was reduced during exercise. Hepatic responses were similar in subjects with and without diabetes (Fig. 20.3). Three additional studies affirm these findings. Martin et al[23] examined the use of plasma glucose by exercising muscle through limb balance measurements that involved the determination of arteriovenous differences across the leg. Individuals with diabetes had higher rates of glucose uptake at equivalent intensity of exercise in comparison to those without diabetes.[23] Similar findings were reported by Kang et al[21] and by Giacca et al,[19] on the basis of isotopic determinations. Thus, these studies indicate that despite insulin resistance, obese patients with type 2 diabetes can have "normal" or even increased utilization of plasma glucose during moderate exercise. The mechanisms that might account for normal or increased glucose utilization in the setting of insulin-resistant diabetes mellitus have also been examined. One of the physiological mechanisms can be increased insulin delivery. While exercise typically causes a fall in insulin levels in those without diabetes, the hyperglycemia and insulin resistance of type 2 diabetes are associated with an elevated fasting insulin level and, typically, there is less or no decline of plasma insulin during exercise. Increased blood flow and capillary recruitment within skeletal muscle leads to increased insulin delivery as well as increased substrate delivery to muscle tissue.

Glucose transport, a process of facilitated transport across the lipid bilayer of sarcolemma, is regarded as the rate-limiting step for glucose metabolism (see review by Goodyear and Kahn).[24] In skeletal muscle, the glucose transport protein isoform, GLUT 4, translocates from a sequestered intracellular vesicle to the cell surface and the region of the transverse tubules in response to insulin. In type 2 diabetes there is impairment of this process and, in fact, this is the putative key defect of reduced insulin-stimulated glucose metabolism in diabetes and obesity-related insulin resistance. However, insulin is not the only mediator of GLUT 4 translocation. Muscle contraction is a potent stimulus for this process, and there is now substantial support for the concept that there are at least two "pools" of GLUT 4, one of which has translocation regulated by insulin and the other primarily regulated by muscle contraction. A study by Kennedy et al[25] found that the translocation of GLUT 4 transporters during exercise was not adversely affected in type 2 diabetes mellitus compared to those without diabetes, while the response to insulin was clearly impaired. These data provide an im-

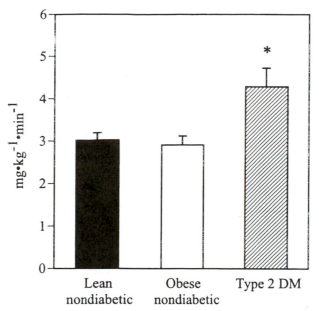

FIGURE 20.3. Rates of glucose utilization during 40 min of mild exercise in lean nondiabetic, obese nondiabetic, and obese diabetic volunteers. Obese diabetic volunteers had significantly greater (p < 0.05) rates of glucose utilization than lean nondiabetic. Adapted with permission *from Colberg SR, Hagberg JM, McCole SD, et al: Utilization of glycogen but not plasma glucose is reduced in individuals with NIDDM during mild-intensity exercise.* J Appl Physiol *81(5):2027–2033, 1996.*

portant clue as to why the uptake of plasma glucose may be increased during exercise in type 2 diabetes, in that the recruitment of glucose transporters in the setting of hyperglycemia would provide a mechanism for mass action effects of increased transport of glucose.

What, if any, are the clinical implications of normal or enhanced glucose uptake during exercise in diabetes mellitus. For the most part, this is probably a positive effect as it helps to reduce hyperglycemia and improve metabolic control. A sustained improvement in metabolic control substantially lowers the risk of end-organ complications in diabetes. However, an acute lowering of plasma glucose could lead to hypoglycemia under certain circumstances. If patients are using medications that further elevate circulating insulin levels, such as injected insulin or oral medications that stimulate insulin secretion (e.g., sul-

fonylureas, repaglinide or netaglinide), then the combination of increased insulin and exercise might produce too great a decline in blood. Without adequate compensation of hepatic glucose production, hypoglycemia could ensue. Typically, in type 2 diabetes, these symptoms are of mild-to-moderate severity, yet patients should be specifically questioned about the occurrence of hypoglycemia symptoms or "weak spells" during exercise that suggests the existence of hypoglycemia. More definite information can be obtained by self-monitoring of blood glucose.

This issue of exercise induced hypoglycemia is even more pertinent for patients with type 1 diabetes, all of whom are receiving insulin injections. If exercise is undertaken concomitant with the peak effects of short-acting insulin preparations, then not only will glucose uptake by tissue be enhanced, but the ability of the liver to produce glucose, and of adipose to release fatty acids will be suppressed and rather marked hypoglycemia can ensue. Thus, as a general concept, exercise for patients with type 1 diabetes should be timed to occur in conjunction with relatively low circulating insulin levels. Typically, these might occur prior to the morning injection or at least 3 h after injection of regular insulin or short-acting insulin analog. Complementary to this is the concept of reducing insulin doses in anticipation of exercise, by 10 to 50% based on prior experience (guided by self-monitoring) and in proportion to the expected intensity and duration of the exercise session.

ACUTE AND CHRONIC EFFECTS OF EXERCISE ON INSULIN RESISTANCE

One of the valuable health benefits of a program of regular physical activity is to improve insulin sensitivity. As previously discussed, an increase in insulin sensitivity denotes that the response to insulin to stimulate glucose utilization is increased in skeletal muscle, and this is most noticeable within the metabolic pathway of glycogen formation. Improved insulin sensitivity can therefore contribute to an overall improvement in glucose control. Moreover, there are other aspects of improved insulin sensitivity and these include lower fasting insulin levels, lower blood pressure, and improvements in lipid profiles. Thus, improved insulin sensitivity may be an important target for overall improvement in cardiovascular health as well as improving glucose control.

The improvement in insulin sensitivity that is induced by exercise can be conceived of as having two aspects, one that is relatively acute and related to each exercise session and another aspect that represents training effects. Among the latter are increased oxidative capacity of skeletal muscle, increased capillary density within muscle, and enhancement of muscle content of GLUT 4 transporters and other biochemical adaptations that improve capacity for substrate utilization. Other chronic factors related to improved insulin

sensitivity include decreased fat mass and increased lean tissue mass. Chronic exercise training results in a multitude of changes consistent with an improved insulin action (Fig. 20.4). Many of these improvements are elicited through the prevention or reversal of the deterioration of metabolic function associated with a sedentary lifestyle. Specifically, changes that may be related to the etiology of type 2 diabetes and prevented by regular exercise include the control of body fat or body composition, capillary perfusion of skeletal muscle, hepatic glucose production, and the bioenergetics within skeletal muscle.

There is a substantial body of data to indicate that even a single session of exercise can ameliorate insulin resistance. The improvement in insulin sensitivity induced by a single exercise session is relatively short-lived, lasting for effectively several days. For example, Devlin and Horton found that a single session of moderate exercise lowered hepatic glucose production for the following day in patients with type 2 diabetes.[26] Rogers et al found that 1 week of daily exercise, at a fairly vigorous intensity (70% of Vo_2 max) had a substantial impact on insulin resistance in patients with type 2 diabetes mellitus and induced marked improvement in glucose tolerance.[27] These are intervals of physical activity that are too brief to induce changes in body composition or to induce changes in oxidative enzyme capacity and capillary density. A single bout of exercise has been demonstrated to increase skeletal muscle sensitivity to insulin and the ability to resynthesize glycogen.[28] The mechanisms responsible for this short-term effect are most likely due to an increase in the number and activity of the GLUT 4 glucose transporters,[29,30] as well as the content and activity of hexokinase[31] in skeletal muscle. In addition, if the exercise is of sufficient intensity, the utilization of muscle glycogen may alter insulin action.

One hypothesis for the acute effects of exercise on insulin sensitivity relate to short-term depletion of muscle glycogen.[21,28] There is "autoregulation" of muscle glycogen content, such that depletion of muscle glycogen leads to en-

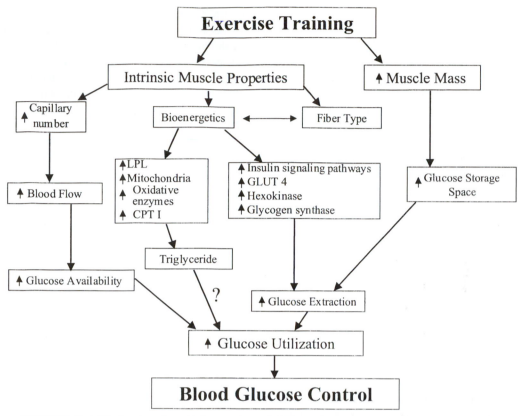

FIGURE 20.4. Mechanisms by which exercise training may improve glucose control through alterations in skeletal muscle.

hanced glucose uptake and repletion of muscle glycogen. The effect of exercise to acutely improve insulin sensitivity may depend on whether there is sufficient utilization of muscle glycogen. This principle was demonstrated in a study by Kang et al[21] Following the experimental paradigm of 7 consecutive days of exercise as used by Rogers et al,[27] Kang et al compared the effect of exercise at 50 versus 70% of Vo_2 max, adjusting the length of exercise at the lesser intensity so that it resulted in equivalent energy expenditure. After 1 week of daily exercise for 50 min at 70% of Vo_2 max, there was an improvement in insulin sensitivity among obese subjects as indicated by lowering plasma insulin responses following ingestion of a standardized glucose load. However, in the same subjects, one week of exercise for 70

min daily at 50% of Vo_2 max did not improve insulin sensitivity despite the expenditure of equivalent calories. During these investigations, Kang et al determined rates of carbohydrate and lipid oxidation and rates of utilization of plasma glucose, the latter performed using isotope dilution methods. At the higher intensity exercise, oxidation of carbohydrates accounts for a higher proportion of energy expenditure than that which occurred at the lesser intensity. However, rates of utilization of plasma glucose were similar and in both cases were less than rates of overall carbohydrate oxidation. The "deficit" between carbohydrate oxidation and use of plasma glucose represents the use of muscle glycogen as a substrate for oxidation. In the studies by Kang et al, the postexercise reductions in insulin were related to the amount of glycogen oxidation, thus providing support for the concept that short-term effects of exercise on insulin sensitivity are related to depletion of muscle glycogen.

There are several potential implications of these findings. First, the positive effects of the more vigorous exercise seem consistent with the epidemiologic data that more vigorous exercise has greater effectiveness in preventing the onset of diabetes mellitus.[7,8] Perhaps periodic depletion of glycogen stores are necessary or at least valuable in providing a metabolic signal to upregulate insulin sensitivity and the attendant capacity for efficient metabolism of glucose. Thus, ideally, one would advocate at least periodic vigorous exercise in order to achieve an optimal effect on insulin sensitivity, and this would be with the purpose of expending muscle glycogen. The principal limitation to implementing this type of plan is whether it is practical for many of the individuals with diabetes or those at risk for diabetes. Previously sedentary individuals may not find it feasible to exercise at a high enough level of intensity or for a long enough interval to attain a sufficient depletion of muscle glycogen. Moreover, and perhaps equally important, many previously sedentary individuals may find this approach to be of unacceptable rigor or too demanding to sustain on a regular schedule. With these important caveats in mind, it is nonetheless worthwhile to implement at least periodic vigorous exercise for those individuals who are able to undertake it.

Another important study also emphasizes the importance of the acute versus the chronic effects of exercise in determining how exercise influences insulin sensitivity. Segal and her colleagues carried out supervised exercise sessions for 12 weeks among previously sedentary lean and obese individuals.[32] Following the 12 weeks of interventions, maximal aerobic capacity was increased significantly, along with other changes in the usual parameters of increased fitness. However, one of the goals of this study was to prevent changes in weight by adjusting calorie intake, and, by design, no changes in body weight

occurred. Moreover, posttraining assessments of insulin action were performed 4 to 5 days following the last exercise session so that sufficient time was permitted for the acute effects to dissipate. Insulin action was measured by the insulin infusion (glucose clamp) procedure, widely regarded as the "gold standard" method to measure insulin resistance and following 12 weeks of aerobic exercise training no change in insulin action was observed. Thus, these findings of Segal et al[32] seem to indicate that either or both the acute effects of exercise and the changes in body composition are of crucial importance in eliciting a positive effect on insulin resistance. Studies such as these reinforce the importance of a regular schedule of exercise and that the program involve physical activity at least 3 times weekly to have an impact upon insulin sensitivity. These data further suggest the importance of collateral effects on body composition.

EFFECTS OF EXERCISE TRAINING ON GLUCOSE CONTROL IN TYPE 2 DIABETES MELLITUS

In general, exercise training has been demonstrated to improve glucose tolerance in glucose-intolerant subjects. Similar effects can be found in patients with type 2 diabetes mellitus, but these findings are less consistent; moreover, the effects of exercise training on glucose control in type 2 diabetes mellitus are equivocal. Schneider et al[33] found that aerobic exercise performed 4 times per week for 1 year reduced fasting plasma glucose in patients with type 2 diabetes. Heath et al[34] found similar results for a similar intervention and duration. Holloszy et al[35] found that 1 year of exercise training in subjects classified as mildly diabetic had an improved glucose tolerance and insulin action concomitant with a normalization of fasting plasma glucose levels. These results are in accordance with those from Reitman et al,[36] who found reduced fasting plasma glucose levels and an improved glucose tolerance following up to 10 weeks of exercise training. Not all exercise training intervention studies, however, have shown improvement in glucose control in subjects with diabetes. Schneider et al[37] found that individuals with type 2 diabetes mellitus engaged in only 6 weeks of aerobic exercise training did not reduce fasting plasma glucose or alter glucose tolerance, although HbA_{1C} was significantly reduced with training, indicating an overall improvement in glucose homeostasis. Dela et al[38] found that 10 weeks of exercise training in individuals with type 2 diabetes resulted in an increase in insulin-stimulated skeletal muscle glucose clearance (Fig. 20.5), but fasting plasma glucose did not change. Segal et al[32] also found no effect of a 12-week supervised aerobic exercise program on fasting plasma glucose. Thus, it appears that improved glucose control can result if regular exercise is maintained for a sufficient period of time. However, short-term exercise in-

tervention studies in which there were little or no changes in body weight have produced less than dramatic results in glucose control. It is not certain then whether the beneficial effects of exercise training on glucose control are due to exercise per se or rather to concomitant changes in body weight or body composition. Another factor concerns the severity of the defect in insulin secretion. In some individuals with severe defects of insulin secretion, there may not be sufficient insulin produced to take advantage of an improved insulin sensitivity and, hence, glucose tolerance may not improve. Nevertheless, a program of regular exercise can indirectly improve glucose control in type 2 diabetes by improving overall energy metabolism and maintaining body weight.

Studies on the effects of resistance training in type 2 diabetes are not available, although one study[39] found that aerobic and resistance training

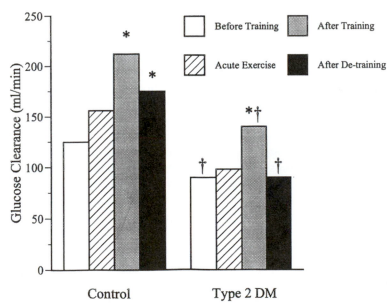

FIGURE 20.5. Insulin-stimulated leg glucose clearance in healthy control subjects and in patients with type 2 diabetes mellitus (DM) before a 10-week one-legged cycling exercise training program, after acute exercise, after training, and after detraining. Significantly different (p < 0.05): * From before training; † from control subjects under the same condition. Detraining values decreased in patients with diabetes mellitus but not in control subjects. *Adapted with permission from Dela F, Larsen JJ, Mikines KJ, et al: Insulin-stimulated muscle glucose clearance in patients with NIDDM.* Diabetes *44:1010–1020, 1995.*

had similar effects on insulin action. This suggests that improvements in insulin action from exercise training can occur without concurrent improvements in cardiorespiratory fitness. This evidence is bolstered by results from short-term exercise training interventions in which no improvements in cardiorespiratory fitness were observed.[27] Thus, questions arise regarding the length of exercise effects and the relative impact of short-term versus long-term exercise training.

UTILIZATION OF LIPID DURING EXERCISE

The use of lipid calories during exercise is also an important and potentially valuable advantage of exercise in patients with diabetes, especially those with type 2 diabetes mellitus. This is important both from the perspectives of weight control and management of dyslipidemias. While exercise alone is generally not as effective as dietary restrictions for achieving weight loss,[40] the combination of exercise and calorie restriction is particularly effective.[41,42] More than one-half of the adult population in the United States is overweight. The prevalence of obesity among patients with type 2 diabetes is even higher than one-half of the adult population, and obesity is a strong risk factor for those with type 2 diabetes, as well as other components of the insulin-resistant syndrome. Moreover, weight loss can have powerful effects in improving metabolic control in type 2 diabetes. One of the principal aspects of modern lifestyles that appear to contribute to the high prevalence of obesity is physical inactivity. Therefore, there is considerable interest in whether exercise should be part of the treatment of obesity, obesity-related insulin resistance, and diabetes complicated by obesity. It is not clear, however, if physical activity, at least by itself, is an effective means to achieve weight loss. Caloric restriction would appear to have greater efficacy for inducing weight loss than would exercise, when the two are compared as isolated treatments. In part, this may be due to the inability of

obese, previously sedentary individuals to engage in exercise of high enough intensity and adequate duration to expend sufficient calories. However, a weight-loss intervention in which exercise is combined with calorie restriction has been found to result in greater weight loss than do diet interventions alone.

The typical pattern of weight loss is that after an interval of several months, an individual begins to find it progressively more difficult to lose more weight and, instead, body weight seems to level off at a new plateau. Among the factors contributing to the response is the decline in resting energy expenditure. A decline in resting energy expenditure by skeletal muscle is a chief contributor to this response. Indeed, a number of homeostatic responses develop following weight loss that either act to prevent additional weight loss or favor weight regain. Inability to maintain a reduced weight is perhaps an even greater challenge than is achieving the initial weight loss. It is in the domain of "weight maintenance" that exercise interventions have proven very useful. Studies based on a weight-loss registry indicate that postobese individuals who have been successful in maintaining a lower body weight than previously typically adhere to a program of regular exercise.

There are several plausible reasons for effectiveness of exercise in maintaining weight, even if exercise per se is not highly effective as a means to initially achieve weight loss. The first explanation relates to achieving a higher level of energy expenditure than normal. Another explanation may relate to the effects of a chronic exercise program to promote the oxidation of fat. At rest, skeletal muscle, like cardiac muscle, normally relies predominately on the oxidation of lipid calories derived from plasma fatty acids, as well as triglycerides stored within muscle fibers. This reliance on lipid oxidation for energy production during fasting conditions is perturbed in obesity[43,44] and type 2 diabetes mellitus.[43] Skeletal muscle in obesity and type 2 diabetes mellitus has a reduced oxidative enzyme activity[45] and, even more specific to the catabolism of fatty acids, a reduced activity of carnitine palmitoyl trans-ferase, regarded as the rate-limiting step for fatty acid oxidation. Rates of fatty acid uptake by muscle are similar in lean and obese subjects, so in the face of reduced lipid oxidation, there is a disposition in obesity for increased fatty acid esterification. In obesity and type 2 diabetes mellitus, there is increased triglyceride deposition within skeletal muscle,[18,46] and there has been increased interest in examining the potentially adverse metabolic associations of increased muscle triglyceride.

Several clinical investigations have demonstrated a potential link between insulin-resistant glucose metabolism and muscle triglyceride.[47–52] Pan and colleagues[49] found that among 38 male Pima Indians without diabetes, an ethnic group with a pronounced disposition for obesity and type 2 diabetes, triglyceride content in skeletal muscle was found to be inversely related to insulin sensitivity. These results are in accordance with others demonstrating a negative association between muscle triglyceride content and insulin-stimulated glucose uptake.[45,51]

Exercise is a key physiological stimulus for the utilization of muscle triglyceride. During contractile activity or exercise, intracellular stores of lipid, or intramuscular triglyceride, can provide up to 25% of energy requirements.[13] These data are affirmed by magnetic resonance spectroscopy (MRS) studies by Boesch et al[53] who found that a single bout of vigorous exercise could lower intramuscular lipid in human volunteers. Collateral studies with biopsy samples using electron microscopy revealed close proximity of lipid droplets to mitochondria within myocytes, supporting the concept that intramuscular triglyceride can be positioned for ready access to oxidative metabolism. Other investigators have made similar observations.[54] Whether the intramuscle lipid in obese and insulin-resistant individuals follows this same cellular distribution is an important question to be addressed, and one might hypothesize that rates of mobilization and access to mitochondria might differ within physically trained muscle as compared to sedentary muscle.

Exercise training increases the oxidative capacity of skeletal muscle[55] and, thus, enhances its capacity for lipid oxidation. A major part of this adaptation appears to be an enhanced capacity to utilize muscle triglyceride.[12] Whether muscle triglyceride content is increased with training is equivocal,[56,57] but the evidence suggests that this energy store can be utilized during exercise. The lack of physical activity in type 2 diabetes could contribute to the accumulation of this substrate within muscle and exacerbate muscle insulin resistance. Thus, the possibility remains that part of the effect of exercise training to enhance insulin sensitivity of skeletal muscle is through the turnover of this storage fuel.

Also, several investigators have begun to evaluate the role of the adenosine monophosphate (AMP) kinase signaling pathway in mediating certain aspects of insulin resistance.[58–61] Interestingly, AMP kinase has a key role both in mediating GLUT 4 translocation in skeletal muscle and in stimulating lipid oxidation. Of additional importance, AMP kinase activity is typically increased sharply by exercise. Thus, this pathway may account for the effects of exercise to promote increased glucose uptake, independent of insulin, while simultaneously increasing fat oxidation—a physiological profile distinct from that of the response to insulin—which promotes glucose uptake while suppressing fat oxidation. While it is clear that there are substantial defects in insulin signaling in relation to type 2 diabetes mellitus, studies suggest that there are also impediments in the AMP kinase pathway. This may be directly relevant to the role of exercise (or sedentary behavior) in relation to type 2 diabetes mellitus.

Another development is that leptin may also help to regulate muscle triglyceride content. Leptin has an overall role to enhance energy expenditure.[62] In skeletal muscle, Shimabukuro et al[52] found that in vivo administration of leptin acted to lower muscle triglyceride in rats. However, exercise does not seem to have a dramatic effect on serum leptin levels,[63,64] thus the effects of exercise to increase insulin sensitivity does not appear to be governed by leptin.

CLINICAL ASPECTS OF EXERCISE IN DIABETES MELLITUS

THE EXERCISE PRESCRIPTION

Constructing and implementing an exercise program begins with a systematic plan. While the fundamental aspects of an exercise prescription involve the type of exercise, duration, frequency, intensity, and timing of activity, the safety of the participant should also be emphasized. Thus, beginning an exercise program should begin with a thorough evaluation, including a medical screening as discussed earlier. The basics of exercise prescription should not be viewed as a rigid regime. Rather, the exercise program should be individualized as much as possible based on the participant's goals and concerns. An obese middle-age patient with type 2 diabetes may be primarily interested in weight control and increased insulin sensitivity, whereas a young patient with type 1 diabetes may be more concerned with improvements in physical fitness and a desire for sports competition. Thus, the following exercise guidelines should be viewed only as guidelines for exercise prescription in order to achieve optimal health benefits from exercise. For a more detailed description of the exercise prescription for the patient with diabetes see Table 20.1.[65,66]

TABLE 20.1. SUMMARY OF EXERCISE PRESCRIPTION FOR PATIENTS WITH DIABETES

Type	Aerobic (e.g., walking, jogging, cycling, or swimming)
Frequency	3–5 times per week
Duration	20–60 min
Intensity	50–75% of maximal aerobic capacity
Timing	Time exercise so that it does not coincide with peak insulin absorption

Adapted with permission from Gordon NF: The Health Professional's Guide to Diabetes and Exercise. Alexandria, VA: American Diabetes Association, 1995, p. 335 and Medicine AC. S. The recommended quantity and quality of exercise for developing and maintaining cardiorespiratory and muscular fitness in healthy adults (position of the American College of Sports Medicine). *Med Sci Sports Exerc* 22:265–274, 1990.

Traditionally, the exercise prescription for patients with diabetes has emphasized, nearly exclusively, forms of physical activity characterized by aerobic activity such as cycling, jogging, and walking. In contrast, resistance training was not given much emphasis. Recent studies have rechallenged these precepts.[67,68] In the first place, recognizing that a minority of patients regularly undertake exercise, it seems counterproductive to discourage virtually any form of exercise unless there are clear adverse effects. Many individuals prefer resistance training. Moreover, studies emphasize the potential positive values of resistance training. Resistance training can maintain skeletal muscle mass and, thus, counter the age-related effects of loss of muscle mass (see review by Evans).[69] Among other positive effects, increased skeletal muscle could potentially increase the capacity for glucose utilization. Increases in insulin sensitivity have been found in response to resistance training in patients with diabetes mellitus (Table 20.2).

The patient with type 1 diabetes (described in Table 20.2) checks his or her blood glucose in the morning before breakfast and injects a combination of slow-acting and fast-acting insulin. He or she waits at least 1 h following breakfast to run to minimize the risk of hypoglycemia. He or she checks his or her glucose again before the run and, in general, if his or her glucose is too high (> 230 mg/dl), he or she injects extra fast-acting insulin. If it is too low (< 110 mg/dl), he or she eats extra carbohydrates. Exercise increases his or her insulin sensitivity so that when he or she is training, his or her insulin demands are substantially reduced. This case demonstrates that good glucose control can result from proper self-monitoring of blood glucose levels prior to and following exercise. The importance of ingesting extra carbohydrates should be emphasized not only in serious athletes or for those participating in strenuous exercise, but also for any patient with type 1 diabetes engaged in physical activity. Thus, this topic deserves special attention.

TABLE 20.2. ADJUSTMENT OF INSULIN DOSE AND BLOOD GLUCOSE LEVELS IN TYPE I DIABETIC RUNNER ON INTENSIVE INSULIN THERAPY

| Day | Insulin Dose (U) (Regular/NPH) | | | | Blood Glucose (mg/dl) | | | | | |
	Breakfast R/NPH	Lunch R	Dinner R	Bedtime NPH	Breakfast	Prerun	Lunch	Dinner	Bedtime	Running
M	4/10	6	4	6	131	120	125	120	135	4 miles
T	4/10	4	4	6	105	125	90	110	145	9 miles
W	4/10	2	4	6	125	131	100	125	122	12 miles
Th	4/10	2	4	6	105	156	125	115	120	Interval running
F	8/10	6	6	6	136	139	114	120	135	No running

NPH, neutral protamine Hagedorn.

SCREENING

Cardiovascular disease is a major cause of mortality in patients with diabetes mellitus and one of the goals of a program of regular exercise is to mitigate the heightened risk of cardiovascular disease associated with diabetes. It is important, however, that patients be evaluated for the presence of cardiovascular disease, in terms of ischemic threshold, propensity for arrhythmias, and left ventricular function. This information can be used to modify the exercise prescription.

Before undergoing an exercise program, all patients with diabetes should undergo a physical examination and history to evaluate cardiovascular function and end-organ complications. In regard to the cardiovascular evaluation, a graded exercise test is needed for patients at high risk for underlying ischemic heart disease. The following criteria for graded exercise testing is recommended:

Type 2 diabetes mellitus with > 10 years duration or all patients > 35 years of age; presence of microvascular disease (retinopathy, nephropathy, or proteinuria); peripheral vascular disease or additional risk factors for coronary artery disease; and presence of autonomic neuropathy.

The exercise test can provide information regarding the initial level of exercise capacity. Exercise of moderate intensity is recommended for patients with known coronary artery disease, being in general targeted at 60 to 80% of maximum heart rate. The target heart rate should be set for at least 10 beats per minute less than the rate of the ischemic threshold. It is also important to attain adequate blood pressure control in patients with hypertension, and, for those patients with moderate or severe hypertension, the blood pressure response to exercise should be monitored initially. The use of a structured and supervised exercise program may be useful in these situations.

For patients with the complication of autonomic neuropathy, exercise must be undertaken with considerable caution. The parasympathetic dysfunction can result in an elevated basal heart rate. However, during exercise there is a blunted heart rate response, perturbated regulation of peripheral vascular resistance, and therefore a decreased cardiac output response during exercise—effects that can be further compounded by left ventricular dysfunction. For those patients with orthostatic hypotension, extra time of warm-up and cool-down should be performed to avoid symptomatic hypotension.

In all patients with diabetes mellitus, one of

the key aspects of the physical examination is an evaluation of the feet with respect to integrity of the skin, adequacy of circulation, and for the presence and severity of neuropathy. Because an exercise program generally involves the use of lower extremities, the value of a careful lower extremity and foot examination is of particular importance to appraise the risk for foot ulceration. Patients who are insensate to monofilament pressure (Semmes-Weinstein 5.07 monofilament) identifies them as being at heightened risk for ulceration. Therefore, exercises such as walking or jogging must be undertaken cautiously, and only after prescription of proper footware. The presence of foot deformities such as Charcot foot makes the risk of ulceration especially high, and alternative exercise should be advocated such as swimming or stationary cycling. Removal of calluses can have a substantial effect on reducing pressure on the foot and thereby lowering the risk of ulceration.

EXERCISE IN TYPE 1 DIABETES MELLITUS

One of the homeostatic responses to exercise is a modest reduction in plasma insulin, and this response is key for the rise in hepatic glucose production (to maintain stable plasma glucose) and for increased rates of lipolysis. In type 1 diabetes mellitus, it is difficult to emulate this decline in insulin. Ideally, exercise is performed when insulin levels are relatively low, as occur in the morning. The caveat is that if the insulin levels are too low, then the rise in catecholamines can trigger hyperglycemia or even ketoacidosis. To avoid hypoglycemia, insulin doses are reduced. For moderate exercise, short-acting insulin doses should be reduced by approximately 33 to 50%, and more if the exercise is of a longer duration. For patients with continuous subcutaneous insulin injections (external pumps), discontinuation of the basal insulin infusion can indeed replicate the normal physiological decline in insulin. While these general concepts are a starting point, the best criterion

is to perform individual monitoring of blood glucose. Patients should be instructed to perform self-monitoring prior to exercise and at the conclusion of exercise. This information can then be used to individualize the insulin adjustments.

Patients should be instructed not to inject insulin in the arms or legs prior to planned exercise since the increased blood flow can increase the rate of insulin absorption and thus increase the risk of a hypoglycemic reaction.

Case Presentation

Exercise for the patient with type 1 diabetes poses special problems because of the risk of hypoglycemia when exercise is combined with insulin therapy. Thus, special consideration should be given to the exercise prescription in these patients, particularly with respect to the timing of exercise and taking steps to avoid hypoglycemia. The importance of altering insulin dose and carbohydrate intake in conjunction with exercise is highlighted in the case presentation of a runner who happens to have diabetes.

A 42-year-old white male was diagnosed with type 1 diabetes mellitus 4 years prior, after complaining of 2 to 3 months of weight loss, blurred vision, fatigue, polydipsia, and polyuria. He had been training for a marathon run prior to admission and attributed his weight loss to his exercise program. At the time of presentation, the following test results were obtained:

Glucose: 539 mg/dl

Bicarbonate: 18

Anion gap: 23

β-hydroxybutyric acid: 5.3 mg/dl
   (normal: < 2.8 mg/dl)

Urine ketones: 80 mg/dl

Glycosylated hemoglobin: 18.8%

C-peptide: < 0.22

Random insulin: 5μU/mL
   (normal: 0.7–9.0 μU)

He was initially started on 70/30 insulin twice a day. He has continued to exercise regularly and is hoping to resume marathon running. He is currently running approximately 35 to 40 miles per week and is following an intensified insulin therapy regimen (described in the following section). He has no complications of diabetes, and HbA_{1C} levels have dropped to 8.9%.

FOOD INTAKE AND EXERCISE IN DIABETES

Ingestion of carbohydrates before, during, and following exercise in healthy individuals can have a dramatic impact on glucose metabolism,[70,71] and it is well known that carbohydrate ingestion during exercise in those without diabetes helps to maintain blood glucose levels.[15,70] However, the risk of hypoglycemia during exercise in type 2 diabetes, particularly for those not on insulin therapy, is low. Therefore, ingestion of excess carbohydrates before, during, or after exercise in these patients should be viewed with caution as it may simply contribute to an excess caloric intake. For the patient with type 1 diabetes or the patient with type 2 diabetes on insulin therapy, some practical considerations should be given with regard to carbohydrate and fluid ingestion in conjunction with exercise:

1. Consume adequate fluids before, during, and following exercise to help prevent dehydration during exercise. During hot and humid weather when greater sweat loss is expected, consider the use of "sport drinks," which contain electrolytes (sodium and potassium) to help restore salt losses. However, realize that most of these products also contain a high amount of sugar, which may affect blood glucose.
2. Eating carbohydrates in the hours before exercise generally does not have adverse effects on exercise capacity. Avoid food with a high fiber or fat content before and during exercise to prevent gastrointestinal problems.
3. During exercise lasting ≥ 45 min, have a carbohydrate drink or snack solution to avoid low

blood glucose and to improve exercise tolerance.
4. Choose carbohydrates ingested before or during exercise that are easily digestible (glucose, sucrose, glucose polymer, etc.) when taken in moderate quantities. Fructose-containing beverages and fruit juice may cause greater gastrointestinal discomfort.
5. Following exercise, ingest modest carbohydrates to minimize the risk of late-acting hypoglycemia induced by an increased insulin sensitivity following exercise.

The preceding section on exercise prescription is meant only to serve as a basic guide to physicians and health professionals who treat or prescribe exercise for the patient with diabetes. Individuals interested in competitive sports should be carefully managed, and those with diabetic complications should receive additional consideration. For more detailed information on exercise prescription for the patient with diabetes and for special diabetic populations, see the guidelines suggested by Gordon.[65]

ADJUSTING MEDICATION IN TYPE 2 DIABETES MELLITUS

In patients with type 2 diabetes mellitus, weight loss and exercise can reduce the need for oral hypoglycemic agents. In the past, virtually the only oral agent used to treat type 2 diabetes mellitus was sulfonylurea, a class of drugs that stimulated insulin secretion. Thus, exercise, even of light-to-moderate intensity, could precipitate hypoglycemic reactions in sulfonylurea-treated patients, though fortunately, most of these reactions were of mild-to-moderate intensity. However, biguanides (metformin) and thiazolidinediones (e.g., troglitazone) increase insulin sensitivity and do not stimulate insulin secretion. There are relatively little data on specific effects of these agents upon glucose homeostasis during exercise. However, one might anticipate that there would not be much risk of hypoglycemia.

SUMMARY

In this chapter we have examined the importance of exercise in type 1 (insulin-dependent) and type 2 (non-insulin-dependent) diabetes mellitus. The incidence of type 2 diabetes is steadily on the rise in the United States and Westernized societies, owing largely to the increase in the prevalence of obesity and the lack of physical activity in these "advanced" cultures. The etiology and pathophysiology of type 2 diabetes are very complex, and, while it is often difficult to distinguish physical activity and obesity as causal factors for the development of diabetes, there is a preponderance of data from large-scale epidemiologic studies suggesting that the lack of physical activity is an independent risk factor for the disease.[6–10] Furthermore, the available evidence suggests that men and women who are at the greatest risk for developing type 2 diabetes are those persons who would derive the greatest benefit from an increase in physical activity. Therefore, getting the most sedentary people to modestly increase their physical activity will probably have the greatest impact on the reduction in the incidence of the disease.

The pathogenesis of type 2 diabetes involves an inability of skeletal muscle to respond to insulin to stimulate glucose uptake, a condition of insulin resistance that normally precedes overt diabetes. While obesity is a major factor in the development of insulin resistance, this condition has been linked to a reduced aerobic capacity, both on a whole-body and skeletal muscle level. There is also an impaired ability to utilize lipid for energy during resting conditions in insulin resistance and in type 2 diabetes, perhaps creating a vicious cycle of inactivity, increased obesity, and further metabolic impairment. Both acute and chronic exercise can have favorable effects on skeletal muscle in improving the insulin-resistant state through their action on energy substrate utilization and storage depots of muscle glycogen and muscle triglyceride. A single exercise session has a dramatic impact on muscle metabolism, so that in many respects there is a "normalization" of metabolism that occurs with each bout of exercise; therefore, at least part of the benefit of an exercise program is derived from single exercise sessions. Chronic exercise is associated with an enhanced metabolic capacity of the muscle to metabolize both lipid and carbohydrate for energy so that there is an effect of exercise training to increase overall energy expenditure and prevent excess fat storage. The strong link between obesity and type 2 diabetes suggests that combining exercise with effective weight-loss and weight maintenance programs is probably the best strategy to maintain caloric balance and to prevent and treat type 2 diabetes. Moreover, given the strong association between obesity, physical activity, and the development of cardiovascular disease, it is clear how exercise may simultaneously reduce the risk for cardiovascular disease and type 2 diabetes. The presence of overt diabetes may provide particular obstacles for exercise, and we have given attention to specific exercise prescriptions for both the patient with type 1 and type 2 diabetes, including special consideration for patients with type 1 diabetes with regard to the timing and doses of insulin.

Now that we have been armed with convincing evidence that exercise is beneficial to prevent and treat type 2 diabetes, what more can we or should we know about the role of exercise in diabetes? First, more research needs to focus on the quantity and intensity of exercise required to elicit improvements in insulin action and glucose control in type 2 diabetes. We need to gain a better understanding of how much or what type of exercise should be performed as a means to prevent the disease versus treat existing disease. We also know little about the interaction of many of the currently popular diabetic medications, particularly newly developed insulin-sensitizing agents, with exercise. Combining these drugs with exercise may indeed be an effective strategy to improve glucose control in many patients with diabetes. There is limited data regarding potential differences with respect to either gender, race, or age on the ability of exercise to improve glucose control. However, the vast majority of evidence indicates that most patients with diabetes should greatly benefit from traditional exercise programs designed to increase cardiovascular and muscular fitness.

REFERENCES

1. Harris MI: Prevalence of non-insulin-dependent diabetes and impaired glucose tolerance, in Harris MI, Hamman RF (eds.): *Diabetes in America.* Washington, DC, U.S. Gov. Printing Office. National Diabetes Data Group, USDHHS, NIH Publication no. 85–1468, 1985, pp. VI, 1–31.
2. Randle PJ, Garland PB, Hales CN, et al: The glucose fatty acid cycle: Its role in insulin sensitivity and the metabolic disturbances of diabetes mellitus. *Lancet* 1:785–789, 1963.
3. Brown MD, Moore GE, Korytkowski MT, et al:

Improvement of insulin sensitivity by short-term exercise training in hypertensive African American women. *Hypertension* 30:1549–1553, 1997.

4. Ruderman N, Chisholm D, Pi-Sunyer X, et al: The metabolically obese, normal-weight individual revisited (Review). *Diabetes* 47:699–713, 1998.

5. Torjesen PA, Birkeland KI, Anderssen SA, et al: Lifestyle changes may reverse development of the insulin resistance syndrome. The Oslo Diet and Exercise Study: A randomized trial. *Diabetes Care* 20:26–31, 1997.

6. Eriksson K-F, Lindgärde F: Poor physical fitness, and impaired early insulin response but late hyperinsulinaemia, as predictors of NIDDM in middle-aged Swedish men. *Diabetologica* 39:573–579, 1996.

7. Helmrich SP, Ragland DR, Leung RW, et al: Physical activity and reduced occurrence of non-insulin-dependent diabetes mellitus. *N Engl J Med* 325:147–152, 1991.

8. Manson JE, Rimm EB, Stampfer MJ, et al: Physical activity and incidence of non-insulin-dependent diabetes mellitus in women. *Lancet* 338:774–778, 1991.

9. Manson JE, Nathan DM, Krolewski AS, et al: A prospective study of exercise and incidence of diabetes among US male physicians. *JAMA* 268(1): 63–67, 1992.

10. Pan XR, Li GW, Hu YH, et al: Effects of diet and exercise in preventing NIDDM in people with impaired glucose tolerance. The Da Qing IGT and Diabetes Study. *Diabetes Care* 20(4):537–544, 1997.

11. Eriksson K-F, Lindgärde F: Prevention of Type 2 (non-insulin-dependent) diabetes mellitus by diet and physical exercise. *Diabetologica* 34:891–898, 1991.

12. Martin WH: Effects of acute and chronic exercise on fat metabolism (Review). *Exerc Sport Sci Rev* 24:203–231, 1996.

13. Romijn JA, Coyle EF, Sidossis LS, et al: Regulation of endogenous fat and carbohydrate metabolism in relation to exercise intensity and duration. *Am J Physiol (Endocrinol Metabol)* 265:E380–E391, 1993.

14. Brooks GA: Importance of the 'crossover' concept in exercise metabolism. *Clin Exper Pharmacol Physiol* 24:889–895, 1997.

15. Coggan AR: Plasma glucose metabolism during exercise: Effect of endurance training in humans

(Review). *Med Sci Sports Exerc* 29(5):620–627, 1997.

16. Coyle EF, Jeukendrup AE, Wagenmakers AJ, et al: Fatty acid oxidation is directly regulated by carbohydrate metabolism during exercise. *Am J Physiol* 273:E268–E275, 1997.

17. Sidossis LS, Gastaldelli A, Klein S, et al: Regulation of plasma fatty acid oxidation during low- and high-intensity exercise. *Am J Physiol* 272: E1065–E1070, 1997.

18. Theriault R, Goodpaster B, Kelley D: Intramuscular lipid content quantified by histochemistry is increased in obesity and type 2 diabetes mellitus. *Diabetes* 47(Supplement):314, #1221, 1998.

19. Giacca A, Groenewoud Y, Tsui E, et al: Glucose production, utilization, and cycling in response to moderate exercise in obese subjects with type 2 diabetes and mild hyperglycemia. *Diabetes* 47: 1763–1770, 1998.

20. Colberg SR, Hagberg JM, McCole SD, et al: Utilization of glycogen but not plasma glucose is reduced in individuals with NIDDM during mild-intensity exercise. *J Appl Physiol* 81:2027– 2033, 1996.

21. Kang J, Robertson RJ, Hagberg JM, et al: Effect of exercise intensity on glucose and insulin metabolism in obese individuals and obese NIDDM patients. *Diabetes Care* 19:341–349, 1996.

22. Minuk HL, Vranic M, Marliss EB, et al: Glucoregulatory and metabolic response to exercise in obese noninsulin-dependent diabetes. *Am J Physiol (Endocrin Metabol)* 240:E458–E464, 1981.

23. Martin IK, Katz A, Wahren J: Splanchnic and muscle metabolism during exercise in NIDDM patients. *American J Physiol (Endocrinol Metabol)* 269:E583–E590, 1995.

24. Goodyear LJ, Kahn BB: Exercise, glucose transport, and insulin sensitivity (Review). *Ann Rev Med* 49:235–261, 1998.

25. Kennedy JW, Hirshman MF, Gervino EV, et al: Acute exercise induces GLUT4 translocation in skeletal muscle of normal human subjects and subjects with type 2 diabetes. *Diabetes* 48: 1192–1197, 1999.

26. Devlin JT, Horton ES: Effects of prior high-intensity exercise on glucose metabolism in normal and insulin-resistant men. *Diabetes* 34:973–979, 1985.

27. Rogers MA, Yamamoto C, King DS, et al:

Improvement in glucose tolerance after 1 week of exercise in patients with mild NIDDM. *Diabetes Care* 11:613–618, 1988.

28. Perseghin G, Price TB, Petersen KF, et al: Increased glucose transport-phosphorylation and muscle glycogen synthesis after exercise training in insulin-resistant subjects. *N Engl J Med* 335:1357–1362, 1996.

29. Houmard JA, Shinebarger MH, Dolan PL, et al: Exercise training increases GLUT-4 protein concentration in previously sedentary middle-aged men. *Am J Physiol* 264:E896–E901, 1993.

30. Houmard JA, Hickey MS, Tyndall GL, et al: Seven days of exercise increase GLUT-4 protein content in human skeletal muscle. *J Appl Physiol* 79: 1936–1938, 1995.

31. Koval JA, DeFronzo RA, O'Doherty RM, et al: Regulation of hexokinase II activity and expression in human muscle by moderate exercise. *Am J Physiol (Endocrin Metabol)* 274:E304–E308, 1998.

32. Segal KR, Edano A, Abalos A, et al: Effect of exercise training on insulin sensitivity and glucose metabolism in lean, obese, and diabetic men. *J Appl Physiol* 71:2402–2411, 1991.

33. Schneider SH, Khachadurian AK, Amorosa LF, et al: Ten-year experience with an exercise-based outpatient lifestyle modification program in the treatment of diabetes mellitus. *Diabetes Care* 15(Suppl 4):1800–1810, 1992.

34. Heath GW, Gavin JRD, Hinderliter JM, et al: Effects of exercise and lack of exercise on glucose tolerance and insulin sensitivity. *J Appl Physiol: Respir Environ Exerc Physiol* 55:512–517, 1983.

35. Holloszy JO, Schultz J, Kusnierkiewicz J, et al: Effects of exercise on glucose tolerance and insulin resistance. Brief review and some preliminary results (Review). *Acta Med Scand* 711(Suppl):55–65, 1986.

36. Reitman JS, Vasquez B, Klimes I: Improvement in glucose homeostasis after exercise training in non-insulin-dependent diabetes. *Diabetes Care* 7:434–441, 1984.

37. Schneider SH, Amorosa LF, Khachadurian AK, et al: Studies on the mechanism of improved glucose control during regular exercise in Type 2 (non-insulin-dependent) diabetes. *Diabetologica* 26: 355–360, 1984.

38. Dela F, Larsen JJ, Mikines KJ, et al: Insulin-stimu-

lated muscle glucose clearance in patients with NIDDM. *Diabetes* 44:1010–1020, 1995.

39. Smutok MA, Reece C, Kokkinos PF, et al: Effects of exercise training modality on glucose tolerance in men with abnormal glucose regulation. *Intern J Sports Med* 15:283–289, 1994.

40. Ballor DL, Keesey RE: A meta-analysis of the factors affecting exercise-induced changes in body mass, fat mass and fat-free mass in obese males and females. *Intern J Obes* 15:717–726, 1991.

41. Ross R, Pedwell H, Rissanen J: Effects of energy restriction and exercise on skeletal muscle and adipose tissue in women as measured by magnetic resonance imaging. *Am J Clin Nutr* 61:1179–1185, 1995.

42. Wing RR, Epstein LH, Paternostro-Balyes M, et al: Exercise in a behavioural weight control programme for obese patients with type 2 (non-insulin-dependent) diabetes. *Diabetologica* 31: 902–909, 1988.

43. Kelley DE, Simoneau J-A: Impaired free fatty acid utilization by skeletal muscle in non-insulin-dependent diabetes mellitus. *J Clin Invest* 94: 2349–2356, 1994.

44. Colberg SR, Simoneau J-A, Thaete FL, et al: Skeletal muscle utilization of FFA in women with visceral obesity. *J Clin Invest* 95:1846–1853, 1995.

45. Simoneau JA, Colberg SR, Thaete FL, et al: Skeletal muscle glycolytic and oxidative enzyme capacities are determinants of insulin sensitivity and muscle composition in obese women. *FASEB J* 9:273–278, 1995.

46. Standl E, Lotz N, Dexel T, et al: Muscle triglycerides in diabetic subjects: Effect of insulin deficiency and exercise. *Diabetologia* 18:463–469, 1980.

47. Oakes ND, Camilleri S, Furler SM, et al: The insulin sensitizer, BRL 49653, reduces systemic fatty acid supply and utilization and tissue lipid availability in the rat. *Metabol: Clin Exper* 46: 935–942, 1997.

48. Oakes ND, Bell KS, Furler SM, et al: Diet-induced muscle insulin resistance in rats is ameliorated by acute dietary lipid withdrawal or a single bout of exercise. *Diabetes* 46:2022–2028, 1997.

49. Pan DA, Lillioja S, Kriketos AD, et al: Skeletal muscle triglyceride levels are inversely related to insulin action. *Diabetes* 46:983–988, 1997.

50. Phillips DIW, Caddy S, Ilic V, et al: Intramuscular

triglyceride and muscle insulin sensitivity: Evidence for a relationship in nondiabetic subjects. *Metabolism* 45:947–950, 1996.

51. Goodpaster BH, Thaete FL, Simoneau J-A, et al: Subcutaneous abdominal fat and thigh muscle composition predict insulin sensitivity independently of visceral fat. *Diabetes* 46:1579–1585, 1997.

52. Shimabukuro M, Koyama K, Chen G, et al: Direct antidiabetic effect of leptin through triglyceride depletion of tissues (see comments). Comment in *Proc Natl Acad Sci USA* 94:4242–4245, 1997. *Proc Natl Acad Sci USA* 94:4637– 4641, 1997.

53. Boesch C, Slotboom J, Hoppeler H, et al: In vivo determination of intra-myocellular lipids in human muscle by means of localized 1H-MR-spectroscopy. *Mag Res Med* 37:484–493, 1997.

54. Vock R, Hoppeler H, Claassen H, et al: Design of the oxygen and substrate pathways. VI. Structural basis of intracellular substrate supply to mitochondria in muscle cells. *J Exper Biol* 199: 1689–1697, 1996.

55. Gollnick PD, Saltin B: Significance of skeletal muscle oxidative enzyme enhancement with endurance training. *Clin Physiol* 2:1–12, 1982.

56. Kiens B, Essén-Gustavsson B, Christensen NJ, et al: Skeletal muscle substrate utilization during submaximal exercise in man: Effect of endurance training. *J Physiol (London)* 469:459–478, 1993.

57. Hurley BF, Nemeth PM, Martin WH, et al: Muscle triglyceride utilization during exercise: Effect of training. *J Appl Physiol* 60:562–567, 1986.

58. Hayashi T, Hirshman MF, Kurth EJ, et al: Evidence for 5′ AMP-activated protein kinase mediation of the effect of muscle contraction on glucose transport. *Diabetes* 47:1369–1373, 1998.

59. Cushman SW, Goodyear LJ, Pilch PF, et al: Molecular mechanisms involved in GLUT4 translocation in muscle during insulin and contraction stimulation (Review). *Adv Exper Med Biol* 441:63–71, 1998.

60. Napoli R, Gibson L, Hirshman MF, et al: Epinephrine and insulin stimulate different mitogen-activated protein kinase signaling pathways in rat skeletal muscle. *Diabetes* 47:1549–1554, 1998.

61. Hayashi T, Hirshman MF, Kurth EJ, et al: Evidence for 5′ AMP-activated protein kinase mediation of the effect of muscle contraction on glucose transport. *Diabetes* 47:1369–1373, 1998.

62. Halaas JL, Gajiwala KS, Maffei M, et al: Weight-reducing effects of the plasma protein encoded by the obese gene (see comments). Comment in *Science* 269:475–476, 1995. *Science* 269:543–546, 1995.

63. Racette SB, Coppack SW, Landt M, et al: Leptin production during moderate-intensity aerobic exercise. *J Clin Endocrinol Metabol* 82:2275–2277, 1997.

64. Perusse L, Collier G, Gagnon J, et al: Acute and chronic effects of exercise on leptin levels in humans. *J Appl Phys* 83:5–10, 1997.

65. Gordon NF: *The Health Professional's Guide to Diabetes and Exercise.* Alexandria, VA: American Diabetes Association, 1995, p. 335.

66. Medicine ACoS: The recommended quantity and quality of exercise for developing and maintaining cardiorespiratory and muscular fitness in healthy adults (position stand of the American College of Sports Medicine). *Med Sci Sports Exerc* 22: 265–274, 1990.

67. Eriksson J, Taimela S, Eriksson K, et al: Resistance training in the treatment of non-insulin-dependent diabetes mellitus. *Intern J Sports Med* 18:242–246, 1997.

68. Eriksson J, Touminen J, Valle T, et al: Aerobic endurance exercise or circuit-type resistance training for individuals with impaired glucose tolerance? *Hormone & Metabol Res* 30: 34–41, 1998.

69. Evans WJ: Reversing sarcopenia: How weight training can build strength and vitality. (Review). *Geriatrics* 51: 46–47, 1996.

70. Coggan AR, Spina RJ, Kohrt WM, et al: Plasma glucose kinetics in a well-trained cyclist fed glucose throughout exercise. *Intern J Sport Nutr* 1: 279–288, 1991.

71. Jeukendrup AE, Saris WHM, Brouns F, et al: Effects of carbohydrate (CHO) and fat supplementation on CHO metabolism during prolonged exercise. *Metabolism* 45:915–921, 1996.

Chapter 21

EXERCISE AND LIPID DISORDERS

J. Larry Durstine, Ph.D.

Great progress has been achieved in defining the beneficial effects of physical activity on plasma lipid and lipoproteins. The many functions of plasma lipids, apolipoproteins (apo), lipolytic enzymes, and lipoprotein receptors are not completely defined but are much clearer than ever before. New knowledge has come from a better understanding of the many factors that influence lipid synthesis and catabolism, the interactions between lipoproteins, apolipoproteins, lipoprotein enzymes, and their impact on the metabolic pathways. This expanded knowledge has come, in part, from a better understanding of the various genetic and environmental influences that alter the lipoprotein metabolic pathways and eventually lipoprotein composition. Environmental factors that modify lipoprotein metabolism and lipoprotein composition include age, body fat distribution, dietary composition, cigarette smoking, medication use, and regular physical activity participation. Intervention programs, such as reducing dietary fat, increasing carbohydrate intake, and increasing daily exercise positively influence plasma lipid and lipoprotein concentrations and reduce coronary artery disease risk. The focus of this chapter is on lipoprotein metabolism, physical activity, and the factors related to exercise required to induce favorable changes in plasma lipids and lipoprotein composition.

LIPOPROTEIN COMPOSITION AND METABOLIC PATHWAYS

LIPIDS

Free fatty acids (FFAs), triglyceride, and cholesterol are the major blood lipids. The FFAs found in the blood are made available for energy metabolism by various means including dietary absorption, adipose tissue lipolysis, and the direct action of lipoprotein lipase (LPL). Triglycerides serve several functions, but are primarily used as a rich energy storage source. A triglyceride molecule consists of 3 FFAs and 1 glycerol molecule.

Although primarily stored in adipose tissue, triglycerides can also be found in all tissues including muscle and are also used in cell membrane construction. Phospholipids are another class of lipids also used in cell membrane construction. In the case of phospholipids, the glycride backbone of the triglyceride molecule remains, but at least 1 fatty acid group is replaced by a phosphate group. Cholesterol is a unique lipid because it contains an alcohol group and is also a building component of all cell membranes. It is also the precursor for all steroids and sex hormones in the body, is degraded to bile acids, and is necessary for vitamin D synthesis.

LIPOPROTEIN COMPOSITION

Triglyceride and cholesterol are not soluble in an aqueous solution and must join with apolipoproteins to form micelle lipid-protein complexes (lipoproteins) to move throughout the body. The resulting water-soluble molecules are spherical in shape with measurable dimensions. They contain phospholipid, triglyceride, free and esterified cholesterol, and various apolipoproteins. Lipoproteins are classified according to their gravitational density (Table 21.1). Chylomicrons are obtained from intestinal absorption of FFAs. Very-low density lipoproteins (VLDLs, or pre-β-lipoprotein), originate in the liver and are involved in the movement of triglyceride to peripheral tissue. Low-density lipoproteins (LDLs, or β-lipoprotein) are the remaining constituent after the catabolism of VLDL. High-density lipoprotein (HDL, or α-lipoprotein) is involved in reverse cholesterol transport. Furthermore, subfractions of each lipoprotein exist including intermediate-density lipoprotein (IDL), an intermediate step in VLDL catabolism; lipoprotein(a) [Lp(a)], an LDL subfraction that is highly related to coronary artery disease; and 2 separate HDL subfractions, HDL_2 and the more dense HDL_3 (Table 21.1).[1]

Lipoproteins have protein or "apolipoprotein" as well as lipid components.[2] Some apolipoproteins are permanently bonded to lipoproteins, while others are free to move among the various

TABLE 21.1.   CHARACTERISTICS OF PLASMA LIPOPROTEINS AND LIPIDS

Lipid/ Lipoprotein	Source	Protein %	Total Lipid %	Percentage of Total Lipid				Apolipoprotein
				TG	Chol	Phosp	Free Chol	
Chylomicron	Intestine	1–2	98–99	88	8	3	1	Major: A-IV, B-48, B-100, H Minor: A-I, A-II, C-I, C-II, C-III, E
VLDL	Major: Liver Minor: Intestine	7–10	90–93	56	20	15	8	Major: B-100, C-III, E, G Minor: A-I, A-II, B-48, C-II, D
IDL	Major: VLDL Minor: Chylomicron	11	89	29	26	34	9	Major: B-100 Minor: B-48
LDL	Major: VLDL Minor: Chylomicron	21	79	13	28	48	10	Major: B-100 Minor: C-I, C-II, (a)
HDL$_2$	Major: HDL$_3$	33	67	16	43	31	10	Major: A-1, A-II, D, E, F Minor: A-IV, C-I, C-II, C-III
HDL$_3$	Major: Liver and intestine Minor: VLDL and chylomicron remnants	57	43	13	46	29	6	Major: A-1, A-II, D, E, F Minor: A-IV, C-I, C-II, C-III
Chol	Liver and diet		100			70–75	25–30	
TG	Diet and liver		100	100				

VLDL, very-low-density lipoprotein; IDL, intermediate-density lipoprotein; LDL, low-density lipoprotein; HDL, high-density lipoprotein; Chol, cholesterol; TG, triglyceride; Phosp, phospolipid.

lipoproteins. At least 17 different apolipoproteins have been identified. More than 1 apolipoprotein can be associated with a specific lipoprotein class.[2,3] Apolipoproteins serve in hormone transport,[4] proteolytic activity, nerve regeneration,[5] and direct and regulate enzymatic function. For example, apo C-II serves as an enzyme cofactor in the activation of LPL, while apo A-I is a cofactor for the lecithin:cholesterol acyltransferase (LCAT) reaction. Apolipoproteins can exist as isoproteins. Examples include apo B, designated apo B-48 and apo B-100, the various forms of Lp(a), and the 3 common apo E variants.[2,6] Apoproteins are also the binding molecules or ligands for interaction with lipoprotein receptors as when apo B-100 and apo E interact with LDL receptors.[2,7]

Most apolipoproteins are synthesized by the liver, intestine, or both while some are produced by other tissues. Although apolipoproteins are necessary for lipoprotein metabolism and en-hance the aqueous solubility of the lipids, some apolipoproteins have been identified as coronary artery disease risk indicators (Table 21.2).[8]

LIPOPROTEIN ENZYMES

Plasma lipoprotein metabolism incorporates several key enzymes. Lipoprotein lipase is an enzyme bound to capillary walls and found in various tissues such as heart, adipose tissue, and skeletal muscle. Its primary function is to hydrolyze the chylomicron and VLDL triglyceride core.[9] Hepatic lipase (HL) is bound to the liver capillary endothelium and participates indirectly in the final conversion of chylomicron and VLDL remnants into LDL.[1] Hepatic lipase also works in conjunction with cholesteryl ester transfer protein (CETP) in the breakdown of HDL$_2$ particles.[10] Cholesteryl ester transfer protein is one of several lipid transfer proteins believed to mediate the movement of esterified cholesterol from HDL$_2$ to

TABLE 21.2. MAJOR HUMAN APOLIPOPROTEINS

Apolipoprotein	Major Function	CAD Risk Factor
A-I	LCAT activator	Inversely related with CAD risk
A-II	LCAT inhibitor and/or activator of heparin releaseable hepatic triglyceride hydrolase	Not associated with CAD risk
B-48	Required for synthesis of chylomicron	Directly associated with CAD risk
B-100	LDL receptor binding site	Directly associated with CAD risk
(a)	Similar characteristics between apo(a) and plasminogen, thus may have a prothrombolytic role by interfering with function of plasminogen, possible acute phase reactant to tissue damage	Directly associated with CAD risk
C-I	LCAT activator	Not associated with CAD risk
C-II	LPL activator	Not associated with CAD risk
C-III	LPL inhibitor, several forms depending on content of sialic acids	Not associated with CAD risk
D	Core lipid transfer protein, possibly identical to the cholesteryl ester transfer protein	Not associated with CAD risk
E	Remnant receptor binding, present in excess in the beta-VLDL of patients with type III hyperlipoproteinemia and exclusively in HDL-C	Not associated with CAD risk

VLDL, very-low-density lipoprotein; IDL, intermediate-density lipoprotein; LDL, low-density lipoprotein; HDL-C, high-density lipoprotein cholesterol; CAD, coronary artery disease; LCAT, lecithin:cholesterol acyltransferase; LPL, lipoprotein lipase.

VLDL and to chylomicron remnants leading to the final transformation of HDL_2 to HDL_3.[11] Lecithin:cholesterol acyltransferase is synthesized by the liver and has been isolated on several lipoprotein fractions. When bound to plasma HDL_3, LCAT catalyzes the esterification of free cholesterol on the HDL surface and eventually promotes the movement of esterified cholesterol into the HDL core, forming the less dense HDL_2.[10,12]

Lipoprotein Metabolic Pathways

Movement of cholesterol and triglyceride between the intestine, liver, and extrahepatic tissue is completed by a complex transport system with plasma lipoproteins as the transport vehicle. Several lipoprotein metabolic pathways have been characterized. One sequence of steps designed for the delivery of cholesterol to extrahepatic tissue is termed the *LDL receptor pathway,* whereas the sequence of steps for returning cholesterol to the liver from peripheral tissue is termed *reverse cholesterol transport.* Both genetic and environmental disturbances of these pathways can alter plasma lipoprotein profiles and modify coronary artery disease risk.

LOW-DENSITY LIPOPROTEIN RECEPTOR PATHWAY

Dietary fat is digested by the small intestine and absorbed as fatty acids and free cholesterol. These absorbed lipids combine with apolipoproteins B-48, A-I, A-II, A-IV, and E and are packaged into large chlyomicrons that enter the blood by the thoracic duct.[12] In the cardiovascular system chylomicrons react with LPL (with apo C-II as an activator) to hydrolyze the lipid core releasing FFAs.[13] During this process, surface remnants from the chylomicrons are transferred to nascent HDL, while the chylomicron remnants acquire other apolipoproteins such as apo C and apo E.[14] Apo E and apo B-48 receptors on the surface of hepatic cells bind to chylomicron remnants and remove them from the circulation.[14,15]

Very-low-density lipoprotein synthesized by the liver is the primary transport vehicle for endogenous lipids.[12,13] As with chylomicrons, LPL hydrolyzes the VLDL triglyceride core releasing FFAs that are then taken up by extrahepatic tissue.[12] Intermediate-density lipoprotein, the remaining particle, interacts with LPL and HL to form LDL.[11,12] The remaining VLDL remnants are removed from circulating blood after binding to hepatic apo E receptors.[7] The LDL particles are the primary cholesterol transport mechanism to extrahepatic tissue where delivery is mediated by LDL receptors located on peripheral tissue cell surfaces.[7] Under normal circumstances, once the LDL particle is recognized by the LDL-apo B-100/apo E receptor, LDL is transported inside the cell and exposed to lysomal digestion.[7,16] Cholesterol is released and used for cellular metabolic needs (Fig. 21.1). Free cholesterol within the cell initiates a negative feedback system causing a reduction in cellular cholesterol synthesis and promoting excess cholesterol storage. At the same

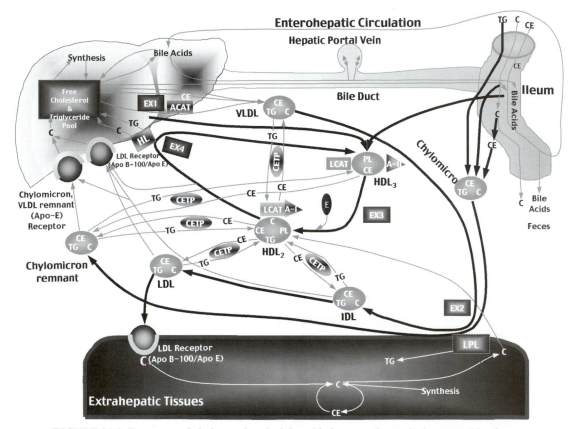

FIGURE 21.1. Transport of cholesterol and triglyceride between tissues in humans. PL, phospholipid; C, free cholesterol; CE, cholesteryl ester; TG, triglyceride; VLDL, very-low-density lipoprotein; IDL, intermediate-density lipoprotein; LDL, low-density lipoprotein; HDL, high-density lipoprotein; ACAT, acyl-CoA:cholesterol acyltransferase; LCAT, lecithin:cholesterol transfer protein; LPL, lipoprotein lipase; HL, hepatic lipase; CETP, cholesteryl ester transfer protein; A-I, apolipoprotein A-I; A-II, apolipoprotein A-II; Apo B-100, apolipoprotein B-100; and Apo E, apolipoprotein E. Heavy dark lines indicate major pathways; lighter lines indicate minor pathways. EX1-4 are points where exercise has a potential impact on lipoprotein metabolism: EX1 is the site for reduced synthesis of triglyceride, EX2 is the site for enhanced activity of LPL, EX3 is the site for enhanced LCAT activity, and EX4 represents enhanced reverse cholesterol transport. Adapted with permission from Durstine JL, Haskell WL: Effects of exercise training on plasma lipids and lipoproteins, in Holoszy JO (ed.): Exercise Sport Science Review, vol. 22. Baltimore: Williams & Wilkins, 1994, pp. 447–521.

time, cellular LDL receptor synthesis is suppressed and further cellular LDL uptake is prevented.[11]

REVERSE CHOLESTEROL TRANSPORT

The process of cholesterol transport by HDL from peripheral tissue back to the liver for catabolism is termed *reversed cholesterol transport* (Fig. 21.2). Several pathways exist for HDL-cholesterol (HDL-C) removal.[10,11] In one pathway, nascent HDL particles secreted by the liver are enriched with free cholesterol and phospho-

lipid derived from LPL-mediated catabolism of chylomicron and VLDL.[11,12] Lecithin:cholesterol acyltransferase, with apo A-I as a cofactor,[8] esterifies the free cholesterol, and the resultant cholesterol ester is shifted into the HDL$_3$ core.[11] The movement of cholesteryl ester into the HDL$_3$ core causes a chemical gradient that allows for a constant cholesterol supply to the LCAT reaction.[17] The influx of cholesteryl ester in the HDL$_3$ core expands the HDL and eventually converts HDL$_3$ to the less dense HDL$_2$ particle. This particular

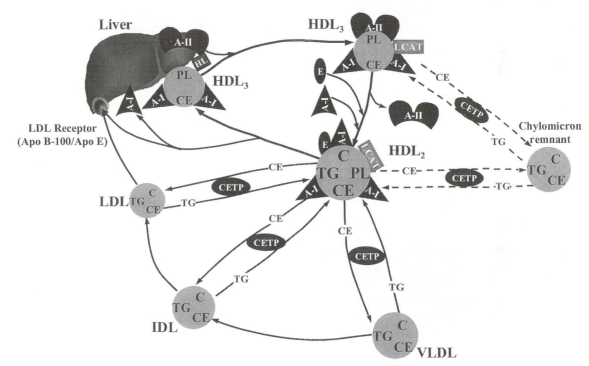

FIGURE 21.2. Reverse cholesterol transport involves the movement of cholesterol and cholesteryl esters by the high-density lipoprotein molecule from the peripheral tissue back to the liver, where they are catabolized. Once the HDL$_2$ molecule becomes cholesterol rich, it can be transported to the liver where the lipids are removed by several pathways. One pathway involves the apo-E-mediated removal of HDL$_2$ by the LDL receptor. PL, phospholipid; C, free cholesterol; CE, cholesteryl ester; TG, triglyceride; VLDL, very-low-density lipoprotein; IDL, intermediate-density lipoprotein; LDL, low-density lipoprotein; HDL, high-density lipoprotein; LCAT, lecithin:cholesterol transfer protein; LPL, lipoprotein lipase; HL, hepatic lipase; CETP, cholesteryl ester transfer protein; A-I, apolipoprotein A-I; A-II, apolipoprotein A-II; and E, apolipoprotein E. Heavy dark lines indicate major pathways, lighter lines indicate minor pathway, and the dotted lines indicate least traveled pathway.

process facilitates 2 other separate sets of chemical reactions. The first set of reactions facilitated by CETP involves the exchange of HDL_2 cholesteryl ester to chylomicron and/or VLDL remnants in exchange for triglyceride. The remaining remnants are transported to the liver where they are removed and metabolized.[10] The second series of reactions involves the HL-mediated removal of triglycerides from the HDL_2 particle, which was enriched with triglyceride by CETP. When HDL_2 triglyceride removal is complete, the end-product is HDL_3, which returns to the circulation to continue the cycle. Two other potential pathways exist for HDL-C removal. One pathway is the direct HDL_2-C exit from circulating blood through liver cells by the action of phospholipase and HL activity.[10] Another pathway is the hepatic apo E receptor-mediated HDL_2 removal.[10,18] Essentially, HDL_2 particles rich with cholesteryl ester and containing apo E are withdrawn from circulating blood by hepatic LDL receptor-mediated endocytosis.[15,18]

LIPIDS, LIPOPROTEINS, AND APOLIPOPROTEINS AS CORONARY ARTERY DISEASE RISK FACTORS

Atherosclerosis is characterized by focal thickening of the arterial intimal wall with accumulations of fat and collagen-like fibers. The genesis and growth of this thickening or arterial plaque occur gradually by a process that involves endothelial injury, connective tissue proliferation, infiltration, and retention of plasma-derived lipids, and tissue necrosis.[19]

The association between blood cholesterol and atherosclerosis is well documented,[20] and the association is both continuous and graded.[21] Early pharmacologic studies evaluating the effect of lowered blood cholesterol on the incidence of a new myocardial infarction are inconclusive,[22,23] but clinical trials lowering blood cholesterol concentration with statin drugs have reduced coronary artery disease mortality and morbidity.[24,25] In addition, lowering plasma cholesterol and

LDL-cholesterol (LDL-C) in patients who have experienced a previous coronary event reduced coronary artery disease mortality.[26] This is also true for patients with normal preintervention blood LDL-C concentrations.[27] Aggressive cholesterol-lowering therapy has also reduced the rate of atherosclerotic disease progression in native coronary arteries[28,29] and in patients with venous coronary artery bypass grafts.[30] Desirable blood cholesterol concentrations for adults are now defined as less than 200 mg/dL,[31] while others suggest that lower plasma cholesterol and LDL-C are necessary to reduce atherosclerotic outcomes.

Though the atherogenic risk of elevated blood total cholesterol is clear, its pathogenicity is also influenced by how cholesterol is distributed among the lipoproteins. Barr[32] was the first to observe the existence of a relative and absolute HDL reduction in the presence of atherosclerosis. Human infants carry a larger plasma cholesterol proportion in HDL as do most animals. Thus, human infants and animals exhibit a high resistance to coronary artery disease. As humans age, the HDL-C proportion is reduced, and the likelihood for coronary artery disease development is increased.[32] These findings were virtually ignored for nearly 2 decades, and most lipid and lipoprotein studies centered on serum total cholesterol and LDL-C. The early focus on LDL-C was a logical outgrowth from the findings that LDL, and not HDL, is the major carrier of cholesterol in humans and plays a major role in the movement of cholesterol to peripheral cells, as well as to arterial plaque sites. Not surprisingly, LDL-C displays a positive relationship with both total serum (or plasma) cholesterol and coronary artery disease. As a result, coronary artery disease risk is often defined in terms of total cholesterol and LDL-C concentrations.[31,33] Moreover, evidence supports the contention that "small" dense LDL particles are more atherogenic than "large" buoyant LDL particles.[34] Another LDL subfraction, Lp(a), contains the glycoprotein apo(a) and is also a strong predictor of premature coronary artery disease[38] (Table 21.3).

Renewed interest in HDL-C concentration and

TABLE 21.3.   PLASMA LIPIDS AND LIPOPROTEINS AND THEIR RELATIONSHIP TO CAD RISK
AND THE EFFECTS OF PHYSICAL ACTIVITY

Lipid/Lipoprotein	Relationship to CAD	Effect of Physical Activity
Chylomicron	Positive	None
VLDL	Somewhat positive	Decreased
IDL	Somewhat positive	Decrease or no change
LDL	Strong positive	Decrease or no change
Lp(a)	Strong positive	Presently, physical activity has no or little impact
HDL$_2$	Strong inverse	Increase
HDL$_3$	Inverse	Decrease
Cholesterol	Strong positive	No change
Triglyceride	Somewhat positive	Decrease

CAD, coronary artery disease; VLDL, very-low-density lipoprotein; IDL, intermediate-density lipoprotein; LDL, low-density lipoprotein; Lp(a), lipoprotein(a); HDL, high-density lipoprotein.

coronary artery disease risk occurred in 1968 when 2815 men and women between the ages of 49 and 82 years were recruited from the Framingham cohort to undergo lipid and lipoprotein analysis. After a 4-year follow-up, serum HDL-C concentrations were inversely related to coronary artery disease incidence.[35] HDL-C level was also the best lipid coronary artery disease risk marker, while LDL-C concentration was only weakly associated with coronary artery disease incidence. Serum HDL-C concentration in the Framingham cohort was also inversely associated with myocardial infarction incidence in a 12-year follow-up.[36] Men with the lowest serum HDL-C concentrations ($\leq$ 46 mg/dl), compared to those with the highest ($\geq$ 67 mg/dl), had a sixfold increased coronary artery disease risk. These findings persisted after adjusting for age and other risk factors. Similar HDL-C effects were found for women. Furthermore, low HDL-C concentrations are predictive of myocardial infarction even in subjects with low total cholesterol concentrations.[37] These data were used to estimate that a 1% lower HDL-C value is associated with a 3 to 4% increased coronary artery disease risk.[39] The strong inverse association between HDL-C and coronary artery disease has been confirmed in other population-based studies.[20,40,41] Finally, the ratios of both total cholesterol to HDL-C and LDL-C to HDL-C are stronger coronary artery

disease risk predictors for both men and women than total cholesterol or HDL-C alone.[40,42]

Other lipoproteins such as the HDL subfraction concentrations HDL$_2$-C and HDL$_3$-C may be useful in quantifying coronary artery disease risk. Women have lower rates of coronary artery disease and higher serum HDL$_2$-C concentrations than do men.[1] An inverse relation between coronary artery disease and both HDL$_2$-C and HDL$_3$-C concentrations has been reported in prospective studies (Table 21.3), and both are negatively associated with myocardial infarction incidence.[34,40,43,44] Elevated triglyceride concentration is also an independent coronary artery disease predictor, especially when considered in light of low HDL-C values.[45,46] Apolipoprotein A-I, the major protein found on HDL, is lower in patients who have suffered an acute myocardial infarction than in those who have not and is a good discriminator of angiographically documented coronary artery disease.[47,48] Similarly, apo B, the major protein associated with LDL, is elevated in coronary artery disease patients (Table 21.2),[49] and the ratio of apo B to apo A-I is a powerful discriminator for the presence and severity of angiographically defined coronary artery disease.[50] Although the apo B/AI ratio is a powerful coronary artery disease risk predictor, this ratio's clinical usefulness is questionable when the LDL-C/HDL-C ratio is known.

EXERCISE TRAINING, LIPIDS, AND LIPOPROTEINS

AEROBIC EXERCISE TRAINING

PLASMA FREE FATTY ACIDS

Plasma FFAs are a primary energy source for prolonged, low-to-moderate intensity exercise.[51–53] Plasma FFA uptake by working tissue is concentration dependent meaning that greater FFA uptake occurs with greater plasma FFA levels.[54] Two facts support the concept that blood FFA uptake is dependent on its rate of use. First, fatty acid uptake by working tissue increases with exercise training.[54,55] Second, plasma FFA concentration plateaus during exercise in sedentary subjects, but the uptake of FFAs in trained subjects increases linearly with increased supply.[56] In addition, because of their essentially unlimited supply, FFAs derived from adipose tissue are an attractive source to increase plasma FFA levels during prolonged endurance activity.[57] However, following exercise training when muscular fat oxidation capacity is increased due to increased mitochondrial volume and enzyme activity levels, evidence suggests a reduction in peripheral FFA mobilization.[58] This discrepancy suggests that following exercise training, blood FFAs are diminished as a fuel source during moderate-to-high intensity exercise in spite of an increased adrenergic-receptor sensitivity to catecholamines.[51,58,59] The latter should increase hormone-sensitive lipase activity and increase lipolysis.

PLASMA TRIGLYCERIDE

Both cross-sectional and exercise training studies indicate that plasma triglyceride concentrations are usually, but not always[60–62] decreased by exercise training, and that the decrease is related to baseline concentrations. Persons with higher baseline triglyceride concentrations often experience a greater reduction in triglyceride concentration with exercise training.[63–67] Previously inactive subjects with triglyceride concentrations of 130 mg/dl had approximately a 10 to 20% lower triglyceride concentration following 3 to 12 months of an exercise intervention.[65,68,69] Subjects with low initial triglyceride concentrations had small triglyceride concentration reductions after similar exercise training programs.[70,71] These studies suggest that exercise training decreases triglyceride concentrations and that those individuals with the highest initial triglyceride values usually have the greatest reductions.

PLASMA CHOLESTEROL

Cross-sectional and exercise training studies of 3-weeks to 1-year duration have observed no change in plasma cholesterol concentration.[63,65,67–69,71,72] Infrequently, decreased cholesterol concentrations have been reported after exercise training.[73–75] Such changes were not related to initial cholesterol concentration or length of the exercise training program. Cholesterol reductions up to 11% have been described after some physical activity interventions, although these were not statistically significant.[67–70,72] Decreased percentage of body fat is observed in some,[74,75] but not all,[73] studies reporting reduced cholesterol. Other investigators observed decreases in body fat without changes in cholesterol.[68,69,71] Consequently, if decreased plasma cholesterol is to occur with exercise training, a decrease in body weight or body fat must accompany the exercise training program.

PLASMA CHYLOMICRON AND VERY-LOW-DENSITY LIPOPROTEIN

Fasting blood VLDL particles, the primary carriers of postabsorptive triglycerides, are generally low in endurance-trained subjects. Chylomicrons are the primary transporter for postprandial triglycerides. The main lipid sources for muscular work come from adipose tissue and intramuscular triglyceride stores, while little is supplied from blood chylomicron and VLDL particles.[51,57] Two reasons exist why these lipoprotein particles are seldom used as substrates during exercise. Chylomicron and VLDL concentrations are elevated only *during* the postprandial period in normal subjects when most people do not exercise, and the total caloric content of these blood lipoproteins is quite small and could only supply a small amount of energy during muscular work.[51] Kiens et al[76] demonstrated that muscle LPL activity is downregulated by physiological concentrations of insulin in contrast to adipose tissue LPL, which is upregulated by insulin. This information supports the concept that the uptake of triglyceride from chylomicron and VLDL during exercise in the postprandial period is limited. Nonetheless, exercise does increase the clearance of postprandial triglycerides.[77,78] This fact supports the potential uptake and oxidation of some triglycerides from chylomicrons and VLDL during muscular work. Finally, regular participation in physical activity is necessary to maintain reduced postprandial triglycerides.[78–80]

PLASMA LOW-DENSITY LIPOPROTEIN

Low-density lipoprotein-cholesterol is a potent predictor of cardiovascular disease (Table 21.3)[81,82] and is increased in individuals who have a high intake of dietary fat, especially saturated fat.[78] Plasma LDL-C is occasionally lower after regular endurance exercise,[78,83] but not always.[63,65,71,72,84–86]

Low-density lipoprotein particles have been divided into different density ranges with each carrying different coronary artery disease risk.[88] The concentration of smaller, denser LDL particles correlates directly with coronary artery disease incidence, but small dense LDL may vary directly with elevated triglyceride concentrations.[88] Williams et al[89,90] examined "small" LDL particle concentrations in healthy mildly overweight men with a mean body mass index (BMI) of 30 after 1 year of exercise training. Although "small" LDL concentrations were not significantly lower after exercise training, both distance run per week and reduced body fat mass correlated significantly with the decrease in small LDL concentrations.[89,90]

Halle et al,[91] using a cross-sectional design, evaluated physically active and inactive hypercholesterolemic (cholesterol > 240 mg/dl) men. Triglyceride and small LDL concentrations were lower in physically active men than they were in nonactive men. Multivariate regression analysis

revealed that the amount of small LDL particles present was related to maximal oxygen consumption ($\dot{V}o_2$ max) and not to BMI.

PLASMA LIPOPROTEIN(a)

Lipoprotein(a) is an LDL subfraction and contains the apolipoprotein apo(a),[81,82,92] which is highly homologous with plasminogen. As a result, the apo(a) portion of Lp(a) competes with plasminogen for binding sites on fibrin[82,92,93] and inhibits fibrinolysis. Moreover, Lp(a) levels > 25 mg/dl are directly correlated to the development of coronary artery disease (Table 21.3).[81,93] Thus, Lp(a) has the same negative coronary artery disease effects as LDL-C and, in addition, inhibits thrombolysis.[92] Lipoprotein(a) is an inherited trait[81,93] and does not appear to respond to regular physical activity participation.[82,92,94,95] A review of the physical activity impact on Lp(a) concentrations has been published by Drowatzky et al[96]

PLASMA HIGH-DENSITY LIPOPROTEIN

High-density lipoprotein-cholesterol is not a substrate that is used for energy metabolism during exercise but has a role in determining coronary artery disease risk. High-density lipoprotein-cholesterol is generally responsive to aerobic training and increases in a dose-dependent manner with increased energy expenditure.[63,84,97] Regular physical activity participation or exercise training that lasts 12 weeks or more *likely* will increase HDL-C levels[65,70,72,75,98] but not always.[69,70,99] Exercise-training-induced increases in HDL-C concentration range from 4 to 22%, whereas the absolute HDL-C increase is more uniform and ranges from 2 to 8 mg/dl. Tran et al[100] performed a meta-analysis and reported an inverse correlation between initial HDL-C concentrations and the change in HDL-C with exercise training. Williams et al[101] found great exercise-induced changes in HDL-C and HDL$_2$-C in overweight subjects (mean BMI of 29). Thompson et al,[65] however, reported no relation between exercise-induced change in HDL-C and baseline HDL-C concentration.

The exercise training volume measured by kilocalories expended during exercise training and the length of the exercise intervention program are important considerations when evaluating HDL-C change. Wood et al[102] observed that only 12 weeks of exercise training produced an increased HDL-C concentration. Nevertheless, there often is no HDL-C change when exercise training programs are 10 weeks or less in duration. Tran et al[100] found a significant correlation between hours spent in exercise training and change in HDL-C. Similarly, others[63,71,84] have observed significant correlations between distance run per week and HDL-C change. These aggregate results provide strong support for the relation between increased physical activity and increases in HDL-C.

Several issues should be considered when comparing different studies. Because of different exercise frequency, intensity, and duration, the quantity of exercise quantified by calories throughout the exercise training program should be considered. Furthermore, time points when blood samples are obtained after exercise training intervention may also have an impact on blood lipid profiles. Crouse et al[103] found a rise in HDL-C and HDL$_2$-C during the 24- to 48-h time period immediately after a single exercise session, whereas the overall effect after the exercise training intervention was an increased HDL$_2$-C and a decreased HDL$_3$-C concentration. Thus, both a single exercise session and exercise training can have independent effects on blood lipid and lipoprotein profiles.

Altered body composition after exercise training can contribute to increased HDL-C concentrations. Wood et al[71] reported a inverse relation between change in body fat and HDL-C. The addition of distance run per week to a multiple regression model did not improve the ability to predict HDL-C change beyond that provided by percentage body fat change alone. Thompson et al used special diets and supplements to maintain body weight and body fat percentage and demonstrated increases in HDL-C of 8 mg/dl[85] and 4 mg/dl.[65] Wood et al[104] employed weight-loss programs using caloric restriction alone or caloric restriction in conjunction with exercise training. Body weight and percentage body fat decreased in both treatment groups, whereas HDL-C concentration increased. Most importantly, the group that combined caloric restriction and exercise training had greater changes in body composition and HDL-C than did the group that did not. Other exercise training studies have found exercise training-induced increased HDL-C both in the presence[68,69,74] and in the absence[70,85] of reduced percentage body fat. These findings collectively suggest that exercise training without altered body weight and/or body composition increases HDL-C and that this increase is augmented by loss of body fat.

The HDL-C subfractions, HDL$_2$-C and HDL$_3$-C, increased after exercise training is some studies,[65,75,85] whereas other studies failed to find exercise-induced change in the HDL subfractions.[69,70] These last 2 studies did not correct lipoprotein concentrations for plasma volume change. Thompson et al[85] found statistically significant changes in HDL$_2$-C and HDL$_3$-C concentrations only after correcting for plasma volume expansion. Therefore, in order to examine change in plasma lipids and lipoproteins due to metabolic factors, exercise-induced changes in plasma volume should be considered.

High-density lipoprotein is also studied by particle diameter. Although most literature suggests that the HDL$_{3b}$ subfraction is directly related to coronary artery disease risk, some studies have reported an inverse relation between coronary artery disease risk and HDL$_{3b}$ subfraction, while HDL$_{2a}$ and HDL$_{2b}$ are associated with reduced coronary artery disease risk. Williams et al[105] reported increased HDL$_{2b}$ and decreased HDL$_{3b}$ after a 1-year exercise intervention program in men who were 20 to 60% above ideal body weight. Nevertheless, when changes in BMI or body fat percentage were included as covariates, neither HDL$_{2b}$ nor HDL$_{3b}$ concentration was significantly different from the initial preexercise training value.

PLASMA APOLIPOPROTEINS

Apolipoprotein A-I is an LCAT activator and is mostly associated with HDL_2-C.[2] Elevated blood levels of apo A-I are associated with reduced coronary artery disease risk.[8] Some investigations have found increases in apo A-I of 1 to 10% after exercise training,[65,73,105] although others have not.[68–71,74,103] Thompson et al[85] found an increased HDL_2-C concentrations with exercise training, but no significant increase in apo A-I. Williams et al[105] reported no statistical change in apo A-I levels when BMI change was included as a covariate. Apolipoprotein A-II is associated with HDL_3-C and is thought to activate HL.[8] After exercise training, apo A-II changes are equivocal. Huttunen et al[68] reported a 10% decrease in apo A-II concentration after a 16-week low-intensity (40% heart rate reserve) exercise intervention program. Thompson et al have reported no change[65] while a 5%[105] and a 21%[85] increase in apo A-II concentrations have also been reported. Williams et al[105] found a significant 7% increase in apo A-II after exercise training and correction for reduced BMI.

Apolipoprotein B is found in 2 forms: B-48 and B-100. Apo B-48 is synthesized by intestinal cells, is the major chylomicron protein, and is required for chylomicron synthesis.[2] The ratio of apo B-48 to apo A-I is a sensitive index of coronary artery disease risk with low ratios indicating low risk.[2] Apolipoprotein B-100 is synthesized in the liver; is associated with plasma chylomicron, VLDL, and LDL; and is necessary for peripheral tissue LDL receptor binding.[2] Whether apo B concentrations decreased[69,74,103] or did not,[70–72] changes in apo B with exercise training parallel changes in LDL-C. Wood et al[71] found no overall change in apo B after a 1-year exercise training program, but did find a significant inverse correlation between distance run and change in apo B concentration.

Apolipoprotein C is found in several forms including apo C-I, apo C-II, and apo C-III; is synthesized by the liver; and is necessary for LCAT (apo C-I) and LPL (apo C-II) activation.[2] Little is known about the impact that exercise has on apo C proteins. Apo C has been examined cross-sectionally with no reported differences between physically active and inactive groups of young and elderly male subjects.[70,106]

Apolipoprotein E is synthesized by most tissues with the liver being the primary production site.[107] Few studies have been published regarding an exercise-induced effect on apo E. The results from these studies are not consistent and have been reviewed by Velliquette et al[107] Marti et al[70] found no apo E differences in current and former runners, whereas others noted higher apo E concentrations in young runners, but not in older runners.[108] Seip et al[69] found a decreased apo E concentration after exercise training for 9- to 12-months duration. Tanabe et al[109] reported an increase in apo E concentrations in men, but not in women after 10 weeks of bicycle ergometer training.

The apo E gene is polymorphic, meaning that the gene exists in 2 or more forms. The common apo E variants are E2, E3, and E4. The 3 common apo E variants produce 6 different phenotypes: E2/2, E2/3, E2/4, E3/3, E3/4, and E4/4.[6] At present, few studies have evaluated phenotype relations and physical activity. Taimela et al[110] in a cross-sectional study of 713 males and 785 females aged 9 to 24 years found no relation between physical activity and apo E phenotype among females. In contrast, there was a significant interaction between physical activity, lipid and lipoprotein concentrations, and apo E phenotypes among males. In males, physical activity was inversely related to total cholesterol and LDL-C. Also physical activity was directly related to the HDL-C:total cholesterol ratio, but only in men with apo E4/3 and E3/2 phenotypes. St-Amand et al[111] reported an inverse association between plasma $\dot{V}O_2$ max and triglyceride concentrations in men and women heterozygous for apo E2 or homozygous for apo E3. These associations were not found for apo E4 phenotypes in either gender. Plasma LDL-C concentrations were inversely associated with $\dot{V}O_2$ max only in women homozygous for apo E3. In men and women who were apo E3 homozygotes,[111] $\dot{V}o_2$ max was positively associated with plasma HDL_2-C concentrations only. These data suggest that the relation between physical activity or $\dot{V}o_2$ max and plasma lipids and lipoproteins is influenced by apo E phenotype.

Two reports further support the concept that apo E polymorphism interacts with the exercise training to influence the ultimate change in serum lipids. Thompson et al examined the impact of 6 to 12 months of exercise training in 18 overweight men.[112] Four men were heterozygous for apo E2, 11 were heterozygous for 3/E3, 2 were for E3/E4, and 1 was for E4/E4. The exercise training changes in the men heterozygous for the E2 gene were compared with the other 3 genetic groups combined. Triglycerides decreased 13% in the apo E2 men, but only 6% in the other subjects. Increases in postheparin LPL activity and fat clearance occurred only in the apo E2 subjects. In fact, postheparin LPL activity increased 39% in the E2 subjects, but only 2% in the other men. None of these changes were statistically significant, possibly because of the small sample size. Nevertheless, the results suggest that apo E genotype affects the lipid response to exercise training. Hagberg et al[113] reported the effect of 9 months of endurance exercise training in 6 men with the E2 allele, 33 homozygous for E3, and 12 men heterozygous for E4. One E2 subject was homozygous for the E2 allele. Triglycerides decreased 23, 16, and 0%, whereas HDL-C increased 22, 9, and 6% in the E2, E3, and E4 groups, respectively. The triglyceride change was significantly greater in the E2 and E3 groups, whereas the HDL-C increase was greater in the E2 subjects. These results make intuitive sense. Apolipoprotein E's major function is to facilitate triglyceride clearance. Apolipoprotein E2 has extremely low affinity for the apo E receptor and in the homozygous form can produce marked hyperlipidemia. Consequently, these results suggest that exercise training is most effective at reducing triglycerides and increasing HDL-C and LPL activity in those individuals whose ability to clear triglycerides and, thereby increase HDL-C, is limited by the presence of the apo E2 gene when these subjects are sedentary.

RESISTANCE EXERCISE TRAINING

The studies considered in this section employed resistance exercise programs that met 3 times weekly. Training protocols consisted of 1 to 3 circuits. One circuit consists of 8 to 14 exercise stations, using 6 to 20 repetitions per exercise with 15 to 120 s rest allowed between each exercise. One circuit would take 12 to 18 min to complete. Quantification of exercise training in kilocalories expended was generally not provided, and most studies did not report lifting resistance as a particular percentage of 1 repetition maximum. However, several investigations reported that at least 1 exhaustive set was included daily with each exercise. Exercise intervention programs were between 8 weeks and 22 months in length. A few studies included a nonexercising control group.

Triglyceride concentrations are not changed after a resistance training program[114,115] even when initial concentrations were mildly elevated (193 mg/dl).[116] Goldberg et al did find a decreased triglyceride concentration in women, but not in men.[117] Reduced total cholesterol and LDL-C concentrations in response to resistance training may depend on body composition change. Thus, when total cholesterol and LDL-C decreased, body fat generally decreased and lean body mass increased.[114,115,119] Conversely, when total body mass, lean body mass, and percentage body fat were unchanged, total cholesterol,[116,118,121] LDL-C,[121] and apo B-100[120] concentrations remained unchanged. Goldberg et al[117] reported decreased sum of skinfolds with nonsignificant reductions in total cholesterol of 7% in men and significant reductions of 10% in women. After a resistance training program, Hurley et al[118] found no change in body weight or body fat, but a 5% decrease in LDL-C. Boyden et al[114] reported no significant relation between changes in percentage body fat, total cholesterol, and LDL-C in premenopausal women.

High-density lipoprotein-cholesterol changes after resistance training have been equivocal. Men have demonstrated no changes in HDL-C[116,117,121] or increases equivalent to those reported after endurance exercise training (5 to 7 mg/dl).[115,118,119] Hurley et al also found an increase in HDL_2-C concentration with resistance training in men.[118] In women, no increased HDL-C concentrations[114,117,120] or apo A-I concentrations[120] were found. Combined assessment of these investigations suggests no consistent relation between resistance-training-induced HDL-C and body composition changes. Furthermore, Ullrich et al[115] reported no correlation between HDL-C, body fat, and lean body mass changes.

A SINGLE EXERCISE SESSION'S IMPACT ON LIPIDS, LIPOPROTEINS, AND APOLIPOPROTEINS

Many changes attributed to regular exercise participation are caused, in part, by a single exercise session, and this topic has received considerable attention. A variety of factors can affect the results obtained with such studies. These include the amount of exercise performed, the preexercise lipid levels, the timing of the blood samples, the length of postexercise follow-up, dietary changes, failure to measure changes in plasma volume, the subjects' exercise training state, and in women menstrual status and oral contraceptive use. These factors have been discussed elsewhere.[1]

PLASMA TRIGLYCERIDE

Immediately after or in the days after an exercise period of short duration and low intensity, triglyceride concentrations are not usually altered.[122–124] In contrast, when subjects exercise for more than 1 h, there is no change immediately after exercise,[125–130] but there is a decrease in triglycerides 24 h after exercise.[125,127,128,130,131] Triglycerides may increase immediately after exercise in women[132] and men,[133] but triglyceride values return to the preexercise concentrations or

are lower than preexercise concentrations 24 h after the exercise session. Following a single session of resistance exercise, triglyceride concentrations are unchanged when the exercise volume was low,[134] or reduced if the work volume was high.[135] Generally, if an exercise session is prolonged and has a large energy requirement, triglyceride concentrations are lower for 2 to 3 days following a single exercise session.

PLASMA CHOLESTEROL

Total plasma cholesterol concentrations for men[122,123,125] and women[136] immediately after and in the days following a single exercise session of short duration are not changed. Total cholesterol immediately after *prolonged* exercise may not change in men[128,131,137] and women,[126,132] but may decrease[127,138] or increase.[129,132] Similarly, on the days after prolonged exercise, total cholesterol may be lower than normal,[127,133,139] increased,[130] or unchanged.[125,126,128,131] Studies evaluating resistance exercise have reported no change in total cholesterol immediately after and in the days following a single exercise session.[134,135] In summary, if a single exercise session is to have an impact on total cholesterol concentrations, the exercise must be prolonged and require a large amount of energy expenditure. Even then, most effects are not observed until 24 h after the exercise.

POSTPRANDIAL LIPEMIA

Postprandial lipid and lipoprotein profiles can provide additional information regarding an individual's coronary artery disease risk. Exaggerated postprandial lipemia is an indication of poor blood triglyceride removal and has been associated with atherosclerosis.[140] A single exercise session 24 h before a high fat meal reduces postprandial lipemia.[77,127,141,142] This reduction in postprandial lipemia is related to the exercise energy expended[127] and the exercise duration.[143] Furthermore, similar energy expenditures at different exercise intensities elicit similar attenuations in postprandial lipemia.[144] The relative contribution of fat or carbohydrate to the energy expended during exercise does not affect the magnitude of the subsequent reduction in postprandial lipemia.[145] Thus, a single exercise session reduces postprandial lipemia and could alter coronary artery disease risk. The magnitude of the reduction appears primarily related to total energy expenditure and not the intensity or energy source during exercise.

Plasma Chylomicron, Very-Low-Density Lipoprotein, and Low-Density Lipoprotein

Short-duration single exercise sessions in men[124] and women[136] have little impact on VLDL and LDL levels immediately after or in the days following exercise. Although not often reported, VLDL-cholesterol (VLDL-C) concentrations immediately after prolonged exercise are lower[127,138,146] or unchanged,[125,126] but may be lower 24 h after exercise.[125] Low-density lipoprotein-cholesterol concentrations can be lower in men[125,127,130,131] and women[132] or are unchanged[126,128,129,138] immediately after prolonged exercise. A single-resistance exercise session does not change VLDL-C or LDL-C concentrations.[134,135] Thus, the duration of a single exercise session should be prolonged and have a large energy expenditure if exercise is to alter VLDL-C or LDL-C concentrations.

Plasma Lipoprotein(a)

Few studies exist that have examined the effects of a single exercise session on Lp(a) concentrations. Durstine et al[122] observed no changes in Lp(a) concentration in trained runners immediately after an exercise session requiring either 50 or 80% $\dot{V}O_2$ max. Dufaux et al[133] found significant increases in Lp(a) in moderately trained males 2 days after a 3-h run, but changes in plasma volume were not considered. In contrast, Hellsten et al[147] reported a large decrease in Lp(a) following an 8-day (10 h per day) skiing event. Yu

et al[138] reported lower Lp(a) concentrations 15 min after completing the Hawaii Ironman Triathlon. Durstine et al[148] found no immediate or delayed changes in Lp(a) in endurance-trained males who completed 2 different exercise sessions both at 70% $\dot{V}O_2$ max. One exercise session required an energy expenditure of 800 kcal (57 min to complete), and the second exercise session required an energy expenditure of 1500 kcal (112 min to complete). Thus, unless exercise is extremely prolonged, Lp(a) concentrations are not affected by a single exercise session.

Plasma High-Density Lipoprotein

Isolated exercise sessions of brief duration and low intensity increase HDL-C immediately after the exercise episode.[123,136] However, Durstine et al[129] noted increases in HDL-C during exercise after 2 h of prolonged walking at 45% of $\dot{V}O_2$ max. This increase persisted to the point of exhaustion at 4.5 h. Davis et al[124] compared exercise at 50 and 75% of $\dot{V}O_2$ max with the energy expenditure for the 2 activities held constant at 950 kcal. Exercise time was 90 and 60 min. There were no changes in HDL-C or any of its subfractions immediately after or in the days following the exercise. In contrast, Gordon et al compared similar low and high intensity exercise sessions and found an increased HDL-C concentration 24 h after the higher intensity exercise.[149] Annuzzi et al[127] found no change in HDL-C after 1.5 h of exercise requiring 77% of maximal heart rate. Generally, prolonged exercise of more than 1.5 h increases HDL-C concentrations immediately after exercise in men[129,133,138] and women,[132] as well as in the days following the exercise.[131–133,146] Ferguson et al[125] suggested that a threshold of energy expenditure is required for HDL-C change. Their data indicate an energy expenditure threshold of 1100 kcal is needed to increase HDL-C concentrations.[125] Trained and sedentary subjects may respond differently to a single exercise session. Kantor et al,[130] using trained subjects, reported elevated HDL-C concentrations immediately after and in the days following the completion of a marathon, whereas sedentary subjects did not show an increase in HDL-C immediately after exercise but did so 24, 48, and 72 h after exercise. A single session of resistance exercise requiring high energy expenditure can increase HDL-C,[135] but a low-volume resistance exercise session does not.[134,135] Consequently, there seems to be a threshold of energy expenditure required to induce HDL-C changes immediately and in the days after a single exercise session. This threshold appears to require a duration of over 1.5 h[129] and/or an energy expenditure of 1100 kcal.[125] This energy expenditure threshold also is likely a function of an individual's state of training and lipid levels. An inactive person with low cardiovascular function and low plasma HDL-C may have lower energy expenditure thresholds for lipid and lipoprotein changes.[87]

PLASMA HIGH-DENSITY LIPOPROTEIN SUBFRACTIONS

Short-duration exercise produces no[124,125] or only modest changes in HDL subfractions[123,136] in the days following exercise. A single prolonged exercise session increases HDL_3-C with no change in HDL_2-C immediately after the exercise period, but both HDL_3-C and HDL_2-C increase in the days following the exercise.[125,131,133] State of training again appears to be an important consideration. Kantor et al[130] noted that exercise increased HDL_2-C, but did not change HDL_3-C in trained subjects in the days following an exercise session, whereas HDL_3-C and not HDL_2-C increased in sedentary subjects. Kiens and Lithell[152] had subjects complete a single exercise session after 8 weeks of 1-leg exercise training. The trained limb produced more HDL_2-C than the untrained limb, suggesting that a limb's or an individual's fitness level may have important effects on the individual acute lipid response to an isolated exercise session.

Diet and an isolated exercise session may also have interactive effects on HDL subfractions. A diet providing 75% of calories as fat when provided in conjunction with exercise increased HDL-C and HDL_2-C concentration, whereas a diet providing 85% of calories as carbohydrate when provided in combination with exercise decreased HDL-C and HDL_3-C.[146] The high fat and exercise protocol also increased HDL_{2b} and decreased HDL_{2a+3a}.

As for the effect of resistance exercise on HDL subfractions, a single high-work volume-resistance exercise session increased HDL-C and HDL_3-C concentrations in the days after exercise, whereas HDL_2-C did not change.[135] A single low-work volume-resistance exercise session had no impact on either HDL_2-C or HDL_3-C.[134,135]

PLASMA APOLIPOPROTEINS

Apolipoprotein A-I and A-II concentrations do not change immediately following a single exercise session;[77,124,131,133] nor does apo B change.[122,131] Annuzzi et al[127] reported no change in apo C-I, C-II, and C-III 24 h after a 1.5-h exercise period, but 24 h after a 3-h exercise period apo C-I was reduced. Plasma apo E concentrations did not change after a 30 min exercise session, whereas VLDL-apo E decreased.[150]

Although plasma concentration of apolipoproteins is not generally affected by a single exercise session, future studies should focus on apolipoprotein metabolism and its impact on intravascular lipid transport. Future studies should also consider how exercise changes apolipoprotein production and clearance. Such studies should be completed before conclusions are made regarding the effect of a single exercise session on apolipoproteins.

MECHANISMS FOR EXERCISE-ALTERED LIPOPROTEIN METABOLISM

LIPOPROTEIN LIPASE

Lipoprotein lipase activity can be measured in muscle from muscle biopsy samples or in plasma after the intravenous injection of fully anticoagulating doses of heparin. Heparin releases LPL from its capillary binding sites and permits its measurement in plasma. The effect of physical activity on skeletal muscle LPL activity has been reviewed by Seip and Semenkovich.[151] Exercise of sufficient volume and intensity to deplete intramuscular triglyceride stores increases secretion and synthesis of muscle LPL.[128] Plasma LPL activity is not usually increased until 4 to 18 h after exercise, but when LPL is increased there is an increased chylomicron and VLDL triglyceride core hydrolysis that results in decreased plasma triglyceride concentrations.[152] Increased chylomicron and VLDL catabolism, mediated in part by LPL, can ultimately increase production of cholesteryl ester remnants that can combine with HDL_3 and yield an increased plasma HDL_2 concentration.[153] This process likely contributes to the increased HDL mass that occurs in the vascular compartments of adipose[90] and muscle tissue[152] after exercise training.

Elevated postheparin plasma LPL activity has often,[154,155] but not always[156] been reported in endurance athletes. Female endurance runners have higher postheparin LPL activity and higher triglyceride clearance, and both are directly correlated with HDL-C concentrations.[154] Seip et al[69] found higher postheparin plasma LPL activity after 9 to 12 months of endurance exercise training, whereas Cedermark et al[157] found increased LPL activity following only 10 days of military physical training requiring marching of 12 to 32 km/day. Following endurance exercise training, sedentary men exhibit significantly higher adipose tissue and postheparin LPL activity.[85] Although Thompson et al[65] found an 11% nonsignificant increase in postheparin LPL activity after 1 year of exercise training, Grandjean et al[62] found no change in body weight and postheparin LPL activity in premenopause and postmenopausal women after 12 weeks of exercise training. Kiens and Lithell[152] trained subjects with a cycle ergometer using only 1 leg. After 8 weeks of training, subjects performed a 2-h exercise session 4 h after exercise. Muscle LPL activity was higher in the trained leg as compared to the untrained leg, suggesting that the higher postheparin LPL after training was at least partly due

to increased LPL in the exercise-trained muscle.[152] Williams et al[90] found increased adipocyte LPL when weight loss occurred in association with endurance exercise training.

Postheparin plasma LPL activity increases after only 1 week of endurance training,[158] but this may be an acute exercise effect. Kantor et al[130] observed increase plasma postheparin LPL activity in trained and sedentary subjects after a single cycling exercise session performed at 80% $\dot{V}O_2$ max. In contrast, Gordon et al[149] found no significant differences in LPL activity in trained runners following a single exercise session requiring an energy expenditure of 800 kcal and performed at either low intensity (60% $\dot{V}O_2$ max) or high exercise intensity (70% $\dot{V}O_2$ max), although the higher exercise intensity tended to increase LPL activity. Shoup et al[134] found increased LPL activity in untrained subjects 24 h after a single high-intensity resistance exercise session requiring only 250 kcal of energy. Ferguson et al[125] observed an increased LPL activity in trained runners 24 h after several treadmill exercise sessions at 70% $\dot{V}O_2$ max requiring energy expenditures of more than 1100 kcal. Sady et al[77] found increased LPL activity and clearance of an artificial lipid emulsion after running a marathon.

The impact of exercise on LPL muscle gene expression has been reviewed.[151] Seip et al[159] had sedentary subjects complete 60 to 90 min of exercise at 55 to 70% peak $\dot{V}O_2$ for 5 consecutive days. Five vastus lateralis biopsies were performed: before the first day of exercise training, immediately before the fifth day of exercise, and 0.2, 4, and 8 h after the fifth session. No changes in muscle LPL mass or LPL messenger ribonucleic acid (mRNA) were found 20 h after exercise on the fourth day. After day 5 of exercise, LPL mRNA increased by 127% at 4 h postexercise and was followed by an increase in LPL mass of 93% at 8 h postexercise. Exercise training (5 to 13 consecutive days) produced increased skeletal muscle LPL mRNA level, LPL protein mass, and total LPL enzyme activity, whereas adipose tissue LPL mRNA, protein mass, and enzyme activity remained unchanged.[160] Hamilton et al[161] reported short-term voluntary run training produced an increased LPL immunoreactive mass and increased total and heparin-releasable LPL enzyme activity in rat white skeletal muscle and in postheparin plasma, but not in white muscle that was not recruited during exercise. Lipoprotein lipase did not increase in red skeletal muscle. These reports suggest that exercise in white skeletal muscle produces an intrinsic stimulus that raises LPL activity by pretranslational mechanisms. In addition, local contractile activity is required for increasing LPL expression during exercise training. (See Table 21.4.)

HEPATIC LIPASE

Resting HL activity is inversely associated with HDL_2-C and directly associated with HDL_3-C.[162,163] Observational studies suggest that resting HL activity is not different between active and inactive individuals.[155] However, Peltonen et al[158] found a decrease in resting HL activity in middle-aged men following 15 weeks of endurance exercise training. Similarly, resting HL activity decreased in elderly subjects following 9 to 12 weeks of endurance exercise training[69] and following weight loss by diet and/or exercise.[65] Nevertheless, when adjusted for plasma volume changes, no changes in resting HL were found after endurance exercise training.[62,85] Finally, a single exercise session has not been associated with significant changes in HL activity.[125,130,131,149] (See Table 21.4.)

CHOLESTERYL ESTER TRANSFER PROTEIN

A decrease in CETP activity may be antiatherogenic by slowing hepatic catabolism of HDL_2 and decreasing the amount of cholesterol-rich particles in the circulation.[164] Gupta et al[165] using a cross-sectional design found higher plasma CETP activity in physically active persons. The method used to measure CETP activity was unusual, however, because the transfer of cholesteryl ester from the solid phase bound HDL to VLDL and LDL was assessed.[166] Seip et el[69] found a decrease in CETP activity after endurance exercise training. This decreased CETP activity is supported by observations that marathon runners have low CETP mass[167] and activity.[168] Low CETP mass and activity were associated with low plasma concentrations of VLDL-C and apo B and with elevated concentrations of HDL-C and apo A-I.[167,168] These decreases in CETP may be an effect of recent exercise and may be transient, because CETP increased after only 1 week of exercise cessation.[167] Föger et al[169] found an increased CETP mass 24 and 48 h after a 230-km cycle race but no significant change in CETP activity. (See Table 21.4.)

TABLE 21.4.   LIPOPROTEIN ENZYME CHANGES ASSOCIATED WITH EXERCISE

Enzyme	Single Exercise Session	Regular Exercise Participation
LPL		
Activity	Delayed change (at least 4 hours)	Increased
Mass	No information	Increased
HL		
Activity	No change	No change (may be reduced with weight loss)
Mass	No information	No information
LCAT		
Activity	Increased/No change	Increased/No change
Mass	No information	No information
CETP		
Activity	No information	No change/increased
Mass	Increased	Increased

LPL, lipoprotein lipase; HL, hepatic lipase; LCAT, lecithin:cholesterol acyltransferase; CETP, cholesteryl ester transfer protein.

Lecithin:Cholesterol Acyltransferase

Increased LCAT has been observed in physically active young[86] and middle-aged men[170] and in endurance-trained sportsmen.[86,165] However, LCAT activity did not change following an exercise-induced weight loss program,[90] an 11-week interval training program,[171] or a 12-week aerobic exercise program.[62] Lecithin:cholesterol acyltransferase may increase[131,172] or remain unchanged[146] after a single exercise session. Since LCAT is not a rate-limiting enzyme for any of the lipoprotein metabolic pathways, a change in LCAT may simply reflect the substrate availability. (See Table 21.4.)

HEALTH CONSIDERATIONS

Present information strongly supports regular physical activity participation as having a positive influence on the plasma lipid and lipoprotein profile. These changes have been studied extensively in men with normal lipid and lipoprotein profiles and to a lesser extent in women. The effect of exercise on dyslipidemic syndromes has received some attention, but diet and drug therapy remain the primary treatment modalities for these disorders, with exercise training used as adjunctive therapy. Several important interactions between exercise, drug, and/or diet therapy can occur. These interactions can further optimize the lipid and lipoprotein profile.

Dietary Intake and Weight Loss

Plasma lipids and lipoproteins are modified by reductions in total dietary energy and cholesterol intake, the percentage of dietary fat, and the type of fat consumed. Dietary fat reductions directly affect plasma cholesterol by decreasing hepatic cholesterol levels. The reduction in blood cholesterol is mediated by an increase in the number of and/or activity of hepatic LDL receptors with an amplified hepatic LDL-C uptake producing a lower total plasma cholesterol concentration. Reductions in dietary fat will reduce plasma HDL-C and increase triglyceride concentrations, but these HDL-C and triglyceride responses are diminished when accompanied by an increase in physical activity. Weight loss achieved by caloric restriction is inversely associated with total cholesterol, LDL-C levels, and HL activity and is directly associated with HDL-C and HDL_2-C concentrations. Even though weight loss increases HDL-C, acute caloric restriction reduces HDL-C concentrations in obese women. In male distance runners, however, HDL-C concentrations are increased by acute caloric restriction. Consequently, reductions in dietary fat and weight loss achieved by caloric restriction should magnify the beneficial changes in blood lipids produced by increased physical activity. Alternatively, exercise can mitigate some of the putatively deleterious changes in HDL-C and triglycerides produced by low-fat and high-carbohydrate diets.

Drug Therapy

Coronary artery disease morbidity and mortality are reduced in dyslipidemic patients with appropriate pharmacologic treatment. Indeed, pharmacologic therapy is the primary means for management of dyslipidemia and dyslipoproteinemia. Nicotinic acid inhibits adipocyte lipolysis, deprives the liver of FFA produced by lipolysis, and thereby suppresses liver VLDL synthesis. Fibric acid derivatives such as clofibrate, gemfibrozil, fenofibrate, and bezofibrate increase LPL activity and increase VLDL and IDL catabolism. The bile acid sequestrants and the HMG CoA reductase inhibitors reduce plasma cholesterol by increasing LDL receptor activity. There are many potential metabolic deficiencies that can produce dyslipidemic profiles. The effect of exercise on these patients may differ substantially from the effect found in other patients. For example, exercise training is not likely to benefit the extremely rare patients with LPL deficiency, or will exercise training increase HDL concentrations in patients with hypoalphalipoproteinemia, a syndrome characterized by the inability to produce normal amounts of the major HDL apoproteins. It is also not know what the effect of exercise will be on individuals with less severe genetic variations in proteins regulating lipid metabolism. Nonetheless, triglyceride reductions after exercise training in men and women with normal triglyceride concentrations and in men with hypertriglyceridemia has been a consistent finding. Moreover, postprandial lipemia is reduced by exercise training and after a single exercise session.

Although exercise is routinely recommended for patients with hypercholesterolemia, there is surprisingly little empirical evidence to support this practice. The few studies completed have presented divergent findings. Specific reasons for these conflicting results remain unclear, but differences in pretraining lipid concentrations, dietary intake during the intervention program, weight loss, exercise training intensity, and exercise training volume may influence the results. Nonetheless, pharmacologic interventions that include restriction of energy intake, decreased dietary fat intake, and reduced percentage of body fat and body mass together with increased physical activity can help in the optimization of the lipid and lipoprotein profile. Total cholesterol and LDL-C concentrations are usually reduced, whereas HDL-C concentrations are often increased by such an intervention. Nevertheless, medications remain the key component of such a treatment regimen except in patients with only mild LDL-C elevations. Bile sequestrant resins often increase triglyceride levels, and this effect can be reduced by aerobic exercise.

PERSONAL PERSPECTIVE

The National Cholesterol Education Program Guidelines promote dietary intake modification, weight loss, and drug therapies, while encouraging the inclusion of regular exercise as part of the medical management of people with lipid and lipoprotein disorders. Although the lipid and lipoprotein profile is positively affected by regular physical activity participation, these exercise-induced changes are augmented by body-weight reduction, body composition change, and dietary fat reduction. The mechanisms responsible for these changes are most clearly related to changes in LPL activity, but changes in LCAT, CETP, and HL enzyme activity may also contribute to an exercise effect. Increased LPL activity enhances the removal of lipids by peripheral tissue for metabolic use and may facilitate the reverse cholesterol transport process. Although we know much about reverse cholesterol transport, the precise mechanisms for HDL-C removal are still not clear. Nonetheless, these exercise-induced lipid and lipoprotein changes occur in both men and women, as well as in many patients with dyslipidemic and dyslipoproteinemic disorders, and are associated with reduced coronary artery disease risk.

At present, the exercise lipid and lipoprotein responses have been scientifically evaluated and as a result we know that in most cases positive changes will occur. Furthermore, we have greater insight into understanding the necessary exercise volume to cause these changes. Though much is known about exercise and LPL activity changes, comparatively less is known about other enzyme changes such as LCAT and CETP activity that are also involved in lipoprotein metabolism. Future research should emphasize evaluation of the interrelations between exercise-induced lipid and lipoprotein changes and these other potential enzyme changes. Initial research is currently underway evaluating the molecular mechanisms responsible for LPL activity change. The study for the molecular basis of other lipid, lipoprotein, and enzymatic change as impacted by exercise should also be completed, because these results could provide new insights for understanding the exercise coronary artery disease protective effect. In addition, further exercise studies are necessary to provide greater comprehension as to why some individuals respond to exercise while others do not. For example, knowing a person's apo E genotype appears very important when evaluating the exercise training response. Another area that should be further evaluated is aging since many physiological changes take place. Present evidence indicates that as some people age there is a likelihood for an increased number of risk factors. This is known as the multiple metabolic syndrome and involves the development of various coronary artery disease risk factors. Our challenge in the future is to better understand the impact that exercise or regular physical activity participation has on optimizing the lipid and lipoprotein profiles in these individuals.

REFERENCES

1. Durstine JL, Haskell WL: Effects of exercise training on plasma lipids and lipoproteins, in Holloszy JO (ed.): *Exercise Sport Science Review,* vol. 22. Baltimore: Williams & Wilkins, 1994, pp. 447–521.

2. Brewer HB, Greg RE, Hoeg JM, et al: Apolipoproteins and lipoproteins in human plasma: An overview. *Clin Chem* 34(Suppl B): B4–B8, 1988.

3. Breslow JL: Genetics of lipoprotein disorders. *Circulation* 87(Suppl III):16–21, 1993.

4. Benvenga S: A thyroid hormone binding motif is evolutionarily conserved in apolipoproteins. *Thyroid* 7:605–611, 1997.

5. Siest G, Pillot T, Regis-Bailley A, et al: Apo E an important gene and protein to follow in laboratory medicine. *Clin Chem* 41:1068–1086, 1995.

6. Zannis VI, Breslow JL, Utermann G, et al: Proposed nomenclature of apo E isoproteins, apo E genotypes, and phenotypes. *J Lipid Res* 23: 911–914, 1982.

7. Brown M, Goldstein JL: A receptor-mediated pathway for cholesterol homeostasis. *Science* 232:34–37, 1986.

8. Leddy J, Horvath P, Rowland J, et al: Effect of a high or a low fat diet on cardiovascular risk factors in male and female runners. *Med Sci Sports Exerc* 29:17–25, 1997.

9. Oscai LB, Essig DA, Palmer WK: Lipase regulation of muscle triglyceride hydrolysis. *J Appl Physiol* 69:1571–1577, 1990.

10. Tall AR: Plasma high density lipoproteins: Metabolism and relationship to atherogenesis. *J Clin Invest* 86:379–384, 1990.

11. Tikkanen MJ: Plasma lipoproteins and atherosclerosis. *J Diabet Complic* 4:35–38, 1990.

12. Shepherd J: Lipoprotein metabolism: An overview. *Ann Acad Med* 21:106–113, 1992.

13. Voutilainen E, Hietanen E: Characterization of lipoproteins and their metabolism: Synthesis and catabolism, in Hietanen E (ed.): *Regulation of Serum Lipids by Physical Exercise.* Boca Raton: CRC Press, Inc., 1982, pp. 1–9.

14. Green PHR, Glickman RM, Sandel CD, et al: Human intestinal lipoproteins: Studies in chyluric subjects. *J Clin Invest* 64:233–242, 1979.

15. Sherrill BC, Innerarity TL, Mahley RW: Rapid hepatic clearance of the canine lipoprotein con-
taining only the E apoprotein by a high affinity receptor. Identity with the chylomicron remnant transport process. *J Biol Chem* 255:1804–1807, 1980.

16. de Duve C: Lysosomes revisited. *Eur J Biochem* 137:391–397, 1983.

17. Deckelbaum RJ, Olivecrona T, Eisenberg S: Plasma lipoproteins in hyperlipidemia: Roles of neutral lipid exchange and lipase, in Carlson LA, Olsson AG (eds.): *Treatment of Hyperlipoproteinemia.* New York: Raven Press, 1984, pp. 85–93.

18. Koo C, Innerarity TL, Mahley RW: Obligatory role of cholesterol and apolipoprotein E in the formation of large cholesterol-enriched and receptor-active high density lipoproteins. *J Biol Chem* 260:11934–11943, 1985.

19. Ross R: The pathogenesis of atherosclerosis: A perspective for the 1990s. *Nature* 362:801–809, 1993.

20. Pekkanen J, Linn S, Heiss G, et al: Ten-year mortality from cardiovascular disease in relation to cholesterol level among men with and without preexisting cardiovascular disease. *N Engl J Med* 322:1700–1707, 1990.

21. Stamler J, Wentworth D, Neaton JD: Is relationship between serum cholesterol and risk of premature death from coronary heart disease continuous and graded? *JAMA* 256:2823–2828, 1986.

22. The Coronary Drug Project Research Group: Clofibrate and niacin in coronary heart disease. *JAMA* 231:360–381, 1975.

23. Report from the Committee of Principal Investigators: A cooperative trial in the primary prevention of ischemic heart disease using clofibrate. *Br Heart J* 40:1069–1118, 1978.

24. Lipid Research Clinics Program: The lipid research clinics coronary primary prevention trial results. I. Reduction in incidence of coronary heart disease. II. The relationship of reduction in incidence of coronary heart disease to cholesterol lowering. *JAMA* 251:351–354, 1984.

25. Shepherd J, Cobbe SM, Ford I, et al: Prevention of coronary heart disease with pravastatin in men with hypercholesterolemia. *J N Engl Med* 333: 1301–1307, 1995.

26. Scandinavian Simvastatin Survival Study Group: Randomized trial of cholesterol lowering in 4444 patients with coronary heart disease: The

Scandinavian Simvastatin Survival Study (4S). *Lancet* 344:1383–1389, 1994.

27. Sacks FM, Pfeffer MA, Maye LA, et al: The effect of pravastatin on coronary events after myocardial infarction in patients with average cholesterol levels. *N Engl J Med* 335:1001–1009, 1996.

28. Blankenhorn DH, Azen SP, Kramsch DM, et al: Coronary angiographic changes with lovastatin therapy: The Monitored Atherosclerosis Regression Study (MARS). *Ann Intern Med* 119: 969–976, 1993.

29. Waters D, Higginson L, Gladstone P, et al: Effects of monotherapy with HMG-CoA reductase inhibitor on the progression of coronary atherosclerosis as assessed by serial quantitative arteriography: The Canadian Coronary Atherosclerosis Intervention Trial. *Circulation* 89:959–968, 1994.

30. The Post Coronary Artery Bypass Graft Trial Investigators: The effect of aggressive lowering of low-density lipoprotein cholesterol levels and low-dose anticoagulation on obstructive changes in saphenous-vein coronary-artery bypass grafts. *N Engl J Med* 336:153–162, 1997.

31. Expert Panel on Detection, Evaluation, and Treatment of High Blood Cholesterol in Adults of the National Cholesterol Education Program: Summary of the second report of the national cholesterol education program (NCEP) expert panel on detection, evaluation, and treatment of high blood cholesterol in adults (adult treatment panel II). *JAMA* 269:3015–3023, 1993.

32. Barr DP: Some chemical factors in the pathogenesis of atherosclerosis. *Circulation* 8:641–654, 1953.

33. National Cholesterol Education Program. Second Report of the Expert Panel on Detection, Evaluation, and Treatment of High Blood Cholesterol in Adults (Adult Treatment Panel II). *Circulation* 89:1331–1445, 1994.

34. Lamarche B, Tchernof A, Moorjani S, et al: Small, dense low-density lipoprotein particles as a predictor of the risk of ischemic heart disease in men. *Circulation* 95:69–75, 1997.

35. Gordon T, Castelli WP, Hjortland MC, et al: High density lipoprotein as a protective factor against coronary heart disease: The Framingham Study. *Am J Med* 62:707–714, 1977.

36. Castelli WP, Garrison RJ, Wilson PW, et al:

Incidence of coronary heart disease and lipoprotein cholesterol levels: The Framingham Study. *JAMA* 256:3835–3838, 1986.

37. Abbott RD, Wilson PW, Kannel WB, et al: High density lipoprotein cholesterol, total cholesterol screening, and myocardial infarction: The Framingham Study. *Arteriosclerosis* 8:207–211, 1988.

38. Bostom AG, Cupples LA, Jenner JL, et al: Elevated plasma lipoprotein(a) and coronary heart disease in men aged 55 years and younger. *JAMA* 276:544–548, 1996.

39. Wilson PW: High-density lipoprotein, low-density lipoprotein and coronary artery disease. *Am J Cardiol* 66:7A–10A, 1990.

40. Stampfer MJ, Sacks FM, Salvini S, et al: A prospective study of cholesterol, apolipoproteins, and the risk of myocardial infarction. *N Engl J Med* 325:373–381, 1991.

41. Jacobs DR, Mebane IL, Bongdiwala SL, et al: High density lipoprotein cholesterol as a predictor of cardiovascular disease mortality in men and women: The follow-up study of the lipid research clinics prevalence study. *Am J Epidemiol* 131:32–47, 1990.

42. Manninen V, Tenkanen L, Koskinen P, et al: Joint effects of serum triglyceride and LDL cholesterol and HDL cholesterol concentrations on coronary heart disease risk in the Helsinki Heart Study. *Circulation* 85:37–45, 1992.

43. Buring JE, O'Connor GT, Goldhaber SZ, et al: Decreased HDL_2 and HDL_3 cholesterol, Apo A-I and Apo A-II, and increased risk of myocardial infarction. *Circulation* 85:22–29, 1992.

44. Lamarche B, Moorjani S, Cantin B, et al: Associations of HDL2 and HDL3 subfractions with ischemic heart disease in men. *Atheroscler Thromb Vasc Biol* 17:1098–1105, 1997.

45. Jeppesen J, Hein HO, Suadicani P, et al: Triglyceride concentration and ischemic heart disease: An eight-year follow-up in the Copenhagen male study. *Circulation* 97:1029–1036, 1998.

46. Gaziano JM, Hennekens CH, O'Donnell CJ, et al: Fasting triglycerides, high-density lipoprotein, and risk of myocardial infarction. *Circulation* 96:2520–2525, 1997.

47. Fager G, Wiklund O, Olofsson S, et al: Serum apolipoprotein levels in relation to acute myocardial infarction and its risk factors. *Arteriosclerosis* 36:67–74, 1980.

48. Maciejko JJ, Holmes DR, Kottke BA, et al: Apolipoprotein A-I as a marker of angiographically assessed coronary-artery disease. *N Engl J Med* 309:385–389, 1983.

49. De Backer G, Rosseneu M, Deslypere JP: Discriminative value of lipids and apoproteins in coronary heart disease. *Atherosclerosis* 42:197–203, 1982.

50. Noma A, Yokosuka T, Kitamura K: Plasma lipids and apolipoproteins as discriminators for presence and severity of angiographically defined coronary artery disease. *Atherosclerosis* 49:1–7, 1983.

51. Martin WH: Effects of acute and chronic exercise on fat metabolism, in Holloszy JO, (ed.): *Exercise Sport Science Review,* vol. 24. Baltimore: Williams & Wilkins, 1996, pp. 203–231.

52. Pendergast DR, Horvath PJ, Leddy JJ, et al: The role of dietary fat on performance, metabolism, and health. *Am J Sports Med* 24:S53–S58, 1996.

53. Nicklas BJ: Effects of endurance exercise on adipose tissue metabolism. *Exerc Sport Sci Rev* 25: 77–103, 1997.

54. Kiens B: Effect of endurance training on fatty acid metabolism: Local adaptations. *Med Sci Sports Exerc* 29:640–645, 1997.

55. Kiens B, Essen-Gustavsson B, Christensen NJ, et al: Skeletal muscle substrate utilization during submaximal exercise in man: Effect of endurance training. *J Physiol* 469:459–478, 1993.

56. Turcotte LP, Richter EA, Kiens B: Increased plasma FFA uptake and oxidation during prolonged exercise in trained vs. untrained humans. *Am J Physiol* 262:E791–E799, 1992.

57. Brouns F, Van der Vusse GJ: Utilization of lipids during exercise in human subjects: Metabolic and dietary constraints. *Br J Nutr* 79:117–128, 1998.

58. Romijn JA, Coyle EF, Sidossis LS, et al: Regulation of endogenous fat and carbohydrate metabolism in relation to exercise intensity and duration. *Am J Physiol (Endocrinol Metabol)* 265:E380–E391, 1993.

59. Phillips SM, Green HJ, Tarnopolsky MA, et al: Effects of training duration on substrate turnover and oxidation during exercise. *J Appl Physiol* 81:2182–2191, 1996.

60. Kokkinos PF, Narayan P, Colleran J: Effects of moderate intensity exercise on serum lipids in African-American men with severe systemic hypertension. *Am J Cardiol* 81:732–735, 1998.

61. Grandjean PW, Oden GL, Crouse SF, et al: Lipid and lipoprotein changes in women following 6 months of exercise training in a worksite fitness program. *J Sports Med Phys Fitness* 36:54– 59, 1996.

62. Grandjean PW, Crouse SF, O'Brian BC, et al: The effects of menopausal status and exercise training on serum lipids and the activities of intravascular enzymes related to lipid transport. *Metabolism* 47:377–383, 1998.

63. Kokkinos PF, Holland JC, Narayan P, et al: Miles run per week and high-density lipoprotein cholesterol levels in healthy, middle-aged men. *Arch Intern Med* 155:415–420, 1995.

64. Williams PT: Relationships of heart disease risk factors to exercise quantity and intensity. *Arch Intern Med* 158:237–245, 1998.

65. Thompson PD, Yurgalevitch SM, Flynn MM, et al: Effect of prolonged exercise training without weight loss on high-density lipoprotein metabolism in overweight men. *Metabolism* 46:217–223, 1997.

66. Gyntelberg F, Brennan R, Holloszy J, et al: Plasma triglyceride lowering by exercise despite increased food intake in patients with Type-IV hyperlipoproteinemia. *Am J Clin Nutr* 30:716–720, 1977.

67. Holloszy JO, Skinner JS, Toro G, et al: Effects of a six month program of endurance exercise on lipids of middle-aged men. *Am J Cardiol* 14: 753–760, 1964.

68. Huttunen JK, Länsimies E, Voutilainen E, et al: Effect of moderate physical exercise on serum lipoproteins: A controlled clinical trial with special reference to serum high-density lipoproteins. *Circulation* 60:1220–1229, 1979.

69. Seip RL, Moulin P, Cocke T, et al: Exercise training decreases plasma cholesteryl ester transfer protein. *Arterioscler Thromb* 13:1359–1367, 1993.

70. Marti B, Suter E, Riesen WF, et al: Effects of long-term, self-monitored exercise on the serum lipoprotein and apolipoprotein profile in middle-aged men. *Atherosclerosis* 81:19–31, 1990.

71. Wood PD, Haskell WL, Blair SN, et al: Increased exercise level and plasma lipoprotein concentrations: A one-year randomized, controlled study in

sedentary middle-aged men. *Metabolism* 32: 31–39, 1983.

72. Després J-P, Moorjani S, Tremblay A, et al: Heredity and changes in plasma lipids and lipoproteins after short-term exercise training in men. *Arteriosclerosis* 8:402–409, 1988.

73. Kiens B, Jörgenson I, Lewis S, et al: Increased plasma HDL-cholesterol and apo A-I in sedentary middle-aged men after physical conditioning. *Eur J Clin Invest* 10:203–209, 1980.

74. Després J-P, Tremblay A, Moorjani S, et al: Long-term exercise training with constant energy intake: Effects on plasma lipoprotein levels. *Int J Obes* 14:85–94, 1990.

75. Wood PD, Stefanick ML, Dreon DM, et al: Changes in plasma lipids and lipoproteins in overweight men during weight loss through dieting as compared with exercise. *N Engl J Med* 319:1173–1179, 1988.

76. Kiens B, Lithell H, Mikines KJ, et al: Effects of insulin and exercise on muscle lipoprotein lipase activity in man and its relation to insulin action. *J Clin Invest* 84:1124–1129, 1989.

77. Sady SP, Thompson PD, Cullinane EM, et al: Prolonged exercise augments plasma triglyceride clearance. *JAMA* 256:2552–2555, 1986.

78. Ziogas GG, Thomas TR, Harris WS: Exercise training, postprandial hypertriglyceridemia, and LDL subfraction distribution. *Med Sci Sports Exerc* 29:986–991, 1997.

79. Bøsheim E, Knardahl S, Høstmark AT: Short-term effects of exercise on plasma very low-density lipoproteins (VLDL) and fatty acids. *Med Sci Sports Exerc* 31:522–530, 1999.

80. Hardman AE, Lawrence JM, Herd SL: Postprandial lipemia in endurance-trained people during a short interruption to training. *J Appl Physiol* 84:1895–1901, 1998.

81. Israel RG, Sullivan MJ, Marks RH, et al: Relationship between cardiorespiratory fitness and lipoprotein(a) in men and women. *Med Sci Sports Exerc* 26:425–431, 1994.

82. Hubinger L, Mackinnon LT: The effect of endurance training on lipoprotein(a) [LP(a)] levels in middle-aged males. *Med Sci Sports Exerc* 28:757–764, 1996.

83. Gaesser GA, Rich RG: Effects of high- and low-intensity exercise training on aerobic capacity and blood lipids. *Med Sci Sports Exerc* 16: 269–274, 1984.

84. Williams PT: Relationship of distance run per week to coronary heart disease risk factors in 8283 male runners: The National Runners' Health Study. *Arch Intern Med* 157:191–198, 1997.

85. Thompson PD, Cullinane EM, Sady SP, et al: Modest changes in high-density lipoprotein concentrations and metabolism with prolonged exercise training. *Circulation* 78:25–34, 1988.

86. Marniemi J, Dahlstrom S, Kvist M, et al: Dependence of serum lipid and lecithin: Cholesterol acyltranferase levels on physical training in young men. *Eur J Appl Physiol* 49: 25–35, 1982.

87. Crouse SF, O'Brien BC, Rohack JJ, et al: Changes in serum lipids and apolioproteins after exercise in men with high cholesterol: Influence of intensity. *J Appl Physiol* 79:279–286, 1995.

88. Coresh J, Kwiterovich PO Jr: Small, dense low-density lipoprotein particles and coronary heart disease risk: A clear association with uncertain implications. *JAMA* 276:914–915, 1996.

89. Williams PT, Krauss RM, Vranizan, KM, et al: Effects of exercise-induced weight loss on low-density lipoprotein subfractions in healthy men. *Arteriosclerosis* 9:623–632, 1989.

90. Williams PT, Krauss RM, Vranizan KM, et al: Changes in lipoprotein subfractions during diet-induced weight lost in moderately overweight men. *Circulation* 81:1293–1304, 1990.

91. Halle M, Berg A, König D, et al: Differences in the concentration and composition of low-density lipoprotein subfraction particles between sedentary and trained hypercholesterolemic men. *Metabolism* 46:186–191, 1997.

92. MacKinnon LT, Hubinger L, Lepre F: Effects of physical activity and diet on lipoprotein(a). *Med Sports Sci Exerc* 29:1429–1436, 1997.

93. Halle M, Berg A, von Stein T, et al: Lipoprotein(a) in endurance athletes, power athletes, and sedentary controls. *Med Sci Sports Exerc* 28:962–966, 1996.

94. Kostka T, Lacour J-R, Berthouze SE, et al: Relationship of physical activity and fitness to lipid and lipoprotein(a) in elderly subjects. *Med Sports Sci Exerc* 31:1183–1189, 1999.

95. Szymanski LM, Durstine JL, Davis PG, et al: Factors affecting fibrinolytic potential: Cardiovascular fitness, body composition, lipoprotein(a). *Metabolism* 45:1427–1433, 1996.

96. Drowatzky KL, Ainsworth BE, Durstine JL: Exercise, lipids and lipoproteins in women. *Clin Kinesiol* 53:28–36, 1999.

97. Durstine JL, Pate RR, Sparling PB, et al: Lipid, lipoprotein, and iron status of elite women distance runners. *Int J Sports Med* 8:119–123, 1987.

98. Stein RA, Michielli DW, Glantz, MD, et al: Effects of different exercise training intensities on lipoprotein cholesterol fractions in healthy middle-aged men. *Am Heart J* 119:277–283, 1990.

99. Stefanick ML, Mackey S, Sheehan M, et al: Effects of diet and exercise in men and post-menopausal women with low levels of HDL cholesterol and high levels of LDL cholesterol. *N Engl J Med* 339:12–20, 1998.

100. Tran ZV, Weltman A, Glass GV, et al: The effects of exercise on blood lipids and lipoproteins: A meta-analysis of studies. *Med Sci Sports Exerc* 15:393–402, 1983.

101. Williams PT, Stefanick ML, Vranizan KM, et al: Effects of weight loss by exercise or by dieting on plasma high-density lipoprotein (HDL) levels in men with low, intermediate, and normal-to-high HDL at baseline. *Metabolism* 43:917–924, 1994.

102. Wood PD, Williams PT, Haskell WL, et al: Physical activity and high density lipoproteins, in Miller NE, Miller GI (eds.) *Clinical and Metabolic Aspects of High-Density Lipoproteins.* Amsterdam: Elsevier, 1984, pp. 133–165.

103. Crouse SF, O'Brien BC, Grandjean PW, et al: Effects of training and single session of exercise on lipids and apolipoproteins in hypercholesterolemic men. *J Appl Physiol* 83:2019–2028, 1997.

104. Wood PD, Stefanick ML, Williams PT, et al: The effects on plasma lipoproteins of a prudent weight-reducing diet, with or without exercise in overweight men and women. *N Engl J Med* 325:461–466, 1991.

105. Williams PT, Krauss RM, Vranizan KM, et al: Effects of weight-loss by exercise and by diet on apolipoproteins A-I and A-II and the particle-size distribution of high-density lipoproteins in men. *Metabolism* 41:441–449, 1992.

106. Tamai T, Nakai T, Takai H, et al: The effects of physical exercise on plasma lipoproteins and apoliproteins metabolism in elderly men. *J Gerontol* 43:M75–M79, 1988.

107. Velliquette RA, Durstine JL, Hand GA, et al: Apolipoprotein E, an important protein involved in triglyceride and cholesterol homeostatsis: Physical activity implications. *Clinical Exercise Physiology* 2:4–14, 2000.

108. Tamai T, Higuchi M, Oida K, et al: Effects of exercise on plasma lipoprotein metabolism, in Sato Y, Poortmans J, Hashimoto I, et al (eds.): *Integration of Sports Sciences. Medical Sports Sciences,* vol 37. Basel: Karger, 1992, pp. 430–439.

109. Tanabe Y, Sasaki J, Urata H, et al: Effects of mild aerobic exercise on lipid and apolipoprotein levels in patients with essential hypertension. *Japan Heart J* 29:199–206, 1988.

110. Taimela S, Lehtimaki T, Porkka AVK, et al: The effect of physical activity on serum total and low-density lipoprotein cholesterol concentrations varies with apolipoprotein E phenotype in male children and young adults: The Cardiovascular Risk in Young Finns Study. *Metabolism* 45:797–803, 1996.

111. St-Amand J, Homme DP, Moorjani S, et al: Apo E polymorphism and the relationships of physical fitness to plasma lipoprotein-lipid levels in men and women. *Med Sci Sports Exerc* 31:692–697, 1999.

112. Thompson PD, Moyna NM, Tsongalis G, et al: The effect of apo E genotype on the lipid response to exercise training. *Med Sci Sports Exerc* 31:S135, 1999.

113. Hagberg JM, Ferrell RE, Katzel LI, et al: Apolipoprotein E genotype and exercise training-induced increases in plasma high-density lipoprotein (HDL)- and HDL$_2$-cholesterol levels in overweight men. *Metabolism* 48:943–945, 1999.

114. Boyden TW, Pamenter RW, Going SB, et al: Resistance exercise training is associated with decreases in serum low-density lipoprotein cholesterol levels in premenopausal women. *Arch Intern Med* 153:97–100, 1993.

115. Ullrich IH, Reid CM, Yeater RA, et al: Increased HDL-cholesterol levels with a weight lifting program. *South Med J* 80:328–331, 1987.

116. Kokkinos PF, Hurley BF, Smutok MA, et al: Strength training does not improve lipoprotein-lipid profiles in men at risk for CHD. *Med Sci Sports Exerc* 32:1134–1139, 1991.

117. Goldberg L, Elliot DL, Schultz RW, et al: Changes in lipid and lipoprotein levels after weight training. *JAMA* 252:504–506, 1984.

118. Hurley BF, Hagberg JM, Goldberg AP, et al: Resistive training can reduce coronary risk factors without altering Vo_{2max} or percent body fat. *Med Sci Sports Exerc* 20:150–154, 1988.

119. Johnson CC, Stone MH, Lopez-SA, et al: Diet and exercise in middle-aged men. *J Am Diet Assoc* 81:695–701, 1982.

120. Manning JM, Dooly-Manning CR, White K, et al: Effects of a resistive training program on lipoprotein-lipid levels in obese women. *Med Sci Sports Exerc* 23:1222–1226, 1991.

121. Smutok MA, Reece C, Kokkinos PF, et al: Aerobic versus strength training for risk factor intervention in middle-aged men at high risk for coronary artery disease. *Metabolism.* 42:177–184, 1993.

122. Durstine JL, Ferguson MA, Szymanski LM, et al: Effect of a single session of exercise on lipoprotein(a). *Med Sci Sports Exerc* 28:1277–1281, 1996.

123. Angelopoulos TJ, Robertson RJ, Goss FL, et al: Effect of repeated exercise bouts on high density lipoprotein-cholesterol and its subfractions HDL_2-C and HDL_3-C. *Int J Sports Med* 14:196–201, 1993.

124. Davis PG, Bartoli WP, Durstine JL: Effects of acute exercise intensity on plasma lipids and apolipoproteins in trained runners. *J Appl Physiol* 72:914–919, 1992.

125. Ferguson MA, Alderson NL, Trost S, et al: Effects of four different exercise volumes on HDL-C and lipoprotein lipase. *J Appl Physiol* 85:1169–1174, 1998.

126. Gordon PM, Fowler S, Warty V, et al: Effects of acute exercise on high density lipoprotein cholesterol and high density lipoprotein subfractions in moderately trained females. *Br J Sports Med* 32:63–67, 1998.

127. Annuzzi G, Jansson E, Kaijser L, et al: Increased removal rate of exogenous triglycerides after prolonged exercise in man: Time course and effects of exercise duration. *Metabolism* 36:438–443, 1987.

128. Cullinane E, Siconolfi S, Saritelli A, et al: Acute decrease in serum triglycerides with exercise: Is there a threshold for an exercise effect. *Metabolism* 31:844–847, 1982.

129. Durstine JL, Miller W, Farrell S, et al: Increases in HDL-cholesterol and the HDL/LDL cholesterol ratio during prolonged endurance exercise. *Metabolism* 32:993–997, 1983.

130. Kantor MA, Cullinane EM, Sady SP, et al: Exercise acutely increases high density lipoprotein-cholesterol and lipoprotein lipase activity in trained and untrained men. *Metabolism* 36:188–192, 1987.

131. Kantor MA, Cullinane EM, Herbert PN, et al: Acute increase in lipoprotein lipase following prolonged exercise. *Metabolism* 33:454–457, 1984.

132. Goodyear LJ, Van Houten DR, Fronsoe MS, et al: Immediate and delayed effects of marathon running on lipids and lipoproteins in women. *Med Sci Sports Exerc* 22:588–592, 1990.

133. Dufaux B, Order U, Muller R, et al: Delayed effects of prolonged exercise on serum lipoproteins. *Metabolism* 35:105–109, 1986.

134. Shoup EE, Durstine JL, Davis JM, et al: Effects of a single session of resistance exercise on plasma lipoproteins and postheparin lipase activity. In review.

135. Wallace MB, Moffatt RJ, Haymes EM, et al: Acute effects of resistance exercise on parameters of lipoprotein metabolism. *Med Sci Sports Exerc* 23:199–204, 1991.

136. Lee R, Nieman D, Raval R, et al: The effects of acute moderate exercise on serum lipids and lipoproteins in mildly obese women. *Int J Sports Med* 12:537–542, 1991.

137. Pay HE, Hardman AE, Jones GJ, et al: The acute effects of low-intensity exercise on plasma lipids in endurance-trained and untrained young adults. *Eur J Appl Physiol* 64:182–186, 1992.

138. Yu HH, Ginsburg GS, O'Toole ML, et al: Acute changes in serum lipids and lipoprotein subclasses in triathletes as assessed by proton nuclear magnetic resonance spectroscopy. *Arterioscler Thromb Vasc Biol* 19:1945–1949, 1999.

139. Ginsburg GS, Agil A, O'Toole M, et al: Effects of a single bout of ultrendurane exercise on lipid levels and susceptibility of lipids to peroxidation in triathletes. *JAMA* 276:221–225, 1996.

140. Miesenböck G, Patsch JR: Postprandial hyperlipidemia: The search for the atherogenic lipoprotein. *Curr Opinion Lipidol* 3:196–201, 1992.

141. Tsetsonis NV, Hardman AE, Mastana SS: Acute effects of exercise on postprandial lipemia: A comparative study in trained and untrained middle-aged women. *Am J Clin Nutr* 65:525–533, 1997.

142. Gill JMR, Murphy MH, Hardman AE: Postprandial lipemia: Effects of intermittent ver-

sus continuous exercise. *Med Sci Sports Exerc* 30:1515–1520, 1998.

143. Tsetsonis NV, Hardman AE: Effects of low and moderate intensity treadmill walking on postprandial lipaemia in healthy young adults. *Eur J Appl Physiol* 73:419–426, 1996.

144. Tsetsonis NV, Hardman AE: Reduction in postprandial lipemia after walking: Influence of exercise intensity. *Med Sci Sports Exerc* 28: 1235–1242, 1996.

145. Malkova D, Hardman AE, Bowness RJ: The reduction in postprandial lipemia after exercise is independent of the relative contribution of fat and carbohydrate to energy metabolism during exercise. *Metabolism* 48:245–251, 1999.

146. Griffin BA, Skinner ER, Maughan RJ: The acute effect of prolonged walking and dietary changes on plasma lipoprotein concentrations and high-density lipoprotein subfractions. *Metabolism* 37:535–541, 1988.

147. Hellsten G, Boman K, Hallmans G, et al: Lipids and endurance physical activity. *Atherosclerosis* 76:93–94, 1989.

148. Durstine JL, Davis PG, Ferguson MA, et al: Effects of short-duration and long-duration exercise on lipoprotein(a). In review.

149. Gordon PM, Goss FL, Visich PS, et al: The acute effects of exercise intensity on HDL-C metabolism. *Med Sci Sports Exerc* 26:671–677, 1994.

150. Klein L, Miller TD, Radam TE, O'Brian T, et al: Acute physical exercise alters apolipoprotein E and C-III concentrations of apo E-rich very low-density lipoprotein fraction. *Atherosclerosis* 97: 37–51, 1992.

151. Seip RL, Semenkovich CF: Skeletal muscle lipoprotein lipase: Molecular regulation and physiologic effects in relation to exercise, in Holloszy JO (ed.): *Exercise Sport Science Review.* Baltimore: Williams & Wilkins, 1998, pp. 191–218.

152. Kiens B, Lithell H: Lipoprotein metabolism influenced by training-induced changes in human skeletal muscle. *J Clin Invest* 83:558–564, 1989.

153. Zhang JQ, Thomas TR, Ball SD: Effect of exercise timing on postprandial lipemia and HDL cholesterol subfractions. *J Appl Physiol* 85: 1516–1522, 1998.

154. Podl TR, Zmuda JM, Yurgalevitch SM, et al: Lipoprotein lipase and plasma triglyceride clear-

ance are elevated in endurance-trained women. *Metabolism* 43:803–813, 1994.

155. Thompson PD, Cullinane EM, Sady SP, et al: High density lipoprotein metabolism in endurance athletes and sedentary men. *Circulation* 84:140–152, 1991.

156. Sady SP, Cullinane EM, Saritelli A, et al: Elevated high-density lipoprotein cholesterol in endurance athletes is related to enhanced plasma triglyceride clearance. *Metabolism* 37:568– 572, 1988.

157. Cedermark M, Froberg J, Lithel lH, et al: Effects of long term heavy exercise on skeletal muscle metabolism in man, in Poortmans J, Niset G (eds.): *Biochemistry of Exercise IV-B.* Baltimore: University Park Press, 1981, p. 117.

158. Peltonen P, Marniemi J, Hietanen E, et al: Changes in serum lipids, lipoproteins and heparin releasable lipolytic enzymes during moderate physical training in man: A longitudinal study. *Metabolism* 30:518–526, 1981.

159. Seip RL, Mair K, Cole TG, et al: Induction of human skeletal muscle lipoprotein lipase gene expression by short-term exercise is transient. *Am J Physiol* 272:E255–E261, 1997.

160. Seip RL, Angelopoulos TJ, Semenkovich CF: Exercise induces human lipoprotein lipase gene expression in skeletal muscle but not adipose tissue. *Am J Physiol* 268:E229–E236, 1995.

161. Hamilton MT, Etienne J, McMclure WC, et al: Role of local contractile activity and muscle fiber type on LPL regulation during exercise. *Am J Physiol* 275:E1016–E1022, 1998.

162. Ehnholm C, Kuusi T: Preparation, characterization, and measurement of hepatic lipase. *Meth Enzymol* 129:716–763, 1986.

163. Lokey EA, Tran ZV: Effects of exercise training on serum lipid and lipoprotein concentrations in women: A meta-analysis. *Int J Sports Med* 10:424–429, 1989.

164. Quintao E: Is reverse cholesterol transport a misnomer for suggesting its role in the prevention of atheroma formation? *Atherosclerosis* 116:1–14, 1995.

165. Gupta AK, Ross EA, Myers JN, et al: Increased reverse cholesterol transport in athletes. *Metabolism* 42:684–690, 1993.

166. Lagrost L: Regulation of cholesteryl ester transfer protein (CEPT) activity: Review of in vitro

and in vitro studies. *Biochim Biophys Acta* 1215:209–236, 1994.

167. Ritsch A, Auer B, Foger B, et al: Polyclonal antibody-based immunoradiometric assay for quantification of cholesteryl ester transfer protein. *J Lipid Res* 34:673–679, 1993.

168. Serrat-Serrat SJ, Ordóñez-Llanos J, Serra-Grima R, et al: Marathon runners presented lower serum cholesteryl ester transfer activity than sedentary subjects. *Atherosclerosis* 101:43–49, 1993.

169. Föger B, Wohlfarter T, Ritsch A, et al: Kinetics of lipids, apolipoproteins, and cholesteryl ester transfer protein in plasma after a bicycle marathon. *Metabolism* 43:633–639, 1994.

170. Marniemi J, Hietanen E: Response of serum lecithin: Cholesterol acyltranferase activity to exercise training, in Hietanen E (ed.): *Regulation of Serum Lipids by Physical Exercise,* Boca Raton: CRC Press, 1982, pp. 116–118.

171. Thomas TR, Adeniran SB, Iltis PW, et al: Effects of interval and continuous running on HDL-cholesterol, apoproteins A-I and B, and LCAT. *Can J Appl Sport Sci* 10:52–59, 1985.

172. Frey I, Baumstark MW, Berg A, et al: Influence of acute maximal exercise on lecithin: Cholesterol acyltransferase activity in healthy adults of differing aerobic performance. *Eur J Appl Physiol* 62:31–35, 1991.

Index

Note: Page numbers followed by letters *f* and *t* refer to figures and tables, respectively.

481